MESOTHELIOMA FROM BENCH SIDE TO CLINIC

MESOTHELIOMA FROM BENCH SIDE TO CLINIC

ALFONSO BALDI
EDITOR

Nova Biomedical Books
New York

For permission to use material from this book please contact us:
Telephone 631-231-7269; Fax 631-231-8175
Web Site: http://www.novapublishers.com

Library of Congress Cataloging-in-Publication Data

Mesothelioma from bench side to clinic / Alphonso Baldi (editor).
p. ; cm.
Includes bibliographical references and index.
ISBN-13: 978-1-60021-789-0 (hardcover)
ISBN-10: 1-60021-789-3 (hardcover)
1. Mesothelioma. I. Baldi, Alphonso.
[DNLM: 1. Mesothelioma. QZ 340 M5825 2007]
RC280.L8M473 2007
616.99'4--dc22

2007024476

Published by Nova Science Publishers, Inc. ✢ New York

Contents

Preface

Malignant mesothelioma is a rare, highly aggressive tumour, accounting for less than 1% of all cancer deaths in the world. Nevertheless, it is becoming a considerable problem internationally, especially for the constant increase in the incidence, due to environmental ambient pollution, and for the lack of effective therapies. Notwithstanding the raise in interest in this disease at scientific, clinical and medico-legal level, there are very few textbooks addressing mesothelioma, and even less books completely dedicated to this malignant tumour. Principal purpose of this book is a comprehensive and up-to-date overview of epidemiology, molecular biology, pathology, animal models, diagnosis and therapy of human mesothelioma. Several authors from different countries have been selected for the contributions, based on their recognized expertise in the different themes covered. It is my hope that the book will serve the needs of mesothelioma investigators for teaching, research and professional reference. Nevertheless, I hope that it could also be an excellent reading for medical and PhD students and anyone that needs a deepening study on this disease.

Alfonso Baldi,
Naples, July 2007

Foreword

Malignant mesothelioma remains a dread disease for patients and their families. It remains a perplexing challenge with pitfalls in both diagnosis and treatment that continue to vex the oncologist. Recently, pharmacologic studies, an aggressive surgical approach, and concentration of patients in mesothelioma treatment centers have begun to generate a small optimism regarding the management of these patients.

Of course, complete removal from our environment of the carcinogens that cause this dread disease would be a first priority. Some progress has been made in eliminating asbestos contamination in the workplace. Progress on this has been much greater in the United States and Europe than it has been in underdeveloped countries. However, even in the most sophisticated environments asbestos exposure to an unknowing individual can occur. This can either be through direct contact or secondary contact especially with children. Unfortunately, most oncologists have very little power to influence the use of asbestos and other possible carcinogens involved in this disease. Our own epidemiologic studies here at the Washington Cancer Institute would suggest that elimination of asbestos from the environment would not eliminate this disease and that a substantial number of patients may have exposure to other unknown carcinogens that cause mesothelioma.

A problem in the past that is only finding a partial solution is rapid and definitive diagnosis. Thoracoscopy and laparoscopy have greatly facilitated accurate diagnosis. Also, immunostains calretinin and CK 5/6 have gone a long way to distinguishing this disease from other cancers that may present with a similar spectrum of signs and symptoms. A molecular diagnosis for this disease may be evident within the near future. Also, more accurate staging both clinically and histopathologically shows promise. An accurate system of prognostic indicators is necessary in order to properly select patients for the broad array of treatment possibilities that exist. Standardization of these assessments between institutions will be difficult but is necessary.

Another development promoting limited optimism in dealing with this cancer concerns the concentration of patients in mesothelioma treatment centers whereby natural history data plus clinical, radiological and histopathological correlates become evident. Only with a well maintained database and sufficient patient accrual can provide the necessary information for progress in patient management to occur.

A great value for the mesothelioma patient in going to a mesothelioma treatment center concerns the increased knowledge and skills of the caregivers at these treatment centers. No longer are patients being cared for by physicians who are only treating one or two patients a year. Treatment centers that are now regularly managing a patient a week are available and should be the site of continued referral. Patients managed in an anecdotal fashion are unlikely to have optimal management. With referral centers this orphan disease fails to be mismanaged as it often is at the community hospital level.

As awareness of the unique features of this disease have become evident, an increased number of global conferences devoted to the new molecular science of mesothelioma and the new and more aggressive treatment strategies are shared between designated treatment centers. Mesothelioma has become a disease that "stands alone" and deserves to have its own basic science cadre, radiologic, medical, and surgical cadre and support staff from nurses and other caregivers. Having these "mesothelioma experts" get together on a regular basis and share their new data has led to an escalation of progress with this disease.

This text on mesothelioma attests to the fact that cooperative efforts in behalf of these patients are occurring. Assembling and disseminating the available information and the identification of "breakthroughs" in understanding this problem can occur. This book should act as an authoritative guide to medical oncologists, radiation oncologists, surgical oncologists, pulmonologists, and basic science individuals who wish to focus on a particular aspect of this disease or to broaden their knowledge concerning its many and varied complexities. These efforts should be taking place in the United States and Europe and need to be carried to the underdeveloped nations. This book can be of help in that regard. Much progress has been made and much more is required.

Paul H. Sugarbaker, MD, FACS, FRCS
Director, Program in Peritoneal Surface Malignancy
Washington Cancer Institute
Washington, DC

Dedication

To Nicoletta, Feliciano and Giulio

In: Mesothelioma from Bench Side to Clinic
Editor: Alfonso Baldi, pp. 1-9
ISBN: 978-1-60021-789-0

Chapter I

Embryology, Histology and Anatomy of Mesothelium

Maria De Falco[1], Michele M. Pisano[2] and Antonio De Luca[3]

[1]Department of Biological Sciences, Section of Evolutionary and Comparative Biology, University Federico II of Naples, Naples, Italy

[2]Birth Defects Center, Department of Molecular, Cellular and Craniofacial Biology, Health Sciences Center, University of Louisville, Louisville, KY, USA

[3]Department of Medicine and Public Health, Section of Clinical Anatomy, Second University of Naples, Naples, Italy

Abstract

The mesothelium consists of an extensive monolayer of flattened mesothelial cells that line the body's serous cavities and the majority of internal organs, playing important roles in maintaining normal serosal integrity and function. This chapter describes the structure and function of the mesothelium and the biology of mesothelial cells.

The mesothelium is formed by a single layer of specialized cells, named mesothelial cells that line serosal cavities such as the peritoneal, pleural, and pericardial cavities, as well as the sac surrounding the testes. The mesothelium lines both the visceral and parietal surfaces of serosal cavities, covering the internal organs and body wall, respectively. The mesothelium plays important roles in maintaining normal serosal integrity and function (Herrick and Mutsaers 2004).

Mesothelium first described by Bichat in 1827 (Whitaker et al. 1982a), who observed that the serous cavities were lined by a monolayer of flattened cells similar to those of the lymphatics. Subsequently, in 1880, Minot referred to this layer as "the epithelial lining of mammalian mesodermic cavities" and then proposed the term "mesothelium" (Minot 1880; Minot 1890; Mutsaers 2002). Mesothelial tissue is composed of a single layer of epithelial-like cells resting on a thin basement membrane supported by sub-serosal connective tissue containing blood vessels, lymphatics, resident inflammatory cells and fibroblast-like cells (Wang 1974; Ishihara et al. 1980; Albertine et al. 1982, Herrick and Mutsaers 2004).

Traditionally, the mesothelium was thought to be a simple tissue with the unique function of providing a slippery, non-adhesive and protective surface to facilitate intracoelomic movements. With the gradual accumulation of information about serosal tissues, the mesothelium is now recognized as a dynamic cellular membrane with many important functions including the control of fluid and solute transport, immune surveillance and the production of extracellular matrix (ECM) molecules, proteases, cytokines and growth factors (Mutsaers 2002; Herrick and Mutsaers 2004).

The mesothelium is bathed in serosal fluid that resembles an ultrafiltrate of plasma and contains blood proteins, resident inflammatory cells, sugars and various enzymes including amylase and lactate dehydrogenase (Dondelinger et al. 1982). The composition and volume of the serosal fluid is indicative of certain pathological states, such as peritonitis, tumorigenesis and endometriosis (Haney 1993), and it is likely that the mesothelial layer responds as a single unit to changes in serosal fluid composition. Indeed, repair of serosal tissue involves increased mesothelial cell proliferation at sites distant to the wound, suggesting diffuse activation of the mesothelium in response to mediators or cells released into the serosal fluid, or via cell-to-cell communication (Mutsaers et al. 1997; Mutsaers et al. 2002; Herrick and Mutsaers 2004).

Embryologically, the mesothelium develops from between 8 and 18 days of gestation depending on the species (Hesseldahl and Larsen 1969; Tiedemann 1976; Moore 1982). In humans, this occurs around day 14 of gestation, with cells gradually differentiating from round or cuboidal cells to elongated flattened cells which line the coelomic cavities (Mutsaers 2004). In addition, the intraembryonic mesoderm on each side of the neural groove differentiates into paraxial, intermediate and lateral mesoderm (Hesseldahl and Larsen 1969; Moore 1982; Herrick and Mutsaers 2004). The lateral mesoderm is continuous with the extraembryonic mesoderm covering the yolk sac and amnion. At the end of week 3 of gestation, small spaces appear in the lateral mesoderm that fuse and divide the mesoderm into two layers: the intraembryonic somatic (parietal) layer and the intraembryonic splanchnic (visceral) layer. The somatic mesoderm and overlying embryonic ectoderm form the embryonic body wall (somatopleure), whereas the splanchnic mesoderm and embryonic endoderm form the embryonic gut wall (splanchnopleure). A continuous mesothelial membrane lines the margin of these two layers and so borders the intraembryonic coelom. Between weeks 5 and 7 of gestation, the coelom is sub-divided by a process of septation into a future pericardial cavity, two pleural cavities and a peritoneal cavity. In this phase of development, the mesothelial and submesothelial layers of the coelom are referred to as the pericardium, pleura, and peritoneum respectively, and together as serous membranes (reviewed by Thors and Drukker 1997). Mesothelial cells are therefore of a primitive mesodermal origin, but share characteristics of both epithelial and mesenchymal cells (Whitaker et al. 1992).

Morphological studies of the mesothelium have demonstrated that it is essentially similar, irrespective of species or anatomical sites (Ishihara et al. 1980; Gaudio et al. 1988; Mutsaers 2002). Histochemical studies have supported these structural findings (Raftery

1973; Whitaker et al. 1980). The mesothelium forms a monolayer of predominantly elongated, squamous-like mesothelial cells, approximately 25 μm in diameter, with characteristic surface microvilli and occasional cilia, with the cytoplasm raised over a central round or oval nucleus (Bloom and Fawcett 1975). Mesothelial cells display many epithelial characteristics including a polygonal cell shape and cytokeratin intermediate filaments (cytokeratins 6, 8, 18 and 19) (Czernobilsky et al. 1985). The cells have the ability to secrete a thin basement membrane, on which they rest, supported by a connective tissue stroma. The biochemical nature of this stroma varies in quantity and quality between the three serous cavities, between visceral and parietal serosa, and between species (Tyler et al. 1971; Ishihara et al. 1980; Albertine et al. 1982). Mesothelial cells also demonstrate features of mesenchymal cells such as the presence of vimentin, desmin and alpha smooth muscle actin (Afify et al. 2002). Although the mesothelium is composed predominantly of squamous-like cells, cuboidal mesothelial cells can be found in various areas including the septal folds of the mediastinal pleura, the parenchymal organs (liver and spleen), the "milky spots" of the omentum, and the peritoneal side of the diaphragm overlying the lymphatic lacunae (Wang 1974; Tsilibary and Wissig 1977; Mironov et al. 1979; Michailova et al. 1999). Cells that are morphologically similar to these cuboidal mesothelial cells also can be identified after injury or stimulation of the serosal surfaces (Whitaker and Papadimitriou 1985; Fotev et al. 1987; Mutsaers et al. 2002).

Ultrastructural analyses of squamous-like and cuboidal mesothelial cells indicate differences between their nuclei and organelles. Squamous-like mesothelial cells have a round or ovoid nucleus, whereas the nuclei of cuboidal cells are larger and contain a prominent nucleolus. (Fukata 1963; Baradi and Hope 1964; Baradi and Campbell 1974; Wang 1974; Mutsaers 2002). Organelles of the squamous-like mesothelial cells are located centrally, close to the nucleus. These cells contain microtubules and microfilaments, glycogen, few mitochondria, a poorly developed Golgi apparatus, and little rough endoplasmic reticulum (RER) (Baradi and Hope 1964; Kluge and Hovig 1967; Baradi and Campbell 1974; Wang 1974; Mutsaers 2002). The microfilaments are located parallel to the cell surface and are situated deep in the cytoplasm (Kluge and Hovig 1967). Alternately, cuboidal mesothelial cells have abundant mitochondria and RER, a well developed Golgi apparatus, and a greater number of microtubules and microfilaments compared with squamous cells – suggesting a more metabolically active state (Fukata 1963; Kluge and Hovig 1967; Baradi and Campbell 1974; Mutsaers 2002; Herrick and Mutsaers 2004).

The luminal surface of the mesothelial cell has a well developed microvillous border, with microvilli varying in length, shape and density. Variations in the concentration of microvilli have been reported on mesothelial cells of different organs (Mutsaers et al. 1996), between adjacent cells, and on the surface of individual cells (Andrews and Porter 1973; Wang 1974; Tsilibary and Wissig 1977; Michailova et al. 1999; Mutsaers 2002). Moreover, the entire population of microvilli is labile, with the number of microvilli present on each cell changing under different physiological conditions (Madison et al. 1979). Differences in the number of microvilli on regenerating mesothelial cells have also been reported and it has been suggested that their concentration reflects functional adaptation (Madison et al. 1979; Wang 1974; Lindic et al. 1993; Mutsaers et al. 1996). These changes are also associated with an alteration in surface charge (Mutsaers et al. 1996). This may reflect changes in the composition of the negatively charged glycocalyx that covers the mesothelial cell surface (Gotloib et al. 1988) or may be due to trapping by microvilli of proteins and other molecules from the serosal fluid (Kluge and Hovig 1967; Fedorko and Hirsch 1971; Andrews and Porter 1973; Wang 1974; Baradi and Rao 1976; Mutsaers et al. 1996; Mutsaers 2002).

Mesothelial cells have a well-developed system of vesicles and vacuoles; most are micropinocytic, but multivesicular bodies and large vacuoles can be found (Whitaker 1984). As with the microvilli, the concentration of these structures varies between cells and sites. Generally, the visceral mesothelium has more vesicles than the parietal mesothelium and the vesicles are more numerous along the luminal cell surface, often in contact with the plasmalemma (Fukata 1963; Kluge and Hovig 1967; Cotran and Karnovsky 1968; Fedorko and Hirsch 1971; Baradi and Campbell 1974; Ishihara et al. 1980). These vesicles are involved in the transport of fluids and particulates across the mesothelium. Experimental studies have shown tracer particles up to 100 nm can traverse the mesothelial cell by pinocytic transport (Fukata 1963; Fedorko and Hirsch 1971; Leak and Rahil 1978; Mutsaers 2002).

The boundaries between mesothelial cells are tortuous, with adjacent cells often overlapping. The mesothelium has well-developed cell–cell junctional complexes including tight junctions (zonula occludens), adherens junctions, gap junctions, and desmosomes (Kluge and Hovig 1967; Whitaker 1984; Pelin et al. 1994; Mutsaers 2002; Herrick and Mutsaers 2004). Tight junctions, located towards the luminal aspect of the mesothelial cell, are crucial for the development of cell surface polarity and the establishment and maintenance of a semipermeable diffusion barrier. Adherens junctions are thought to form the structural and adhesive support of the mesothelial cell layer, and gap junctions function as aqueous intercellular channels. Mesothelial cells express E-, N- and P-cadherins, although, unlike the epithelium, N-cadherin predominates (Simsir et al. 1999). Furthermore, membrane-associated expression of zonula occludens (ZO)-1 has been demonstrated in intact sheets of normal mesothelium (Foley-Comer et al. 2002; Mutsaers 2002; Herrick and Mutsaers 2004).

Von Recklinghausen, in 1863, described the presence of ‘stomata’ (cavities at the junction of two or more mesothelial cells) which he postulated allowed movement of fluid and particulate matter to and from the serous cavities. Scanning and transmission electron microscopy studies combined with tracer studies have clearly documented their existence, although there is still much debate about their location, density and function (Wang 1975; Baradi and Rao 1976; Tsilibary and Wissig 1977; Bettendorf 1978; Leak and Rahil 1978; Mironov et al. 1979; Leak 1983; Moalli et al. 1987; Fukuo et al. 1990; Negrini et al. 1991; Shaw et al. 1991; Li 1993; Ohtani et al. 1995; Michailova et al. 1999; Miura et al. 2000). Stomatal openings, 3–12 μm in diameter, are generally found in those regions where cuboidal mesothelial cells are present, such as on the peritoneal side of the diaphragm or over the omental “milky spots”. These openings provide direct access to the underlying submesothelial lymphatic system, allowing rapid removal of fluid, cells, bacteria and particles from the serosal cavities (Fukuo et al. 1990; Ohtani et al. 1995; Nakatami et al. 1996; Shao et al. 1998; Miura et al. 2000). It also has been proposed that stomata provide a direct link between the pleural and peritoneal cavities (Ohtani et al. 1995; Ohtani and Ohtani 1997). This may explain how inhaled materials, such as asbestos, can enter the peritoneal cavity and cause asbestos-induced fibrosis or malignant mesothelioma (Mutsaers 2002).

Classically, the two main functions attributed to the mesothelium are to provide a protective barrier and a frictionless interface for the free movement of apposing organs and tissues. Mesothelial cells are firmly bound together by tight junctions, thereby providing a protective barrier against physical damage and invading organisms. Mesothelial cells secrete surface proteoglycans, such as hyaluronan, which are assembled into hyaluronan-containing pericellular matrixes ("coats") around microvilli that protect the cells from abrasive damage and infective agents. An increase in the concentration of hyaluronan is associated with the presence of activated cuboidal mesothelial cells in pleural effusions (Satoh et al. 1987; Wang and Lai-Fook 1998; Mutsaers 2002). Mesothelial cells also secrete phosphatidylcholine, the major constituent of lamella bodies and pulmonary surfactant that functions as a lubricant to reduce friction between serosal surfaces (Mutsaers 2002; 2004). The mesothelium is involved in the transport and movement of fluid and particulate matter across the serosal cavities by pinocytic vesicles (Fukata 1963; Fedorko and Hirsch 1971; Leak and Rahil 1978; Mutsaers 2002). It has been demonstrated that resting mesothelium is primarily involved in with membrane transport; whereas cuboidal mesothelial cells have a wider spectrum of functional activities. Moreover, it has been suggested that flat resting mesothelial cells can become metabolically active cuboidal cells (Mutsaers 2002). In recent years, it has been discovered that this tissue also plays important roles in the initiation and resolution of inflammation, tissue repair, and lysis of fibrin deposits, thereby preventing serosal adhesion formation and affording protection against invading microorganisms and tumour dissemination. Mesothelial cells participate in serosal inflammation by secreting various pro-, anti- and immunomodulatory mediators such as prostaglandins and prostacyclin, chemokines, nitric oxide (NO) and reactive nitrogen/oxygen species, anti-oxidant enzymes, cytokines and products of the coagulation cascade. These mediators are released in response to bacterial endotoxins and cytokines (Antony et al. 1993), asbestos (Boylan et al. 1992), or instilled agents (Antony et al. 1995) with the purpose of restoring normal serosal architecture and function (Mutsaers 2002). Moreover, several studies have demonstrated that mesothelial cells have the capacity to secrete a variety of growth factors and ECM molecules known to be involved in inflammation and tissue repair (Mutsaers 2002). Mesothelial cells also play an important role in regulating the turnover of ECM that follows serosal injury, by secreting metalloproteinases (MMP) and tissue inhibitors of metalloproteinases (TIMP) (Marshall et al. 1993; Rougier et al. 1997; Ma et al. 1999). The state of differentiation of these cells seems to have a marked influence on MMP and TIMP expression, such that cells with an epithelioid morphology demonstrate a more ECM-degradative phenotype (Marshall et al. 1993). A precise balance between MMP and TIMP activities is therefore important for the outcome of serosal injury, resulting in both tissue regeneration and re-establishment of normal function, or fibrosis and serosal adhesion (Mutsaers 2002). Furthermore, mesothelial cells demonstrate both procoagulant and fibrinolytic activity, and play an important role in local fibrin deposition as well as fibrin clearance within serosal cavities. As with metalloproteinase regulated ECM biosynthesis/degradation, a fine balance exists between fibrin deposition and breakdown in serosal cavities, which, if inappropriately regulated, can cause reduced fibrin clearance and result in adhesion formation (Holmdahl et al. 1998).The fibrinolytic activity of mesothelial cells is a key factor in the prevention and removal of fibrin deposits that form following mechanical injury, hemothoraces and infection. In the thorax, pleural loculation and adhesions can impair lung function (Mutsaers 2002).

Although the mesothelium was first described about 180 years ago, only in the past 25 years has the role of mesothelium in maintaining normal serosal membrane integrity and function come to be understood and appreciated. This knowledge provides the foundation upon which to examine the contribution of altered mesothelial integrity and function to various disease states.

References

Afify, AM; Al-Khafaji, BM; Paulino, AF; Davila, RM. Diagnostic use of muscle markers in the cytologic evaluation of serous fluids. *Appli. Immunohistochem. Mol. Morphol.*, 2002, 10, 178–182.

Albertine, KH; Wiener-Kronish, JP; Roos, PJ; Staub, NC. Structure, blood supply, and lymphatic vessels of the sheep's visceral pleura. *Am. J. Anat.*, 1982, 165, 277–294.

Andrews, PM; Porter, KR. The ultrastructural morphology and possible functional significance of mesothelial microvilli. *Anat. Rec.*, 1973, 177, 409–426.

Antony, VB; Godbey, SW; Kunkel, SL; Hott, JW; Hartman, DL; Burdick, MD; Strieter, RM. Recruitment of inflammatory cells to the pleural space. Chemotactic cytokines, IL-8, and monocyte chemotactic peptide-1 in human pleural fluids. *J. Immunol.*, 1993, 151, 7216–7223.

Antony, VB; Hott, JW; Kunkel, SL; Godbey, SW; Burdick, MD; Strieter, RM. Pleural mesothelial cell expression of C-C (monocyte chemotactic peptide) and C-X-C (interleukin 8) chemokines. *Am. J. Respir. Cell Mol. Biol.*, 1995, 12, 581–588.

Baradi, AF; Campbell Jr, WG. Exudative peritonitis induced in mice by bovine serum albumin. *Arch. Pathol.*, 1974, 97, 2–12.

Baradi, AF; Hope, J. Observations on ultrastructure of rabbit mesothelium. *Exp. Cell Res.*, 1964, 34, 33–44.

Baradi, AF; Rao, SN. A scanning electron microscope study of mouse peritoneal mesothelium. *Tissue Cell,* 1976, 8, 159–162.

Bettendorf, U. Lymph flow mechanism of the subperitoneal diaphragmatic lymphatics. *Lymphology,* 1978, 11, 111–116.

Bloom, W; Fawcett, DW (eds). *A Textbook of Histology.WB Saunders*, Philadelphia, 1975.

Boylan, AM; Ruegg, C; Kim, KJ; Hebert, CA; Hoeffel, JM; Pytela, R; Sheppard, D; Goldstein, IM; Broaddus, VC. Evidence of a role for mesothelial cell-derived interleukin 8 in the pathogenesis of asbestos-induced pleurisy in rabbits. *J. Clin. Invest.*, 1992, 89, 1257–1267.

Cotran, RS; Karnovsky, MJ. Ultrastructural studies on the permeability of the mesothelium to horseradish peroxidase. *J. Cell Biol.*, 1968, 37, 123–137.

Czernobilsky, B; Moll, R; Levy, R; Franke, WW. Co-expression of cytokeratin and vimentin filaments in mesothelial, granulosa and rete ovarii cells of the human ovary. *Eur. J. Cell Biol.*, 1985, 37, 175–190.

Dondelinger, RF; Boverie, JH; Cornet, O. Diagnosis of pancreatic injury: a need to improve performance. *JBR-BTR*, 1982, 83, 160–166.

Fedorko, ME; Hirsch, JG. Studies on transport of macromolecules and small particles across mesothelial cells of the mouse omentum. I. Morphologic aspects. *Exp. Cell Res.*, 1971, 69, 113–127.

Foley-Comer, AJ; Herrick, SE; Al-Mishlab, T; Prele, CM; Laurent, GJ; Mutsaers, SE. Evidence for incorporation of free-floating mesothelial cells as a mechanism of serosal healing. *J. Cell Sci.*, 2002, 115, 1383–1389.

Fotev, Z; Whitaker, D; Papadimitriou, JM. Role of macrophages in mesothelial healing. *J. Pathol.*, 1987, 151, 209–219.

Fukata, H. Electron microscopic study on normal rat peritoneal mesothelium and its changes in absorption of particulate iron dextran complex. *Acta Pathol. Jpn.*, 1963, 13, 309–325.

Fukuo, Y; Shinohara, H; Matsuda, T. The distribution of lymphatic stomata in the diaphragm of the golden hamster. *J. Anat.*, 1990, 169, 13–21.

Gaudio, E; Rendina, EA; Pannarale, L; Ricci, C; Marinozzi, G. Surface morphology of the human pleura. A scanning electron microscopic study. *Chest*, 1988, 93, 149–153.

Gotloib, L; Shostack, A; Jaichenko, J. Ruthenium-redstained anionic charges of rat and mice mesothelial cells and basal lamina: The peritoneum is a negatively charged dialyzing membrane. *Nephron*, 1988, 48, 65–70.

Haney, AF. Endometriosis, macrophages, and adhesions. *Progr. Clin. Biol. Res.*, 1993, 381, 19–44.

Hesseldahl, H; Larsen, JF. Ultrastructure of human yolksac: Endoderm, mesenchyme, tubules and mesothelium. *Am. J. Anat.*, 1969, 126, 315–335.

Herrick, SE; Mutsaers, SE. Mesothelial progenitor cells and their potential in tissue engineering. *Int. J. Biochem. Cell Biol.*, 36, 621-642.

Holmdahl, L; Eriksson, E; Eriksson, BI; Risberg, B. Depression of peritoneal fibrinolysis during operation is a local response to trauma. *Surgery*, 1998, 123, 539–544.

Ishihara, T; Ferrans, VJ; Jones, M; Boyce, SW; Kawanami, O; Roberts, WC. Histologic and ultrastructural features of normal human parietal pericardium. *Am. J. Cardiol.*, 1980, 46, 744–753.

Kluge, T; Hovig, T. The ultrastructure of human and rat pericardium. II. Intercellular spaces and junctions. *Acta Pathos. Microbiol. Scand.*, 1967, 71, 547–563.

Leak, LV. Interaction of mesothelium to intraperitoneal stimulation. I. Aggregation of peritoneal cells. *Lab. Invest.*, 1983, 48, 479–491.

Leak, LV; Rahil, K. Permeability of the diaphragmatic mesothelium: The ultrastructural basis for 'stomata'. *Am. J. Anat.*, 1978, 151, 557–593.

Li, J. Ultrastructural study on the pleural stomata in human. *Funct. Dev.Morph.*, 1993, 3, 277–280.

Lindic, J; Psenicnik, M; Bren, A; Gucek, A; Ferluga, D; Kveder, R. The morphology of parietal peritoneum: A scanning electron micrograph study. *Adv. Perit. Dial.*, 1993, 9, 36–38.

Ma, C; Tarnuzzer, RW; Chegini, N. Expression of matrix metalloproteinases and tissue inhibitor of matrix metalloproteinases in mesothelial cells and their regulation by transforming growth factor-beta1. *Wound Repair Regen.*, 1999, 7, 477–485.

Madison, LD; Bergstrom-Porter, B; Torres, AR; Shelton, E. Regulation of surface topography of mouse peritoneal cells. Formation of microvilli and vesiculated pits on omental mesothelial cells by serum and other proteins. *J. Cell Biol.*, 1979, 82, 783–797.

Marshall, BC; Santana, A; Xu, QP; Petersen, MJ; Campbell, EJ; Hoidal, JR; Welgus, HG. Metalloproteinases and tissue inhibitor of metalloproteinases in mesothelial cells. Cellular differentiation influences expression. *J. Clin. Invest.*, 1993, 91, 1792–1799.

Michailova, K; Wassilev, W; Wedel, T. Scanning and transmission electron microscopic study of visceral and parietal peritoneal regions in the rat. *Anat. Anz.*, 1999, 181, 253–260.

Minot, CS. A sketch of comparative embyology. *Am. Nat.*, 1880, 14, 871–880.

Minot, CS. The mesoderm and the coelom of vertebrates. *Am. Nat.*, 1890, 24, 877–898.

Mironov, VA; Gusev, SA; Baradi, AF. Mesothelial stomata overlying omental milky spots: Scanning electron microscopic study. *Cell Tissue Res.*, 1979, 201, 327–330.

Miura, T; Shimada, T; Tanaka, K; Chujo, M; Uchida, Y. Lymphatic drainage of carbon particles injected into the pleural cavity of the monkey, as studied by video-assisted thoracoscopy and electron microscopy. *J. Thorac. Cardiovasc. Surg.*, 2000, 120, 437–447.

Moalli, PA; MacDonald, JL; Goodglick, LA; Kane, AB. Acute injury and regeneration of the mesothelium in response to asbestos fibers. *Am. J. Pathol.*, 1987, 128, 426–445.

Moore, KL (ed.). *The Developing Human*, 3rd edn. WB Saunders, Philadelphia, 1982.

Mutsaers, SE; Whitaker, D; Papadimitriou, JM. Changes in the concentration of microvilli on the free surface of healing mesothelium are associated with alterations in surface membrane charge. *J. Pathol.*, 1996, 180, 333–339.

Mutsaers, SE; Bishop, JE; McGrouther, G; Laurent, GJ. Mechanisms of tissue repair: from wound healing to fibrosis. *Int. J. Biochem. Cell Biol.*, 1997, 29, 5–17.

Mutsaers, SE. Mesothelial cells: their structure, function and role in serosal repair. *Respirology*, 2002, 7, 171–191.

Mutsaers, SE; Whitaker, D; Papadimitriou, JM. Stimulation of mesothelial cell proliferation by exudates macrophages enhances serosal wound healing in a murine model. *Am. J. Pathol.*, 2002, 160, 681–692.

Mutsaers, SE. The mesothelial cells. *Int. J. Biochem. Cell Biol.*, 36, 9-16.

Nakatani, T; Ohtani, O; Tanaka, S. Lymphatic stomata in the murine diaphragmatic peritoneum: The timing of their appearance and a map of their distribution. *Anat. Rec.*, 1996, 244, 529–539.

Negrini, D; Mukenge, S; Del Fabbro, M; Gonano, C; Miserocchi, G. Distribution of diaphragmatic lymphatic stomata. *J. Appl. Physiol.*, 1991, 70, 1544–1549.

Ohtani, Y; Ohtani, O. Obliteration of the lymphatic trunks draining diaphragmatic lymph causes peritoneal fluid to enter the pleural cavity. *Arch. Histol. Cytol.*, 1997, 60, 503–510.

Ohtani, Y; Ohtani, O; Nakatani, T. Microanatomy of the rat diaphragm with special reference to the lymphatics and mesothelial stomata. *Ital. J. Anat. Embryol.*, 1995, 100, 143–153.

Pelin, K; Hirvonen, A; Linnainmaa, K. Expression of cell adhesion molecules and connexins in gap junctional intercellular communication deficient human mesothelioma tumour cell lines and communication competent primary mesothelial cells. *Carcinogenesis*, 1994, 15, 2673–2675.

Raftery, AT. An enzyme histochemical study of mesothelial cells in rodents. *J. Anat.*, 1973, 115, 365–373.

Rougier, JP; Moullier, P; Piedagnel, R; Ronco, PM. Hyperosmolality suppresses but TGF beta 1 increases MMP9 in human peritoneal mesothelial cells. *Kidney Int.*, 1997, 51, 337–347.

Satoh, K; Arai, H; Nagai, H; Ito, M; Sato, H; Motomiya, M; Konno, K. Acid glycosaminoglycans in experimental pleural effusions. *Lung*, 1987, 165, 191–199.

Shao, XJ; Ohtani, O; Saitoh, M; Ohtani, Y. Development of diaphragmatic lymphatics: The process of their direct connection to the peritoneal cavity. *Arch. Histol. Cytol.*, 1998, 61, 137–149.

Shaw, RJ; Benedict, SH; Clark, RA; King Jr, TE. Pathogenesis of pulmonary fibrosis in interstitial lung disease. Alveolar macrophage PDGF (B) gene activation and up-regulation by interferon gamma. *Am. Rev. Respir. Dis.*, 1991, 143, 167–173.

Simsir, A; Fetsch, P; Mehta, D; Zakowski, M; Abati, A. E-Cadherin, N-cadherin, and calretinin in pleural effusions: The good, the bad, the worthless. *Diagn. Cytopathol.*, 1999, 20, 125–130.

Thors, F; Drukker, J. Serous membranes and their development, structure and topography. *Peritoneal adhesions* (pp. 3–13). Berlin: K.-H. Treutner, and V. Schumpelich (Eds.) Springer-Verlag.; 1997.

Tiedemann, K. On the yolk sac of the cat. Endoderm and mesothelium. *Cell Tissue Res.*, 1976, 173, 109–127.

Tsilibary, EC; Wissig, SL. Absorption from the peritoneal cavity: SEM study of the mesothelium covering the peritoneal surface of the muscular portion of the diaphragm. *Am. J. Anat.*, 1977, 149, 127–133.

Tyler, WS; Gillespie, JR; Nowell, JA. Modern functional morphology of the equine lung. *Equine Vet. J.*, 1971, 3, 84–94.

Von Recklinghausen, FV. Zur fettresorption. *Arch. Pathol. Anat.*, 1863, 24, 172–208.

Wang, NS. The regional difference of pleural mesothelial cells in rabbits. *Am. Rev. Respir. Dis.*, 1974, 110, 623–633.

Wang, NS. The preformed stomas connecting the pleural cavity and the lymphatics in the parietal pleura. *Am. Rev. Respir. Dis.*, 1975, 111, 12–20.

Wang, PM; Lai-Fook, SJ. Effects of ventilation on hyaluronan and protein concentration in pleural liquid of anesthetized and conscious rabbits. *Lung*, 1998, 176, 309–324.

Whitaker, D; Papadimitriou, JM; Walters, MN. The mesothelium: A histochemical study of resting mesothelial cells. *J. Pathol.*, 1980, 132, 273–284.

Whitaker, D; Papadimitriou, JM; Walters, MN. The mesothelium and its reactions: A review. *Crit. Rev. Toxicol.*, 1982; 10, 81–144.

Whitaker, D. *The mesothelium of the rat and its response to injury*. PhD Thesis, University of Western Australia, Perth. 1984.

Whitaker, D; Papadimitriou, J. Mesothelial healing: morphological and kinetic investigations. *J. Pathol.*, 1985, 145, 159–175.

In: Mesothelioma from Bench Side to Clinic
Editor: Alfonso Baldi, pp. 11-23
ISBN: 978-1-60021-789-0

Chapter II

Signaling Involved in Epithelial-Mesenchymal Transitions: From Embryogenesis to Cellular Pathogenesis

***Maria De Falco*[1]*, Michele M. Pisano*[2] *and Antonio De Luca*[3]**

[1] Department of Biological Sciences, Section of Evolutionary and Comparative Biology, University Federico II of Naples, Naples, Italy

[2]Birth Defects Center, Department of Molecular, Cellular and Craniofacial Biology, Health Sciences Center, University of Louisville, Louisville, KY, USA

[3]Department of Medicine and Public Health, Section of Clinical Anatomy, Second University of Naples, Naples, Italy

Abstract

Epithelial-mesenchymal transition (EMT) is an important mechanism during morphogenesis and is a remarkable example of cellular plasticity. EMT regulates important processes during the early stages of development of most organisms, but also has a role in adult organisms, as it has been shown to contribute to the pathology of certain diseases. This chapter discusses the molecular basis of EMT involved both in developmental processes and in pathological situation.

The Cellular and Molecular Basis of Epithelial-Mesenchymal Transitions

Normal epithelia possess cell-to-cell contacts that account for both the proper development of these tissues during embryonic life and for the maintenance of homeostasis and architecture of epithelial structures during adult life (Boyer et al. 2000). Epithelia serve several fundamental, related purposes: they serve as a barrier to the external environment, allowing the embryo to create an internal, physiologically controlled environment free from other organisms and debris; they potentially regulate patterning by forming barriers and limiting the diffusion of signaling molecules within the embryonic cavity; they also serve to polarize signaling and patterning within a two-dimensional sheet, through the planar cell polarity pathway (Adler, 2002; Shook and Keller 2003). Moreover, cells organized as an epithelium may provide more mechanical integrity than mesenchymal cells in the early embryo, and thus serve as the first line of defence of the embryo against mechanical disruption (Shook and Keller 2003). Epithelial-mesenchymal transition (EMT) is an integral component of several morphogenetic and organogenetic processes (Boyer et al. 2000). Gastrulation in many species, the emigration of neural crest cells from the neural tube, and the formation of cardiac valves are but a few of the critical developmental processes that proceed by EMT events (Duband et al. 1995; Hay 1995; Viebahn 1995; Boyer et al. 2000). Internalization of cells provides a mechanism for generating a new cell type, the mesenchymal cell, and results in an increase in embryonic complexity from diploblastic to triploblastic grades of organization (Buss 1987; Shook and Keller 2003). Release from the epithelial layer may have facilitated the evolution of the phenotypic plasticity of the mesenchymal cell type, in particular its ability to actively migrate individually, and thereby supporting further evolutionary diversification (Perez-Pomares and Munoz-Chapuli 2002). One advantage mesenchymal cells have over epithelial cells is that they are free to rearrange themselves or move about in three dimensions. Accordingly, EMT is used as a mechanism for reorganizing groups of progenitor cells into a more complex set of juxtaposed tissues, thereby allowing new inductive interactions (Behringer et al. 2000; Tam et al. 2001). The molecular mechanisms that regulate EMT are considerably overlapping with those that control cell adhesion, motility invasion, survival and differentiation (Thiery and Sleeman 2006). Consequently, it is important that EMTs occur in the correct spatial-temporal progression, such that progenitor cells are distributed in the appropriate patterns necessary for their further migration and differentiation.

Numerous cellular changes are associated with EMT. A primary EMT involves loss of the epithelial phenotype, or de-epithelialization, which would leave non-epithelial, or nominal "mesenchymal" cells, in place of what was an epithelium, and also leave a surrounding epithelium with free edges where the process of de-epithelialization had terminated (Shook and Keller 2003). Specification toward a mesenchymal phenotype involves many important changes in gene expression and protein function that must all work in concert for an EMT to occur correctly. Such changes may initiate withdrawal from the cell division cycle so that the cytoskeleton can be used to drive the cell shape changes and cell migration needed for EMT (Shook and Keller 2003). Therefore, cells must continue the process of turning off epithelial characteristics and turning on mesenchymal characteristics. This requires a major reorganization of the cell, including completely dismantling the apical junctional "scaffold" that is thought to regulate discrimination between apical and basal-lateral surfaces (Rashbass and Skaer 2000) by vesicular traffic, and organization of the cytoskeleton. This, in conjunction with the removal of the apical membrane, results in the loss of the cell's apical-basal polarity. The basal-lateral membrane also must be remodelled, including the removal of epithelial adhesive molecules, perhaps by endocytosis, and replacement by mesenchymal-type adhesion molecules (cadherins) and matrix receptors (integrins) (Shook and Keller 2003). In some cases, cells undergoing EMT start synthesizing extracellular matrix (ECM) molecules such as fibronectin, collagen I, vimentin, and tenascin (Hulboy et al. 2001;Prindull and Zipori 2004), as well as ECM metabolizing molecules such as stromelysin-1 (a matrix metalloproteinase) and other proteolytic enzymes involved in matrix degradation that contribute to cell motility and invasiveness (Boyer et al. 2000; Hulboy et al. 2001). During EMT, cell scattering consists of at least two biological events, which appear to occur simultaneously or synchronously in the cells: (a) cell-cell dissociation, resulting from the breaking apart of intercellular adhesion complexes, and (b) cell movement, driven by rearrangement of the cytoskeleton and formation of new cell-substratum contacts. The two responses can occur independently. Moreover, cell scattering appears as a non-cell-autonomous process, requiring external stimuli to be activated (Boyer et al. 2000).

The primary mode of induction of EMT is provided by specific growth factors or extracellular matrix components binding to their cognate cellular receptors. With the exception of transforming growth factor beta (TGF-β), which is involved in EMTs during developmental morphogenetic events (Runyan et al. 1990), the majority of growth factors exert their scattering effect trough receptors with ligand-inducible intrinsic receptor tyrosine kinase (RTK) activity (Boyer et al. 2000). It has been demonstrated that any growth factor binding to a tyrosine kinase receptor is a potential scatter factor, provided that its cognate receptor is expressed and that the responding cell is equipped with the machinery needed for cell scattering. This idea is reinforced by the finding that a large number of growth factors that bind to RTK are endowed with scattering activity. The prototype of scattering factors is the hepatocyte growth factor/scatter factor (HGF/SF) binding to its receptor c-Met, a member of the RTK family (Boyer et al. 2000). Activation of RTKs by their cognate ligands generates cascades of cytoplasmic events initiated by the autophosporylation of specific tyrosines on the activated receptors. RTKs have a pivotal role in the regulation of a variety of biological functions which are associated with changes in cell morphology, including malignant transformation (Parsons and Weber 1989), epithelial plasticity (Warren and Nelson 1987), and modulation of intercellular adhesion (Volberg et al. 1991; Boyer et al. 2000).

The oncogene Src belongs to a family of cytoplasmic tyrosine kinases. The Src family is composed of nine members, all of which contain one SH2 and one SH3 domain. In this family, Src, Fyn and Yes are ubiquitously expressed while the other members have a more restricted pattern of expression. Src and Yes have redundant functions during cell scattering, probably by phosphorylating common substrates important for signaling, and by binding the same target proteins (Boyer et al. 1997; Boyer et al. 2000). Although the mechanisms whereby Src kinases exert their functions are still unclear, three hypotheses have emerged: 1) Src phosphorylates specific substrates which are mainly cytoskeletal-based components, and molecules localized in cell-cell and cell-substratum adhesion complexes (Kellie et al. 1991; Wu et al. 1991; Clark and Brugge 1993; Okamura and Resh 1995), the tyrosine phosphorylation of which could in turn alter the cellular architecture; 2) Src participates in entry into S-phase by inducing Myc via a specific signal transduction pathway (Barone and Courtneidge 1995); 3) Src activity interacts with other signaling pathways, for example, activated Src can bind Shc, an early element of the Ras cascade, leading to the activation of this pathway (McGlade et al. 1992; Nagai et al. 1995; Boyer et al. 2000). The SH2-SH3 domain-containing adaptor protein Grb2 that connects activated RTK to the Ras pathway participates in HGF-induced cell scattering (Gay et al. 1999). Among the different Ras effectors, the best characterized is the serine/threonine kinase Raf that initiates a series of phosphorylation reactions resulting in the activation of mitogen activated protein kinase (MAPK). The regulation by MAPKs has been implicated in a wide variety of biological processes, including cell proliferation, integrin-mediated cell adhesion, secretion, neuronal cell differentiation and others. A role of the MAPK pathway has been demonstrated in HGF/SF-induced scattering (Herrera 1998; Potempka and Ridley 1998; Tanimura et al. 1998). MAPK may also act in cell scattering by activating transcription factors other than the Jun/Fos complex or by phosphorylating cytoplasmic substrates that remain to be identified. p38, another member of the MAPK family, also has been implicated in cell motility stimulated by platelet-derived growth factor (PDGF) and it is activated via a Ras-dependent pathway (Matsumoto et al. 1999). Moreover, Ras has been implicated in the activation of other signaling molecules involved in EMT (Boyer et al. 2000). The phosphatidylinositol 3-kinase (PI3K) is likely to be involved in cell motility by activating the small GTPase Rac (Stephens et al. 1996; Hooshmand-Rad et al. 1997; Sander et al. 1998), whose role in cell migration and invasiveness is well established (Keeley et al. 1997; Arber et al. 1998; Jones et al. 1998; Gimond et al. 1999). Rac may in turn stimulate the p21 (cdc42/Rac)-activated kinase Pak1, which could induce the phosphorylation of myosin light chain, thus linking the Rac-induced pathway to proteins directly affecting cell movement (Knaus and Bokoch 1998; Sells et al. 1999). Rac also has been shown unambiguously to strengthen cell–cell adhesion, thereby preventing tumor cell invasiveness (Hordijk et al. 1997; Takaishi et al. 1997). Moreover, activities of both Rac and Rho are required for the formation of cellular adherens junctions (Braga et al. 1997; Takaishi et al. 1997; Braga et al. 1999). The apparent discrepancy between the two antagonistic roles attributed to Rac may well be related to the finding that the type of response following Rac activation depends on the cell substratum. On substrata permissive for locomotion, under conditions preventing the formation of adherens junctions, expression of active Rac promotes motile behaviour. Whereas, on substrata impeding cell motility, Rac-dependent cell-cell adhesion is favoured (Sander et al. 1998). Rho, another small GTPase of the Rho family, has complex functions in cell scattering, probably related to its attributed role in the assembly of focal adhesion contacts and actin stress fibers formation in fibroblast cells (Ridley and Hall 1992). The mechanism whereby Rho regulates cytokinesis and cell motility is likely due to its ability to stimulate the phosphorylation of the myosin light chain (Amano et al. 1996) and/or adducin, an actin-binding protein (Fukata et al. 1999). In contrast to the promotion of cell motility by Rho-mediated signaling, Rho activity may antagonize epithelial cell scattering signals (Ridley et al. 1995) by reinforcing cell-cell adhesion complexes (Boyer et al. 2000).

Because Since EMT events require the coordinated expression of numerous genes, it is of pivotal importance to identify the molecular components of signaling pathways which mediate the transcriptional regulation of these genes. Among these, several transcription factors have been considered as master genes, capable of controlling the entire EMT process. Such a role may be attributed to the Fos transcriptional activator (Reichman et al. 1992; Fialka et al. 1996), which induces an EMT process by activating a Wnt-like pathway initiated by β-catenin nuclear localization (Eger et al. 2000). The Fos transcriptional dimerization partner, Jun, exerts its effect in EMT by mediating the translocation of Rac to the plasma membrane, which is a prerequisite for its activation and the subsequent cytoskeletal rearrangements required for cell motility (Malliri et al. 1998). Other transcription factors also are capable of inducing EMTs. The Snail family has been implicated in EMTs during embryogenesis and in tumor progression by inducing a dramatic epithelial to mesenchymal conversion, concomitant with the loss of E-cadherin, and thereby promoting the acquisition of invasive and migratory behaviour (Batlle et al. 2000; Cano et al. 2000). The adhesion molecule E-cadherin localizes to cell-cell boundary regions and is regulated by integrins (Somasiri et al. 2001; Avizienyte et al. 2002; Prindull and Zipori 2004). Another Snail family member, Slug, does not appear to participate in E-cadherin down-regulation, but has been demonstrated to contribute to the maintenance of the mesenchymal phenotype (Ros et al. 1997). In addition to the above-mentioned transcription factors, members of the Ets family also have been suggested to play a role in EMTs. The Ets family members participate in EMT by controlling urokinase-type plasminogen activator (uPA) activity, which facilitates cell migration by degrading extracellular matrix components (Delannoy-Courdent et al. 1998). Ets also may regulate the transcription of other genes that remain to be identified (Boyer et al. 2000).

Dissociation of cell-cell contacts, an integral step in EMTs, occurs through several distinct mechanisms. Down-regulation of E-cadherin, the transmembrane adhesion molecule that participates in the establishment of adherens junctions, is well documented and may account for a number of EMTs (Takeichi 1993; Birchmeier and Behrens 1994; Perl et al. 1998). As E-cadherin levels become limiting, E-cadherin-mediated sequestering of β-catenin in the cytoplasm is abolished (Thiery and Sleeman 2006). As a result, ß-catenin localizes to the nucleus and feeds into Wnt signalling pathway by activating transcriptional regulation through LEF/TCF4 (lymphoid-enhancer-binding factor/T-cell factor-4) (Thiery and Sleeman 2006). As an early step in EMTs, E-cadherin–mediated adhesion of epithelial cells decreases to allow for mesenchymal motility (Prindull and Zipori 2004). In the majority of cases, the absence of E-cadherin can be correlated to either silencing mutations in the E-cadherin gene or transcriptionally mediated down-regulation of its expression, occurring at the transcriptional level Henning et al. 1996). Cell-cell dissociation, occurring in EMT processes in which E-cadherin-dependent adhesion is not a direct target of EMT signals, also can result from the perturbation of intercellular junctions other than cellular adherens junctions. The component of cell-cell junctions, p120 catenin, participates in regulation of cell motility by being a link between the formation and disruption of cadherin-mediated contacts (Grosheva et al. 2001; Prindull and Zipori 2004). Ephrins, cell surface receptor tyrosine kinases, reversibly signal cell boundaries in developmental cell recognition, synergize with E-cadherin, and, likewise, have been implicated in a variety of EMTs during embryogenesis (Orsulic and Kemler 2000; Prindull and Zipori 2004). Cell-cell dissociation has also been associated with epidermal growth factor (EGF)-mediated desmososmal internalization and down-regulation (Boyer et a. 1989)

The disruption of intercellular junctions may not be sufficient to promote the entire set of morphological changes, including acquisition of cell motility, that accompany EMT processes. Therefore, even though intercellular junctions appear as primary targets in epithelial cell scattering, other cellular events, independent of cell-cell dissociation, could contribute to the initiation and completion of the EMT process. For instance, cytoskeletal remodelling and simultaneous acquisition of cell motility are not likely to depend directly on cell-cell dissociation. Rather, they are governed by cell–substratum adhesion sites, in which integrins represent the transmembrane receptors for extracellular components (Sarkar 1999). Activation of α2β1 integrins by collagen is sufficient to drive a growth factor-independent EMT process, during which cell-cell dissociation appears as a consequence of the mechanical forces exerted on cell-cell adhesion sites by cells in motion (Tucker et al. 1990). Integrins have an important role in EMTs because they mediate intercellular communication by binding to the ECM and signaling information from the ECM, through an extensive network of cytoskeletal molecules (Darribere et al. 2000; Prindull and Zipori 2004). Extensive crosstalk between integrin signalling and pathways that regulate EMTs has been observed. For example, the TGF-β signalling through p38 MAPK that is required for EMT is dependent on signalling by β1 integrin (Bhowmick et al. 2001). Conversely, TGF-β-induced expression of disabled-2 (DAB2), an adaptor molecule that binds to β1 integrin, is required for integrin activation, the formation of cellular focal adhesions and cell survival during EMTs (Prunier and Howe 2005). Similarly, α2β1 integrin is required for aspects of collagen and fibroblast growth factor 1 (FGF1)-induced EMT (Valles et al. 1996).The mechanism by which the EMT signal is converted into cell motility is likely to involve the actin/myosin motility machinery, which can be a direct target of several growth factor-induced signaling pathways. The Rho family of small G proteins may be the link between the growth factor signal and the cytoskeletal reorganization which is necessary for cell motility. An alternate, yet not exclusive hypothesis is that cell motility is triggered by integrins activated by the EMT signal. Indeed, several effector molecules of integrin-mediated signalling have been demonstrated to affect the actin cytoskeleton (Keeley et al. 1998; Schoenwaelder and Burridge 1999; Boyer et al. 2000).

EMTs and Tumorigenesis

In addition to the critical role of EMTs in the development of many tissues during embryogenesis, similar cellular changes, as occur in EMTs, are recapitulated during pathological processes such as fibrosis and cancer. A common spectrum of EMT-associated changes in morphology and gene-expression patterns are associated with embryogenesis and tumorigenesis, and recent studies have shown a remarkable similarity between the signalling pathways that regulate EMT in these apparently disparate processes (Thiery and Sleeman 2006). EMT is believed to be activated during the later stages of tumor progression but does not seem to play a major role in the initiation of neoplasms. Phenotypic EMT may represent an early indication that a cell no longer recognizes or respects its neighbours, is no longer subject to contact inhibition and coordinating synergism, and may serve as a vehicle for tumor dissemination. Forced expression of N-cadherin leads to EMT. The extracellular repeat portion of N-cadherin was shown to be necessary and sufficient to promote EMT and cell motility (Kim et al. 2000). Snail triggers EMT-associated tumor progression by virtue of its strong suppressor effects on E-cadherin gene expression (Cano et al. 2000). Epithelial cells, ectopically expressing snail, adopt a fibroblast phenotype and acquire tumorigenic and invasive properties. Clinically, Snail is expressed in all ductal carcinomas with lymph node metastases, including breast tumors. The intensity of Snail expression correlates inversely with the degree of cellular differentiation (Carver et al. 2001) Since β-catenin is an E-cadherin–associated protein and a key component of the Wnt signaling pathway, it is not surprising that mutated β-catenin is a pathogenetic factor in the transition of premalignant to neoplastic cancer and in invasion and metastases in several types of cancer (Reya et al 2001). Target genes of β-catenin include matrix metalloproteinase 7 (MMP-7), urokinase-type plasminogen activator (uPA), as well as the cell adhesion molecule NrCAM (Conacci-Sorrell et al. 2002). During promotion of EMT in several premalignant and malignant human carcinomas, members of the EGF/CfC gene family, such as Cripto, suppress β-catenin function. Expression of Cripto is increased several-fold in EMT, not only in human tumors such as colon, gastric, pancreas, lung, and breast carcinoma, but also is detectable in premalignant lesions of some of these neoplasms (Saloman et al 2000). TGF-β, which interfaces with other signalling pathways such as the Wnt and EGF/Cripto pathways, indeed promotes EMT in late stage tumors. *In vitro* treatment of several human carcinoma cell lines with TGF-β-neutralizing antibody results in loss of invasiveness (Oft et al. 1998). The capacity of TGF-β to mediate EMT is dependent on cooperation with Ras signaling. Ha-Ras and TGF-β cause sustained EMT and a metastatic phenotype that is mediated through the activation of Raf/MAPK. However, phosphatidylinositol 3-kinase (PI3K) activation has a complementary function in promoting tumorigenesis, e.g. proliferation (Janda et al. 2002a; Janda et al. 2002b). Elevated H-ras expression induces nuclear accumulation of Smad-2 which promotes EMT and subsequent invasiveness and metastatic dissemination (Oft et al. 2002). EMT may be a reversible phenomenon, even in aggressive tumor cell lines such as small cell lung cancer, if the cells are allowed to re-establish E-cadherin-mediated cellular adhesion contacts. Exposure of small cell lung carcinoma to 5-bromodeoxyuridine leads to reversion back to a normal cell phenotype, with re-establishment of cell-cell and cell-to-matrix adhesions, down-regulation of vimentin, up-regulation of cytokeratin, and redistribution of the actin cytoskeleton (Gilchrist et al. 2002). The high level of cell plasticity, inherent in both embryonal development and tumor progression, suggests that various aspects of tumorigenesis could be a recapitulation of stages of embryogenesis. Indeed, a comparison between Snail-induced E-cadherin repression in undifferentiated mesoderm and in tissues undergoing EMT, in early mouse development versus tumor cell lines, lead to the conclusion that "the same molecules are used to trigger epithelial-mesenchymal transition during embryonic development and in tumor progression" (Cano et al. 2000) It is possible that the tumor stroma contains mesenchymally transformed epithelial cancer cells – generated by EMT – that participate with the physiologic stroma cells in creating a nascent tumor's microenvironment (Prindull and Zipori 2004). Although EMT seems to be closely associated with, and probably functions as a basic mechanism in, cancer progression, more detailed information is needed on the properties of EMT-transformed epithelial cells and on the sequence of steps that take place during cancer progression.

References

Adler, PN. Planar signaling and morphogenesis in Drosophila. *Dev. Cell*, 2002, 2, 525–535.

Amano, M; Ito, M; Kimura, K; Fukata, Y; Chihara, K; Nakano, T; Matsuura, Y; Kaibuchi, K. Phosphorylation and activation of myosin by Rho-associated kinase (Rho-kinase). *J. Biol. Chem.,* 1996, 271, 20246–20249.

Arber, S; Barbayannis, FA; Hanser, H; Schneider, C; Stanyon, CA; Bernard, O; Caroni, P. Regulation of actin dynamics through phosphorylation of cofilin by LIM-kinase. *Nature*, 1998, 393, 805–809.

Avizienyte, E; Wyke, AW; Jones, RJ; McLean, GW; Westhoff, MA; Brunton, VG; Frame, MC. et al. Src-induced de-regulation of E-cadherin in colon cancer cells requires integrin signalling. *Nat. Cell Biol.*, 2002, 4, 632-638.

Barone, MV; Courtneidge, SA. Myc but not Fos rescue of PDGF signalling block caused by kinase-inactive Src. *Nature*, 1995, 378, 509–512.

Batlle, E; Sancho, E; Franci, C; Dominguez, D; Monfar, M; Baulida, J; Garcia de Herreros, AG. The transcription factor snail is a repressor of E-cadherin gene expression in epithelial tumour cells. *Nat. Cell Biol.*, 2000, 2, 84–89.

Bhowmick, NA; Zent, R; Ghiassi, M; McDonnell, M. Moses, HL. Integrin □1 signaling is necessary for transforming growth factor-□ activation of p38MAPK and epithelial plasticity. *J. Biol. Chem.*, 2001, 276, 46707–46713.

Birchmeier, W; Behrens, J. Cadherin expression in carcinomas: Role in the formation of cell junctions and the prevention of invasiveness. *Biochim. Biophys. Acta*, 1994, 1198, 11–26.

Boyer, B; Tucker, GC; Valles, AM; Franke, WW; Thiery JP. Rearrangements of desmosomal and cytoskeletal proteins during the transition from epithelial to fibroblastoid organization in cultured rat bladder carcinoma cells. *J. Cell Biol.*, 1989, 109, 1495–1509.

Boyer, B; Roche, S; Denoyelle, M; Thiery, JP. Src and Ras are involved in separate pathways in epithelial cell scattering. *EMBO J.,* 1997, 196, 5904–5913.

Boyer, B; Valles, AM; Edme, N. Induction and regulation of epithelial–mesenchymal transitions. *Biochem. Pharmacol.*, 2000, 60, 1091–1099.

Braga, VM; Machesky, LM; Hall, A; Hotchin, NA. The small GTPases Rho and Rac are required for the establishment of cadherin-dependent cell– cell contacts. *J. Cell Biol.*, 1997, 137, 1421–1431.

Braga, VM; Del Maschio, A; Machesky, L; Dejana, E. Regulation of cadherin function by Rho and Rac: Modulation by junction maturation and cellular context. *Mol. Biol. Cell*, 1999, 10, 9–22.

Buss, LW.. *The Evolution of Individuality*. Princeton University Press, Princeton, NJ. 1987.

Cano, A; Perez-Moreno, MA; Rodrigo, I; Locascio, A; Blanco, MJ; del Barrio, MG; Portillo, F; Nieto, MA. The transcription factor snail controls epithelial-mesenchymal transitions by repressing E-cadherin expression. *Nat. Cell Biol.*, 2000, 2, 76–83.

Carver, EA; Jiang, R; Lan, Y; Oram, KF; Gridley, T. The mouse snail gene encodes a key regulator of the epithelial-mesenchymal transition. *Mol. Cell Biol.*, 2001, 21, 8184-8188.

Clark, EA; Brugge, JS. Redistribution of activated pp60csrc to integrin-dependent cytoskeletal complexes in thrombin-stimulated platelets. *Mol. Cell Biol.*, 1993, 13, 1863–1871.

Conacci-Sorrell, ME; Ben-Yedidia, T; Shtutman, M; Feinstein, E; Einat, P; Ben-Zeev, A. Nr-CAM is a target gene of the beta-catenin/LEF-1 pathway in melanoma and colon cancer and its expression enhances motility and confers tumorigenesis. *Genes Dev.*, 2002, 16, 2058-2072.

Darribere, T; Skalski, M; Cousin, HL; Gaultier, A; Montmory, C; Alfandari, D. Integrins: regulators of embryogenesis. *Biol. Cell*, 2000, 92, 5-25.

Delannoy-Courdent, A; Mattot, V; Fafeur, V; Fauquette, W; Pollet, I; Calmels, T; Vercamer, C; Boilly, B; Vandenbunder, B; Desbiens, X. The expression of an Etsl transcription factor lacking its activation domain decreases uPA proteolytic activity and cell motility, and impairs normal tubulogenesis and cancerous scattering in mammary epithelial cells. *J. Cell Sci.*, 1998, 111, 1521–1534.

Duband, JL; Monier, F; Delannet, M; Newgreen, D. Epithelium–mesenchyme transition during neural crest development. *Acta Anat.* (Basel), 1995, 154, 63–78.

Eger, A; Stockinger, A; Schaffhauser, B; Beug H; Foisner, R. Epithelial mesenchymal transition by c-Fos estrogen receptor activation involves nuclear translocation of betacatenin and upregulation of beta-catenin/lymphoid enhancer binding factor-1 transcriptional activity. *J. Cell Biol.*, 2000, 148, 173–188.

Fialka, I; Schwarz, H; Reichmann, E; Oft, M; Busslinger, M; Beug, H. The estrogen-dependent c-JunER protein causes a reversible loss of mammary epithelial cell polarity involving a destabilization of adherens junctions. *J. Cell Biol.*, 1996, 132, 1115–1132.

Fukata, Y; Oshiro, N; Kinoshita, N; Kawano, Y; Matsuoka, Y; Bennett, V; Matsuura, Y; Kaibuchi, K. Phosphorylation of adducin by rho-kinase plays a crucial role in cell motility. *J. Cell Biol.*, 1999, 145, 347–361.

Gay, B; Suarez, S; Weber, C; Rahuel, J; Fabbro, D; Furet, P; Caravatti, G; Schoepfer, J. Effect of potent and selective inhibitors of the Grb2 SH2 domain on cell motility. *J. Biol. Chem.*, 1999, 274, 23311–23315.

Gilchrist, AJ; Meuser, R; Turchinsky, J; Shaw, AR; Pasdar, M; Dixon, WT. Cell adhesion-mediated transformation of a human SCLC cell line is associated with the development of a normal phenotype. *Exp. Cell. Res.* 2002, 276, 63-78.

Gimond, C; van der Flier, A; van Delft, S; Brakebusch, C; Kinkman, I; Collard, JG; Fasler, R; Sonnenberg, A. Induction of cell scattering by expression of b1 integrins in b1-deficient epithelial cells requires activation of members of the Rho family of GTPases and downregulation of cadherin and catenin function. *J. Cell. Biol.*, 1999, 147, 1325–1340.

Grosheva, I; Shtutman, M; Elbaum, M; Bershadsky, AD. p120 catenin affects cell motility via modulation of activity of Rho-family GTPases: a link between cell-cell contact formation and regulation of cell locomotion. *J. Cell. Sci.*, 2001, 114, 695-707.

Hay, ED. An overview of epithelio-mesenchymal transformation. *Acta Anat.* (Basel), 1995, 154, 8–20.

Hennig, G; Lowrick, O; Birchmeier, W; Behrens, J. Mechanisms identified in the transcriptional control of epithelial gene expression. *J. Biol. Chem.*, 1996, 271, 595–602.

Herrera, R. Modulation of hepatocyte growth factor-induced scattering of HT29 colon carcinoma cells. *J. Cell. Sci.*, 1998, 111, 1039–1049.

Hooshmand-Rad, R; Claesson-Welsh, L; Wennstrom, S; Yokote, K; Siegbahn, A; Heldin, CH. Involvement of phosphatidylinositide 39-kinase and Rac in platelet-derived growth factor-induced actin reorganization and chemotaxis. *Exp. Cell. Res.*, 1997, 234, 434–441.

Hordijk, PL; ten Klooster, JP; van der Kammen, RA; Michiels, F; Oomen, LC; Collard, JG. Inhibition of invasion of epithelial cells by Tiam1-Rac signaling. *Science*, 1997, 278, 1464–1466.

Hulboy, DL; Matrisian, LM; Crawford, HC. Loss of JunB activity enhances stromelysin 1 expression in a model of the epithelial-to-mesenchymal transition of mouse skin tumors. *Mol. Cell. Biol.*, 2001, 21, 5478-5487.

Janda, E; Lehmann, K; Killisch, I; Jechlinger, M; Herzig, M; Downward, J; Beug, H; Grunert, S. Ras and TGF cooperatively regulate epithelial cell plasticity and metastasis: dissection of Ras signaling pathways. *J. Cell. Biol.*, 2002, 156, 299-313.

Janda, E; Litos, G; Grunert, S; Downward, J; Beug, H. Oncogenic Ras/Her-2 mediate hyperproliferation of polarized epithelial cells in 3D cultures and rapid tumor growth via the PI3K pathway. *Oncogene,* 2002, 21, 5148-5159.

Jones, GE; Allen, WE; Ridley, AJ. The Rho GTPases in macrophage motility and chemotaxis. *Cell. Adhes. Commun.*, 1998, 6, 237–245.

Keely, P; Parise, L; Juliano, R. Integrins and GTPases in tumour growth, motility and invasion. *Trends Cell. Biol.*, 1998, 8, 100–106.

Keely, PJ; Westwick, JK; Whitehead, IP; Der, CJ; Parise, LV. Cdc42 and Rac1 induce integrin-mediated cell motility and invasiveness through PI(3)K. *Nature*, 1997, 390, 632–636.

Kellie, S; Horvath, AR; Elmore, MA. Cytoskeletal targets for oncogenic tyrosine kinases. *J. Cell. Sci.,* 1991, 99, 207–211.

Kim, JB; Islam, S; Kim, YJ; Prudoff, RS; Sass, KM; Wheelock, MJ; Johnson, KR. N-Cadherin extracellular repeat 4 mediates epithelial to mesenchymal transition and increased motility. *J. Cell. Biol.*, 2000, 151, 1193-1206.

Knaus, UG; Bokoch, GM. The p21Rac/Cdc42-activated kinases (PAKs). *Int. J. Biochem. Cell. Biol.,* 1998, 30, 857–862.

Malliri, A; Symons, M; Hennigan, RF; Hurlstone, AF; Lamb, RF; Wheeler, T; Ozanne, BW. The transcription factor AP-1 is required for EGF-induced activation of rho-like GTPases, cytoskeletal rearrangements, motility, and in vitro invasion of A431 cells. *J. Cell. Biol.*, 1998, 143, 1087–1099.

Matsumoto, T; Yokote, K; Tamura, K; Takemoto, M; Ueno, H; Saito, Y; Mori, S. Platelet-derived growth factor activates p38 mitogen-activated protein kinase through a Ras-dependent pathway that is important for actin reorganization and cell migration. *J. Biol. Chem.*, 1999, 274, 13954–13960.

McGlade, J; Cheng, A; Pelicci, G; Pelicci, PG; Pawson, T. Shc proteins are phosphorylated and regulated by the v-Src and v-Fps protein-tyrosine kinases. *Proc. Natl. Acad. Sci. USA*, 1992, 89, 8869–8873.

Nagai, K; Takata, M; Yamamura, H; Kurosaki, T. Tyrosine phosphorylation of Shc is mediated through Lyn and Syk in B cell receptor signaling. *J. Biol. Chem.*, 1995, 270, 6824–6829.

Oft, M; Akhurst, RJ; Balmain, A. Metastasis is driven by sequential elevation of H-ras and Smad2 levels. *Nat. Cell Biol.*, 2002, 4, 487-494.

Oft, M; Heider, KH; Beug, H. TGFbeta signaling is necessary for carcinoma cell invasiveness and metastasis. *Curr. Biol.*, 1998, 8, 1243-1252.

Okamura, H; Resh, MD. p80/85 cortactin associates with the Src SH2 domain and colocalizes with v-Src in transformed cells. *J. Biol. Chem.*, 1995, 270, 26613–26618.

Orsulic, S; Kemler, R. Expression of Eph receptors and ephrins is differentially regulated by E-cadherin. *J. Cell. Sci.*, 2000, 113, 1793-1802.

Parsons, JT; Weber, MJ. Genetics of src: Structure and functional organization of a tyrosine protein kinase. *Curr. Top. Microbiol. Immunol.*, 1989, 147, 79–127.

Perez-Pomares, JM; Munoz-Chapuli, R. Epithelial–mesenchymal transitions: a mesodermal cell strategy for evolutive innovation in metazoans. *Anat. Rec.*, 2002, 268, 343–351.

Perl, AK; Wilgenbus, P; Dahl, U; Semb, H; Christofori, G. A causal role for E-cadherin in the transition from adenoma to carcinoma. *Nature*, 1998, 392, 190–193.

Potempka, S; Ridley, AJ. Activation of both MAPK and phosphatidylinositide 3-kinase by Ras is required for hepatocytes growth factor/scatter factor-induced adherens junction disassembly. *Mol. Biol. Cell*, 1998, 9, 2185–2195.

Prindull, G; Zipori, D. Environmental guidance of normal and tumor cell plasticity: epithelial mesenchymal transitions as a paradigm. *Blood*, 2004, 103, 2892–2899.

Prunier, C; Howe, PH. Disabled-2 (Dab2) is required for transforming growth factor □-induced epithelial to mesenchymal transition (EMT). *J. Biol. Chem.*, 2005, 280, 17540–17548.

Rashbass, P; Skaer, H. Cell polarity: nailing crumbs to the scaffold. *Curr. Biol.*, 2000, 10, R234–R236.

Reichman, E; Schwarz, H; Deiner, EM; Leitner, I; Eilers, M; Berger, H; Busslinger, M; Beug H. Activation of an inducible c-FosER fusion protein causes loss of epithelial polarity and triggers epithelial-fibroblastoid cell conversion. *Cell,* 1992, 71, 1103–1116.

Reya, T; Morrison, SJ; Clarke, MF; Weissman, IL. Stem cells, cancer, and cancer stem cells. *Nature*, 2001, 414, 105-111.

Ridley, AJ; Hall, A, The small GTP-binding protein rho regulates the assembly of focal adhesions and actin stress fibers in response to growth factors. *Cell*, 1992, 70, 389–399.

Ridley, AJ; Comoglio, PM; Hall, A. Regulation of scatter factor/hepatocyte growth factor responses by Ras, Rac, and Rho in MDCK cells. *Mol. Cell. Biol.*, 1995, 15, 1110–1122.

Ros, M; Sefton, M; Nieto, MA. Slug, a zinc finger gene previously implicated in the early patterning of mesoderm and the neural crest, is also involved in chick limb development. *Development*, 1997, 124, 1821–1829.

Runyan, RB; Potts, JD; Sharma, RV; Loeber, CP; Chiang, JJ; Bhalla, RC. Signal transduction of a tissue interaction during embryonic heart development. *Cell, Regul.*, 1990, 1, 301–313.

Saloman, DS; Bianco, C; Ebert, AD; Khan, NI; De Santis, M; Normanno, N; Wechselberger, C; Seno, M; Williams, K; Sanicola, M; Foley, S; Gullick, WJ; Persico, G. The EGF-CFC family: novel epidermal growth factor related proteins in development and cancer. *Endocr. Relat. Cancer*, 2000, 7, 199-226.

Sander, EE; van Delft, S; ten Klooster, JP; Reid, T; van der Kammen, RA; Michiels, F; Collard, JG. Matrix-dependent Tiam1/Rac signaling in epithelial cells promotes either cell– cell adhesion or cell migration and is regulated by phosphatidylinositol 3-kinase. *J. Cell. Biol.,* 1998, 143, 1385–1398.

Sarkar, S. Focal adhesions. *Curr. Biol.* 1999, 9, 428–430.

Schoenwaelder, SM; Burridge, K. Bidirectional signaling between the cytoskeleton and integrins. *Curr. Opin. Cell. Biol.*, 1999, 11, 274–286.

Sells, M; Boyd, J; Chernoff, J. p21-activated kinase 1 (Pak1) regulates cell motility in mammalian fibroblasts. *J. Cell. Biol.*, 1999, 145, 837–849.

Shook, D; Keller, R. Mechanisms, mechanics and function of epithelial-mesenchymal transitions in early development. *Mech. Dev.*, 2003, 120, 1351–1383.

Somasiri, A; Howarth, A; Goswami, D; Dedhar, S; Roskelley, CD. Overexpression of the integrinlinked kinase mesenchymally transforms mammary epithelial cells. *J. Cell. Sci.*, 2001, 114, 1125-1136.

Stephens, L; Hawkins, PT; Eguinoa, A; Cooke, F. A heterotrimeric GTPase-regulated isoform of PI3K and the regulation of its potential effectors. *Philos. Trans. R. Soc. Lond. B Biol. Sci.,* 1996, 351, 211–215.

Takaishi, K; Sasaki, T; Kotani, H; Nishioka, H; Takai, Y. Regulation of cell– cell adhesion by rac and rho small G proteins in MDCK cells. *J. Cell. Biol.*, 1997, 139, 1047–1059.

Takeichi, M. Cadherins in cancer: Implications for invasion and metastasis. Curr. Opin. Cell. Biol., 1993, 5, 806–811.

Tam, PP; Gad, JM; Kinder, SJ; Tsang, TE; Behringer, RR. Morphogenetic tissue movement and the establishment of body planduring development from blastocyst to gastrula in the mouse. *Bioessays*, 2001, 23, 508–517.

Tanimura, S; Chatani, Y; Hoshino, R; Sato, M; Watanabe, S; Kataoka, T; Nakamura, T; Kohno, M. Activation of the 41/43kDa mitogen-activated protein kinase signaling is required for hepatocyte growth factor-induced cell scattering. *Oncogene*, 1998, 17, 57–65.

Thiery, JP; Slleman, JP. Complex networks orchestrate epithelial-mesenchymal transitions. *Nat. Rev.*, 7, 131–142.

Tucker, GC; Boyer, B. Gavrilovic J; Emonard H and Thiery JP, Collagen-mediated dispersion of NBT-II rat bladder carcinoma cells. *Cancer Res.*, 1990, 50, 129–137.

Valles, A. M; Boyer, B; Tarone, G; Thiery, JP. α2 β1 integrin is required for the collagen and FGF-1 induced cell dispersion in a rat bladder carcinoma cell line. *Cell. Adhes. Commun.,* 1996, 4, 187–199.

Viebahn, C. Epithelio-mesenchymal transformation during formation of the mesoderm in the mammalian embryo. *Acta Anat.* (Basel), 1995, 154, 79–97.

Volberg, T; Geiger, B; Dror, R; Zick, Y. Modulation of intercellular adherens-type junctions and tyrosine phosphorylation of their components in RSV-transformed cultured chick lens cells. *Cell. Regul.*, 1991, 2, 105–120.

Warren, SL; Nelson, WJ. Nonmitogenic morphoregulatory action of pp60v-src on multicellular epithelial structures. *Mol. Cell. Biol.*, 1987, 7, 1326–1337.

Wu, H; Reynolds, AB; Kanner, SB; Vines, RR; Parsons, JT. Identification of a novel cytoskeleton-associated pp60c-src substrate. *Mol. Cell. Biol.*, 1991, 11, 5113–5124.

In: Mesothelioma from Bench Side to Clinic
Editor: Alfonso Baldi, pp. 25-66

ISBN: 978-1-60021-789-0

Chapter III

Epidemiology of Mesothelioma: The Role of Asbestos

Massimo Menegozzo[1], Roberto Pasetto[2], Simona Menegozzo[1] and Pietro Comba[2]

[1] Campania Regional Operating Center (COR) of the National Mesothelioma Registry (ReNaM), Experimental Medicine Department, Second University of Naples, Naples, Italy

[2] Department of Environment and Primary Prevention, Istituto Superiore di Sanità, Rome, Italy

Abstract

Mesothelioma is a rare but lethal disease. This chapter provides an explanation of the disease and descriptive epidemiological data: incidence, mortality, survival, temporal trends and geographical distribution. It also presents etiological data on asbestos and asbestos-type fibers and delves into the effects of the duration and intensity of exposure and the dose-response relation. It describes the contexts of occupational risk in general terms, details on exposure and the risks associated with specific work sectors. The report then goes on to illustrate multiple scenarios of environmental exposure. Finally, it elaborates on the contribution of the epidemiology of mesothelioma to Public Health initiatives: environmental reclamation, identification of groups at risk and the prevention of asbestos related pathologies in developing countries.

Definition

Malignant mesothelioma is a rare and very severe form of cancer of the serous membranes of mesothelial origin, with an unfortunate prognosis and a highly limited survival time [1, 2, 3].

Malignant mesothelioma attacks the serous membranes originating from the embryonal mesodermal folium and has the following clinical manifestations:

- pleural mesothelioma
- peritoneal mesothelioma
- pericardial mesothelioma
- mesothelioma of the tunica vaginalis testis

From a histological perspective, it appears in three primary forms:

- epithelial
- sarcomatoid
- biphasic or mixed

This classification is approximate as the availability of wide ranging samples of mesothelioma determines a significant variability of the histological picture.

Nevertheless, classification in the three istotypes is sufficiently correlated both with the prognosis and with the evaluation criteria for surgery: epitheliomorphic mesotheliomas have a better prognosis and are susceptible to a therapeutic approach with an improved probability of survival.

Diagnosis of a malignant pleural mesothelioma involves numerous difficulties relating to possible superimposition of such clinical contexts as carcinoma of the lung in a juxtapleural location, pleural metastasis of the extra-pulmonary primary carcinomas, reactive pleuritis.

Peritoneal mesothelioma is also associated with problems of differential diagnostics relative to peritoneal metastasis of primary carcinomas, with peritoneal localization of TBC.

Mesotheliomas of the pericardium and of the tunica vaginalis testis are rare.

The principal etiological agent of malignant mesothelioma is asbestos [4,5,6], although other agents cannot be excluded for a limited percentage of cases, such as environmental exposure to other types of complex silicates found in nature [7,8] and previous exposure to ionizing radiation.

Diagnosis of mesothelioma is currently based on several basic parameters:

(a) patient's clinical history: (work anamnesis with special regard to evaluation of a previous exposure to asbestos, clinical outcome, course of the illness, temporal evolution up to exitus);
(b) imunohistochemical assessment: based on the availability of a set of markers that allow for a differential diagnosis between pleural mesothelioma and pulmonary adenocarcinoma [9]. The best set of biomarkers consists of:

    - positive biomarkers per MM: calretinina and cytokeratine 5/6 and WT 1;
    - negative biomarkers per MM: CEA and MOC-31

(c) image diagnostics using standard chest x-rays (I.L.O. ' 80) [10] and new imaging techniques:

    - TC [11]
    - PET [12]

- Magnetic Resonance [13]

(d) serum markers capable of acting as precocious biomarkers for the onset of mesothelioma:

- SMRP (Serum Mesothelin-Related Protein) [14]
- Auto antibodies P53 [15]
- N-ERC/mesothelin [16]
- Osteopontina [17]

(e) profile of gene expression: [18,19,20]

Numerous studies have been conducted since 1999 to assess the presence of any specific profiles of gene expression (micro-array analysis) to define the criteria for differential diagnostics between pleural mesothelioma and lung cancer. A set of genes has consequently been identified that accompany the transformation of the mesothelial cell into a cancerous cell by modifying its activity by means of gene over-expression for some and of under-expression for others. The study of gene expression has proven useful not only for the differential diagnosis of pleural mesothelioma, but also for an evaluation of the prognosis.

Descriptive Epidemiology of Mesothelioma

Incidence

Mesothelioma may be considered as a rare disease. The incidence of "natural" pleural mesothelioma, of background type (no exposure to asbestos), is estimated to be less than 1 case per million per year [7], but the number of cases is much higher in populations that are exposed to asbestos. An assessment of the distribution of cases of mesothelioma conducted using a database with indices of the proportion of workers exposed to carcinogenic agents and their level of exposure by region, throughout the world, has led to the following distribution of the 43,000 deaths estimated for the year 2000: Eastern Mediterranean 2,300, Africa 3,100, Americas 3,200, Europe 7,000, Southeast Asia 11,100, Western Pacific 16,300 [21].

During the 20th century asbestos was part of the industrialization process. According to the data provided by the U.S. Geological Survey between 1900 and 2003, approximately 182 million tons of asbestos were extracted [22], reaching a production peak of 5 million tons in the 70s. In 2003, 2.15 million tons of chrysotile (white asbestos) were extracted, with the principal producers being, in decreasing order: Russia (878,000 tons), Kazakhstan, China, Canada, Brazil (195,000 tons).

The causal relationship between exposure to asbestos and mesothelioma is a consolidated one and in many countries a relation has been observed between the pattern of mortality/incidence by mesothelioma and the consumption curves of asbestos, with a lag time of approximately 30-40 years [23,24] (table 1).

An estimate of the incidence in different countries can be made starting with the data of the International Association of Cancer Registries (IACR). It must first be pointed out that many countries have no cancer registries and so the estimates of incidence based on such registries are not complete. Furthermore, even in countries that may have one or more registries, the surveys are based on local compilations and generally cover a limited section of territory. The data found in the most recent IACR publication of the series "Cancer Incidence in Five Continents", refer to 186 registries from 57 countries for the years 1993-1997 [25]. The estimated incidence varies between a minimum corresponding to the limit of detection of rates, a number of registered cases of less than 5, equaling an incidence of slightly higher than 1 case per one million per year, in poorer countries and with an inferior coverage of the population, to a standardized rate (using as reference the age structure of the world population) of 6 cases per 100,000 per year among men in regions of Australia and in Italy. Cases observed in women are an average of 3 to 4 times less than those observed in men. The crude rates, indicating the extent of the disease by country, without considering age incidence, have higher values (between 4 and 12 cases per 100,000 men per year) in the western countries of Europe, in Australia and in the United States.

Mortality

Mortality from pleural mesothelioma, according to the International Classification of Diseases (ICD), is considered within the category of malignant tumors of the pleura (ICD IX edition, 163.0-163.9). This category includes, in addition to mesotheliomas of the pleura, other primary tumors located in the pleura, prevalently sarcomas, which are very rare, and erroneously classified secondary tumors, for the most part metastatic carcinomas of primary tumors originating in the breast and lung.

Mesotheliomas in other sites are not categorized separately. Furthermore, the percentage of pleural mesotheliomas present in cancer registries is generally greater than 80% of the total number of mesotheliomas and exceeds 90% in more numerous case series [25].

Mortality from pleural mesothelioma is, on the epidemiological level, a reasonable approximation of the incidence of pleural mesothelioma. The quality of the registration of causes of death by pleural mesothelioma has been assessed on a limited number of cases in Australia [26], the United States [27], Italy [28] and France [29]. The percentage of pleural mesotheliomas correctly classified in the category of death from malignant tumor of the pleura varied, in the years preceding 1990, between 23% and 76% considering different periods of study, different stages and different sub-groups analyzed (i.e. by sex). An estimate of 40% of false positives and 18% of false negatives was recently reported on the basis of a regional, Italian, registry of mesothelioma cases [30]. There is a general consensus that the misclassification of individual cases attains a sort of compensation at the level of population, making the mortality data usable for analyses of descriptive epidemiology.

Mesothelioma of the pleura is a lethal pathology with a median survival rate of less than one year from diagnosis [2,31,32]. In addition, while the incidence data are based on cancer registries, with consequent limitation of the population covered by the survey, mortality data are often available for large populations and are based on current data flows that are temporally stable and standardized. For these reasons mortality data are used for an indirect estimate of the incidence of pleural mesothelioma. In addition to being the only type of evaluation possible for frequency of pathology in nations without cancer registries, this estimate may be better than the estimate obtained from real incidence data, especially for countries with cancer registries that have insufficient population coverage and geographic heterogeneity for frequency of disease. Mortality data are generally used for geographic type descriptions and for predictions of temporal trends.

Survival

Mesothelioma is currently an incurable disease. Survival does not appear to have changed substantially over time, reflecting both the gravity of the disease and the inefficacy of therapies used to date. The average survival rate for peritoneal mesothelioma is less than that of pleural mesothelioma, about 6 months from diagnosis, and the two genders differ greatly [32]. This difference, in favor of women, is probably attributable to a misclassification of female tumors of the genital tract [2]. Recognized prognostic factors are age, histological type and diagnostic certainty [2, 33, 34].

There is an inverse relation between age and survival, with survival being less at an advanced age [32]. The risk from fibrous mesotheliomas is approximately three times that of epithelial and biphasic mesotheliomas [32, 33, 34]. Finally, diagnostic certainty also appears to be a predictive factor. Mesotheliomas classified as suspect are attributed a higher risk factor than those classified as certain. This may be linked to the tendency to avoid invasive diagnostic procedures for patients in an advanced stage of the illness and in generally precarious conditions [32].

Temporal Trends

The epidemic of mesotheliomas is increasing in countries that have made vast use of asbestos in the past. The epidemic curve, in fact, follows that of consumption over time. It has been estimated that there have been more than 20,000 asbestos-related lung tumors and 10,000 mesotheliomas per year in the period immediately preceding the year 2000 in the populations of Western Europe, Scandinavia, North America, Japan and Australia [35]. The complete ban on the importation, manufacture, sale and use of asbestos or its restriction was applied successively in these countries beginning at the end of the 80s and a complete ban on asbestos was adopted by a progressively increasing number of states worldwide (www.ibas.btinternet.co.uk).

On the basis of incidence and mortality trends, we deduce that the epidemic curve of mesothelioma has already reached its peak in the United States, at least among men [36] and the "plateau" is expected to be reached in the period 2010-2020 in Great Britain [37], France [38], Holland [39], Finland [40], Sweden [41], New Zealand [42] and Australia [31]. In Italy, the maximum level of the epidemic may follow a year or so later, using as reference the peak of consumption leading up to the 80s [43].

While the use of asbestos has been prohibited or reduced in some countries, it is increasing in Asia, Latin America and in the Commonwealth of Independent States (Byelorussia, Russian Federation, Ukraine) [44]. The first 5 countries for asbestos consumption in the year 2000 were, in order of priority: Russia (447,000 tons), China, Brazil, India, Thailand (121,000 tons) [45] .

These data lead to the reasonable supposition that a decline in preventable mesothelioma related deaths in industrialized countries will be followed by a growth in developing countries.

Geographic Distribution

The "macro" geographic distribution of mesothelioma has already been described in the paragraph concerning incidence. In respect of individual countries, epidemiological monitoring systems based on specific registries of the pathology or on assessments of mortality data, provide a more refined description and a detailed distribution of mesotheliomas on a national level [46, 47, 48, 49, 50, 51]. These types of analyses indicate that clusters of mesotheliomas are concentrated in areas of the country with major industrial plants in which in the asbestos is extracted (quarries and milling plants), processed as a primary raw material (i.e. production of asbestos cement), used as a component of the production process (i.e. used for insulation in shipyards) and is widely found in the structures of industrial systems (i.e. insulation in heating pipes for chemical plants).

Table 1. Cases of mesothelioma in the 90s and consumption of asbestos in the 70s. Countries listed by decreasing order of cases observed (modified by Tossavainen 2004 [45])

Country	Cases (year)	Asbestos tons (year)
United States	2,800 (2000)	552,000 (1975)
Great Britain	1,595 (1999)	170,000 (1970)
Germany	1,007 (1997)	230,000 (1975)
Italy	930 (1995)	140,000 (1975)
France	750 (1996)	143,000 (1970)
Australia	490 (2000)	70,000 (1970)
Netherlands	377 (1997)	49,000 (1976)
Sweden	105 (1996)	20,000 (1970)
Finland	74 (1999)	11,000 (1970)
New Zealand	50 (1996)	8,000 (1970)
Norway	48 (1995)	8,000 (1970)

These systems allow us to verify, in space and time, those areas of the country that are most dangerous and thus requiring the implementation of medical surveillance systems for subjects previously exposed and centers of excellence for treatment of asbestos related diseases. Generally, epidemiological monitoring draws attention to situations in which asbestos exposure is already known but, in some cases, it may highlight situations of non-recognized occupational exposure (i.e. non-asbestos textile factories [52]) or special conditions such, for example, as those resulting from a natural contamination of the soil by asbestos-type fibers (exposure to fluoro-edenite in a town in Sicily [53]).

Etiological Role of Asbestos and Other Fibers

Asbestos

Asbestos consists of a series of fibrous minerals found in nature and is easy to extract and process.

The different types of asbestos found in nature are classified into two large families:

- serpentines in which the principal mineral is *chrysotile*
- amphyboles, encompassing several different species:
    - *crocidolite*
    - *amosite*
    - *anthophyllite*
    - *tremolite*
    - *actinolite*

The fibrous structure of asbestos makes it almost indestructible, non-flammable, resistant to acids and corrosives, highly flexible, resistant to stress, and has excellent properties for absorbing heat and noise.

Because of its extraordinary characteristics, it is estimated that asbestos was used in more than 3,000 products and objects during the XX century. Possible negative effects of this mineral on human health began to appear just a few years after it began to be extensively used, especially in the textile industry.

As indicated in the book "Late lessons from early warnings" [54], the first observation of possible harm to human health caused by exposure to asbestos may be attributed to Lucy Deane, one of the first Women Inspectors of Factories in the UK. Writing in 1898, Deane included asbestos work as one of the four dusty occupations which came under observation that year. She went on to observe that: '*the evil effects of asbestos dust have also instigated a microscopic examination of the mineral dust by HM Medical Inspector. Clearly revealed was the sharp glass-like jagged nature of the particles, and where they are allowed to rise and to remain suspended in the air of the room in any quantity, the effects have been found to be injurious as might have been expected.*'[55]

The pathological consequences of occupational exposure to asbestos are amply recognized in international medical literature (the first works are all in English medical literature) and bear the following dates:

- 1907: recognition of the first cases of asbestosis in workers of textile plants in Great Britain [56];
- 1927: Cooke coins the term asbestosis for the pulmonary fibrosis induced by inhalation of asbestos fibers [57];
- 1930: recognition of asbestosis as an occupational disease caused by occupational exposure to asbestos [58];
- 1931: first regulation on the use of asbestos in Great Britain through issue of the “Asbestos Industry Regulations “ [59];
- 1935: initial studies on the possibility of bronchial carcinomas caused by occupational exposure to asbestos [60];
- In 1943 Wedler cites the presence of “pleural carcinomas” in his German statistics on the onset of tumors of the respiratory system in individuals suffering from asbestosis [61];
- In 1947 Mallory presents a case of pleural mesothelioma in a worker exposed to asbestos [62];
- 1955: the inquiries carried out by Doll demonstrate in an incontrovertible manner that exposure to asbestos leads to a significant incidence of death by pulmonary cancer [63];
- 1960: Wagner’s studies of workers in the asbestos mines of South Africa identify pleural mesothelioma as a typical tumor caused by occupational exposure to asbestos [64];
- subsequent studies conducted by Wagner’s group in South Africa and by Selikoff in the U.S. confirm this data, extending the risk of mesothelioma not only to the pleura but to all mucosa of mesothelial origin (peritoneum [65], pericardium, tunica vaginalis testis);

In spite of the fact that the negative effects on human health were already known in the 60s, it was only at the beginning of the 80s that a decrease in the world production of asbestos begins to be noted, going from 4.7 million tons in 1980 to 1.5 million tons in the year 2000.

However, this decrease is not homogeneously distributed world wide. In this sense it is paradoxical that Canada, though prohibiting the use of asbestos within its own territory, continues to extract asbestos from its mines and to export it widely, accompanied by a capillary propaganda campaign on the safe use of chrysotile asbestos.

Other Mineral Fibers Implicated in the Etiopathogenesis of Mesotheliomas

In addition to asbestos in its serpentine and amphybole varieties, other minerals with a fibrous structure have been recognized as causal factors of incidence of mesothelioma in the populations exposed.

Specifically, we refer to the data provided by literature on two mineral species:

- *erionite:* this fibrous mineral is found in the regions of Anatolia and is considered responsible for the epidemic of mesotheliomas registered in those regions [66].
- *fluoro-edenite:* a new mineral species only recently identified in the vicinity of the town of Biancavilla in Sicily, responsible for the epidemic of mesotheliomas among the inhabitants of the town [67].

Both these mineral fibers and related epidemiological findings are dealt with in the section on environmental exposure to asbestos and other mineral fibers.

Duration and Intensity of Exposure to Asbestos and Dose-Response Relation

A dose-response relation between the level of exposure to asbestos, estimated according to the work performed, and the inception of mesothelioma, was initially described by Newhouse [68] and by Newhouse and Berry [69] among workers in the textile industry. In 1979 Seidman et al [70] wrote "*using the duration of work activity in an amosite plant as a measure of the dose of asbestos, we noted that in general the lower the dose the greater the time required for onset of the adverse experience of mortality, and even when this does appear it is less severe. This fact has important implications in controlling cancer: if it is not possible to completely avoid exposure to carcinogenic agents, a reduced exposure can delay the onset of adverse effects and the frequency of their occurrence*". The issue was taken up by other authors such as Armstrong et al. [71] who described the relationship between cumulative exposure to asbestos and mortality by mesothelioma among crocidolite miners in Australia. Tuomi et al. [72] and Rogers et al. [73], respectively in Finland and Australia, also wrote of the significant relation between the risk of mesothelioma and the concentration of asbestos fibers in the pulmonary tissues.

Of particular importance is the contribution made by Iwatsubo et al. [74] who conducted a case-control study demonstrating that a dose-response relation already existed at an exposure of 0.5 ff/ml/year (fibers per milliliter per year). And finally it should be noted that the risk associated with continuous exposure is higher than the risk associated with intermittent exposure [64].

In a comment on this work, Siemiatycki and Boffetta [75] examined the study in detail, concluding that the inquiry is valid, even though the quantitative aspects require further replication.

In another contribution, Boffetta [76] reviewed the quantitative aspects of asbestos induced cancer, suggesting that the incidence of mesothelioma may vary according to latency period, exposure expressed in fibers/milliliter, to the constant that expresses the specific carcinogenic power per type of fiber and type of industry, to the minimum latency required to reveal an increase in mesothelioma and to the effect of the latency period. The significance of this model lies in the fact that each brief period of exposure leads to an addition to the subsequent risk, proportionate to the concentration of dust at that time, multiplied by the p-th power of the time that has passed since that moment.

Berry et al [77] found a significant exposure/response relation for pleural mesothelioma in a cohort of 5,000 subjects exposed to asbestos in the city of London between 1933 and 1980.

Hodgson and Darnton [5], demonstrate how pleural mesothelioma increases sublinearly with the cumulative dose, even though a linear relation is compatible with the data, and do not believe they can assume the existence of a threshold.

In accordance with the above, it should be noted that there is a correlation between the duration of exposure to asbestos and the quantity of asbestos bodies found in lung tissue and between the duration of exposure and the total quantity of fibers in the lungs [78].

In the monograph by the World Health Organization [79] on the medical effects of chrysotile, observations on mesothelioma indicate that in the mining sector, which has the greatest number of mesotheliomas, there were no cases associated with exposures of less than two years while it appeared that there was a clear dose-response relation, with crude rates (in terms of cases /1000 persons-year) between 0.15 (for lower cumulative exposure) and 0.95 (for cumulative exposures three times greater).

Finally, the American Conference of Governmental Industrial Hygienists (ACGIH)[80] recently re-confirmed the existence of a dose-response relation for pleural mesothelioma.

Thus prolonged exposure to asbestos is not a mandatory condition for the onset of mesothelioma. There is an appreciable increased risk of mesothelioma also as a result of brief exposure to asbestos, as documented by Seidman et al. [70] and subsequently confirmed by other authors, including Roggli [78], Neumann et al [81] and Leigh et al [31]. The latter two works are of special interest as they refer to two rather extensive case series, respectively the mesothelioma registries for Germany and for Australia. In Germany, Neumann et al examined 1,605 cases of mesothelioma, identifying an occupational history of exposure to asbestos in 70% of the subjects studied. The average duration of exposure was 17.5 years, with a range of between 1 month and 56 years. In Australia, Leigh et al studied 6,329 cases of mesothelioma diagnosed between 1945 and 2000, for 82% of whom there was documented exposure to asbestos. Three percent (3%) of the cases had been exposed for less than 3 months.

To be noted is the fact that there are dose-response relations in connection with occupational exposure and also for non-occupational environmental exposure [82,83]. Hansen's study in particular, conducted on a community residing near a crocidolite mine, demonstrates that for subjects not occupationally asbestos exposed the incidence of mesothelioma increases in relation to the period of latency, the duration of exposure and the cumulative exposure.

Concerning the periods of latency, understood as the time between the beginning of exposure and manifestation of the disease, tumors generally follow normal or log-normal distributions [84]. This means that the probability of discovering very high or very low individual data increases with increased observations.

Estimates on the latency of mesothelioma were provided by Prof. Selikoff's group as part of the extensive study conducted on a cohort of asbestos workers [85]. For the 356 cases of pleural mesothelioma observed, the average latency was 33.8 years, with a standard derivation of 8.9 years. Subsequently, additional data were provided by other authors. Shorter latency periods are normally around 15 years and the longer ones around 60-70 years [86,87].

With reference to asbestos caused cancer, a final observation concerns the role played by the size of the fibers. Some authors have measured the length and diameter of the fibers that, surpassing the lung-pleura barrier, were deposited on the parietal pleura near the sites in which the mesothelioma develops. The majority of these fibers are particularly short (less than 5 μm) and thin (diameter less than 0.25 μm), as observed by various authors [88,89,90,91]. This observation has led some to maintain that only ultrafine fibers play an etiologic role in mesothelioma [92]. In actual fact, the issue is more complex, as there are elements supporting the theory that the pleura-pulmonary barrier may also be exceeded by larger particles and fibers [93,94], and that fibers may reach areas distant from the lung by migration or diffusion [95,96]. The most commonly held opinion is that asbestos fibers of any length can provoke a pathological response [97,98].

Occupational Exposure

The enormous quantity of asbestos produced during the course of the past century, in spite of the progressive decrease in production beginning in the 80s, is a strong risk factor for humans on a global scale because since it is non biodegradable, it has an injurious potential for an unlimited period of time.

The etiological role of asbestos in determining mesotheliomas is characterized by a correlation between the cumulative dose [74] and the incidence of mesotheliomas in the exposed population, without defining a threshold to exclude the induction of mesothelioma.

From the data available in literature on mesothelioma registries, based on an evaluation of exposure to asbestos obtained through the indirect method of interviews, we note that in reference to occupational and non occupational contexts, exposure is present in up to approximately 80% of the cases [99,100,101].

Thus we can state that, in terms of human health, asbestos as such, or asbestos as part of complex materials, represented and may still represent a significant occupational risk characterized by different methods of action:

a) Direct Occupational

- Miners tasked with direct extraction of the mineral, in serpentine and amphybole form (an increasingly decreasing cohort in western countries, but still present in countries that still carry out mineral extraction).
- Miners tasked with extraction of minerals other than asbestos, but exposed to the presence of asbestos minerals contaminated by the rocks extracted..
- Workers in the production of materials containing asbestos at different levels of friability, according to the matrix used (i.e. asbestos cement, asbestos glues, asbestos resins, braking systems).
- Workers in the sector of application of materials containing asbestos for the insulation of buildings, means of transportation, etc. (i.e. ships, trains, buses, trams, airplanes).

- Workers in the sector of maintenance and demolition of buildings insulated with asbestos, means of transportation, systems (i.e. heating plants, insulated pipes), equipment (i.e. contactors), other devices (i.e. vehicle braking systems, cranes) containing material with an asbestos content.
- Workers tasked with removing insulation from materials containing asbestos (an important activity during the present phase of radical elimination of the asbestos risk).

b) Indirect Occupational

- Workers who do not perform activities requiring the handling or manipulation of materials containing asbestos, but who work alongside other departments that are not adequately separated and in which processes take place using materials containing asbestos. This situation in particular is found inside large industrial hangars with unseparated work units, in which there is no effective form of primary prevention to trap asbestos fibers at the source nor adequate industrial cleaning of the departments.

c) Environmental Occupational

- Workers exposed to inhalation of asbestos fibers not from direct occupational exposure but from contamination by airborne fibers issuing from sprayed application of asbestos, or from roofs of industrial hangars containing asbestos cement and/or other asbestos material found in the work environment;

Obviously there are some work environments in which there may exist more than one type of occupational exposure to asbestos fibers, such as:

- insulation of railway carriages applied using a sprayed mixture of crocidolite, water and glue, in an occupational environment where there occur simultaneous activities such as molding of asbestos cartons, in hangars covered with segments of Eternit in an unsatisfactory state of preservation;
- seamen working in engine rooms insulated with asbestos and who live in rooms-cabins insulated with materials containing asbestos.

We must not forget that asbestos fibers dispersed in the work environment may lead to forms of *extra occupational risk in living environments*, in two ways:

- diffusion to nearby living environments, when the dispersion of asbestos fibers in the work environment is such that it can be transmitted to the nearby ecosystem by air currents. This can lead to significant contamination, especially if the production plant is in a highly urbanized area;
- diffusion to domestic living environments and to family members of workers occupationally exposed to the asbestos risk, through contamination of work clothes brought into the home for cleaning;

Numerous epidemiological studies have identified significant excessive rates of mortality by mesothelioma in many productive sectors that involve occupational exposure to asbestos [4].

The risk of mesothelioma resulting from occupational risk to asbestos varies according to the different occupational sectors in which asbestos is used.

This variability refers to the different types of asbestos used (serpentines and/or amphyboles), intensity of exposure (estimated both as average concentration of airborne asbestos fibers and as time of exposure), environmental and individual prevention measures implemented.

In respect of the intensity of exposure required to produce a significant incidence of mesothelioma in an exposed working population, studies based on the fiber content in lungs of unexposed subjects, subjects who have died from asbestosis and subjects deceased from mesothelioma, have demonstrated that the level of exposure to asbestos fibers for individuals dying of mesothelioma is significantly greater that the level of exposure of subjects who have not been exposed (background) but also significantly lower than the average level of exposure for subjects who have died of asbestosis [102].

As to latency (time between the initial exposure to asbestos and the insurgence of mesothelioma) the Consensus Panel for 1997 [103] has determined that a minimum latency of 10 years from initial exposure is required to attribute a nexus between exposure to asbestos and mesothelioma.

Recent data relative to the second report of the National Registry of Mesotheliomas in Italy (ReNaM) [47], dealing with a total of 5,173 cases during the period 1993 – 2001 and reconstructing exposure by means of interviews, indicate that:

- In 77.2% of the cases of mesothelioma, exposure to asbestos was distributed as follows:
    - 67.4% from occupational exposure (certain, probable, possible)
    - 4.3% from familial exposure
    - 4.2% from environmental exposure
    - 1.3% from exposure to an extra occupational leisure activity or hobby

- An average latency of 43.6 years between the beginning of the exposure and appearance of the disease

Data indicates a tendentially decreasing risk in the mining sector, while the impact seems to be much greater in the sector of secondary processes.

The productive sectors most affected are construction, shipbuilding, the mechanical and metallurgical industry, the sector of construction and repair of railways and the asbestos cement industry.

Along with these traditional sectors, the ReNaM study also highlights sectors in which there is no direct processing of materials containing asbestos but whose work environment does contain asbestos as an insulation material (sugar refineries, chemical, oil extraction and refining industries, production of electrical energy).

All data is reported in the table contained in the aforementioned ReNAM 2006 Report:

Table 2. Number of exposures per economic sector of exposure (ReNaM recodification) and period of diagnosis for cases of malignant mesothelioma caused by certain, probable or possible occupational exposure (period of incidence 1993 – 2001)

Category	1993-1995	%	1996-1998	%	1999-2001	%	Total	%
Metallurgical and mechanical industry	21	5.5	59	7.2	111	7.1	191	6.9
Metallurgical industry	17	4.5	35	4.3	64	4.1	116	4.2
Oil extraction and refining	6	1.6	10	1.2	15	1.0	31	1.1
Extraction of minerals	3	0.8	2	0.2	10	0.6	15	0.5
Manufacturing of metal products	23	6.0	36	4.4	88	5.6	147	5.3
Textile industry	2	0.5	30	3.7	103	6.6	135	4.9
Non metallurgical mineral industry (excluding asbestos cement)	7	1.8	10	1.2	18	1.2	35	1.3
Asbestos cement industry	21	5.5	26	3.2	54	3.5	101	3.7
Railways	21	5.5	45	5.5	63	4.0	129	4.7
Shipyards	65	17.0	150	18.4	161	10.3	376	13.6
Production and maintenance of means of transportation; vehicle and motor vehicle repair shops (excluding ship and railway yards)	11	2.9	32	3.9	63	4.0	106	3.8
Food and beverage industry (excluding sugar refineries)	9	2.4	8	1.0	39	2.5	56	2.0
Sugar refineries	10	2.6	9	1.1	22	1.4	41	1.5
Chemical and plastics industry	15	3.9	20	2.5	62	4.0	97	3.5
Rubber industry	5	1.3	8	1.0	23	1.5	36	1.3
Wood and wood products industry	0	0.0	2	0.2	5	0.3	7	0.3
Tobacco industry	0	0.0	0	0.0	1	0.1	1	0.0
Tanning and curing industry, manufacturing of leather and fur products	0	0.0	1	0.1	3	0.2	4	0.1
Clothes manufacturing	1	0.3	0	0.0	10	0.6	11	0.4
Glass and ceramics industry	3	0.8	12	1.5	24	1.5	39	1.4
Paper and paper products (including publishing)	3	0.8	2	0.2	8	0.5	13	0.5
Other manufacturing industries (furniture, jewelry, musical instruments, sports items, etc.)	5	1.3	12	1.5	26	1.7	43	1.6

Table 2. (Continued)

Category	1993-1995	%	1996-1998	%	1999-2001	%	Total	%
Construction	50	13.1	105	12.9	252	16.1	407	14.7
Production of electrical energy and gas	7	1.8	13	1.6	21	1.3	41	1.5
Re-cycling	0	0.0	1	0.1	7	0.4	8	0.3
Agriculture and husbanding industry	1	0.3	8	1.0	13	0.8	22	0.8
Fishing	0	0.0	1	0.1	2	0.1	3	0.1
Hotels, restaurants, bars	0	0.0	3	0.4	4	0.3	7	0.3
Sales (wholesale and retail)	15	3.9	20	2.5	37	2.4	72	2.6
Marine transportation	13	3.4	25	3.1	37	2.4	75	2.7
Ground and air transportation	9	2.4	24	2.9	62	4.0	95	3.4
Maritime cargo movements	13	3.4	27	3.3	34	2.2	74	2.7
Public administration	2	0.5	7	0.9	17	1.1	26	0.9
Education	1	0.3	0	0.0	9	0.6	10	0.4
Military Defense	16	4.2	42	5.1	49	3.1	107	3.9
Banks, insurance, postal system	0	0.0	5	0.6	5	0.3	10	0.4
Health and social services	4	1.0	8	1.0	26	1.7	38	1.4
Other	3	0.8	17	2.1	16	1.0	36	1.3
Non Classified	0	0.0	1	0.1	0	0.0	1	0.0
Total	*382*	*100*	*816*	*100*	*1.564*	*100*	*2.762*	*100*

Description of Types of Exposure and Risk in Various Occupational Sectors

The following section contains detailed information on exposure to asbestos and its health consequences for individual occupational sectors. They are only a part of the work activities affected by the asbestos risk, but are nevertheless representative of the various types of exposure, according to the categories previously defined.

Production of Asbestos Cement

Asbestos cement has surely been one of the most widely used products among those containing asbestos. It is estimated that approximately 70% of asbestos is used for this product.

Factories for the production of asbestos cement products have been located throughout the world, since the first was established in Austria (Vocklabruck) in 1895 [104].

Other locations were Casale Monferrato - Italy (1907), Lund (1907) Sweden, Salonit Anhovo (1921) Slovenia, Split (1920) Croatia, Aalborg (1927) Denmark, Chongqin (1939) China, Osasco (1941) Brazil, Slemmestad (1942) Norway, Toronto (1948) Ontario – Canada, Acco (1952) Israel, Tyler (1954) Texas – U.S., Tarnow (1959) Poland, Pusan (1969) South Korea, Mina-Abdulla (1977) Kuwait.

Numerous epidemiological studies have been conducted on the injurious effects on humans of exposure to asbestos fibers released by the manufacture of asbestos cement, as reported in a review conducted by Magnani and Colleagues [105].

It is interesting to note that various types of asbestos are used in the asbestos cement mixture, the principal one being chrysotile.

Studies of mortality for cohorts exposed to asbestos cement have involved more general aspects relating to the carcinogenic nature of chrysotile, denied by some authors who maintain that cancer from asbestos (and specifically mesothelioma) is to be attributed to contamination by amphybole asbestos (tremolite) [106].

In contrast to this theory of a potentially safe use of chrysotile, the study by Yano and colleagues [107], conducted on a cohort of asbestos cement workers in Chongquin, China, demonstrates that this cohort, exposed to chrysotile lacking any tremolite contamination, also had a significant incidence of mesotheliomas.

It should also be noted that epidemiological studies have frequently highlighted the incidence of cases of mesothelioma caused by extra occupational environmental pollution from contamination of the ecosystem located near the cement/asbestos companies (para-occupational exposure) [108,109,110] or contamination of the domestic environment when washing work clothes at home [111].

Insulation and Maintenance Activities of Insulated Industrial Plants

The insulation of industrial plants and means of marine and rail transportation has often been assigned to companies that performed solely this activity, both for the application of insulation using materials containing asbestos (to install panels and/or spray applications using mixtures of amphyboles – water – glue), and subsequent maintenance and removal of deteriorated insulation material.

These groups of workers are high risk cohorts because of the intensity of exposure and the prevalence of amphyboles (crocidolite and amosite), considered the most dangerous type of asbestos for the insurgence of mesotheliomas.

The first great epidemiological study was conducted by Selikoff who investigated a cohort of approximately 17,800 insulation workers registered with the International Association of Heat and Frost Insulators and Asbestos Workers (AFL-CIO-CLC) operating in the U.S. and Canada. This same group was also the subject of a follow-up epidemiological study beginning in 01.01.1967.

The results of this study published over various dates, were an extraordinary contribution not only to further knowledge of the incidence of mesothelioma in a cohort of insulation workers, but also because they cleared up a great many issues relating to the effects on human health caused by occupational exposure to asbestos [85,112]. Overall, up to 1992, 457 workers died of malignant mesothelioma, with an uncommon prevalence of deaths by peritoneal mesothelioma in respect of pleural mesothelioma.

Additional epidemiological studies of cohorts of insulators have confirmed the high incidence of mesothelioma [113,114], and in particular the high prevalence of peritoneal mesothelioma [115].

Construction, Maintenance, Restoration and Repair of Ships

Since the 1940s numerous studies have been published, in different countries, on the neoplastic risks in the shipyard industry. The wealth of data available is proof of the magnitude of asbestos consumption in ship construction since the beginning of the 1900s, as a result of the conversion from sails to the steam engine, and the subsequent introduction of iron and steel hulls. Up to the 1970s there has always been an increasingly greater demand for new ships and an uninterrupted increase and expansion of navigation companies. A significant increase in the number of ships under construction was provided by the Second World War: we saw a forced development of military fleets in Germany, Japan, Great Britain, Italy and an even greater one with the participation of the United States in the conflict and the American decision to rapidly equip a fleet that would allow the U.S. to be present simultaneously in the European and in the Asiatic theatre.

It is only in the past few decades that naval construction has retrenched: in the Europe of 15 nations the number of employees was approximately 350,000 in 1975, decreasing to 85,000 in 2002 with the disappearance of almost two thirds of the shipyards (in Italy marine employees were 36,260 in 1975 and 13,438 in 2002).

The first indication of pleural mesotheliomas among shipyard workers in Italy was provided by Zanardi and colleagues [116]: it refers to 8 lung tumors and 1 case of mesothelioma observed in Liguria.

In 1972 Zannini stated that in examining "several *thousand workers from all the shipyards of Liguria* " he found "*approximately 700 cases of pleura-pulmonary asbestosis, some of which were associated with pulmonary and pleural neoplasia - 6 cases of pulmonary neoplasia and 3 cases of pleural mesothelioma; it is important to specify that 5 of these neoplasias were found in workers in the insulation sector and 4 in subjects performing other work*" [117]. The authors state that they found *"a greater incidence of pleurapulmonary neoplasia (ship repair workers in the port of Genova) compared to other port workers and the population of the rest of the city ".*

During this same period the first data was published on the incidence of cases of mesothelioma in shipyard workers of Trieste and Monfalcone [118]. The progressive study of these cases indicates that in the period between 1968 and 2000, the number of mesotheliomas observed increased from 20 to 557, and that the majority of the afflicted had undergone occupational exposure in a shipyard [100].

A study of mortality on 3,890 shipyard workers (construction and repair) of Genova, using the mortality of the general population of Genova for comparison [119], indicates an increased general mortality (SMR – Standardized Mortality Ratio – 108.8) from tumors (SMR 122.6), and an excessive mortality for all the different sites of the respiratory system: SMR of 148.2 – 442 – 138.6 for lung tumors, primary pleural tumors, tumors of the larynx.

Also important was a mortality study of 893 employees of the Davidson Company of Genova, which carries out insulation work using materials containing asbestos, including sprayed applications, in shipyards, railway carriage construction companies and in the building construction sector [114].

The assessment of mortality, compared with that of the Italian population, is based on 97 deaths. These exceed the rate of total mortality by 41%, for tumors by 65% and for respiratory tumors by 102%. There is a marked excess of mortality by primary pleural tumors (based on 4 deaths) and by primary peritoneal tumors (based on 2 cases).

In recent years we have become aware of a serious public health problem: ships insulated with asbestos and scheduled to be demolished are being sent to the "southern part of the world", particularly to India [120]. Of the approximately 45,000 ocean-going ships in the world, about 700 are taken out of service every year. In the early 1970s, shipbreaking was a highly mechanized industrial operation carried out in the shipyards of Great Britain, Taiwan, Mexico, Spain, and Brazil. Rigorous environmental and health and safety standards have shifted this activity to poorer Asian nations. It is estimated that over 100,000 workers are employed at shipbreaking yards worldwide. By the end of the 1990s, 70% of ships were being scrapped in India.

Studies conducted in the area of Hamburg, Germany, site of the asbestos textile industries and civilian and military shipyards, have identified progressively greater cases of mesothelioma [121], dozens of which are related to shipyards. Cases of mesothelioma in subjects not directly exposed have been noted also in family members of asbestos insulators.

In Holland, in 1958, Van der Schoot published a study of three cases of malignant mesothelioma in individuals working in the sector of shipyard insulation [122].

Stumphius [123] writes that he has identified asbestos corpuscles in approximately 60% of the employees of a shipyard on the isle of Walcheren whom he had examined. He presents a case study of 25 cases of mesothelioma, identified in the period 1962-1968, for which he reconstructs the work place and the presence of exposure to asbestos: these are subjects who lived near the shipyards and 22 had worked in the naval shipyard of Royal Schelde in some capacity.

Concerning Great Britain, an initial survey of cases of mesothelioma in shipyards dates to 1958 [124] and refers to 13 mesotheliomas, observed in the shipyards of Belfast. The author reports of an increase in the problem and in a subsequent article the cases had become 45 [125]. The deceased had asbestos corpuscles in the lungs while the presence of pulmonary asbestosis was infrequent.

Examples of other cases of mesotheliomas are provided by McEwen, who reports on 83 cases of mesothelioma observed during the period 1950-1967 in Scotland [126] and the extensive study by Wagner on 622 cases of mesothelioma, with exposure to asbestos occurring prevalently in shipyards [127].

Construction, Maintenance, Restoration and Repair of Railway Carriages

The evaluation of cases of mesothelioma in this sector can benefit from previous studies on the use and methods of use of asbestos in the rail sector and the results of several epidemiological studies. [64, 128, 129, 130, 131, 132, 133, 134, 135, 136, 137, 138, 139, 140, 141, 142, 143].

The most extensive description of cases of mesothelioma resulting from the use of asbestos in steam locomotives was conducted by Mancuso and colleagues on railway workers in the United States during the 20s.

During the period between the two world wars, the asbestos used in railway carriages in Italy was contained in objects: belts, ropes and cartons containing chrysotile asbestos in steam coupling devices (pipes bringing the steam from the boiler or heater to the wagon), in the pipes used to convey steam located in the underlying steam boxes and, in the interior of the wagons, to the hot air vents (heating vents) located under the passenger seats or to the backrest in some types of wagons. In electrical locomotives, asbestos was present in the contactors, in the rheostats, as sheathing for the cables subject to heat stress and in the heaters located in the conductor's cabin.

This first exposure to asbestos in Italy therefore took place in the sites in which the locomotives and wagons were built. Only later did the railway company use asbestos for repairs and maintenance requiring small, medium and major interventions. The great change in Italy occurred with the decision of the State Railway System in 1956 (FFSS), that would later lead to similar decisions by private railway companies, to use trains with a body insulated with crocidolite mixed with water and vinyl glue, applied by sprayer.

It is interesting to note that the use of asbestos in railroads was not limited only to Italy. in fact cases of mesothelioma or epidemiological studies report on its use and describe its effects in several European countries (Switzerland [144], Scandinavia [145], England [51],

Germany [81], Holland [146]) and non European countries (Australia [50], South Africa [64]).

What is original is that the consequences of the decision to insulate using spray applied crocidolite were not evaluated in Italy until the 80s, an aspect that differentiates Italy from other countries.

A useful comparison in this respect is found in England. Descriptions of environmental surveys indicate that railways in England began to be insulated using spray applied asbestos from the end of the 30s, a technique that was simultaneously much used in ship construction.

Spray applied insulation was patented and immediately implemented upon issue of the first English law protecting from asbestos in 1931. This method of application however was not governed by any regulation. The English Labor Inspectorate (HSE) responsible for monitoring enforcement decided to undertake environmental measurements to assess the intensity of exposure considered to be high and ordered employers to provide safety devices for the respiratory system not only for insulation workers but also for other workers located in their proximity. The extension of the safety measures to "*bystanders*" worried employers and led to a contrast that would be resolved only with new legislation on asbestos in 1969 [147].

Regarding work with the risk of exposure to asbestos in the field of transportation, railway machinists were among the first subjected to exposure of sprayed insulation easily accessible from the interior of the conductor's cabin.

Among those tasks with the most direct exposure in rail construction and repair are those of boiler operator and pipe-fitters, employees who worked on the steam pipes extending from the boiler wagon to the passenger wagon. Riggers, pipe-fitters and electricians were involved in the systems installation and furnishings of new trains. Panel installers, carpenters, upholsterers, plumbers and electricians were all subject to direct exposure during maintenance and repair operations. As for indirect exposure the list is much longer, as work sites in which rail repair and maintenance operations were conducted had no separations or measures to contain exposure, thus leading to widespread contamination of the entire hangars in which the work took place, a judgment confirmed by the results of some environmental measures.

Personnel Travelling in Means of Transportation Insulated with Asbestos: Ships and Trains

The exposure to asbestos suffered by embarked personnel is a consequence of the vast use of asbestos for several decades by the ship building industry undertaking marine construction, repair and restoration.

Occupational exposure to asbestos by embarked naval personnel coincides with the beginning of the industrial use of asbestos, at the end of the 1800s.

More specifically, the modern era of asbestos use can be dated to an article appearing in the prestigious review *The Engineer* on 22 June 1883, titled "*Asbestos and its applications*" [148]. In this article the writer refers to an initial industrial application of asbestos introduced by John Bell in 1879, by insulating steam engines with material containing asbestos. This application found immediate use in the navies of Great Britain and Germany.

The use of asbestos was extensive in ship building since the end of the 1800s. It was especially widespread in the navies because of its thermal insulation and fireproofing properties.

Asbestos made it possible to create areas inside ships that could be insulated in case of fire, by using special firewalls; other objectives were also attained, such as thermal and acoustic insulation of engine rooms and related heating systems [149].

During the First World War the use of asbestos greatly increased in the navies and merchant marine worldwide.

It should finally be noted that exposure to asbestos by seamen was prolonged and went beyond simple occupational exposure since work environments were the same as living environments, providing a 24hours exposure.

Concerning the installation of asbestos in the hull of the ship, with the consequent risk of occupational exposure, we refer to the Italian document developed by the *Coordinamento per la Prevenzione nei luoghi di lavoro delle Regioni e delle Province Autonome di Trento e Bolzano* dated 30 August 2000 [150].

Table 3 illustrating the distribution of materials containing asbestos in the structure of the ship shows the vast extent of its use within the entire ship:

Specifically, embarked personnel were subjected to the greatest exposure in the following compartments:

(a) Lodgings for on board personnel: upon conclusion of work hours embarked naval personnel remained exposed to the risk of asbestos even in the “living environment”.
(b) Engine room: particularly significant exposure due to the massive use of materials containing asbestos as insulation for engines and also because of the generally confining and insufficiently ventilated space of the engine room. It should also be borne in mind that the vibrations typical of an engine room is a factor that strongly conditions the dispersion of asbestos fiber from the matrix.
(c) Passenger lounges: the activity of steward could also expose to the risk of occupational inhalation of airborne asbestos fibers.

The first indications of the risk of asbestos for seamen in Italy are attributed to Puntoni et al [151] as part of a study of port workers in Genova and to Bianchi et al [152]. These writers describe three cases of pleural mesothelioma in embarked subjects on different types of ships, and in discussing the cases point out three aspects: exposure takes place especially during the phases of inspection, maintenance and repair; the fact that exposure is not massive nor continuous does not eliminate the risk; engine room personnel are the most exposed.

In the U.S., Jones et al [153] examined the chest x-rays of over 5,000 naval machinists, observing pleural alterations caused by asbestos in 12% of the subjects; the prevalence of these contexts was higher (27%) among those who had been embarked for a greater number of years. Also in the U.S., Selikoff et al [154] studied more than 3,000 seamen and observed pleural or pulmonary alterations caused by asbestos in 35% of the subjects.

The prevalence of these alterations was greater in engine room personnel, intermediate in deck workers and lesser among stewards. Confirmation was provided by a smaller study conducted in Greece [155]: in a group of 141 seamen, 41% had at least one radiological sign of damage from asbestos.

Table 3. Material with the possible presence of asbestos inside ships [150]

Area	Material, equipment, furnishings	Type of material containing asbestos
GARAGE	Ceiling and/or covering of room and perimeter walls	Flocks, Sprayed, Panels
	Pipes	Cement mixture, Fabric, Gaskets, Cushions
	Conduits for electrical lines	Plaits, Packing, Stucco, Cement mixture
	Doors	Panels, Cement mixture
CORRIDORS AND STAIRS	Walls	Sprayed, Panels, Cement mixture
	False ceiling	Sprayed, Panels, Cement mixture
	Doors	Panels, Cement mixture
	Ventilation ducts	Gaskets, Plastering
	Pipes	Cement mixture, Gaskets
LODGING FOR EMBARKED PERSONNEL	Cabin walls	Sprayed, Panels, Cement mixture
	False ceiling	Sprayed, Panels, Cement mixture
	Doors	Panels, Cement mixture
	Ventilation ducts	Gaskets, Stucco
	Pipes	Cement mixture, Fabric, Gaskets
	Conduits for electrical lines	Plaits, Packing, Stucco, Cement mixture
PASSENGER LOUNGES	Walls	Sprayed, Panels, Cement mixture
	Ceilings and false ceilings	Sprayed, Panels, Cement mixture
	Doors	Panels, Cement mixture
	Ventilation ducts	Gaskets, Stucco
	Pipes (hot water, washing, fire prevention, etc..)	Cement mixture, Fabric, Gaskets
	Conduits for electrical lines	Plaits, Packing, Stucco, Cement mixture
ENGINE ROOMS AND AUXILIARY MOTORS	Engine gas exhaust collectors	Insulation cushions, Fabric, Mattresses, Cement mixture, Gaskets
	Smoke exhaust pipes for boilers and incinerators	Insulating cushions, Fabric, Mattresses, Cement mixture, Gaskets
	Pipes (steam, hot water, fire prevention, etc..)	Cement mixture, Fabric, Plaits, Gaskets
	Conduits for electrical lines	Plaits, Packing, Stucco, Cement mixture
	Ventilation ducts	Gaskets, Stucco
MISCELLANEOUS	Reefer cells	Sprayed, Panels, Mattresses, Cement mixture
	Kitchen	Sprayed, Panels, Cement mixture
	Ovens and stoves	Panels, Plaits, Stucco, Slabs of asbestos cement
	Ventilation ducts	Gaskets, Stucco
	Pipes	Cement mixture, Gaskets

The first quantitative sign of the risk of mesothelioma among seamen is based on the seven cases observed in a study of an English cohort of 13,000 officers and seamen of the Navy, versus two expected cases [156].

In Italy a study of a cohort of 984 seamen in Civitavecchia, embarked at least once between 1936 and 1975, displayed a significant increase in mortality by lung tumors, with a trend associated with the duration of employment as seaman; one subject died of mesothelioma of the pleura [157].

On the basis of all the data that emerged during the decade 1980-90, Greenberg [158] affirmed that the massive quantities of materials containing asbestos on ships, also subjected to continuous vibrations and mechanical stress, was the cause of the frequent radiological alterations observed in seamen and of the increased risk of cancer that was beginning to become obvious.

The Australian Registry of Mesotheliomas (1945-2000) reports 224 cases of seamen out of a total of 3,008 activities involving exposure to asbestos [31].

In Finland [159], a case-control study of 10 cases of mesothelioma observed in a cohort of 30,000 seamen embarked during the period 1960-80, revealed a significant increase in the risk associated with the activity of machinist (OR –Odds Ratio- 7.50, conf. int. 95% 1.53-36.7 with a 10 year latency; OR 9.75, conf. int. 95% 1.88-50.6 with a 20 year latency). In Sweden [160], the Standardized Incidence Ratio (SIR) for pleural mesothelioma for seamen in the period 1961-1998 was 2.83 (conf. int. 95% 1.41-5.09).

Industrial and Civilian Construction Work

The use of asbestos in the construction sector came about because of its thermal and acoustic insulation properties and the fact that it was fireproof.

This particular use was extensive in North America (Canada and U.S.) and was applied using the crocidolite spray method [161]. The percentage of asbestos used in construction products varied from approximately 20% for floors to approximately 80% for insulation of heating pipes [162].

The considerable quantity of material containing asbestos in the Twin Towers of the WTC in New York caused significant environmental contamination from asbestos fibers after the September 11 attacks. [163]

Epidemiological studies have progressively highlighted the risk of mesothelioma in workers in the construction sector [164]: we must note in fact that the significance of this occupational exposure is also in relation to the large number of construction workers, even though the concentration of asbestos fibers does not reach the same levels as in the shipyard and railway sectors.

We estimate that in the U.S. construction workers form the largest group of workers occupationally exposed to asbestos. Baker assessed that in 1980 the number of construction workers exposed to asbestos was approximately 7,500,000. [165].

Additional epidemiological studies conducted by Robinson et al [166] on a cohort of 31,068 electricians in the construction sector revealed an excessive level of mortality by mesotheliomas.

Similar data was found by Peto in the United Kingdom, who also indicated that this category will have the greatest increase of mesothelioma cases in the near future [167].

Textile Sector

An assessment of the risk associated with occupational exposure considered potentially carcinogenic is provided by the *International Agency for Research on Cancer* (IARC). The IARC included the activity of the textile sector in group 2B [168] on the basis of the limited evidence of carcinogenicity provided by available studies. This assessment is based on the increased incidence of bladder cancer among dyers and millers (azoic dyes) and of carcinoma of the paranasal sinuses among weavers (dust from fibers and fabric). A case review by the Sloan-Kettering Cancer Center in 1982 evidences the appearance of mesotheliomas in textile workers that is not, however, associated with a possible exposure to asbestos [169];

In the past, with the exception of the infrequent production of fireproof fabrics (containing asbestos), the asbestos risk in the textile industry has never been sufficiently studied.

Eventually, however, some studies began to document a possible risk of occupational exposure to minerals for workers of this sector:

- studies conducted in the city of Prato (Tuscany) drew attention to an increased risk of lung cancer among the fabric sorters (exposed in the 50s) and weavers (employed in the 70s), suggesting asbestos and mineral oils, respectively, as carcinogenic factors [170] and to an observable cluster of mesothelioma cases associated with re-use of asbestos bags [171];
- some cases of malignant mesothelioma (MM) appearing among silk spinners in Lombardy may have been caused by exposure to asbestos dispersed into the air by the insulation and fittings on pipes [172];
- in Piedmont there was a case of mesothelioma in a worker assigned to maintenance of pipes bringing water and steam to the dying and finishing sections in the textile industry [173];
- the Mesotheliomas Registry for Tuscany indicated the need to further study possible exposure in the textile department, as subjects who perform different tasks may be affected [174];
- some parts of textiles machinery (ferrules, gaskets) may be points of potential dispersion [175].

A recent review of cases was conducted by the Mesothelioma Registry for Lombardy [176].

The ReNaM archives contain 90 cases of malignant mesothelioma from occupational exposure in the textile sector, excluding workers in weaving and spinning of fireproof materials containing asbestos. The anatomic location of the disease that is most involved is the pleural area with 88 cases (97.8%). There are also 2 cases involving the peritoneum (2.2%) and none for the pericardium and the tunica vaginalis testis. The clinical diagnosis according to the ISPESL criteria [177] was certain in 80 cases (88.9%), probable in 7 cases (7.8%) and possible in 3 cases (3.3%). Occupational etiology was certain in 49 cases (54.4%), probable in 15 cases (16.7%) and possible in 26 cases (28.9%).

Installation and Repair of Lifts

The braking systems on lifts have lining with an asbestos content. When in operation, asbestos fibers are released and collect on the floor of the elevator booth.

There is exposure to asbestos during the installation and maintenance and repair phase of lifts.

Cases of mesotheliomas among lift workers were observed by Huncharek [178] and colleagues and by Tonut [179]. Epidemiological studies showing a significant incidence of malignant mesothelioma in lift workers were conducted by Bruno and colleagues in 1999 [180].

Environmental Exposure

Even since the initial indication [64] of a relationship between asbestos and malignant mesothelioma (MM) the substantial risk of exposure linked to the environment in a wider sense has also emerged. This includes:

- *paraoccupational exposure* from matter released into the surrounding environment by mining and processing systems;
- *residential exposure* from the presence in the immediate vicinity of the house or inside the house of materials contaminated by asbestos, co-habitation with workers exposed to asbestos, the performance of daily activities, including play by children, using items containing contaminated materials.

In the original series of 33 cases of mesothelioma observed by Wagner and colleagues, circumstances of non-occupational exposure were the only ones present in the anamnesis of 14 cases. Since that time, the epidemic of mesotheliomas in the crocidolite mining areas of South Africa has provided additional proof of the consequences of environmental exposure [181]; furthermore, the mining area of Wittenoom Gorge in Australia, where crocidolite is extracted, was the object of extensive studies to investigate the dose-response relation at different levels of environmental exposure, thanks to the availability of environmental measures [82].

In a completely different context, the inquiry conducted in London a few years after Wagner's report used a case-control approach to highlight the high risk of MM from exposures defined as "neighboring" [182]. Overall, 9 of the 76 cases for which a complete history was available had as the sole significant condition a relative who had worked in the asbestos industry, and an additional 11 had lived within half a mile from an asbestos industry.

The description of the epidemic of MM linked to environmental exposure to erionite, in the villages of Karain in central Anatolia, Turkey [183,184] became a turning point in the perception of the problem of non occupational exposure to asbestiform fibers. In the case of erionite, a mineral without any commercial or industrial use, the cases observed could not be etiologically attributed to occupational conditions. Almost simultaneously another group of cases was described in the population of Tuzkoy, about 50 km from Karain [185], in an area also contaminated by erionite, and another aggregate in the population of Cermik, in south-east Anatolia [186], this time in relation to the use of local materials strongly contaminated by fibrous tremolite, used as plaster.

More recently, numerous works [187,188,189,190] have allowed for updating of the incidence of mesothelioma by environmental exposure to asbestos, in the areas of eastern Anatolia.

Epidemics with characteristics very similar to the above have been described in Greece [191], Cyprus [192], Corsica [193], New Caledonia [194], China [195], Italy [196], Montana and California [197].

Three systematic reviews [7,198,199] have recently summarized the current state of knowledge, even though the results of the study on the residents of Wittenoom, cited above, are not included. These reviews emphasized the part played by today non occupational exposure in explaining a significant number of the cases of MM observed, and the fact that the strong association between these exposures and the risk of MM is not a modest one. It was also pointed out that lacking appropriate countermeasures the exposures could prolong the epidemic of MM in countries in which there is no longer any industrial use of asbestos.

The contribution of environmental and familial exposure to the overall incidence of malignant mesothelioma is certainly not a negligible one, especially among women [111]. The risk to which subjects are exposed can reach levels comparable to those of occupational cohorts [200].

Of the 5,173 cases found in the ReNaM Archive [201] there is currently sufficient information to evaluate the exposure for 3,552 cases, approximately 69%. In 302 cases, equal to approximately 9% of cases with defined exposure, a familial or environmental exposure has been determined, in the absence of any occupational exposures.

Of a total of 187 cases of environmental exposure attributed to the cases classified as having an environmental etiology, one third (76) are attributable to proximity to plants that produce asbestos cement items. There are also various periods of habitation in the proximity of shipyards and ports (16 periods), iron and steel industries/foundries, chemical/petrochemical plants, electrical plants (15), railway lines (12), asbestos textile industries (9).

In general, the production sectors most frequently associated with environmental cases of MM have also used amphyboles (amosite and crocidolite). Nevertheless, the most widely used type of asbestos was certainly chrysotile and we cannot ignore that there is epidemiological evidence of an increased risk of mesotheliomas caused by environmental contamination induced by the extraction and processing of chrysotile [202].

One highly important case was discovered in the town of Biancavilla, Italy, where there was such a high concentration of deaths by malignant tumor of the pleura that an investigation was conducted, confirming many cases as MM and identifying the etiology of the epidemic in the exploitation of materials from a local quarry, contaminated by a fibrous asbestiform mineral not previously known, fluoroedenite [203].

The potential of injury to one's health caused by exposure to asbestos linked to natural sources in the living environment, when such sources are disturbed by some anthropical activity, was also demonstrated by two inquiries conducted on a small aggregate of cases in two areas distant from each other, one in Piedmont and one in Basilicata, but associated by the presence of serpentinites contaminated by tremolite [202,204].

The latency, measured between the beginning of the first exposure and diagnosis, goes from a minimum of 6 years up to 84 years, with an average of 46.5 (±14.7). The duration of exposure varies from 2 to 84 years, with an average of 32.1 (±19.6).

Of 144 cases, 137 (67 men and 70 women) had a pleural localization, 6 (3 men and 3 women) peritoneal, and one pericardium. Cases with a non pleural localization are rare and analytic studies to determine environmental risk have not been conducted, even though there are well documented cases [205].

In many, if not all, areas in which a significant share of environmental etiology has been noted, there have also been cases of domestic origin, caused by one or more family members working in the asbestos industry and bringing fibers into the home, on their work clothes or other items [111].

In the ReNaM Archives their number is equivalent to the number of environmental contaminations. However, there is a clear predominance of women among the familial cases, compared with the substantial equilibrium between the two sexes in the environmental cases. Another characteristic of familial exposures is the wider range of work processes to which they are associated: production of asbestos cement (22 work periods), asbestos weaving (9), naval construction and repair (21), railway construction and repair (11). More than half of the work periods involving exposure referred to activities and tasks in which asbestos was not present as a raw material, but was installed on systems, such as in the chemical, rubber and sugar refining industry (10 periods of work), in the production of electrical energy (6), in iron and steel industries and foundries (9), in textiles (8), railways (8), and in material or objects of more or less widespread use, as in construction (18 periods of work), installation and maintenance of electrical or hydraulic machinery and systems (11) and vehicle production (5).

Latency, measured from the beginning of the initial exposure to actual diagnosis, extends from a minimum of 19 years to 86 years, with an average of 47.8 (±14.6). The duration of exposure varies from less than one year to 78 years, with an average of 21.6 (±13.5).

Of 150 cases, 146 (23 men and 123 women) had pleural localization and 4 (1 man and 3 women) peritoneal. The cases with peritoneal localization all have a histologically confirmed diagnosis, with certain mesothelioma in two cases and probable mesothelioma in another two. The occupation of the relatives exposed were, respectively, a cast iron foundry, forging, construction and glassworks. Latency could be estimated only for two cases, and was very long: 49 and 70 years.

Urban Environment

Some authors have debated the existence of an "urban factor" for mesothelioma (Hemminki et al 2003 [206], Polednak 2003 [207]) in light of the extensive use of asbestos in construction over the past decades, the aging of buildings, the increased release of fibers from the cement matrix caused by the deterioration of the structures, and especially the massive release of spray applied fibers (Marconi et al 1987 [208]). In a large city like Rome, there are more cases of mesothelioma without occupational exposure to asbestos than in the surrounding areas, with a greater proportion of women, compared to the rest of the Latium Region (Ascoli et al 2004 [209]). This observation could be explained by the greater number of subjects exposed to asbestos in the homes and offices of a metropolitan area compared with the surrounding territory.

Contribution of the Epidemiology of Mesothelioma to Public Health Initiatives

In light of the above, we believe epidemiological studies of mesothelioma serve a dual purpose, in accordance with the evolution of prevention policies in the different countries. The two circumstances to be kept separate are those in countries that have stopped using asbestos and those that still use it. Unquestionably, epidemiological surveillance of mesothelioma as a whole and consequent ascertainment of the medical impact of asbestos are more evolved in countries that have banned this agent compared to those that still allow its extraction and use in work places and in daily life. [210].

In the more advanced countries that had made wide use of asbestos in the course of the XX century and banned it in the past few decades, epidemiological studies of mesothelioma determine the priorities to be followed in environmental reclamation and identify the groups at high risk who require greater protection.

Environmental Reclamation and Identification of Groups at Risk

Determination of priorities for environmental reclamation must generally consider the foreseeable number of cases, estimated according to the number of subjects exposed, the level of exposure and the course of exposure over time, as well as the different types of exposure, in other words, identification of those sections of the population experiencing the highest level of exposure in the absence of appropriate mechanisms providing legal and social protection or simply, access to information [211]. This establishes a link between identification of groups at risk through epidemiological observation, and the consequent implementation of environmental reclamation procedures. This course of action requires a high level of integration among medical and environmental operators, cooperation between scientists and administrators and the involvement of the communities affected, leading to less arbitrary decision-making processes founded on scientific evidence and, in the end, appreciably more equitable.

Prevention of the Asbestos Pathology in Developing Countries

The role of epidemiology in countries that still allow the use of asbestos, mostly located in developing areas of the world, is more complex. Here the medical impact of asbestos is often denied, or underestimated, for two principal reason: the active role played by the asbestos industry in influencing the scientific community, government bodies and workers' organizations, including through the contrived re-proposition of scientific controversies of little significance for the implementation of appropriate preventive measures [212], and the inadequacy of epidemiological surveillance systems considering the relatively brief time that has passed since the initial widespread diffusion of asbestos and the consequent non attainment of sufficient latency [213]. Nonetheless, there is such a huge amount of epidemiological studies and prognostic models of the epidemic curve, that it is possible to imagine future scenarios even in these regions of the world. If current methods of using asbestos remain in effect and only limited measures of prevention are implemented, the medical impact for workers and for the general population will be dramatic. There are no alternatives to a complete ban on the use of asbestos [214].

This conclusion, advocated by minority, though highly qualified, voices in the past (Collegium Ramazzini 2004) [215] has also recently been reached by the World Health Organization [216], whose strategy to eliminate asbestos pathologies includes banning the use of this agent, encouraging the use of alternative materials, prevention of exposure during reclamation and the improvement of early diagnostic procedures, medical treatment, rehabilitation and social support to the afflicted. To this end, the WHO recommends the implementation of national plans to eliminate diseases caused by asbestos by promoting training, cooperation among the institutions involved and, in the final analysis, an increased awareness of the problem.

References

[1] Robinson, BW; Musk, AW; Lake, RA. Malignant mesothelioma. *Lancet,* 2005, 366, 397-408.

[2] Spirtas, L; Connelly, RR; Tucker, MA. Survival patterns for malignant mesothelioma: the SEER experience. *Int. J. Cancer*, 1988, 41, 525-530.

[3] Gangemi, M; Bertolotti, M; Mirabelli, D; Gennaro, V; Viarengo, P; Merler, E; Roberti, S; Magnani, C. La sopravvivenza per i casi di mesotelioma maligno: review degli studi pubblicati. *Roma: ISPESL*; Registro Nazionale Mesoteliomi, II Rapporto; 2006; 71-79.

[4] Doll, R; Peto, J. Asbestos. *Effects on health of exposure to asbestos*. Health and Safety Commission. London, Her Majesty's Stationery Office, 1985.

[5] Hodgson, J; Darton, A. The quantitative risk of mesothelioma and lung cancer in relation to asbestos exposure. *Ann. Occup. Hyg.*, 2000, 44, 565-601.

[6] Muhle, H; Pott, F. Asbestos as reference material for fibre-induced cancer. *Int. Arch. Occup. Environ. Health,* 2000, 73, 653-659.

[7] Hillerdal, G. Mesothelioma: cases associated with non occupational and low dose exposures. *Occup. Environ. Med.*, 1999, 56, 505-513.

[8] Pasetto R; Comba P; Marconi A. Mesothelioma associated with environmental exposure. *Med. Lav.*, 2005, 96, 330-337.

[9] Ordonez, NG. The immunoistochemical diagnosis of mesothelioma: a comparative study of epithelial mesothelioma and lung adenocarcinoma. *Am. J. Surg. Pathol.*, 2003, 27, 1031-1051.

[10] ILO international classification of radiographs of pneumoconiosis: occupational safety and health series. Geneva, International Labour Office, 1980, no. 22 revised.

[11] Armato, SG 3rd; Oxnard, G; Kocherginsky, M; Vogelzang, N; Kindler, H; MacMahon, H: Evaluation of semiautomated measurements of mesothelioma tumor thickness on CT scans. *Acad. Radiol.*, 2005, 12, 1301-1309.

[12] Schneider, DB; Clary-Macy, C; Challa, S; Sasse, KC; Merrick, SH; Hawkins, R; Caputo, G; Jablons, D. Positron emission tomography with f18-fluorodeoxyglucose in the staging and preoperative evaluation of malignant pleural mesothelioma. *J. Thorac Cardiovasc. Surg.*, 2000, 120, 128-133.

[13] Heelan, RT; Rusch, VW; Begg, CB; Panicek, DM; Caravelli, JF; Eisen, C. Staging of malignant pleural mesothelioma: comparison of CT and MR imaging. *Am. J. Roentgenol.*, 1999, 172, 1039-47.

[14] Robinson Bruce, WS; Creaney, J; Lake, R; Nowak, A; Musk, AW; de Klerk, N; Winzell, P; Hellstrom, KE; Hellstrom, I. Mesothelin-family proteins and diagnosis of mesothelioma. *Lancet*, 2003, 362, 1612-1616.

[15] Creaney, J; McLaren, BM; Stevenson, S; Musk, AW; de Klerk, N; Robinson, BW; Lake, RA. p53 autoantibodies in patients with malignant mesothelioma: stability through disease progression. *Br. J. Cancer*, 2001, 84, 52-56.

[16] Shiomi, K; Miyamoto, H; Segawa, T; Hagiwara, Y; Ota, A; Maeda, M; Takahashi, K; Masuda, K; Sakao, Y; Hino, O. Novel ELISA system for detection of N-ERC/mesothelin in the sera of mesothelioma patients. *Cancer Sci.*, 2006, 97, 928-932.

[17] Pass, HI; Lott, D; Lonardo, F; Harbut, M; Liu, Z; Tang, N; Carbone, M; Webb, C;Wali, A. Asbestos exposure, pleural mesothelioma, and serum osteopontina levels. *N. Engl. J. Med.*, 2005, 353, 1564-1573.

[18] Ramos-Nino, ME; Testa, JR; Altomare, DA; Pass, HI; Carbone, M; Bocchett,a M; Mossman, BT. Cellular and molecular parameters of mesothelioma. *J. Cell Biochem.*, 2006, 98, 723-734.

[19] Gordon, GJ; Rockwell, GN; Jensen, RV; Rheinwald, JG; Glickman, JN; Aronson, JP; Pottorf, BJ; Nitz, MD; Richards, WG; Sugarbaker, DJ; Bueno, R. Identification of novel candidate oncogenes and tumor suppressors in malignant pleural mesothelioma using large-scale transcriptional profiling. *Am. J. Pathol.*, 2005, 166, 1827-1840.

[20] Gordon, GJ; Rockwell, GN; Godfrey, PA; Jensen, RV; Glickman, JN; Yeap, BY; Richards, WG; Sugarbaker, DJ; Bueno, R. Validation of genomics-based prognostic tests in malignant pleural mesothelioma. *Clin. Cancer Res.*, 2005; 11, 4406-4414.

[21] Driscoll, T; Nelson, DI; Steenland, K; Leigh, J; Concha-Barrientos, M; Fingerhut, M; Prüss-Üstün, A. The global burden of disease due to occupational carcinogens. *Am. J. Ind. Med.*, 2005, 48, 419-431.

[22] Virta, RL. *Worldwide asbestos supply and consumption trends 1900 to 2000.* Restov, Virginia: US Geological Survey; 2003.

[23] McDonald, JC. Health implications of environmental exposure to asbestos. *Environ. Health Persp.*, 1985, 62, 319-328.

[24] Selikoff IJ; Hammond EC; Seidman H. Latency of asbestos disease among insulation workers in the United States and Canada. *Cancer,* 1980, 46, 2736-2740.

[25] IARC. *Cancer incidence in five continents* vol. VIII. Lyon: IARC Scientific publications n. 155; 2002.

[26] Xu, Z; Armstrong, BK; Blundson, BJ; Rogers, JM; Musk, AW; Shilkin, KB. Trends in mortality from malignant mesothelioma of the pleura, and production and use of asbestos in Australia. *Med. J. Aust.*, 1985, 143, 185-187.

[27] Connely, RR; Spirtas, R; Myers, MH; Percy, CL; Fraumeni, JF. Demographic patterns for mesothelioma in the United States. *J. Natl. Cancer Ist.*, 1987, 78, 1053-1060.

[28] Bruno, C; Comba, P; Maiozzi, P; Vetrugno, T. Accuracy of death certification of pleural mesothelioma in Italy. *Eur. J. Epidemiol.*, 1996, 12, 421-423.

[29] Iwatsubo, Y; Matrat, M; Michel, E; Boutin, C; Galateau-Salle, F; Jougla, E; Bignon, J; Pairon, JC; Brochard, P. Estimation of the incidence of pleural mesothelioma according to death certificates in France. *Am. J. Ind. Med.*, 2002; 42, 188-199.

[30] Gorini, G; Merler, E; Chellini, E; Crocetti, E; Costantini, AS. Is the ratio of pleural mesothelioma mortality to pleural cancer mortality approximately unity for Italy? Considerations from the oldest regional mesothelioma register in Italy. *Br. J. Cancer,* 2002, 86, 1970-1971.

[31] Leigh, J; Davidson, P; Hendrie, L; Berry, D. Malignant mesothelioma in Australia, 1945 to 2000. *J. Occup. Health Safety-Aust N.Z.*, 2001, 17, 453-470.

[32] Marinaccio, A; Nesti M; Regional Operational Centers. Analysis of survival of mesothelioma cases in the Italian register (ReNaM). *Eur. J. Cancer*, 2003, 39, 1290-1295.

[33] Van Gelder, T; Damhuis, RAM; Hoogsteden, HC. Prognostic factors and survival in malignant pleural mesothelioma. *Eur. Respir. J.*, 1994, 7, 1035-1038.

[34] Beer, TW; Buchanan, R; Matthews, AW; Stradling, R; Pullinge,r N; Pethybridge, RJ. Prognosis in malignant mesothelioma related to MIB 1 proliferation index and histological subtype. *Num. Pathol.*, 1998, 29, 246-251.

[35] Tossavainen, A. International export meeting on new advances in the radiology and screening of asbestos related diseases. Consensus report. *Scand. J. Work Environ. Health,* 2000, 26, 449-454.

[36] Price, B; Ware, A. Mesothelioma trends in the United States: and update based on surveillance, epidemiology, and results program data for 1973 through 2003. *Am. J. Epidemiol.*, 2004, 159, 107-112.

[37] Hodgson, JT; McElvenny, DM; Darnton, AJ; Price, MJ; Peto, J. The expected burden of mesothelioma mortality in Great Britain from 2002 to 2050. *Br. J. Cancer*, 2005, 92, 587-593.

[38] Banaei, A; Auvert, B; Goldberg, M; Gueguen, A; Luce, D; Goldberg, S. Future trends in mortality of French men from mesothelioma. *Occup. Environ. Med.*, 2000, 57, 488-494.

[39] Segura, O; Burdof, A; Looman, C. Update of predictions of mortality from pleural mesothelioma in the Nederlands. *Occup. Environ. Med.*, 2003, 60, 50-55.

[40] Karjalainen, A; Pukkala, E; Mattson, K; Tammilehto, L; Vainio, H. Trends in mesothelioma incidence and occupational mesothelioma in Finland in 1960-1995. *Scand. J. Work Environ. Health*, 1997, 23, 266-270.

[41] Hemminki, K; Li, X. Mesothelioma incidence seems to have levelled off in Sweden. *Int. J. Cancer*, 2003, 103, 145-146.

[42] Kjellstrom, T; Smartt, P. Increased mesothelioma incidence in New Zealand. N.Z. *Med. J.,* 2000, 133, 485-490.

[43] Marinaccio, A; Montanaro, F; Mastrantonio, M; Uccelli, R; Altavista, P; Nesti, M; Seniori Costantini, A; Gorini, G. Predictions of mortality from pleural mesothelioma in Italy: a model based on asbestos consumption figures supports results from age-period-cohort models. *Int. J. Cancer*, 2005, 115, 142-147.

[44] Kazan-Allen, L. Asbestos and mesothelioma: worldwide trends. *Lung Cancer*, 2005, 49 Suppl 1, S3-S8.

[45] Tossavainen, A. Global use of asbestos and the incidence of mesothelioma. *Int. J. Occup. Environ. Health*, 2004, 10, 22-25.

[46] Goldberg, M; Imbernon, E; Rolland, P; Gilg Soit Ilg, A; Savès, M; de Quillacq, A; Frenay, C; Chamming's, S; Arveux ,P; Boutin, C; Launoy, G; Pairon, JC; Astoul, P; Galateau-Sallé, F; Brochard, P. The Frech national mesothelioma surveillance program. *Occup. Environ. Med.*, 2006, doi:10.1136/oem.2005.023200.

[47] Marinaccio, A; Cauzillo, G; Chellini, E; De Zotti, R; Gennaro, V; Gorini, G; Iavicoli, S; Magnani, C; Menegozzo, M; Mensi, C; Merler, E; Mirabelli, D; Montanaro, F; Musti, M; Pannelli, F; Romanelli, A; Scarselli, A; Silvestri, S; Tosi, S; Tumino, R, Nesti, M; Gruppo di Lavoro ReNaM. *"II Rapporto del Registro Nazionale dei Mesoteliomi"*. Roma Edizioni: ISPESL; 2006.

[48] Bang, KM; Pinheiro, GA; Wood, JM; Syamlal, G. Malignant mesothelioma mortality in the United States, 1999-2001. *Int. J. Occup. Environ. Health*, 2006, 12, 9-15.

[49] Kanazawa, N; Ioka, A; Tsukuma, H; Ajiki, W; Oshima, A. Incidence and survival of mesothelioma in Osaka, Japan. *Jpn. J. Clin. Oncol.*, 2006, 36, 254-257.

[50] Leigh, J; Driscoll, T. Malignant mesothelioma in Australia, 1945-2002. *Int. J. Occup. Environ. Health*, 2003, 9, 206-217.

[51] McElvenny, DM; Darnton, AJ; Price, MJ; Hodgson, JT. Mesothelioma mortality in Great Britain from 1968 to 2001. *Occup. Med.*, 2005, 55, 79-87.

[52] Pesatori, AC; Mens,i C. Peculiar features of mesothelioma occurrence as related to exposure patterns and circumstances in the Lombard Region, Italy. *Med. Lav.*, 2005, 96, 354-359.

[53] Bruno, C; Comba, P; Zona, A. Adverse health effects of fluoro-edenitic fibers: epidemiological evidence and public health priorities. *Ann. N.Y. Acad. Sci.*, 2006, 1076, 778-783.

[54] Gee, D; Greenberg, M. Asbestos: from "magic" to malevolent mineral. In: Harremoës, P; Gee, D; MacGarvin, M; Stirling, A; Keys, J; Wynne, B; Guedes Vaz, S (Eds.). European Environmental Agency. Late lessons from early warnings: the precautionary principle 1896-2000. Environmental issue report n. 22. *EEA, Copenhagen: Office for Official Publications of the European Communities*. 2001, 52-63.

[55] Deane, L 1898. Report on the health of workers in asbestos and other dusty trades. Chief Inspector of Factories and Workshops, 1899. London: HMSO, *Annual Report for 1898*, pp.171-172.

[56] Murray, HM. *Report of the Departmental Committee*. London: HM Stationery Office, 1907.

[57] Cooke, WE. Pulmonary asbestosis. *Br. Med. J.,* 1927, 2, 1024-1025.

[58] Vigliani, EC. Asbestosi polmonare. *Rassegna Med. Ind.*, 1939, 6.

[59] Asbestos Industry Regulations. London: HMSO, 1931 .(S.I. 1931 no. 1140).

[60] Lanza, AJ; Mc Connell, WJ; Fehnel, JW. Effects of the inhalation of asbestos dust on the lung of asbestos workers. *Public Health Rep.*, 1935, 50, 1-12.

[61] Wedler, HW. Asbestose und Lungenkrebs. *Dtsch. Med. Woch.*, 1943, 69, 575-576.

[62] Mallory, TB; Castleman, B; Parris, EE. Case records of the Massachusetts General Hospital - Case 33111. *N. Engl. J. Med.*, 1947, 236, 407-412.

[63] Doll, R. Mortality from lung cancer in asbestos workers. *Br. J. Ind. Med.*, 1955, 12, 81-86.

[64] Wagner, JC; Sleggs, CA; Marchand, P. Diffuse pleural mesothelioma and asbestos exposure in the north Western Cape Province. *Br. J. Ind. Med.*, 1960, 17, 260-271.

[65] Keal, EE. Asbestosis and abdominal neoplasma. *Lancet,* 1960, 2, 1211-1216.

[66] Selcuk, ZT; Coplu, L; Emri, S; Kalyoncu, AF; Sahin, AA; Baris, YI. Malignant pleural mesothelioma due to environmental mineral fiber exposure in Turkey. Analysis of 135 cases. *Chest*, 1992, 102, 790-796.

[67] Comba, P; Gianfagna, A; Paoletti, L. Pleural mesothelioma cases in Biancavilla are related to a new fluoro-edenite amphibole. *Arch. Environ. Health*, 2003, 58, 229-232.

[68] Newhouse, ML. A study of the mortality of workers in an asbestos factory. *Br. J. Ind. Med.*, 1969, 26, 294-301.

[69] Newhouse, ML; Berry, G. Patterns of mortality in asbestos factory workers in London. *Ann. N.Y. Acad. Sci.*, 1979, 330, 53-60.

[70] Seidman, H; Selikoff, IJ; Hammond, EC. Short-term asbestos work exposure ad long-term observation. *Ann. N.Y. Acad. Sci.*, 1979, 330, 61-89.

[71] Armstrong, BK; de Klerk, NH; Musk, AW; Hobbs, MST. Mortality in miners and millers of crocidolite in Western Australia. *Br. J. Ind. Med.*, 1988, 45, 5-13.

[72] Tuomi, T; Huuskonen, MS; Virtamo, M; Tossavainen, A; Tammilehto, L; Mattson, K; Lahdensuo, A; Mattila, J; Karhunen, P; Liippo, K; et al. Relative risk of mesothelioma associated with different levels of exposure to asbestos. *Scand. J. Work Environ. Health,* 1991, 17, 404-408.

[73] Rogers, AJ; Leigh, J; Berry, G; Ferguson, DA; Mulder, HB; Ackad, M. Relationship between lung asbestos fiber type and concentration and relative risk of mesothelioma. *Cancer,* 1991, 67, 1912-1920.

[74] Iwatsubo, Y; Pairon, JC; Boutin, C; Menard, O; Massin, N; Caillaud, D; Orlowski, E; Galateau-Salle, F; Bignon, J; Brochard, P. Pleural mesothelioma: dose-response relation at low levels of asbestos exposure in a French population-based case-control study. *Am. J. Epidemiol.*, 1998, 148, 133-142.

[75] Siemiatycki, J; Boffetta, P. Invited commentary: is it possible to investigate the quantitative relation between asbestos and mesothelioma in a community-based study? *Am J. Epidemiol.*, 1998, 148, 143-147.

[76] Boffetta, P. Health effects of asbestos exposure in humans: a quantitative assessment. *Med. Lav.*, 1998, 89, 471-480.

[77] Berry, G; Newhouse, ML; Wagner, JC. Mortality from all cancers of asbestos factory workers in east London 1933-80. *Occup. Environ. Med.*, 2000, 57, 782-785.

[78] Roggli, VL. Malignant mesothelioma and duration of asbestos exposure: correlation with tissue mineral fibre content. *Ann. Occup. Hyg.*, 1995, 39, 363-374.

[79] World Health Organization. Chrysotile asbestos. Geneva: *WHO. Environmental Health Criteria* 203; 1998.

[80] ACGIH. Documentation on the threshold limit values and biological exposure indices. *American Conference of Governmental Industrial Hygienists*. Seventh edition; 2001; 4-6.

[81] Neumann, V; Günther, S; Müller, KM; Fischer, M. Malignant mesothelioma - German mesothelioma register 1987-1999. *Int. Arch. Occupat. Environ. Health*, 2001, 74, 383-395.

[82] Hansen, J; de Klerk, NH; Musk, W; Hobbs, MS. Environmental exposure to crocidolite and mesothelioma. *Am. J. Resp. Crit. Care Med.*, 1998, 157, 69-75.

[83] Magnani, C; Agudo, A; Gonzalez, CA; Andrion, A; Calleja, A, Chellini, E; Dalmasso, P; Escolar, A; Hernandez, S; Ivaldi, C; Mirabelli, D; Ramirez, J; Turuguet, D; Usel, M; Terracini, B. Multicentric study on malignant pleural mesothelioma and non-occupational exposure to asbestos. *Br. J. Cancer*, 2000, 83, 104-111.

[84] Hayes, RB; Vineis, P. Time dependency in human cancer. *Tumori,* 1989, 75, 189-195.

[85] Ribak, J; Lilis, R; Suzuki, Y; Penner, L; Selikoff, IJ. Malignant mesothelioma in a cohort of asbestos insulation workers: clinical presentation, diagnosis, and causes of death. *Br. J. Ind. Med.*, 1988, 45, 182-187.

[86] Lanphear, BP; Buncher, CR. Latent period for malignant mesothelioma of occupational origin. *J. Occup. Med.*, 1992, 34, 718-721.

[87] Bianchi, C; Giarelli, L; Grandi, G; Brollo, A; Ramani, L; Zuch, C. Latency periods in asbestos-related mesothelioma of the pleura. *Eur. J. Cancer Prev.*, 1997, 6, 162-166.

[88] Paoletti, L; Falchi, M; Batisti, D; Zappa, M; Chellini, E; Biancalani, M. Characterization of asbestos fibres in pleural tissue from 21 cases of mesothelioma. *Med. Lav.*, 1993, 84, 373-378.

[89] Boutin, C; Dumortier, P; Rey, F; Vialat, JR; De Vuyst, P. Black spots concentrate oncogenic asbestos fibres in the parietal pleura. Thoracoscopic and mineralogical study. *Am. J. Respir. Crit. Care*, 1996, 153, 444-449.

[90] Suzuki, Y; Yuen, SR. Asbestos fibers contributing to the induction of human malignant mesothelioma. *Ann. N.Y. Acad. Sci.*, 2002, 982, 160-176.

[91] Suzuki, Y; Yuen, SR; Ashley, R. Short, thin asbestos fibers contribute to the development of human malignant mesothelioma: pathological evidence. *Int. J. Hyg. Environ. Health,* 2005, 208, 201-210.

[92] Chiappino, G. Mesotelioma: il ruolo delle fibre ultrafini e conseguenti riflessi in campo preventivo e medico legale. *Med. Lav.,* 2005, 96, 3-23.

[93] Gibbs, AR; Stephens, M; Griffiths, DM; Blight, BJN; Pooley, D. Fibre distribution in the lungs and pleura of subjects with asbestos related diffuse pleural fibrosis. *Br. J. Ind. Med.*, 1991, 48, 762-770.

[94] Mitchev, K; Dumortier, P; De Vuyst, P. "Black Spots" and hyaline pleural plaques on the parietal pleura of 150 urban necroscopy cases. *Am. J. Surg. Pathol.*, 2002, 26, 1198-1206.

[95] Dodson, RF; Williams, MG; Corn, CJ. A comparison of asbestos burden in lung parenchyma, lymphoodes and plaques. *Ann. N.Y. Acad. Sci.*, 1991, 643, 53-60.

[96] Dodson, RF; O'Sullivan, MF; Huang, J; Hiliday, DB; Hammar, SP. Asbestos in extrapulmonary sites - omentum and mesentery. *Chest*, 2000, 117, 486-493.

[97] Dodson, RF; Atkinson, MA; Levin, JL. Asbestos fiber length as related to potential pathogenicity: a critical revue. *Am. J. Ind. Med.*, 2003, 444, 291-297.

[98] Tomatis, L; Cantoni, S; Carnevale, F; Merler, E; Mollo, F; Ricci, P; Silvestri, S; Vineis, P; Terracini, B. Il ruolo della dimensione delle fibre da amianto nella patogenesi e nella prevenzione del mesotelioma. *Epidemiol. Prev.*, 2006, 30, 289-294.

[99] van Gelder, T; Hoogsteden, HC; Versnel, MA; van Hezik, EJ; Vandenbroucke, JP; Plateydt, HAT. Malignant pleural mesothelioma in the Southwestern part of the Netherlands. *Eur. Respir. J.,* 1989, 2, 981-984.

[100] Bianchi, C; Brollo, A; Ramani, L; Bianchi, T; Giarelli, L. Asbestos exposure in malignant mesothelioma of the pleura: a survey of 557 cases. *Ind. Health*, 2001, 39, 161-167.

[101] Spirtas, R; Heineman, EF; Bernstein, L; Beebe, GW; Keehn, RJ; Stark, A; Harlow, BL; Benichou, J. Malignant mesothelioma: attributable risk of asbestos exposure. *Occup. Environ. Med.,* 1994, 51, 904-811.

[102] Carbone, M; Kratzke, R; Test,a JR. The pathogenesis of mesothelioma. Semin. *Oncol.*, 2002, 29, 2-17.

[103] Finnish Institute of Occupational Health. Asbestos, Asbestosis, and cancer: the Helsinki criteria for diagnosis and attribution. *Consensus Report. Scand. J. Work Environ. Health,* 1997, 23, 311-316.

[104] Neuberger, M; Kundi, M. Individual asbestos exposure: smoking and mortality - a cohort study in asbestos cement industry. *Br. J. Ind. Med.*, 1990, 47, 615-620.

[105] Magnani, C; Terracini, B; Ivaldi, C; Mancin,i A; Botta, M. Mortalità per tumori ed altre cause tra i lavoratori del cemento amianto a Casale Monferrato. *Med. Lav.*, 1996, 87, 133-146.

[106] McDonald, JC; McDonald, AD. Chrysotile, tremolite and carcinogenicity. *Ann. Occup. Hyg.*, 1997, 41, 699-705.

[107] Yano, E; Wang, ZM; Wang, ZR; Wang, MZ; Lan, YJ. Cancer mortality among workers exposed to amphybole-free chrysotile asbestos. *Am. J. Epidemiol.*, 2001, 154, 538-543.

[108] Magnani, C; Bellis, D; Borgo, C; Botta, M; Ivaldi, C; Mollo, F; Terracini, B. Incidence of mesotheliomas among people environmentally exposed to asbestos. *Eur. Respir. Rev.*, 1993, 3, 105-107.

[109] Berry, M. Mesothelioma incidence and community asbestos exposure. *Environ. Res.*, 1997, 75, 43-40.

[110] Szeszenia-Dabrowska, N; Wilczynska, U; Szymczak, W; Laskowicz, K. Environmental exposure to asbestos in asbestos cement workers: a cause of additional exposure from indiscriminate use of industrial wastes. *Int. J. Occup. Med. Environ. Health*, 1998, 11, 171-177.

[111] Magnani, C; Terracini, B; Ivaldi, C; Botta, M; Budel, P; Mancini, A; Zanetti, R. A cohort study on mortality among wives of workers in the asbestos cement industry in Casale Monferrato, Italy. *Br. J. Ind. Med.*, 1993, 50, 779-784.

[112] Ribak, J; Selikoff, IJ. Survival of asbestos insulation workers with mesothelioma. *Br. J. Ind. Med.*, 1992, 49, 732-735.

[113] Ulvestad, B; Kjaerheim, K; Martinen, JI; Mowe, G; Andersen, A. Cancer incidence among members of the Norvegian trade union of insulation workers. *J. Occup. Environ. Med.,* 2004, 46, 84-89.

[114] Menegozzo, M; Belli, S; Borriero, S; Bruno, C; Carboni, M; Grignoli, M; Menegozzo, S; Olivieri, N; Comba, P. Studio di mortalità di una coorte di coibentatori. *Epidemiol. Prev.*, 2002, 26, 71-75.

[115] Jarvholm, B; Sanden, A. Lung cancer and mesothelioma in the pleura and peritoneum among Swedish insulation Workers. *Occup. Environ. Med.*, 1998, 55, 766-770.

[116] Zanardi, S; Fontana, L. Osservazioni su possibili rapporti tra amianto e tumori pleuropolmonari in Liguria. *Med. Lav.*, 1971, 62, 336-343.

[117] Tannini, D; Bogetti, B; Ottenga, F. Il rischio e la prevenzione dell'asbestosi nelle lavorazioni navali. *Med. Lav.*, 1972, 63, 221-244.

[118] Bianchi, C. Esposizione lavorativa all'amianto in 20 casi di mesotelioma diffuso della pleura. *Min. Med.*, 1973, 64,1724-1727.

[119] Merlo, F; Reggiardo, G; Garrone, E; Ceppi, M; Puntoni, R.. Cancer risk among 3890 workers employed at the industrial branch of the shipyard of Genoa, Italy: a retrospective cohort. *Proceedings of the 9th International Symposium in Epidemiology and Occupational Health*, Cincinnati, USA 23-25 September 1992: 229-232.

[120] Joshi, TK; Bhuva, UB; Katoch, P. Asbestos ban in India - challenges ahead. *Ann. N.Y. Acad. Sci.*, 2006, 1076, 292-308.

[121] Dalquen, P; Dabbert, AF; Hinz, I. Zur Aetiologie der Pleuramesotheliome. *Prax Pneumol.*, 1969, 23: 547-558.

[122] Van der Schoot, HCM. *Asbestosis en pleuragezwellen*. Nedijdschr. Geneeskd., 1958,102, 1125-1126.

[123] Stumphius, J. Epidemiology of mesothelioma on Walcheren Island. *Br. J. Ind. Med.*, 1971, 28, 59-66.

[124] McCaughey, WTE. Primary tumours of the pleura. *J. Path. Bact.*, 1958, 76, 517-529.

[125] McCaughey, WTE; Vade, OL; Elmes, PC. Exposure to asbestos dust and diffuse pleural mesothelioma. *Br. Med. J.*, 1962, 2, 1397.

[126] McEwen, J; Finlayson, A; Mauir, A; Gibson, AA. Mesothelioma in Scotland. *Br. Med. J.,* 1970, 4, 575-578.

[127] Wagner, JC; Gilson, JC; Berry, G; Timbrell, V. Epidemiology of asbestos cancers. *Br. Med. Bull.*, 1971, 27, 71-76.

[128] Battista, G; Belli, S; Comba, P; Fiumalbi, C; Grignoli, M; Loi, F; Orsi, D; Paredes, I. Mortality due to asbestos-related causes among railway carriage construction and repair workers. *Occup. Med.*, 1999, 49, 536-539.

[129] Blasetti, F; Bruno, C; Comba, P; Fantini, F; Grignoli, M. Studio di mortalità relativo agli addetti alla costruzione di carrozze ferroviarie a Colleferro. *Med. Lav.*, 1990, 81, 407-413.

[130] Gerosa, A; Ietri, E; Belli, S; Grignoli, M; Comba, P. Alto rischio di morte per mesotelioma pleurico in un'Officina Grandi Riparazioni delle Ferrovie dello Stato. *Epidemiol. Prev.*, 2000, 24, 117-119.

[131] Magnani, C; Cardini, I; Governa, M; Serio, A. Uno studio di coorte degli addetti ad una officina grandi riparazioni (OGR) delle ferrovie dello stato. *Med. Lav.*, 1986, 77, 154-161.

[132] Magnani, C; Ricci, P; Terracini, B. A mortality historical cohort study in the Verona repair workshop of Italian railways. *Acta Oncol.*, 1989, 10, 201-207.

[133] Maltoni, C; Pinto, C; Dominaci, R. Mesoteliomi tra i meccanici delle ferrovie in Italia: un problema di attualità. *Med. Lav.*, 1989, 80, 103-110.

[134] Menegozzo, M; Belli, S; Bruno, C; Canfora, V; Costignola, A; Di Cintio, P; Di Lello, L; Grignoli, M; Palombo, F; Sapio, P; et al. La mortalità per cause correlabili all'amianto in una coorte di addetti alla costruzione di carrozze ferroviarie. *Med. Lav.*, 1993, 84, 193-200.

[135] Merler, E; Ricci, P; Carnevale, F; et al. Identificazione dei casi di mesotelioma insorti in Italia per l'esposizione ad amianto usato nella coibentazione di mezzi ferroviari. *Rass. Med. Lav.*, 1990, 16, 1-25.

[136] Seniori-Costantini, A; Ercolanelli, M; Silvestri, S; Innocenti, A; Ciapini, C. Studio di coorte sugli addetti ad una azienda di costruzione e riparazione di rotabili ferroviari (Breda): aggiornamento del follow-up del precedente studio al 31/12/2000. In: *L'intervento sanitario per gli ex esposti ad amianto della ditta Breda. Regione Toscana: Servizio Sanitario della Toscana;* 2002, 10-20.

[137] Tessari, R; Canova, C; Limonato, L. Indagine epidemiologica sullo stato di salute degli addetti alla produzione e riparazione carrozze ferroviarie: uno studio prospettico di mortalità. *Med. Lav.*, 2004, 95, 381-391.

[138] Mancuso, TF. Mesothelioma among machinists in railroad and other industries. *Am. J. Ind. Med.*, 1983, 4, 501-513.

[139] Mancuso, TF. Relative risk of mesothelioma among railroad machinists exposed to chrysotile. *Am. J. Ind. Med.*, 1988, 13, 639-657.

[140] Mancuso, TF. Mesothelioma among railroads workers in the United States. *Ann. N.Y. Acad. Sci.*, 1991, 643, 333-346.

[141] Ohlson, CG; Klaesson, B; Hogstedt, C. Mortality among asbestos-exposed workers in a railroad workshop. *Scand. J. Work Environ. Health*, 1984, 10, 283-291.

[142] Schenker, MB; Garshick, E; Munoz, A; Woskie, SR; Speizer, FE. A population-based case-control study of mesothelioma deaths among US railroad workers. *Am. Rev. Respir. Dis.*, 1986, 134, 461-465.

[143] Comba, P; Merler, E; Pasetto, R. Asbestos related diseases in Italy: epidemiologic evidence and public health issues. *Int. J. Occup. Environ. Med.*, 2005, 11, 36-44.

[144] Rüttner, JR; Reber, P; Schüler, G; Srpycher, MA; Stolkin, P; Wälchi, P. Endemie von Pleuramesotheliomen in Eisenbah-waggonbau- und-reparaturarbeiten. Arbetismed. *Sozialmed. Präventivmed.*, 1986, 20, 128-131.

[145] Malker, HS; Laughlin, JK; Malker, BK; Stone, BJ; Weiner, JA; Erickson, JL; Blot, WJ. Occupational risks for pleural mesothelioma in Sweden, 1961-79. *J. Natl. Cancer Inst.*, 1985, 74, 61-66.

[146] Burdof, A; Dahhan, M; Swuste, P. Occupational characteristics of cases with asbestos-related diseases in the Netherlands. *Ann. Occup. Hyg.*, 2003, 47, 485-492.

[147] Tweendale, G. Magic mineral to killer dust. London, Oxford University Press, 2000.

[148] Murray, R. Asbestos: a chronology of its origin and health effects. *Br. J. Ind. Med.*, 1990, 47, 361-365.

[149] Vallestrisco, M; Casadio, S (1997). *Materiali a base di amianto*. Torino, Italy: Giappichelli Editore.

[150] Coordinamento per la prevenzione nei luoghi di lavoro delle Regioni e delle Province Autonome di Trento e Bolzano: Prime linee di indirizzo per l'attuazione dell'art. 1 del DM 20 Agosto 1999 "Ampliamento delle normative e delle metodologie tecniche per gli interventi di bonifica, ivi compresi quelli per rendere innocuo l'amianto, previsti dall'art. 5, comma 1, lettera f), della Legge 27 marzo 1992, n. 257, recante norme relative alla cessazione dell'impiego dell'amianto". 30 Agosto 2000.

[151] Puntoni, R; Valerio, FE; Sanit, L. Il mesotelioma pleurico fra i lavoratori di Genova. *Tumori,* 1976, 62, 205-210.

[152] Bianchi, C; Brollo, A. Mesoteliomi maligni della pleura e del peritoneo: tumori professionali dei marittimi. Roma: Atti della Sezione Studi, Centro Internazionale Radio Medico; 1991; 5-12.

[153] Jones RN; Diem, JE; Ziskand, MM; Rodriguez, M; Weill, H. Radiographic evidence of asbestos effects in american marine engineers. *J. Occup. Med.*, 1984, 26, 281-284.

[154] Selikoff, IJ; Lilis, R; Levin, G. Asbestotic radiological abnormalities among United States merchant marine seamen. *Br. J. Ind. Med.*, 1990, 47, 292-297.

[155] Velonakis, EG; Tsorva, A; Tzonou, A; Trichopoulos, D. Asbestos-related chest X-ray changes among Greek merchant marine seamen. *Am. J. Ind. Med.*, 1989, 15, 511-516.

[156] Darby, SC, Muirhead, CR, Doll, R, Kendall, GM, Thakrar, B. Mortality among Unit Kingdom servicemen who served abroad in the 1950s and 1960s. *Br. J. Ind. Med.*, 1990, 47, 793-804.

[157] Rapiti, E; Turi, E; Forastiere, F; Borgia, P; Comba, O; Peducci, CA; Axelson, O. A mortality cohort study of seamen in Italy. *Am. J. Ind. M*ed., 1992, 21, 863-872.

[158] Greenberg, M. Cancer mortality in merchant seamen. *Ann. N.Y. Acad. Sci.*, 1991, 643, 321-332.

[159] Saarni, H; Pentti, J; Pukkala, E. Cancer at sea: a case-control study among male Finnish seafarers. *Occup. Environ. Med.*, 2002, 59, 613-619.

[160] Hemminki, K; Li, X. Time trends and occupational risk factors for pleural mesothelioma in Sweden. *J. Occup. Med.*, 2003, 45, 456-463.

[161] Reitze, WB; Nicholson, WJ; Holaday, DA; Selikoff, IJ. Application of sprayed inorganic fiber containing asbestos: occupational health hazards. *Am. Ind. Hyg. Assoc. J.,* 1972, 33, 178-191.

[162] Oliver, LC. Asbestos in buildings: management and related effects. *Adv. Modern Environ. Toxicol.* 1994; 22: 175-188.

[163] Landrigan, PJ; Lioy, PJ; Thurston, G; Berkowitz, G; Chen, LC; Chillrud, SN; Gavett, SH; Georgopoulos, PG; Geyh, AS; Levin, S; Perera, F; Stephen Rappaport, SM; Small, C; NIEHS World Trade Center Working Group. Health and environmental consequences of the World Trade Center disaster. *Environ. Health Persp.*, 2004, 112, 731-739.

[164] Huncharek, M. Changing risk groups for malignant mesothelioma. *Cancer,* 1992, 69, 2704-11.

[165] Baker, EL; Dagg, T; Greene, A. Respiratory illness in the construction trades. *J. Occup. Med.*, 1985, 27, 483-489.

[166] Robinson, CF; Petersen, M; Palu, S. Mortality patterns among electrical workers employed in the U.S. construction industry, 1982-1987. *Am. J. Ind. Med.*, 1999, 36, 630-637.

[167] Peto, J; Hodgson, JT; Matthews, FE; Jones, JR. Continuing increase of mesothelioma mortality in Britain. *Lancet*, 1995, 345, 535-539.

[168] IARC. Monographs on the evaluation of the carcinogenic risks of chemicals to humans. Lyon, *IARC scientific publication*, vol. 48, 1990.

[169] Brenner, J; Sordillo, PP; Magill, GB; Golbey, RB. Malignant mesothelioma of the pleura: review of 123 patients. *Cancer*, 1982, 49, 2431-2435.

[170] Paci, E; Buiatti, E; Geddes, M. A case-referent study of lung tumors in non-asbestos textile workers. *Am. J. Ind. Med.*, 1987, 11, 267-273.

[171] Paci, E; Dini, S; Buratti, E; Seniori Costantini, A; Lenzi, S; Zappa, M. Malignant mesothelioma in non-asbestos textile workers in Florence. *Am. J. Ind. M*ed., 1987, 11, 249-254.

[172] Barbieri, PG; Migliori, M; Merler, E. Incidenza del mesotelioma maligno (1977-1996) ed esposizione ad amianto nella popolazione di un'area limitrofa al Lago d'Iseo, Nord Italia. *Med. Lav.*, 1999, 90, 762-775.

[173] Colli, G; Terzi, M; Vinci, L; Terzi, R; Caldura, SM. Un caso di mesotelioma pleurico da inusuale esposizione professionale ad amianto nell'industria della lana. G. *Ital. Med. Lav. Ergon.*, 2001, 23, 18-20.

[174] Gorini, G; Silvestri, S; Merler, E; Chellini, E; Cacciarini, V; Seniori Costantini, AS. La valutazione dell'esposizione ad amianto in Toscana attraverso i dati dell'Archivio Regionale Toscano dei Mesoteliomi Maligni (1988-2000). *Med. Lav.*, 2002, 93, 507-518.

[175] Yu, IJ; Choi, JK; Kang, SK; Chang, HK; Chung, YH; Han, JH; Song, KS; Lee, YM; Chung, HK. Potential source of asbestos in non-asbestos textile manufacturing company. *Environ. Int.*, 2002, 28, 35-39.

[176] Chiappino, G; Pellissetti, D; Moretto, O; Picchi, O. Il rischio amianto nel settore tessile: i sistemi frenanti delle macchine di penultima generazione. *Med. Lav.*, 2005, 96, 250-257.

[177] ISPESL. Linee Guida per la rivelazione e la definizione dei casi di mesotelioma maligno e la trasmissione delle informazioni all'ISPESL da parte dei Centri Operativi Regionali. Seconda edizione. Roma: *ISPESL,* 2003.

[178] Huncharek, M; Muscat, J; Capotorto, JV. Pleural mesothelioma in a lift mechanic. *Br. J. Ind. Med.*, 1989, 46, 500-501.

[179] Tonut, S. Il mesotelioma della pleura e la manutenzione degli ascensori. *SNOP*, 1990, 14/15, 29.

[180] Bruno, C; Belli, S; Redaelli, ML; Corno, O; Simonetto, R; Comba, P. Tumori dell'apparato respiratorio in una coorte di addetti alla produzione ed alla manutenzione /riparazione di ascensori (abstract). In: *Atti Conferenza Nazionale sull'Amianto*. Roma: Presidenza del Consiglio dei Ministri, Ministero della Sanità; 1999, 42.

[181] Rees, D; Myers, JE; Goodman, K; Furie, E; Blignaut, C; Chapman, R; Bachmann, MO. Case-control study of mesothelioma in South Africa. *Am. J. Ind. Med.*, 1999, 35, 213-222.

[182] Newhouse, ML; Thompson, H. Mesothelioma of pleura and peritoneum following exposure to asbestos in the London area. *Br. J. Ind. Med.*, 1965, 22, 261-269.

[183] Baris, YI; Sahin, AA; Ozesmi, M; Kerse, I; Ozen, E; Kolacan, B; Altinors, M; Goktepeli, A. An outbreak of pleural mesothelioma and chronic fibrosing pleurisy in the village of Karain/Urgup in Anatolia. *Thorax*, 1978, 33, 181-192.

[184] Baris, YI; Saracci, R; Simonato, L; Skidmore, JW; Artvinli, M. Malignant mesothelioma and radiological chest abnormalities in two villages in central Turkey. *Lancet,* 1981, 1, 984-987.

[185] Artvinili, M; Baris, YI. Malignant mesotheliomas in a small village in the Anatolian region of Turkey: an epidemiologic study. *J. Natl. Cancer. Inst.,* 1979, 63, 17-22.

[186] Yazicioglu, S; Ilçayto, R; Balci, K; Sayli, BS; Yorulmaz, B. Pleural calcification, pleural mesotheliomas, and bronchial cancers caused by tremolite dust. *Thorax*, 1980, 35, 564-569.

[187] Zeren, EH; Gumurdulu, D; Roggli, VL; Zorludemir, S; Erkisi, M; Tuncer, I. Environmental malignant mesothelioma in Southern Anatolia: a study of fifty. cases. *Environ. Health Perspect.*, 2000, 108, 1047-1050.

[188] Senyigit, A; Babayigit, C; Gokirmak, M; Topcu, F; Asan, E; Coskunsel, M; Isik, R; Ertem, M. Incidence of malignant pleural mesothelioma due to environmental asbestos fiber exposure in the southeast of Turkey. *Respiration*, 2000, 67, 610-614.

[189] Metintas, S; Metintas, M; Ucgun, I; Oner, U. Malignant mesothelioma due to environmental exposure to asbestos: follow-up of a Turkish cohort living in a rural area. *Chest,* 2002, 122, 2224-2229.

[190] Hasanoglu, HC; Yildirim, Z; Ermis, H; Kilic, T; Koksal, N. Lung cancer and mesothelioma in towns with environmental exposure to asbestos in Eastern Anatolia. *Int. Arch. Occup. Environ. Health,* 2005, published on-line 30 august 2005.

[191] Costantopoulos, SH; Goudevenos, JA; Saratzis, N; Langer, AM; Selikoff, IJ; Moutsopoulos HM. Metsovo lung: pleural calcification and restrictive lung function in Northwestern Greece. Environmental exposure to mineral fiber as etiology. *Environ. Res.* 1985, 38, 319-331.

[192] Mc Connochie, K; Simonato, L; Mavrides, P; Christofides, P; Pooley, FD; Wagner, JC. Mesothelioma in Cyprus: the role of tremolite. *Thorax,* 1987, 42, 342-347.

[193] Steinbauer, J; Boutin, C; Viallat, JR; Dufour, G; Gaudichet, A; Massey, DG; Charpin, D; Mouries, JC. Plaques pleurales et environnement asbestosique en Corse du Nord. *Rev. Mal. Resp.*, 1987, 4, 23-27.

[194] Goldberg, P; Luce, D; Billon-Galland, MA; Quénel, P; Salomon-Nekiriai, C; Nicolau, J; Brochard, P; Goldberg, M. Role potentiel de l'exposition environnementale et domestique à la trémolite dans le cancer de la plèvre en Nouvelle Caledonie. *Rev. Epidemiol.* Santé Publ., 1995, 43, 444-450.

[195] Pan, XL; Day, HW; Wang, W; Beckett, LA; Schenker, MB. Residential proximity to naturally occurring asbestos and mesothelioma risk in California. *Am. J. Respir. Crit. Care Med.*, 2005, 172, 1019-1025.

[196] Magnani, C; Terracini, B; Ivaldi, C; Botta, M; Mancini, A; Andrion, A. Pleural malignant mesothelioma and non-occupational exposure to asbestos in Casale Monferrato, Italy. *Occup. Environ. Med.*, 1995, 52, 362-367.

[197] Maynard, C. Asbestos problem in Montana e California. *Environ. Sci. Technol.* 2004, 1, 38, 46.

[198] Valérie, B; Boffetta, P; Pisani, P. Environmental exposure to asbestos and risk of pleural mesothelioma: review and meta-analysis. *Eur. J. Epidemiol.*, 2000, 16, 411-417.

[199] Magnani, C; Dalmasso, P; Biggeri, A; Ivaldi, C; Mirabelli, D; Terracini, B. Increased risk of malignant mesothelioma of the pleura after residential or domestic exposure to asbestos: a case-control study in Casale Monferrato, Italy. *Environ. Health Perspect.*, 2001, 109, 915-919.

[200] Silvestri, S; Magnani, C; Calisti, R; Bruno, C. The experience of the Balangero chrysotile asbestos mine in Italy: health effects among workers mining and milling asbestos and the health experience of people living nearby. *Can. Mineral.*, 2001, 5, 177-186.

[201] Mirabelli, D; Cavone, D; Merler, E; Mensi, C; Magnani, C; Musti, M. I casi di mesotelioma maligno ad eziologia ambientale e familiare: considerazioni generali ed analisi dei dati ReNaM. II Rapporto ReNaM. *Roma: ISPESL*; 2006; 91-104.

[202] Mirabelli, D; Cadum, E. Mortality from pleural and peritoneal malignancies in the Upper Susa Valley. *Epidemiol. Prev.*, 2002, 26, 284-286.

[203] Biggeri, A; Pasetto, R; Belli, S; Bruno, C; Di Maria, G; Mastrantonio, M; Trinca, S; Uccelli, R; Comba, P. Mortality from chronic obstructive pulmonary disease and pleural mesothelioma in an area contaminated by natural fiber (fluoro-edenite). *Scand. J. Work Environ. Health*. 2004, 30, 249-252.

[204] Pasetto, R; Bruni, B; Bruno, C; Cauzillo, G; Cavone, D; Convertini, L; De Mei, B; Marconi, A; Montagano, G; Musti, M; Paoletti, L; Comba, P. Pleural mesothelioma and environmental exposure to mineral fibres: the case of a rural area in the Basilicata region, Italy. *Ann. Ist. Super. Sanità*, 2004, 40, 251-265.

[205] Rosenthal, R; Langer, I; Dalquen, P; Marti, WR; Oertli, D. Peritoneal mesothelioma after environmental asbestos exposure. *Swiss Surg.*, 2003, 9, 311-314.

[206] Hemminki, K; Li, X. Mesothelioma is a killer of urban men in Sweden. *Int. J. Cancer*, 2003, 105, 144-146.

[207] Polednak, AP. Geographic distribution of incident mesothelioma in Connecticut men, 1990-99. *Int. J. Cancer*, 2003, 107, 509-510.

[208] Marconi, A; Rossi, L; Migliaccio, G; Di Girolamo, P; Scaccia, M; Galoppini, P; Barbieri, M. Environmental fibers contamination related to fibrous mineral materials: results from an investigation in a big office building. *G. Ig. Ind.*, 1987, 12, 25-63.

[209] Ascoli, V; Comba, P; Pasetto R. Urban mesothelioma: is there an emerging risk of asbestos in Place. (letter to the Editor). *Int. J. Cancer*, 2004, 111, 975-976.

[210] Bianchi, C; Bianchi, T. Asbestos and globalization. Eur. J. Oncol., 2005, 10, 169-172.

[211] Comba, P; Magnani, C; Botti, C. L'individuazione delle priorità per il risanamento ambientale dall'amianto: aspetti etici. *Epidemiol. Prev.*, 2000, 24, 85-86.

[212] Braun, L; Greene, A; Manseau, M; Singhal, R; Kisting, S; Jacobs, N. Scientific controversy and asbestos: making the disease invisibile. *Int. J. Occup. Environ. Health*, 2003, 9, 194-205.

[213] Terracini, B. Additional features of the worldwide double standards in the prevention of asbestos-related diseases. *Ann. Ist. Super. Sanità*, 2006, 42, 174-177.

[214] Terracini, B. The scientific basis of a total asbestos ban. *Med. Lav.*, 2006, 97, 383-392.

[215] Collegium Ramazzini. Call for an international ban on asbestos: Statement update. Richiesta di messa al bando internazionale dell'amianto: Aggiornamento della posizione del Collegium Ramazzini. *Eur. J. Oncol.*, 2005, 10, 5-8.

[216] WHO. Elimination of asbestos-related diseases. Geneva: 2007.02.01. Available from: www.WHO.int/occupational_health/publications/asbestosrelateddiseases.PDF.

In: Mesothelioma from Bench Side to Clinic
Editor: Alfonso Baldi, pp. 67-104

ISBN: 978-1-60021-789-0

Chapter IV

Non-Asbestos Causes of Mesothelioma

John H. Lange[1], John A. Hoskins and Giuseppe Mastrangelo
[1]Envirosafe Training and Consultants,
P.O. Box 114022 Pittsburgh, PA 15239 USA
[2]Haslemere, Surrey GU27 2JH, UK
[3]Department of Environmental Medicine and Public Health,
University of Padova, Padova, Italy

Abstract

Mesothelioma is considered by most a fatal cancer with its causative agent often associated with asbestos. There have been a large number of reports indicating that the only agent responsible for this disease is airborne exposure to asbestos, and this exposure results from both environmental and occupational sources. Historically, mesothelioma was considered to be a marker or signal disease for asbestos exposure with a high relationship to the occupational environment. Recent reports have suggested that not all mineralogical forms of asbestos are equal in capability of causing this disease, as well as other asbestos-related diseases (e.g. lung cancer). Numerous investigations have suggested that there are other exposure agents/substances that appear to be causative for this disease along with idiopathic and familial relationships. There also appears to be a "natural" background level of this disease, in part, indicating that it arises spontaneously. Some of the agents that have been reported in causing/contributing to mesothelioma are: ionizing radiation, chemicals, metals, non-asbestos fibrous substances (e.g. erionite), smoking, genetic factors, inflammation. There are also studies that suggest infectious disease agents (e.g. SV40 virus) can cause or contribute to this disease. It has been estimated that around 5-30% of all cases of mesothelioma are a result of non-asbestos event(s); although, a higher percentage has been suggested (0-87%). A discussion is presented on some of the current thought regarding non-asbestos causes of mesothelioma and presents agents that may be responsible for this disease besides asbestos.

Abbreviations

AOS	active oxygen species
BC	before Christ
CI	confidence interval
DMM	diffuse malignant mesothelioma
DNA	deoxyribonucleic acid
GSTM1	glutathione-S-transferase M1
Gy	Gray
HEI-AR	Health Effects Institute – Asbestos Research
IARC	International Agency for Cancer Research
PPV	Inactivated polio vaccine (Salk)
JCV	Jamestown Canyon virus
MM	malignant mesothelioma
MMMF	man-made mineral fiber(s)
MMVF	man-made vitreous fibers
MPM	malignant pleural mesothelioma
NAT1	N-acetyltransferase 2
NAT2	N-acetyltransferase 2
NF2	neurofibromatosis 2
NHL	non-Hogkins lymphoma
NTP	National Toxicology Program
OPV	oral polio vaccine
OR	odds ratio
PCR	polymerase chain reaction
PMM	pleural malignant mesothelioma
RCF	refractory ceramic fibers
RNS	reactive nitrogen species
ROS	reactive oxygen species
RReg	simian virus regulatory primer
SD	standard deviation
SV40	simian virus40
T Ag or Tag	T antigen (for SV40 virus)

Introduction

Exposure to asbestos has been associated and related to various pulmonary diseases (Abraham, 1983; Rom, 1983; Berry et al., 2000). These diseases became evident shortly after asbestos industry developed into a commercial business around the 1880's. Before that time period asbestos had limited use (Rom, 1983) and its exposure was not common; thus, the occurrence of related diseases would have mostly gone unnoticed. However, there is the suggestion of diseases that are now associated with asbestos, including mesothelioma, as early as the 1700's, but at that time it was uncertain as to the cause and origin and if these were truly asbestos-related (McDonald and McDonald, 1996). The first noted case of disease (asbestosis) was reported in 1899 involving an Englishman that worked in an asbestos factory.

Diseases reported to be associated with asbestos exposure include asbestosis, lung cancer, pleural plaques, pleural effusion and mesothelioma. Some have also indicated that gastrointestinal cancer is associated with inhalation and ingestion of asbestos, but occurrence of this "disease" in study populations is more likely related to dietary habits and other social economic factors (e.g. smoking) (Gamble, 1994).

The word asbestos comes from the Greek language, meaning inextinguishable, indestructible not quenchable, depending on the exact translation inferred (Browne and Murray, 1990; Greenberg, 1997; Ross and Nolan, 2003). Various reports (Browne, 2003) indicate it was used as far back as ancient times (circa 2000-3000 BC), for example in napkins and clay pots. However, use appears to not have been limited to the Greeks and Romans, but Native Americans and Europeans as well (Browne and Murray, 1990; Browne, 2003). Apparently such use was not limited to cooking and textile items in the early civilizations, the Egyptians used asbestos in embalming; although, its modern use did not begin until around the 1880's when it begin to be mined for incorporation into textiles and other products. It is interesting to note that an Amerinicidian "Magic" purse, made of chrysotile, was bought in 1724 by Benjamin Franklin and sold to Sir Hans Sloane whose collection formed the basis of the British Museum in London. This suggests that those in North American had also used these minerals in some way; although, such use was minor. Other uncommon uses are still encountered in the twentieth century. In the film "The Wizard of Oz", the Wicked Witch of the West appeared on a besom broom with "twigs" made of chrysotile and this mineral was also used in the studios as artificial snow. For an even more modern use it should be noted that the solid fuel boosters of the Space Shuttle are insulated with chrysotile from the Jeffrey mine in Southern Quebec.

The industrial exploration of asbestos began over 100 years ago with the discovery of large deposits of these minerals in Canada and Southern Africa. In 1847, a geological survey discovered deposits in Quebec and serious commercial mining began in 1878 near the town of Thetford. Mining activity spread and some 60 miles away the mining town of Asbestos was founded. Some time after the usefulness of these minerals were realized the quantities employed expanded dramatically and many other deposits were found in other countries and commercially exploited.

The first recorded observations of occupational related diseases were by the early Greeks and Romans, which may have included incidences related to asbestos. Later, around the beginning of the 1900's asbestos began to be incorporated in a variety of building and construction materials, paper products, and textiles. After World War II, its use dramatically expanded. Certainly at this time, the hazards of exposure, especially at high levels, were incompletely known in modern medical science. The group of minerals known as asbestos had been found to be excellent in a number of ways: as for example, fire control, acoustic insulation, friction resistance, heat and cold insulation, chemical resistance, and electrical insulation. There has been an estimated that this mineral has been incorporated into over 3,600 different building type materials or products. This use included almost all facets of the construction and maritime industries.

Although its use has been curtailed in many of the developed nations, it is still commonly used in many locations through out the world and mining occurs in a variety of locations, especially the underdeveloped nations. It is still mined in Canada; although now only in southern Quebec, which was a major supplier of the one mineralogical form chrysotile to the United States. Approximately 95% of all asbestos used in the US was of the chrysotile variety (Ilgren and Wagner, 1991). Although it is still mined, its use has dramatically diminished in developed nations; although, some have suggested that chrysotile lacks the health hazards associated with the name asbestos and legislation against this specific mineral is extreme example of the precautionary principle (Lange, 2002; Yarborough, 2006; Bernstein and Hoskins, 2006). In the US, the peak year of use was around 1973 (Price and Ware, 2004) with stringent regulations regarding use, abatement and control beginning around 1987 (Lange et al., 1987). These regulations began to focus on the relationship of asbestos and public health. Although regulations before this time existed, they were mostly focused on the occupational environment. In 1997, it was estimated that about 2 million tons of asbestos were mined worldwide, a figure similar to that produced today (Buckingham and Virta, 2005), with the vast majority used for asbestos cement. Thus, in many ways its use is still common.

A few literature reports (Lange, 2001) have even suggested that use of asbestos in some situations may carry benefits over risks; although, comparison of risks in this way has never been determined. Continued use is supported, in part, by the lack of disease associated with some forms of asbestos (Yarborough, 2006) and in industries such as that associated with asbestos-cement (Neuberger and Vutuc, 2003; Hoskins and Lange, 2004). However, others have called for a worldwide ban and its complete elimination of use and mining (Maltoni, 2000).

Health Effects

The only practical route of exposure to asbestos is through its inhalation. However, it has been suggested (Van Kesteren et al., 2004) that ingestion of asbestos can result in disease; although, current investigations (Browne et al., 2005; Lange and Hoskins, 2004) do not support such claims and the present acceptable concentration of asbestos in drinking water for the US is 7 million fibers per liter.

The major disease hazard related to asbestos is lung cancer (Lee, 2001; Britton, 2002). This is primarily due to the high smoking rates associated with workers in this industry (Lange et al., 2004). Smoking can also influence the rates of other cancers such as that associated with the gastrointestinal system (Gamble, 1994; Homa et al., 1994). Previous studies have shown that exposure to cigarette smoking and asbestos result in a synergistic effect in the incidence of lung cancer (Hammond et al., 1979). Since a large number of today's asbestos abatement workers smoke or are frequently associated with secondhand smoke (environmental tobacco smoke), this factor will act as a major confounder to many diseases, especially lung cancer. Thus, there will likely continue to be elevated rates of "asbestos" related diseases, especially lung cancer, in those exposed (Lange et al., 1987). The smoking rates for asbestos workers in the US have been estimated to be between 50% and

80%, depending on whether management and related persons (e.g. air sampling technicians) were included in the study (Lange, 1992, 2006). If only those performing the work are included in the analysis (e.g. asbestos abatement workers), the percent of smokers is about 80%. Recently studies have reported a potential association between smoking and mesothelioma (Hirao et al., 2002). Similarly for asbestosis (De Vuyst et al., 1995), there is a suggested interaction with smoking, which might be explained by changes in fiber clearance (Churg et al., 1992; Churg and Stevens, 1995).

Historically, the primary agent reported in causing mesothelioma has been asbestos (Rom, 1983); although, recent reports have indicated that other agents/substances (Lange, 2004) are contributing to this cancer as well along with its occurrence being spontaneous (Hubbard, 1997; Huncharek, 2002).

The other commonly associated disease of asbestos, besides lung cancer is asbestosis. This disease is diagnosed based on the occupational history and occurrence of parenchymal fibrosis that may exist with or without pleural fibrosis. As mentioned, the first noted case of this disease was reported in 1899 involving an Englishman that worked in an asbestos factory. The common diagnosis for this disease is through radiographic appearance. In some cases, the existence of this disease state is necessary for compensation for injury that has been suggested to have occurred from asbestos exposure. Smoking appears to influence in lung fibrosis; thus, can be classified as contributory in asbestosis (De Vuyst et al., 1995).

Pleural plaques (circumscribed and localized) and pleural effusion have often been reported to be associated with asbestos exposure. However, these can also be a result of other events and causes (e.g. tuberculosis) (Cugell and Kamp. 2004; Mutsaers et al., 2004). Pleural plaques are well-demarked areas of fibrosis, usually bilateral, which are localized on the inner surface of the diaphragm and or ribcage. Commonly these plaques are calcified and are detected by radiographs. Pleural effusion is the accumulation of fluid in the pleural space. While this may be a sign of past asbestos exposure pleural effusions have no specific prognostic implications with respect to the subsequent development of pleural plaques or mesothelioma (Caugell and Kamp, 2004). Some authors have considered them, especially pleural plaques, to be a precursor to mesothelioma (Bianchi et al., 1997). A recent study has indicated that these pathologies are not an indicator of cumulative exposure (Van Cleeput et al., 2001). Thus, there is some controversy as to the actual relation of these pulmonary events and asbestos exposure. In most cases they are considered of little clinical importance.

Mesothelioma has been called a marker disease for asbestos exposure. This is based on the large number of cases associated with those occupationally employed in industries that used and had asbestos within their facilities (Robinson and Lake, 2006). However, there are a large number of other agents as well as spontaneous occurrences that contribute to this disease (Lange, 2004). The percent of mesothelioma cases that are not a result of asbestos exposure widely varies from publication to publication; although, the actual percent is likely around 5-30 (Lange, 2004). Since mesothelioma is a rare cancer, the distribution of cases by cause is difficult and often requires judgment on an individual basis. Some have suggested that a threshold-level exists (Cugell and Kamp. 2004; Hoskins and Lange, 2004) in causation, even though some still hold on to the one-fiber theory. The one-fiber theory represents a no-threshold exposure concept. If background levels of exposure to asbestos are examined, there exists no support for the one-fiber theory since if this hypothesis were correct a dramatic increased rate of disease in populations not exposed to asbestos occupationally would be occurring, which is not being observed (Price and Ware, 2004). In addition asbestos use since the 1900's has dramatically increased, especially between the 1940's and 1970's, and the rate of mesothelioma's in women and their lifetime probability of risk, in the US, for this disease has remained steady (Price and Ware, 2004). Since exposure to women are mostly environmental and consumption has increased, up to about the 1970's, resulting in a higher environmental exposure level, the background level of this disease should have increased as well if its incidence were related to low concentrations and no threshold existed. That the sexes are equally affected is shown by the few cohorts of women who were occupationally exposed, notably those who were involved in making military gas-masks containing crocidolite (Acheson et al., 1982). In addition, the rate of this disease in men is now declining, in the US, which should not occur if low doses of asbestos were responsible for mesothelioma. Thus, if the one-fiber theory were correct, then there would be a stead increase in this environmentally exposed population (e.g. women), which has not occurred in the US. Thus, support is lacking for the one-fiber theory (Hoskins and Lange, 2004). Certainly asbestos can cause disease, but as with any substance, there exists from a realistic and practical measure, a dose-response relationship. Most appear to forget this basic toxicological principle.

Anatomical and Histological Characteristics of Mesothelioma

Mesothelioma is a rare cancer that occurs in various locations (organ sites) of people and other multicellular organisms and arises from tissue called mesothelium. The mesothelium is part of serous membranes which lines the cavities of various internal organs. This membrane (serous) consists of three components, which include a layer of simple squamous epithelium (mesothelium), a basement membrane, and a delicate layer of loose connective tissue. These cancers are most commonly associated with the pleura (pleural) (outer lining of the lungs, peritoneum (or peritoneal) (lining of the abdominal cavity) or pericardium (or pericardial) (lining of the heart). The tissue that is formed by these mesothelial cells is called mesothelium. Mesothelium helps protect the organs by producing a lubricating fluid that lets organs move around. This fluid makes it easier for the lungs to expand and move around inside the chest during breathing. Mesothelium tissue exists at other locations within organisms and has been associated with malignancy at these sites (adenomatoid mesothelioma, testis mesothelioma) (Ilgren and Wagner, 1991; Mishra and Shet, 2004; Lanneau et al., 2005). Malignant mesothelioma (MM) has been traditionally associated with asbestos exposure with most forms being a diffuse malignant mesothelioma (DMM). The DMM is different from a begin solitary type tumor which remains localized. Since most cases involve the pleura this type of mesothelioma is commonly called malignant pleural mesothelioma (MPM) or pleural malignant mesothelioma (PMM). Related to asbestos, there are two basic locations where mesothelioma is said to arise, from the peritoneal and the pleural locations.

The term mesothelioma was first made popular by Klemperer and Rabin in 1931 (Rom, 1983; Hughes, 2005). These two are given credit with coining the term mesothelioma and establishing it as a tumor entity (Hughes, 2005). However, there was confusion at this time about the accurate classification of these diseases and it was not until 1960 when Wagner et al. (1960) that a clear association between asbestos and this disease emerged.

MM consists of three different histological types: (monophasic) epithelioid, sacromatous (/fibroblastic or desmoplastic) (spindle cell) and mixed (biphasic) (Hughes, 2005). It has been reported that the frequency of these cell types is about 40:20:40 (Wagner et at., 1960). The mean survival time, in months, is about 16.2 for epitheliod, 14.7 for mixed and about 10.1 for sarcomatous (Yates et al., 1997). In another study (Gorini et al., 2005) the median survival time for a cohort population of 381 MPM cases from Tuscan, Italy was 11.1 months, which is similar to that reported by Yates. However, there does not appear to be any differences the in the frequency of metastasis among the histological types (Yates et al., 1997). It is interesting to note that right sided tumors are more common than those on the left (Yates et al., 1997), which could be a result of the right lung being larger in size. In many cases initial determination is made by histology with confirmation accomplished by immunohistochemical techniques (Hughes, 2005; King et al., 2006).

Asbestos as a Cause of Disease

Historically, it has been recognized that asbestos exposure is an important cause of mesothelioma (Robinson and Lake, 2006). However, it has become known that all minerals identified as asbestos are actually not the same in disease causation potential.

The types or forms of asbestos and its potential in causing mesothelioma are of great interest and have been discussed considerably in the literature (Hoskins and Bernstein et al., 2003; Lange, 2004; Bernstein and Hoskins, 2006). It has been suggested for some time that chrysotile is not a mesothelioma producer (Bernstein and Hoskins, 2006); although, this is controversial (Robinson and Lake, 2006). Studies reporting chrysotile as a causative agent of this lung disease is actually a result of a mixture effect that included exposure to amphiboles. This is supported by an epidemiological study (McDonald et al., 1993) that found little association between chrysotile exposure and disease in a Quebec chrysotile cohort (number about 11,000) of miners born between 1891 and 1920. On the other hand, exposure to amphiboles, especially crocidolite has been well associated with mesothelioma (Weill et al., 2004; Yarborough, 2006).

Other Agents besides Asbestos, Including Those Naturally Occurring

As mentioned, numerous reports (Dog, 2003; Dogan, 2003; Lange, 2004) have indicated that asbestos is not the only agent (e.g. erionite) associated with the occurrence of mesothelioma. One of the best investigated and documented fibrous agents besides asbestos that causes mesothelioma are the zeolites. These are naturally occurring minerals that exist in many locations throughout the world. Most studies associated with these minerals are from Turkey, with erionite being considered the most import of these agents in the cause of mesothelioma, including MPM or PMM (Baris et al., 1996). This agent has also been suggested to be more potent than asbestos in causing this disease (Emri and Demir, 2004), and may be responsible for many cases of this disease that are suggested to have been caused by asbestos. Study of mesothelioma in areas of Turkey where high erionite concentrations exists have also reveled a genetic predisposition for the occurrence of this disease (Emri et al., 2002; Dogan et al., 2006), indicating that genetics may have an important role in its occurrence. Mesothelioma has also been shown to occur spontaneously, without any history of exposure to suspect causative agents (Fraire et al., 1988). There are also a large number of other agents (e.g. chemicals) that have been implicated in the causation of this disease as well.

Non-Asbestos Causes of Mesothelioma

Commonly it is presented that the cause of this disease is asbestos. However, it has become well known that asbestos is not the only causative factor (Lange, 2004; Hughes, 2005). Numerous publications (Lange, 2004) have reported cases of this disease where there was little or no exposure of asbestos (Table 1). In additional, there are reports of this disease where the latency period is too short for the cause to be asbestos-related resulting in the suggestion that this disease can occur spontaneously, have a genetic predisposition (familial relationship) or result from a non-asbestos related cause (e.g. ionizing radiation). A virus, the Simian Virus 40 (SV40), an infectious disease agent, has been implicated in association with MM, and is of great debate regarding this disease. Various estimates have been published on the percent of these cancers that are non-asbestos-related (0-87% (Peterson et al., 1984); although; the general value is probably in the range of 5-30% (Lange, 2004). In many ways studies that evaluate the history of asbestos exposure provide some of the strongest evidence for the existence of non-asbestos cases in that exposure levels are insufficient as an explanation.

Yates et al., (1997) provided information on the exposure history of 272 mesothelioma patients from south east England. These results indicate that 11% of the population had no asbestos exposure while if the possible/probable/unclassified are included in this category, the percent increased to 22. In a case-control study (Cristaudo et al., 2005), data were collected on the subject population regarding exposure to asbestos and a similar result was observed (Table 2); although, the percent of non-exposed cases was higher (about 32%). This investigation also evaluated the relationship of SV40 and MM. In this study a control population was employed for determining primer sequences in another cancer, urothelioma. Urothelioma was the control cancer, which is a cancer of the kidney and appears to be unrelated to asbestos. The Odds ratio (OR) for the association involving Simian Virus regulatory primer (RReg) and SV40/asbestos exposure was 12.6 (CI 95% - confidence interval, 1.2-133.9) (asbestos positive and RReg positive) supporting the existence of a relationship with this infectious disease agent.

Table 1. Agents, other than asbestos, reported to cause mesothelioma

Agent	Reference
Natural occurring agents[1]	Wagner et al., 1985; Dogan, 2003
Ionizing Radiation	Lerman et al., 1991
Sugar Cane	Das et al., 1976
Pleural Scars	Hillerdal and Berg, 1985; Hubbard, 1997
Familial/genetic	Risberg et al., 1980
Spontaneous	Fraire et al., 1988
Infectious agents[2]	Cristaudo et al., 2005
Dietary factors	Huncharek, 2002
Man-made mineral fibers	Health Effects Institute-Asbestos Research, 1991
Metals[3]	Ilgren and Wagner, 1991
Chemicals[4]	National Toxicology Program - NTP, 2000
Synthetic agents[5]	Ilgren and Wagner, 1991
Polymers[6]	Ilgren and Wagner, 1991
Hydrocarbons[7]	Ilgren and Wagner, 1991
Hormones[8]	Ilgren and Wagner, 1991
Inflammation[9]	Ilgren and Wagner, 1991
Smoking	Hirao et al., 2002

1 – erionite; 2 – like Simian Virus 40 – SV40; 3 – beryllium; 4 – o-nitrotoluene; 5 – glass dust; 6 – polyurethane; 7 - benzo[a]pyrene; 8 – stilbesterol; 9 – recurrent pneumothorax.

Table 2. Characteristics of the study subjects. (Asbestos exposure vs. non-asbestos exposure, with a comparison population - urothelioma)

	Mesothelioma	Urothelioma
Sex		
Male	13 (68.42%)	15 (83.3%)
Female	6 (31.58%)	3 (16.7%)
Age (mean +/- SD)	56.6 +/-10.9	71.3 +/-9.2
Asbestos exposure		
No	6 (31.58%)	14 (77.8%)
Yes	13 (68.42%)	4 (22.2%)
Total	19	18

From Cristaudo et al., 2005, with permission from American Association for Cancer Research.

Using data from Cristaudo et al., (2005) for mesothelioma without asbestos exposure (31.6%), the percent of non-asbestos related cases fall within the range suggested by Lange (2004) supporting the occurrence of non-asbestos cases. However, these values are probably also highly dependent on the geographical location and the type of asbestos commonly used in that area along with exposure to other chemicals/substances (e.g. erionite, o-nitrotoluene). Each of the agents listed in Table 1 are discussed as to their relevance in causing this disease. Probably the most extensively evaluated agent is a virus known as the SV40, which has raised considerable controversy as to its relationship with this disease (Crisaudo et al., 2005).

However, strong support now exists, some may even say conclusive evidence, for ionizing radiation (Richie, 2006), erionite (Emri et al., 2002) and genetic/spontaneous (Huncharek, 2002) in causation of mesothelioma, as well as SV40.

Erionite

Erionite is a fibrous zeolite mineral that occur throughout the world. This mineral has been extensively studied in Turkey where it exists as volcanic tuffs and is used in the construction of buildings. However, this mineral does occur in other locations of the world as well (e.g. Oregon). Numerous epidemiological studies (Baris et al., 2006; Emri et al., 2002) have indicated that this mineral is a strong mesothelioma producer, one that appears to be more potent than asbestos (crocidolite). It is reported to be the only zeolite that has these properties. A recent investigation (Baris et al., 2006) indicated that exposure to erionite in Turkey (central and southern Anatolia region) has an incidence rate of mesothelioma from 200 to 700/100,000 inhabitants. Genetics also appears to play a major importance in relation to this mineral and the occurrence of mesothelioma (Dogan et al., 2006).

These epidemiological investigations are supported by animals studies that eriorite can produce mesothelioma (Dogan et al. 2003). In some experiments, greater than 90% of the animals exposed developed mesothelioma, which is consistent in that one epidemiological investigation in Turkey reported that 50% of the total deaths were due to this disease (Emri et al., 2002). These results, although some what limited, demonstrate the potency of this zeolite mineral in causation of disease. This suggests that the cause of mesothelioma is greatly related to the fiber structure, as has been previously indicated for asbestos (Bernstein and Hoskins, 2006). Thus, asbestos is not the only naturally occurring mineral fiber that is associated with this disease. It is likely that there are numerous other fibrous materials that are mesothelioma producers, but have not been fully recognized, possibly due to most cases being identified as a result of asbestos. Since erionite exists in a wide variety of locations through out the world (e.g. Oregon), consideration of this and possibly other fibers and substances (Table 1) as causative agents for this disease must be evaluated. Other zeolites have been shown to cause peritoneal mesothelioma when administered by an intraperitonal route, further illustrating concerns with these (e.g. eriorite) agents. Overall, this zeolite illustrates the occurrence of a non-asbestos material that is a known mesothelioma producer. Dogan et al., (2006) in a study of genetics and erionite has indicated that the individual genetic predisposition is of major important in relation to mineral fibers carcinogenicity, which probably also true for asbestos. Thus, the importance of genetics, which is only now being investigated, may be of greater influence than previously considered (Emri et al., 2002).

Man-Made Mineral Fibers

The term man-made mineral fiber(s) (MMMF) is a generic term used to identify a large number of fibrous (inorganic) agents/substances. These agents are most commonly made from clay, glass, rock or slag (Health Effects Institute – Asbestos Research – HEI-AR, 1991). The most common of these, in general, are the fibrous wools, which are vitreous or fibrous glass materials that have been treated and in some way, including heat, by flame-blowing/drawn-air into a fibrous material. This results in a uniform sized fiber. Sometimes these products are also called man-made vitreous fibers (MMVF). Due to the fibrous nature of these materials, they have been evaluated for cancerous properties, including that as a potential mesothelioma producer. Studies on fiberglass (glass), slag and rock wool have suggested they are not strong mesothelioma producers in man (De Vuyst et al., 1995; Marsh et al., 2001). However, animal studies have indicated that MMMF are highly carcinogenic, at least based on some studies (HEI-AR, 1991). For refractory ceramic fibers (RCF), the most recent data also indicate that they fall within the categorization of these other MMMF regarding mesothelioma; however, overall insufficient data exists for conclusive findings (Brown et al., 2005). There is an indication of increased of pleural plaques for those exposed to RCF, suggesting that a risk may exist, and the latency period has not been sufficient in studies to adequately determine carcinogenicity (Brown et al., 2005). Evaluation of RCF in animals do indicate that they can cause this disease; thus, must be considered suspect (Brown et al., 2005). It is likely that some categories of MMMF do result in mesothelioma. It appears that the important factor for causing such disease is related to its biopersistence and other characteristics of the fiber (Bernstein et al., 2003; 2005; 2006; Brown et al., 2005). If this is considered, along with animal studies of MMMF, and the precautionary principle "criteria" that is used with chrysotile included (Yarborough, 2006), these agents/substances must be considered as potential hazards. Further studies on the various types of MMMF are warranted to better evaluate each as a potential mesothelioma producer. It should be noted that there are no epidemiological data on fibers classified as superfine (< 1 um in diameter), which are more likely to be of a carcinogenic nature (De Vuyst et al., 1995).

Ionizing Radiation/Radionuclides/Radionucleotides

It is well known that there is an association between radiation, both ionizing (Hill, 1997; Hofmann et al., 1994) and radionucleotide particles (e.g. Plutonium oxide - PuO_2) (Sanders and Jackson 1972) and mesothelioma. A large number of studies (Shannon et al. 1995) have reported on radiation exposure and occurrence of mesothelioma; although, most only provide information on one or two cases in their report. These investigations have shown that there is a relationship between radiation and this disease, which has been additionally supported by experimental investigations (Sanders and Jackson., 1972).

Babcock et al. (1976) was the first to report on a case of external radiation induced mesothelioma in man; although, previous cases (Mauer and Egloff, 1975) of this cancer have been related to treatments involving thorotrast. Mauer and Egloff (1975) reported on a single case of peritoneal mesothelioma (mesothelioma in the abdominal area) that was caused by internal and external radiation for a carcinoma of the cervix. This tumor appeared 7 years after treatment. It has been proposed that radiation causes deoxyribonucleic acid (DNA) breaks in cells of the mesothelium that have a defective or non-functioning p53 gene (or protein product) (Marsella et al., 1997). This mechanism may also be how asbestos causes this disease as well; although, other tumor suppressor systems and pathways are probably also related and involved (Hirao et al., 2002). It has been shown that MM's are frequently aneuploid and exhibit cytogenetic abnormalities (Taquchi et al., 1993), which may be a result of a defective p53 gene. For asbestos, macrophages release reactive oxygen and nitrogen species (e.g. active oxygen species - AOS, reactive oxygen - ROS, reactive nitrogen - RNS) that react with the DNA causing an abnormality in the cell cycle and resistance to the occurrence of apoptosis. The SV40 virus may also act in this way by binding to p53 proteins and inactivating normal functions (Ko and Prives, 1996). Thus, radiation and asbestos in many ways could be acting in a similar manner regarding mechanisms of carcinogenesis. It should be noted that comparison studies have reported mutations of suppressor genes in both asbestos and non-asbestos related mesothelioma's (Mayall et al., 1999).

Park et al., (1970) was the first investigator to indicate a link between mesothelioma and radionuclides/radionucleotides (Huncharek, 2002). These investigators (Park et al., 1970) exposed dogs to PuO_2 using an inhalation (respiratory) route, which resulted in 22 out of the 35 animals developing mesothelioma in the lung. The histological type reported for this mesothelioma was epithelial, which is common in humans. Later another investigator, Sanders and Jackson, (1972), conducted similar experiments except they used rats; although, in this investigation the PuO_2 was administered by intraperitoneal injection. Again, tumors developed in some of the experimentally treated animals that were reported to be mesothelioma. In addition, other types of cancers also occurred, which are common in radiation experiments, indicating that this agent is a strong tumor former, including for mesothelioma. It also appears based on autoradiograms that the plutonium concentrated in "hotspots" (Sanders and Jackson, 1972), suggesting that this agent, radionucleotide, become localized. Additional experiments by Sanders (1992) confirmed his initial finding and that of Park et al., (1970) providing good experimental evidence that radionucleotides are mesothelioma inducing agents. Although there is some confusion about the localization of this agent by different routes of exposure, the formation of mesothelioma is clear. A study (Priest and Giannola, 1980) of distribution of plutonium has shown that this nucleotide is taken up by macrophages and osteoclasts and would therefore be in the local area of the lung pleura after intraperitoneal injection. However, the high does administered are not necessarily comparable to what most people would receive. Regardless, since most people do not develop the disease as rapidly as the animals, under experimental situations, the inclusion of additional time, as associated with most cases of MM, make these experiments in some ways relatable to man. Although the histological type for these studies was identified, this may be subject to some bias and the type of tumor may actually be a mixed form or one that is related, mostly due to the current information that immunohistochemistry (staining) is important for accurate differentiation (Lucas et al., 2003).

There is one human report (Gold and Kathren, 1998) that mentions the occurrence of mesothelioma in workers exposed to radionucleotides, although these workers also appear to have been exposed to asbestos. The authors' in this investigation contributed these cases to the asbestos; however, when evaluated with that of the experimental reports, some suggestion to one or more of these cases being related to radionucleotides must be considered. However, when these data are evaluated in comparison to control populations, there does not appear to be an increase in the disease rate. In addition, many facilities have been historically "contaminated" with asbestos, confounding results.

Another investigator, Hahn and Lundgren (1992) evaluated inhaled cerium, a beta-emitter, with rats. They used cesium oxide that was stable and non-exposed animals as controls. These animals were administered one to multiple doses of the radionucleotides, resulting in an exposure dose of 0.26 Gray (Gy) to 250 Gy. These animals developed a number of different types of cancer, including mesothelioma. The animals receiving the highest dose of radiation developed the largest number of tumors in the lung. Osteocarcinoma also developed in the ribs, supporting previous studies (Priest and Giannola, 1980) that radionucleotides are taken up by the osteoclasts and most likely osteoblasts as well; thus, concentrating the agent in the subpleural region of the lung. Although this does not directly support uptake by macrophages, this is also likely occurring; further suggesting that these cells are depositing some of the radionucleotide in locations or hotspots that result in the mesothelioma and possibly other cancers. When these data, along with that previously discussed, are taken together with reports of mesothelioma's in nuclear workers, the suggestion can be made that radionucleotides can result in the occurrence of this disease in man.

The first evidence in man associating radiation with mesothelioma comes from the use of thorotrast that involved a 59 year old patient (Mauer and Egloff, 1975). This patient developed peritoneal mesothelioma after thorotrast was used in the peritoneal cavity. This treatment agent, which is no longer used, remains in the body for an extremely long period of time, with one estimate of its half-life being 400 years. It was initially used in 1931 and continued through the 1940's and 50's as a contrast medium for X-rays. It was an excellent medium because it a high opacity to X-rays; thus, allowing well observed images. Today barium sulfate is used instead of this agent. Thorotrast ($^{232}ThO_2$ – thorium dioxide) is an alpha-emitter that is retained in various organs, including the liver, as well as mesothelial surfaces of these organs (Andersson et al., 1995). Andersson reported that patients who received a larger amount of this agent (e.g. 20 ml) had a dramatically higher rate of MM (7.8%) when compared to those receiving a lower concentration (1.4%). Although this is a small study population (999 patients) and the number of cases is also small, it indicates that there is a dose-response relationship with thorotrast and the induction of MM. However, this rate of disease for MM has not been reported in other studies that evaluated thorotrast (Ishikawa et al., 1995). Here a dose-response relationship was not seen; although, the frequency of MM was greater than that expected when compared to a control population. However, as previously noted, the small populations involved in these studies (370) and the few cases of MM (1 case), limits the analysis of these data. However, these investigations have been supported by others that provide good evidence that thorotrast is a MM producer (Van Kaick, 1999). In this paper by van Kaick, (1999) 9 cases of MM was observed in thorotrast patients while none were observed in controls, providing strong supportive evidence for the previous studies and the experimental investigations of radionucleotide induced MM.

Similar finding, although not as dramatic have been reported for patients receiving radiation treatment and the occurrence of MM (Babcock et al., 1976; Hill, 1997). As mentioned previously, most reports on MM and radiation therapy involve only a single case report making epidemiological analysis difficult. In addition, not all cases of mesothelioma reported involve the lung. For example, Stock et al (1979) reported a case of peritoneal mesothelioma in a patient 16 years after radiation therapy. This patient was treated for seminoma of the right testicle and had no reported documented exposure to asbestos. Other case studies have reported similar findings (Gilks et al.,1988; Tassile et al., 1998; Sato et al., 2000; Amin et al., 2001) and have indicated that there is some concern for the occurrence of cancer resulting from therapy, including mesothelioma. Gilks, Sato and Tassile also reported on mesothelioma that was related to radiation therapy of testicular seminoma. Amin et al., (2001) made a similar report on two cases of DMM in the peritoneum that were suggested to have arisen from treatment of testicular tumors, with these data supported in a cohort of 40,576 (Travis et al., 2005). Travis et al., (2005) reported a statistical increase of mesothelioma in patients that were treated for testicular cancer and that this increase represents a risk to survivors from radiotherapy. Most recently, this treatment has been shown to also result in an increased risk of pleural mesothelioma (Richie, 2006). Richie reported a relative risk of 3.4 (95% CI of 1.7 – 5.9) in the cohort described by Travis for pleural mesothelioma. This indicates a "significant" risk of MM can result from radiotherapy and that radiation can be considered effective in the induction of this disease. Thus, mesothelioma represents a secondary cancer from radiotherapy treatment of testicular cancer and that this occurrence is not an artifact. These cases were initially considered to have resulted from the radiotherapy administered in cancer treatment and are in some ways isolated, but supportive of the cause of radiotherapy in causation of MM. However, the recent finding of Travis and Richie are highly supportive of radiation's role in MM. Most of the other reports involving radiotherapy are associated with four different tumor types: Wilm's tumor, Hodgkin's disease, breast or cervical cancer and the occurrence of MM is considered a secondary cancer. Investigations involving these cancers and their treatments using radiation have not involved the population size that was examined for testicular cancer; however, based on those studies (Richie, 2006), and case reports relating to other cancers that result in secondary events of MM, in total they must be considered supportive. Overall, these investigators (Richie, 2006) indicate that cancer, including mesothelioma, is a risk in relation to radiotherapy treatment.

There are several reports of mesothelioma arising from the treatment of Wilm's tumor in children. Wilm's is a rare cancer of the kidney that is most common in children under the age of 5; although, can as a more rare event, occur in older children and adults. However, this type of tumor is not restricted to man and has been reported in animals as well (e.g. dogs) (Sato et al. 2005). In one investigation of MM in relationship to treatment of Wilm's, Austin et al., (1986), reported that this secondary cancer arose in the pulmonary area where the person had previously received radiation therapy. Additional case reports by Antman et al. (1983) and Anderson et al. (1985), support this initial finding of radiation induced MM in relation to treatment of Wilm's tumor. It is interesting to note that in a veterinary case of a dog (Sato et al., 2005), it presented at necropsy both MM and Wilm's tumor. This raises the question as to whether some relationship exists between the two tumors. Since a number of cases of radio-induced MM exist in regard to treatment of Wilm's tumor, chance in these associations must be considered.

A relationship with the radiotreatment of breast cancer and MM has also been reported (Shannon et al.1995). These findings are consistent with published reports that radiation treatment in the chest area can result; although rare, in the occurrence of MM and has been identified as a complication of such treatment (Mesurolle et al., 2000). The first to report an association was Shannon, who described two patients that were treated for breast cancer and later developed MM 10 and 35 years following their radiotherapy. This is supported by the findings of Hill et al., (1997) that radiotherapy can result in MM.

Neugut et al. (1997) conducted a retrospective cohort study on 251,750 women that were registered in a breast carcinoma study. In this study 6 cases of mesothelioma (MPM) were observed with 2 in the breast cancer group that were treated with radiotherapy of the thorax. The other 4 cases were not treated with radiotherapy, supporting other causative agents (e.g. chemotherapeutics). It is interesting to note that there were no mesothelioma cases in the Hodgkin's disease patients. A single case report on a woman that underwent radiotherapy for breast cancer and later developed mesothelioma was reported by Rustemeyer et al., (1997). In this report, the patient was 63 years old at the time of diagnosis for MM and the radiotherapy occurred 21 years ago with an irradiation dose of 132 Gy. The authors' indicated that this was a radiation induced malignancy and the latency for this causative agent is similar to that reported in the literature. Melato and Rizzardi (2001) also reported on a single case of MM in a 42 year old woman that was treated using radiotherapy for breast cancer. In this case there was no history of asbestos exposure and the occurrence of the MM had a very short latency period. These authors report that this is the first case of MM in a breast cancer patient whose treatment consisted of only radiotherapy and did not include chemotherapy. The young age of the person also suggests that the disease was unlikely a result of environmental asbestos exposure.

A number of investigators have reported case studies involving the treatment of Hodgkin's disease with radiotherapy and the occurrence of MM (Flachero et al. 1996; de la Pena and Lucas, 1997; Das et al., 2005). However, one study (Neugut et al., 1997) of Hodgkin's disease patients did not find any cases of MM. Most of the cases reported in relation of radiotherapy of Hodgkin's disease involve the occurrence of MM after a considerable period of time. Many of these cases were also treated with chemotherapy, making it difficult as to which or combination of treatment is the likely causative agent for MM (Warren et al., 1981). Chemotherapeutic agents may also be mesothelioma producers (Neugut et al., 1997).

One of the earliest case-reports of treatment for Hodgkin's disease and occurrence of MM is from Ladero-Quesada et al. (1991). Here a patient was treated with radiotherapy and chemotherapy and developed MM 14 years after successful treatment as well as a heart condition. The MM developed in a location that did not have direct radiation exposure. Since the MM did not develop in the radiation area, suspicion that this case is a result of radiation therapy must be considered. This was later followed by Weissman et al., (1996) who reported on 4 cases of MM at the Dana-Farber Cancer Institute that occurred after radiotherapy for Hodgkin's disease. These authors' also described a fifth patient based on their literature review. The mean time period between treatment of the disease and the occurrence of MM was 15 years, which is shorter than the average latency period for asbestos induced MM. These patients were reported to have had no exposure to asbestos and this finding was supported through evaluation of lung tissue in one patient for ferruginous bodies. In this case, the concentration of ferruginous bodies was 250 bodies per gram, which is consistent for no "significant" prior exposure to asbestos. Others have used the value of 200 ferruginous bodies per gram in disguising light from heavy asbestos exposure (Hirao et al., 2002).

In 1996, Cavazza et al. (1996) provided evidence of MM in patients that had received radiation therapy for cancer. In this report the histological classification of the mesothelioma was reported, increasing the likelihood that there were in fact mesothelioma cases. They identified 8 patients that received radiotherapy and developed mesothelioma at the site of this therapy. The mean age and latency period for mesothelioma, as with other reports, was generally less than the average latency period for asbestos induced disease. They reported an average (mean) age of 45 with a latency period of 21 years. Three of these patients were also reported to have received chemotherapy. In their review, they identified 142 patients that were treated for cancer and later developed mesothelioma. These patients were located through tumor registries of the National Cancer Institute and Connecticut. The majority of cases involved men (89%) with a higher mean age than that of the original 8 (68.5 years); although, the median latency period between the initial cancer and mesothelioma was only 4.3 years. It is interesting to note that the latency period range was 2 months to 29.3 years, strongly suggesting that at least some of these cases were not asbestos related, and that the mesothelioma was in fact a secondary cancer to the treatment.

Lerman et al. (1991) reported on the occurrence of MM in a 24 year old woman that was treated for Hodgkin's disease 20 years earlier. They reported that the histological type of mesothelioma was epithelial. This finding is supported by a single case reported by Hofmann et al. (1994) on pleural mesothelioma after successful treatment for Hodgkin's disease. They also reported that other cancers (e.g. sarcomas) arise as a result of radiotherapy. In 1996, Falchero et al. (1996) also reported on a single case similar to that by Lerman and Hofmann. In this report, a case of pleural mesothelioma occurred 17 years after radio- and chemotherapy for Hodgkin's disease. The author's suggested that this is a secondary cancer resulting from the treatment and described 14 other cases that had been reported in the literature. These cases are further supported by Pappo et al., (1997) and de la Pena and Lucas, (1997).

In 2000, Kramer et al., (2000), reported the occurrence of PMM 24 years after a patient was treated with thoracic radiotherapy for Hodgkin's disease. Most recently, Das et al., (2005) also reported on the occurrence of mesothelioma in Hodgkin's disease patients. These studies overall indicate that there is a risk of secondary cancers from radiotherapy, including mesothelioma. This supports the suggestion that radiation can induce mesothelioma and can be considered a causative agent or factor for this disease.

There is only one case study report on treatment of cervical cancer using radiotherapy and MM (Kinutani et al., 1994). Recently a case of pericardial mesothelioma was described (Velissaris et al., 2001) in a patient (49 year-old woman) undergoing field radiotherapy for Hodgkin's disease. This study appears to follow the concept of the others that exposure to radiation can result in MM.

One of the first suggestions that radiation, chemicals and its combination could result in mesothelioma is from Warren et al. (1981). These investigators reported and increased rate of mesothelioma in rats that were treated with radiation and a chemical (methycholanthrene). When animals were also exposed to asbestos and these agents there was a dramatic increase in mesothelioma. This study indicates that there is a strong effect with asbestos, chemicals and radiation in the induction of mesothelioma.

Most cases of radiation induced mesothelioma have been associated with radiotherapy of other cancers (Hofmann et al., 1994; Saggia et al., 2004); although, others have been reported in relation to environmental exposures, such as that associated with the atomic bomb in Nagasaki (Mizuki et al., 1997). Most of the reports that involve ionizing radiation are related to radiotherapy of Hodgkin's disease (Mauch et al., 1996). It appears that therapy of this nature can induce mesothelioma as well as other forms of cancer, which are identified as secondary cancer. Some of the cases of mesothelioma may also be a result of the chemicals used in treating cancer (e.g. chemotherapeutic agents). Thus, both radiation and chemotherapetic agents together can result in mesothelioma, and in most cases the actual causative agent can not be determined. The strongest evidence to date for radiation induction of mesothelioma comes from Richie (2006) on Hodgkin's disease where significance was observed in the induction of this secondary cancer. Regarding animal studies, inhalation or injection (implantation) of plutonium has been shown to cause cancer associated with epithelial and mensenchymal tissues (Huncharck, 2002). This is supported by an investigation using rats that when injected with plutonium oxide with 77% developing peritoneal mesothelioma in rats (Huncharck, 2002).

Nutrition (Dietary Factors)

It has become well established that nutrition is very important in cancer prevention. Epidemiological studies have shown that a diet "rich" in vegetables and fruits result in a lower risk of cancer, including that associated with the lung (Mayne et al., 1994). From this prospective, it is not surprising that various nutritional or dietary characteristics are associated with changes in rates of mesothelioma (Steinmetz and Potter, 1991). In many ways, nutrition is probably also related to the genetics of the person and the two factors separately and together have importance in occurrence of this disease. Influence of various nutrients is probably related to an increase in anti-oxidants which provide protection against free radicals. Since mesothelioma may be greatly influenced by oxidative radical species (e.g. ROS's), diet may be of more importance than in other cancers, especially since many of the workers associated asbestos are from socio-economic groups (Lange et al., 1987; Lange, 1992) that have high fat and low vegetable diets. Unfortunately most cohorts of mesothelioma patients are not sufficiently large enough to provide definitive study data on various relationships of disease, including nutritional factors. Currently, there have been two studies that investigated the impact of nutrition and mesothelioma (Schiffman et al., 1988; Muscat and Huncharek, 1996).

Schiffman et al., (1988) performed a case-control investigation of mesothelioma cases in Louisiana in attempt to determine if there is a relationship with diet and this disease. As with any study of this nature, although attempts were made to evaluate occupational exposure to asbestos, the potential of unknown exposure must be considered. However, since current evidence indicates that there is a dose-response effect for mesothelioma (Ilgren, 2001), low levels of asbestos exposure may not be that great of importance, especially when evaluated against a control population. This study reported that those consuming cruciferous vegetables, growing their own vegetables and all vegetables combined had a lower rate of mesothelioma. Although this population is small (58 cases), it does suggest that an increased consumption of vegetables provides protection against mesothelioma. Another issue with this study is the high rate of cancer in Louisiana (Steineck et al., 1983), which in itself may be a confounder.

Muscat and Hunchareh (1996) had a slightly larger population (94 cases) in a case-control study that examined mesothelioma and diet. However, in this study the number of controls was 64, which is smaller than the number of cases, and possibly creates bias in the findings. Although the results in this study were non-significant, these findings do indicate that tomatoes and tomato juice consumption reduced the risk for mesothelioma. However, there was significance of reduced risk for those that consumed carrots (0.2, CI 95% 0.1-0.8), while no association existed for broccoli, cabbage, cantaloupe, cauliflower, spinach, sweat potatoes, orange juice, and red meat. It is likely that the association with carrots, tomatoes and juice is spurious; although, these results are somewhat similar to that reported by Schiffman et al., (1988).

The studies on nutrition and diet suggest that there is some relationship with mesothelioma. However, due to the limited size of the study populations and only a few studies being conducted, conclusions of any association must be tempered with caution. As with other studies of fruits and vegetables and cancer, there is likely an association in general, but due the rare nature of mesothelioma, it is unlikely that a detailed study would be feasible. However, a multi-center case-control investigation could be conducted, with the understanding that its power would be limited. Thus, based on the present data and that from other cancer studies, only generalities can be made, which overall can be said that there is likely some association with consumption of fruits and vegetables and a reduced rate of mesothelioma. It is also likely that some vitamins and related micronutrients (e.g. selenium), especially those that have anti-oxidant properties may also reduce risks associated with this cancer.

Genetic Predisposition

Importance of individual genetic factors in the occurrence of this disease has been known for sometime (Huncharek, 2002). As with most forms of cancer, there is limited information on the genetic characteristics; although, many of the genes associated with cancer are commonly placed in three categories: proto-oncogenes (damaged version called oncogenes), DNA repair genes and tumor suppressors. In addition, there are genes associated with energy production/metabolism and regulatory control, which may not be directly related to development of cancer, but may be necessary for growth and expansion. Two genes in particular have been reported to be related to mesothelioma: (GSTM1 (glutathione-S-transferase M1) and NAT2 (N-acetyltransferase 2). GSTM1 is important in the detoxification of carcinogens and NAT2 is involved with the biotransformation of carcinogens, aromatic amines and hydrazine drugs. Since existence of the null genotype (absence of the gene) results in an increased risk for mesothelioma, twofold for GSTM1 and sevenfold for

GSTM1+/NAT2+, this would suggest a mechanism of carcinogenicity associated with agents/substances that have been previously identified as non-asbestos mesothelioma producers (e.g. chemicals, non-asbestos fibers) (Hughes, 2005). Thus, these genes, and likely others like NAT1 (N-acetyltransferase 1), which is related to NAT2, are intrinsically associated with cancer; although, in many cases through indirect mechanisms or pathways. Mutations for both these genes have been associated with other cancers as well.

Loss of tumor suppressor genes has also been associated with mesothelioma. It has been indicated that loss of tumor suppressor genes $P16^{INK4a}$, $P16^{/CDKN2A}$, and P^{14ARF}, and neurofibromatosis 2 (NF2) are suggested to be major confounders in the disease (Jaurand and Fleury-Feith, 2005; Robinson et al., 2005). These loci are important in the cell cycle and changes can disrupt this system, which in part, may be responsible for the occurrence of a cancerous state in a cell (Le Frere-Belda et al., 2004). Historically, many cancers loss the tumor suppressor genes p53 and Rb, which are of importance, but that does not appear to be true for this type of cancer (Kelsey et al., 1986), except as related to the SV40 virus (De Luca et al., 1997). However, other studies have suggested that down regulation of these tumor suppressor systems are of importance, which may have involvement with the INK4 locus (Hirao et al., 2002). For example, protein kinases (Lopez-Rios et al., 2006) have been suggested to be important in relation to the aggressiveness of this disease. Changes in the chromosome structure also appear to be important in this disease (Musti et al., 2002). It appears that in mesothelioma deletions have been reported on chromosomes which include 1p, 3p, 9p, 6q, 9p, 13q, 14q and 22q (Ascoli et al., 2001; Hirao et al., 2002; Robinson and Lake, 2006). Much of the information on the genetics of mesothelioma has been gained from studying tumor cells in culture and family clusters.

The initial suggestion that genetics has some effect on occurrence of mesothelioma came from a study by Newhouse and Thompson (1965, 1965a). In this study the authors' reported on mesothelioma among family members.

In one study (Musti et al., 2002) of a family of three sisters and one brother, all exposed to environmental-related asbestos, there was a loss of chromosomal structure at the 9p region, and this is suggested to be related to tumor suppression and occurrence of MM. Such loss, which can exist in genetically related populations, may result in increased susceptibility for this disease. A similar suggestion had been reported for the p16, specifically at two reading frames of $p16^{INK4a}$ and $p14^{ARF}$, which alteration at these sites may make the individual more susceptible to the disease (Hirao et al., 2002). A similar report has been published by (Ascoli et al., 1998); although, information on chromosome abnormalities were not included. Thus, a subpopulation may be at greatest risk of this disease.

From epidemiological data, it has been suggested that these genetic factors are also important in regard to fiber clearance and residence time (Roushdy-Hammaly et al., 2001), further indicating the importance of the type of asbestos associated with exposure. It is likely, as suggested for mesothelioma related to erionite exposure that genetic factors are in play regardless of whether the disease is directly related to asbestos or another substance/material (Kelsey et al., 1986). These associations of genetics and mesothelioma have been supported in family clusters (Risberg et al., 1980; Musti et al., 2002) and sibling cases (Picklesimer et al., 2005).

Spontaneous/Children

As with any cancer, the occurrence of spontaneous mesothelioma has been shown to arise in both man (Grundy and Miller, 1972) and animals (Kang et al., 2004). Much of the evidence for such occurrences in man comes from those that are generally young in age and there has been an insufficient latency period to associate this diseases event with asbestos. There have been cases of this disease in adults where there has been no documented exposure to asbestos (Law et al., 1983; Peterson et al., 1984). Since most case references as related to spontaneous events involve children, generally; exposure to asbestos has been limited or minimal. However, the latency period for this disease; although long, has been reported to exhibit a wide range (e.g. 6-67 years) (Yeung et al., 1999), when examining occupational populations. It is likely that the shorter time periods where asbestos is likely involved are a result of past unknown exposure or events; thus, not being the true latency period reported and/or extremely high exposure to asbestos being related to the event. These populations where the range is reported are also older individuals (e.g. 50's and above); thus, in a somewhat different situation than that of children as well. In addition, where latency periods are short, these involve occupational groups and not children or environmentally exposed populations. The other issue in spontaneous cases is the low frequency which disease occurs overall (0.4/100,000 for woman). Thus, those that develop this disease even at a younger age would be lower than that for background making the disease even rarer. To further complicate this scenario, most studies involve a single case event; thus, not allowing an epidemiological analysis. It is also interesting to note that many cases where there is no asbestos exposure reported, the time of survival is often less than that for cases associated with asbestos (Law et al., 1983) and these cases are generally more resistant to treatment (Huncharek, 2002).

A review of 45,000 death certificates for children and young adults in the US by Grundy and Miller (1972) revealed 31 cases of this disease. However, only 13 cases were confirmed as being mesothelioma. As with any retrospective study, information associated in the cause of mesothelioma is difficult and in most cases incomplete. In the classic study by Hillerdal of 4710 cases of MM he found 9 cases of mesothelioma of the *tunica vaginalis* in boys (Hillerdal, 1983). However, the general young age of these cases support that at least some MM's reported can be considered to have resulted as a spontaneous event.

Other investigators (Brenner et al., 1981) have conducted similar studies as Grundy and Miller and reported like findings. This investigation (Brenner et al., 1981) was at the Sloan-Kettering Memorial Hospital in New York, where many of the patients would have been from that local area. This study reported on 7 patients that were treated at this hospital since 1953 to about publication date. Thus, for these cases environmental contribution in the cause of the disease must be considered along with prior radiation, medications and family cancer history (Cooper et al., 1989), as well as being a potential spontaneous case event. Since cities are historically more polluted than other locations, and asbestos and other reported mesothelioma producers (e.g. chemicals) are at higher concentrations, it is possible that some of these cases are more environmentally related, in part. In this investigation, the authors' did not report family-related exposures of asbestos, further indicating that these are non-asbestos related mesotheliomas. Although this report by Brenner presents information on childhood mesothelioma cases, it primary focus was on treatment of this disease in younger patients. However, it does support the concept of spontaneous cases and cases arising that do not involve asbestos exposure, especially as related to occupational events or exposures that would be considered heavy (Hirao et al., 2002).

In another study (Fraire et al., 1988), similar findings were reported as mentioned previously that support the occurrence of spontaneous cases of this disease in children. As previously, these children were not likely exposed to asbestos, at least at elevated concentrations, and could be classified as a non-asbestos exposed group (Fraire et al. 1988). However, like the other studies in general, histological and other confirmatory testing, for the cases were incomplete. Although some cases where histology was evaluated, the mesothelioma was identified as being either mixed (biphasic) or of the epitheloid type. Again, as in other studies, these cases overall do not have documented exposure to asbestos, as exists for those in industrial situations.

Cases of childhood related mesothelioma continue to appear in the literature (Kovalivker and Motovic, 1985; Mutafoglu-Uysal et al., 2002). Overall, these cases support the spontaneous occurrence of this disease, which is best illustrated by the insufficient "latency" period normally associated with occupational cases of the disease, which is commonly attributed to asbestos exposure.

One report (Kannerstein and Churn, 1980) suggested that experimental studies of mesothelioma in animals are similar to that seen in man. Since spontaneous cases have been reported in animals, as well as chemically induced (National Toxicology Program - NTP, 2002), this evidence supports the occurrence of spontaneous events and non-asbestos associated cases in man (Peterson et al., 1984). Although the number of mesothelioma cases resulting from spontaneous events, as compared to asbestos and other non-asbestos causes, is unknown, the events reported in children indicate that they do occur.

Sugarcane

Epidemiological studies (Das et al., 1976; Steineck et al., 1983) have indicated that sugarcane farming/workers may be at risk for mesothelioma. However, other studies (Miller et al., 1993) have not confirmed these findings and little research has been conducted on risks associated with agricultural occupations and MM's. It has been hypothesized that the burning of sugarcane, which occurs prior to harvest, results in fibers that are similar to asbestos (Newman, 1986). This hypothesis suggests that these biogenic silica fibers act in a similar manner as that of asbestos fibers. Sugarcane farming has been associated with an increased risk of lung cancer (Brooks et al., 1992; Miller et al., 1993; Wong and Foliart, 1993). One explanation given for the reports of increased rates of mesothelioma in these occupational groups is due to chance (Miller et al., 1993). In the Louisiana study (Steineck et al., 1983), the cases of mesothelioma have been suggested to be a result of asbestos that was associated with the refining facility (Miller et al., 1993). An association with asbestos in the refining facility may certainly have some merit, but the five cases reported by Das et al., (1976) in an agricultural community where exposure to asbestos and other non-asbestos causing mesothelioma agents are unlikely do not support the act of chance. Although the evidence is limited, there does appear to be some relationship between sugarcane and the occurrence of this disease and fibers (e.g. biogenic), or other substances/chemicals, of this nature.

Pleural Scars/Inflammation

Chronic injury (scares and inflammation have been suggested to cause mesothelioma (Ilgren and Wagner, 1991). MM has been observed in relation to scars in the pleura that resulted from chronic emphysema or therapeutic activities/events or recurrent pneumothorax (Hillerdal and Berg, 1985). This is supported by a more recent case (Shieh et al., 2004) where cutaneous mesothelioma developed after about 14 months following surgery for visceral mesothelioma. In this case, the mesothelioma was histologically identified as being an epithelioid tumor and was confirmed with immunohistochemistry. Although, such occurrences are generally rare, these case studies do indicate that such events can result from scars/inflammation. It is likely that the mesothelioma is arising from inflammation associated with the scar area. There are other studies in the literature reporting similar events (Prieto et al., 1997); although, as indicated they are not all restricted to the chest cavity. For example, Prieto et al., (1997) reported mesothelioma associated with the dermis in a patient that had a history of this disease in the pleural cavity. In this case, the patient was previously treated with pneumonectomy and radiotherapy. It is also possible that some cases are a result of multiple factors, such as scaring and radiotherapy, as indicated in the case report by Prieto et al., (1997). Certainly a relationship between chemotherapy/drug treatment related to these patients must also be considered.

Smoking

Numerous investigations have reported a synergistic relationship with smoking (e.g. cigarettes) and asbestos in the cause of lung cancer, but not mesothelioma (Hammond et al., 1979). However, recent information suggests that there may be an association between smoking and mesothelioma in subpopulations (Hirao et al., 2002). These investigators found an association between alteration of p16 and smoking history in mesothelioma patients. In this study patients that had methylation of p16 promotor region (INK4 locus) were smokers, which was statistically significant. Since the population evaluated was small 11 non-smokers and 32 smokers, the association of smoking may be a confounder as well. However, as indicated by the authors', this effect may exist "only in a subpopulation" and due to the small size may be obscured in larger studies. It has been shown that the longer the smoking the greater the methylation (hyper) of p16 (Kim et al.,2001), suggesting that a dose-response effect may exist. Based on these data; although limited, smoking does appear to have some impact on the occurrence of mesothelioma. Thus, tobacco smoke may be a contributor to this disease and can be considered a co-carcinogen. Since alteration of other chromosomes commonly occur in MM, it is possible that such events are occurring elsewhere and a combination of methylations or epigenetic interactions may be acting on or influencing this cancer. This includes impact to other gene systems (e.g. NAT2). Since the SV40 virus has an effect on tumor suppressor systems, there may even be interaction between smoking and this virus related to mesothelioma. Thus, smoke, including second hand tobacco smoke, may be a non-asbestos related factor in this disease.

SV40

The SV40 virus is a polyomavirus that causes asymptomatic infections in several species of monkeys and was reported in 1959 to exist as a contaminant in the inactivated polio vaccine (Salk polio vaccine) (IPV) (Hillman, 1998). This virus was discovered by Sweet and Hillerman and is just one of 40 or more viruses infecting Rhesus monkey kidney cells. It is a single stranded DNA virus and is about 5kb in length (Vilchez and Butel, 2004). This virus has been reported to be associated with a number of different tumors/cancers (e.g. brain tumors, non-Hogkins lymphoma (NHL), MM, and bone tumors). A common source of the virus originated from the polio vaccine being grown in Rhesus monkey kidney cells (cell culture), where it exists as a "contaminant". However, it is also found in people that were never vaccinated with the "contaminated" polio vaccine as well (Vilchez and Butel, 2004). In 1961 researchers observed that the virus causes abnormal development (transformation) in hamster cells. There are other related viruses, such as BKU and Jamestown Canyon (JCV), which may also have oncogenic properties. Polio vaccine (Salk) that was contaminated with this virus was used during the time period 1955 to 1963, resulting in millions of people being accidentally inoculated with SV40. The SV40 virus does share about 70% of its genetic sequence with other human viruses; although, one of its viral proteins, T antigen (T Ag or Tag), which binds to tumor suppressor proteins, such as p53 and pRb (including Rb family proteins) appears to be of importance for cellular transformation (Gazdar et al., 2002). Recently, it has been suggested that the oral polio vaccine (Sabin) (OPV) was also contaminated with this virus, with contaminated vaccine used from the time period 1960's to 1978 (Cutrone, 2005). Adenovirus vaccines used during the time period 1957-1960 for the general public and that used for the military (1961-1975) were contaminated with SV40 as well (Rollison et al., 2004). So, contamination in vaccines appears to have been more widespread than previously considered (Gazdar et al., 2002). In addition, since this virus has similar genetic sequences with other viruses, some of these other organisms, including viruses, besides SV40, may also be acting as a co-carcinogens with asbestos or carcinogens themselves in the induction of mesothelioma.

The presence of this virus in tissues is determined by using primers followed by amplification of the DNA through PCR (polymerase chain reaction) (Huncharek, 2002). Studies have varied as to whether they are able to identify the primer sequence in tissue samples from a mesothelioma patient. Based on this information, claims are made as to whether the virus was present in the case. This has resulted in considerable controversy (Lopez-Rios and Ladanyi, 2006; Robinson and Lake, 2006) in that some investigators find a high rate of the SV40 (primer) (Gaarfar and Eldin, 2005) and others do not (Manfredi et al., 2005), resulting in various claims of a relationship. It has become apparent using this technique that there are different sensitivities with these primers and this sensitivity changes with the exact methodology employed (Elmishad et al. 2006). By changing the detection method and using the same immuno-precipitation/western blot method, for 20 mesothelioma specimens, the positive rate varied from 2/20 to 7/20. This provides a strong explanation for the variability in results observed.

The oncogenic activity of the SV40 virus is suggested to be related to interaction of its large T Ag and tumor suppressor gene products. There are two suppressor proteins that appear to be involved with the SV40 virus (p53 and pRb) (Hughes, 2005). These regulator proteins (systems) prevent or down regulate cell proliferation, with p53 in particular acting in response to cellular stress. T Ag can act as a stimulator for growth of mesothelioma cells. For pRb, T Ag appears to relax growth controls on cells, resulting in an increase of cell growth (Hughes, 2005).

The question as to whether SV40 can cause or contribute to cancer, including mesothelioma. Based on the most recent investigations, there does appear to be "conclusive" support that this virus can cause or result in a number of different cancers/tumors, including mesothelioma (Gazdar et al., 2002; Cristaudo et al., 2005). This issue is of great medical-legal importance (Kops, 2000) because of the numerous and frequent lawsuits relating to asbestos and mesothelioma. Defense lawyers have attempted to substantiate that this virus is the cause of the disease in some legal cases or as a contributory negligence or defect in the causation and direct liability away from asbestos. There appears to be two variations of the concept, one that provides evidence that there is no oncogenic effect of SV40 (Engels et al., 2003; Manfredi et al., 2005) and the other which indicates that it has a role (Cristaudo et al., 2005).

Engels et al., (2003) suggested that the virus is not a causative agent of cancer, including mesothelioma, based on examination of a birth cohort of children in the Denmark population that were exposed to the polio vaccine (contaminated with SV40) and found that there was no difference in cancer rates for those receiving the contaminated vaccine and those not receiving it. For mesothelioma, the rates in all cohorts examined were statistically similar. However, since there is now evidence that some of the oral polio vaccine was contaminated and there also appears transmission among the population (Gazdar et al., 2002), these studies may be biased in that comparisons may include cases involving both the Salk (IPV) and Sabin (OPV) vaccines; although, the exposure was by different routes (injection verse oral), and person to person/animal to person transmission exists/occurs. Others have suggested that using birth cohorts for evaluating cancer rates for SV40-contaminated vaccines are not adequate in establishing a close-casual relationship (Vilchez et al., 2003, 2003a).

Other studies have reported an association of populations having this virus and increased rates of cancer, including mesothelioma. Vilchez and Butel, (2004) evaluated brain cancer, NHL and mesothelioma in relation to SV40. In 13 studies published from 1975 to 2002 in a meta-analysis for brain cancer reported a combined OR of 3.9 (95% CI 2.6-5.8). For mesothelioma, they included 15 studies and the OR was 16.8 (95% CI 10.3-27.5). While for NHL, they included 3 studies, reporting a combined OR of 5.4 (95% CI 3.1-9.3). These data suggest that the virus is influencing not only mesothelioma, but other types of cancer as well. Other studies have reported an association between the contaminated vaccine and occurrence of mesothelioma (Vilchez et al., 2003; Cristaudo et al., 2005). These data, along with recent information supporting an association of the disease and vaccination (Vilchez et al., 2003; Cristaudo et al., 2005), provide very strong evidence that SV40 does cause cancer in humans, including mesothelioma, and that vaccination is a contributory cause in this disease. When examining both the epidemiological and experimental data, a close-casual relationship exists. It is interesting to note that a geographic difference exists for SV40-related tumors. Where the contaminated polio vaccine was not used, Finland, Turkey and Austria, SV40-postive tumors have not been reported (Gazdar et al., 2002). In addition, before this vaccine, the occurrence of MM was rare and in review of 47 thousand autopsies at the Massachusetts General Hospital from 1896 to 1947 no cases were observed (Mark and Yokoi, 1991).

Some have suggested that this virus should be identified by the International Agency for Cancer Research (IARC) within the classification of a group 2 carcinogen. Other viruses, such as the Epstein-Barr virus, are identified as carcinogens. This classification (group 2) is dependent on sufficient epidemiological and animals evidence, which clearly exists (Gazdar et al., 2002). Although, there is controversy, from a scientific basis, SV40 and asbestos are co-carcinogens in the transformation of mesothelial cells (Cristaudo et al., 2005); although, this is a difficult acceptance for those in the legal professions that represent parties having this disease, especially plaintiff attorney's (Kops, 2002). This concept of SV40 being related to MM has been seized upon by defense attorney's and remains as a controversial issue, especially from a legal prospective. However, from a scientific prospective, evidence is clear that this virus, and most likely others that are related, are carcinogens.

The virus has been reported at high concentrations in sewage in India (Gazdar et al., 2002). This suggests that transmission from animal to human and human to human is occurring. It appears that both horizontal and vertical transmission is occurring, based on those that did not receive the contaminated vaccine(s). This complicates epidemiological studies that examine comparisons of vaccinated verse non-vaccinated. Thus, transmission of the virus may now be going from person to person. The percent sero-positive for this virus varies from geographical region to region, with many of those positive never given contaminated vaccine. For example, in Hungary the percent prevalence of those sero-positive is 9 (Vilchez and Butel, 2004). This supports the concept of transmission from person/animal to person/animal and that infection may be more wide spread than previously considered.

Overall, current data indicate that the SV40 virus is a co-carcinogen/carcinogen with asbestos and can transform cells. It ability to transform cells suggests that the virus may be a mesothelioma producer of its own with-out asbestos or another agent/substance. Although it is not possible to determine the exact cause of mesothelioma in relationship to this virus, in general, it is well supported that this virus alone and in combination can cause of mesothelioma (Gazdar et al., 2002). Regardless, SV40 is an oncogenic virus. Much of the criticism against this virus being identified as a carcinogenic agent arises from legal disputes relating to mesothelioma (Kops, 2002).

Chemicals

Numerous chemical (organics) have been implication as causative agents of mesothelioma (Ilgren and Wagner, 1991). Much of this evidence arises from animal studies (National Toxicology Program - NTP, 2000). However, there are a few epidemiological investigations (Gamble et al., 2000; Burns et al., 2005) that allude to an association with chemicals; although, exposure to asbestos is indicated to have occurred in these populations confounding the findings. In some cases (Burns et al., 2005) an increased incidence of mesothelioma exists while the same does not for lung cancer, providing an inference of a causative agent for this disease (MM). Since workers in most industrial facilities (e.g. petrochemical plants, paint plants) are exposed to a large number of substances, including asbestos, separation of the causation of a cancer is difficult if not impossible; thus, requiring reliance on animal investigations in establishing an association. There have also been suggestions of this cancer being associated with mineral oil (mineral oil aspiration pneumonia), glass dust and isoniazid - a drug commonly used to treat tuberculosis) (Truman et al., 1980; Ilgren and Wagner, 1991).

Currently several animal studies (Kim et al., 2006; NTP, 2000, 2002; Dunnick, 1993) have reported the occurrence of mesothelioma's in mice and rats that were exposed to different chemicals. Chemicals identified in studies as mesothelioma producers are shown in table 3. If the NTP database is examined, there are a large number of tested agents where mesothelioma's have been reported; although, in many cases the numbers are not significantly different from controls. These data; although limited, support the suggestion that chemicals are causative agents of mesothelioma. However, since historically most epidemiological studies on workers exposed to various chemicals are in locations where asbestos has existed or still exists, separation of the contributory cause is impossible. A recent study by Kim et al., (2006) on the genetic relationship of chemically induced mesothelioma in animals as a model for that of man support the findings in table 3. It is likely that there is a wide variety of chemicals (e.g. benz[a]pyrene) (Ilgren and Wagner, 1991) that can induce mesothelioma that have not yet been identified. Hydrocarbons (e.g. benzene) (Sorahan et al., 2005) have also been suggested as possible agents of mesothelioma (Ilgren and Wagner, 1991). It should also be noted that the occurrence of mesothelioma's in control animals support epidemiological data of this disease occurring spontaneously or naturally. These animal data are supported to some extent in patients receiving chemotherapy for cancer (Warren et al., 1981; Neugut et al., 1997) in that MM arises as a secondary cancer as a result of treatment.

Table 3. Chemicals reported to be associated with the causation of mesothelioma in animal studies

Chemical	Study
Bromochloracetic acid	Kim et al., 2006
Ferric saccharate+	Okadaet al., 1997
o-nitrotoluene sulfone	National Toxicology Program - NTP, 2002
o-nitrotoluene	NTP, 2000
o-toluidine	NTP, 2000
m and p nitrotoluene	Dunnick, 1993; Dunnick et al., 1994
ethylene/propylene oxide	Lynch et al., 1984
Methylchoanthrene	Warren et al., 1981
methyleugenol	NTP, 2000
pentachlorophenol	NTP, 1999

+ also discussed as a metal.

Metals

There have been limited reports on metals causing mesothelioma (Ilgren and Wagner, 1991). These reports do suggest beryllium exposure can cause this disease (Oels et al., 1971); although, support is limited. Other metals, such as arsenic, iron, nickel, cadmium and chromium may also be mesothelioma producers, but again this is somewhat speculative at this time (Gottshall, 2002). Iron as ferric saccharate has been shown to "cause" mesothelioma "in the serosa of tunica vaginalis or the length of spermatic cord" and peritoneal in rats when this chemical/metal was administered by injection (Okada et al., 1997). Metals have been shown to be carcinogenic agents (e.g. arsenic). Epidemiological studies (Becker, 1999; Vecker, 1999) that evaluated welders reported an elevated number of mesothelioma cases in this population as compared to a control group. Although this study does not directly access the relationship between metals and this disease, it does suggest that there may be some relationship. However, in these studies overall, the role of asbestos and other agents can not be completely excluded.

Other Substances

A large number of other substances/compounds/agents have been identified as possibly causing mesothelioma (Ilgren and Wagner, 1991). A few agents/substances listed in table 1 were not presented as a separate section. This is due to the limited information currently available. Other agents/substances that have been suggested to cause or contribute to this disease are synthetic compounds (e.g. glass dust), polymers (e.g. polyurethane) and hormones (e.g. stilbesterol). However, reports (Ilgren and Wagner, 1991) have indicated occurrence of mesothelioma in relation to these various and can be said to provide descriptive evidence of a relationship. Since there are many confounding factors in the occurrence of mesothelioma, it is difficult to separate out the various causes. This is one of the reasons why little information exists, especially beyond animal studies. In addition, the regulatory push on the hazards of asbestos has resulted in a blinding of other factors in this disease. This alone has limited and deterred research on other factors. There is clearly a need for additional research on these less well known factors, both epidemiological and experimental.

Conclusion

There a large number of substances and event occurrences related to induction of mesothelioma in man and animals. Based on the number of studies reported on non-asbestos causes of this disease, asbestos is not the only factor to be considered when such an event arises. Future studies are needed to better evaluate agents in the cause of mesothelioma. As asbestos is removed in the US and other countries (e.g. United Kingdom), these other agents/substances will likely become more important as causes of this disease, and their role will become better recognized and investigated.

References

Abraham JL. (1983). Environmental pathology of the lung., In Environmental and Occupational Medicine, Rom WN, editor, *Little, Brown and Company*, Boston, MA, Pages 123-155.

Acheson ED, Gardner MJ, Pippard EC, Grime LP. (1982). Mortality of two groups of women who manufactured gas masks from chrysotile and crocidolite asbestos: a 40-year follow-up. *British Journal of Industrial Medicine* 39:344-348)

Amin AM, Mason C, Rowe P. (2001). Diffuse malignant mesothelioma of the peritoneum. *European Journal of Surgical Oncology* 27:214-5.

Anderson M, Hurley WC, Hurley BT, Ohrt DW. (1985). Malignant pleural mesothelioma following radiotherapy in a 16 year old boy. *Cancer* 56:273-6.

Andersson M, Wallin H, Jonsson M, Nielsen LL, Visfelt J, Vyberg M, Bennett WP, De Benedetti VM, Travis LB, Storm HH. (1995). Lung carcinoma and malignant mesothelioma in patients exposed to Thorotrast: incidence, histology and p53 status. *International Journal of Cancer* 63:330-6.

Antman KH, Ruxer RL, AIsner J, Vawter G. (1984). Mesothelioma following Wilm's tumor. *American Journal of Clinical Pathology* 86:227-30.

Ascoli V, Scalza CC, Bruno C, Facciolo F, Lopergolo M, Granone P, Nardi F. (1998). Familial pleural malignant mesothelioma: clustering in three sisters and one cousin. *Cancer Letters* 130:203-7.

Ascoli V, Aalto Y, Carnovale-Scalzo C, Nardi F, Falzetti D, Mecucci C, Knuutila S. (2001). DNA copy number changes in familial malignant mesothelioma. *Cancer Genetics and Cytogenetics* 127:80-2.

Austin MB, Fechner RE, Roggli VL. (1986). Pleural malignant mesothelioma following Wilm's tumor. *American Journal of Clinical Pathology* 86:227-30.

Babcock TL, Powell DH, Bothwell RS. (1976). Radiation-induced peritoneal mesothelioma. *Journal of Surgical Oncology* 8:369-72.

Baris YI, Grandjean P. (2006). Prospective study of mesothelioma mortality in Turkish villages with exposure to fibrous zeolite. *Journal of the National Cancer Institute* 98:414-417.

Becker N. (1999). Cancer mortality among arc welders exposed to fumes containing chromium and nickel. Results of a third follow-up: 1989-1995. *Journal of Occupational and Environmental Medicine* 41:294-303.

Bernstein DM, Rogers R, Smith P. (2003). The biopersistence of Canadian chrysotile asbestos following inhalation. *Inhalation Toxicology* 15:247-274.

Bernstein DM, Chevalier J, Smith P. (2005). Comparison of Calidria chrysotile asbestos to pure tremolite: final results of the inhalation biopersistence and histopathology examination following short-term exposure. *Inhalation Toxicology* 17:427-49.

Bernstein DM, Rogers R, Smith P, Chevalier J. (2006). The toxicological response of Brazilian chrysotile asbestos: a multidose subchronic 90-day inhalation toxicology study with 92-day recovery to assess cellular and pathological response. *Inhalation Toxicology* 18:313-32.

Bernstein DM, Hoskins JA. (2006) The health effects of chrysotile: current perspective based on recent data. *Regulatory Toxicology and Pharmacology*. (in press).

Berry G, Newhouse ML, Wagner JC. (2000). Mortality from all cancers of asbestos factory workers in east London: 1933-80. *Occupational and Environmental Medicine* 57:782-5.

Bianchi C, Brollo A, Ramani L, Zuch C. (1997). Pleural plaques as risk indicators for malignant pleural mesothelioma: a necropsy-based study. *American Journal of Industrial Medicine* 32:445-9.

Brenner J, Sordillo PP, Magill GB. (1981). Malignant mesothelioma in children: report of seven cases and review of the literature. *Medical and Pediatric Oncology* 9:367-73.

Britton M. (2002). The epidemiology of mesothelioma. *Seminars in Oncology* 29:18-25.

Brooks S, Stockwell H, Pinkham P. (1992). Sugarcane exposure and the risk of lung cancer and mesothelioma. *Environmental Research* 58:195-203.

Browne C. (2003) Salamander's wool: the historical evidence for textiles woven with asbestos fibre. *Textile History* 34:64-73.

Brown RC, Bellmann B, Muhle H, Davis JM, Maxim LD. (2005). Survey of the biological effects of refractory ceramic fibres: overload and its possible consequences. *Annals of Occupational Hygiene* 49:295-307.

Browne K, Murray R. (1990). *Asbestos and the Romans*. (letter). Lancet 336:445.

Browne ML, Varadarajula D, Lewis-Michl EL, Fitzgerald EF. (2005). Cancer incidence and asbestos in drinking water, Town of Woodstock, New York, 1980-1998. Environmental Research 98:224-32.

Buckingham DA, Virta RL. (2005). Asbestos Statistics. http://minerals.usgs.gov/ds/2005/140 /asbestos.pdf)

Burns C, Harrison K, Jammer B, Zaccarini D, Lafrance B. (2005). A cancer incidence and mortality study of Dow chemical Canada, Inc., manufacturing sites. *Occupational Medicine* (London) 55:618-24.

Cavazza A, Travis LB, Travis WD, Wolfe JT, Foo ML, Gillespie DJ, Weidner N, Colby TV. (1997). Post-irradiation malignant mesothelioma. *Cancer* 79:192-3.

Churg A, Wright JL, Hobson, J, Stevens, B (1992). Effects of cigarette smoke on the clearance of short asbestos fibres from the lung and a comparison with the clearance of long asbestos fibres. *International Journal Experimental Pathology*. 73: 287-97.

Churg A, Stevens B. (1995). Enhanced retention of asbestos fibers in the airways of human smokers. *American Journal Respiratory Critical Care Medicine* 151:1409-1413.

Cooper SP, Fraire AE, Buffler PA, Greenberg SD, Langston C. (1989). Epidemiologic aspects of childhood mesothelioma. *Pathology Immunopathology Research* 8:276-86.

Cristaudo A, Foddia R, Vivaldi A, Buselli R, Gattini V, Guglielmi G, Cosentino F, Ottenga F, Ciancia E, Libener R, Filoberti R, Neri M, Betta PG, Tognon M, Mutti L, Puntoni R. (2005). SV40 enhances the risk of malignant mesothelioma among people exposed to asbestos: a molecular epidemiologic case-control study. *Cancer Research* 65:3049-52.

Cugell DW, Kamp DW. (2004). Asbestos and the pleura. *Chest* 125:1103-1117.

Cutrone R, Lednicky J, Dunn G, Rizzo P, Bocchetta M, Chumakov K, Minor P, Carbone M. (2005). Some oral poliovirus vaccines were contaminated with infectious SV40 after 1961. *Cancer Research* 65:10273-9.

Das PB, Fletcher AG, Deodhare SG. (1976). Mesothelioma in an agricultural community of India: a clinicopathological study. *Australian New Zealand Journal of Surgery* 47:218-26.

Das PB, Ng AG, Stevenson MA, Mauch PM. (2005). Clinical course of thoracic cancers in Hodgkin's disease survivors. *Annals of oncology* 16:793-7.

De la Pena A and Lucas I. (1997). Malignant peritoneal mesothelioma as al ate complication of radiotherapy for Hodgkin's disease. *Annals de Medicina Interna* 14:319 (Spanish).

De Luca A, Baldi A, Esposito V, Howard CM, Bagella L, Rizzo P, Caputi M, Pass HI, Giordano GG, Baldi F, Carbone M, Giordano A. (1997). The retinoblastoma gene family pRb/p105, p107, pRb2/p130 and simian virus-40 large T-antigen in human MMs. *Nature* 3:913-6.

De Vuyst P, Dumortier P, Swaen GM, Pairon JC, Brochard P. (1995). Respiratory health effects of man-made vitreous (mineral) fibres. *European Respiratory Journal* 8:2149-73.

Dog M. (2003). Sources and types of mineral dust in regions of turkey with endemic malignant mesothelioma. *Indoor and Built Environment* 12:377-83.

Dogan AU, Baris YI, Dogan M, Emri S, Steele I, Elmishad AG, Carbone M. (2006). Genetic predisposition to fiber carcinogenesis causes a mesothelioma epidemic in turkey. *Cancer Research* 66:5063-8.

Dogan AU. (2003). Mesothelioma in Cappadocian villages. *Indoor and Built Environment* 12:367-75.

Dunnick JK. (1993). NTP technical report on the toxicity studies of ortho-,meta, and para-nitrotoluenes (CAS Nos. 88-72-2, 99-08-1,99-99-0) administered in dosed feed to F344/N rats and B6C3F1 mice. *Toxicological Reporting Service* 23:1-E4.

Dunnick JK, Elwell MR, Buncher JR. (1994). Comparative toxicities of o-, m-, and p-nitrotoluene in 13 week feed studies in F344 rates and B6C3F1 mice. *Fundamentals of Applied Toxicology* 22:411-21.

Elmishad AG, Bocchetta M, Pass HI, Carbone M. (2006). Polio vaccines, SV40 and human tumors: an update on false positive and false negative results. *Developmental Biology* (Basal) 123:109-17.

Emri S, Demir A, Dogan M, Akay H, Bozkurt B, Carbone M, Baris I. (2002). Lung diseases due to environmental exposures to erionite and asbestos in Turkey. *Toxicological Letters* 28:251-7.

Emri S, Demir AU. (2004). Malignant pleural mesothelioma in Turkey, 2000-2002. *Lung Cancer* 45 (Suppl): 1:S17-20.

Engels EA, Katki HA, Nielsen NM, Winther JF, Hialgrim H, Gjerris F, Rosenberg PS, Frisch H. (2003). Cancer incidence in Denmark following exposure to poliovirus vaccine contaminated with simian virus 40. *Journal of the National Cancer Institute* 95:532-9.

Falchero L, Coiffier B, Guibert B, Souquet PJ, Issac-Pinet S, Trillet-Lwnoir V. (1996). Mesotheliome malin de la plevre après irradiation pour maladie de Hodgkins. *Bulletin of Cancer* 83:964-8.

Fraire AE, Cooper S, Greenberg SD, Buffler P, Langston C. (1988). Mesothelioma of childhood. *Cancer* 62:838-47.

Gaarfar RM, Eldin NH. (2005). Epidemic of mesothelioma in Egypt. *Lung Cancer* 49 (Suppl) 1:S17-20.

Gamble JF. (1994). Asbestos and colon cancer: a weight-of-the-evidence review. *Environmental Health Perspective* 102:1038-50.

Gamble JF, Lewis RJ, Jorgensen G. (2000). Mortality among three refinery/petrochemical plant cohorts: II retires. *Journal of Occupational and Environmental Medicine* 42:730-7.

Gazdar AF, Butel JS, Carbone M. (2002). SV40 virus and human tumours: myth, association or causality. *Nature Reviews* 2:957-964.

Gilks B, Hegedus C, Freeman H, Fratkin L, Chung A. (1988). Malignant peritoneal mesothelioma after remote abdominal radiation. *Cancer* 61: 2019-21.

Gold B and Kathren RL. (1998). Causes of death in a cohort of 260 plutonium workers. *Health Physics* 75:236-40.

Gorini G, De Gregorio G, Silvestri S, Chellini E, Cupelli V, Costantini AS. (2005). Survival of malignant mesothelioma cases in the Tuscan mesothelioma register, 1988-2000: a population-based study. *European Journal of Cancer Prevention* 14:195-199.

Gottschall EB. (2002). Occupational and environmental thoracic malignancies. Journal of Thoracic Imaging 17:198-97.

Greenberg M. (1997). History of Mesothelioma. *European Respiratory Journal* 10:2690-1.

Grundy GW, Miller RW. (1972). Malignant mesothelioma in childhood: report of 13 cases. *Cancer* 30:1216-8

Hahn FF, Lundgren DL. (1975). Pulmonary neoplasms in rats that inhaled cerium-144 dioxide. *Toxicological Pathology* 20:169-78.

Hammond EC, Selikoff IJ, Seidman H. (1979). Asbestos exposure, cigarette smoking and death rates. *Annals of the New York Academy of Science* 330:473-90.

Health Effects Institute – Asbestos Research. (1991). *Asbestos in public and commercial buildings: a literature review and synthesis of current knowledge.* HEI-AR, Cambridge, MA..

Hill JK, Heitmiller RF, Askin FB, Kuhlman JE. (1997). Localized benign pleural mesothelioma arising in a radiation filed. *Clinical Imaging* 21:189-94.

Hillerdal G. (1983). Malignant mesothelioma 1982: review of 4710 published cases. *British Journal of Diseases of the Chest* 77: 321-343.

Hillerdal G, Berg J. (1985). Malignant mesothelioma secondary to chronic inflammation and old scars. *Cancer* 55:1968-72.

Hillerdal G, Berg J. (1985). Malignant mesothelioma secondary to chronic inflammation and old scares. Two new cases and review of the literature. *Cancer* 55:1968-72.

Hillman M. (1998). Discovery of simian virus 40 (SV40) and its relationship to poliomyelitis virus vaccines. *Developmental Biology Standard* 94:183-90.

Hirao T, Bueno R, Chen C-J, Gordon GJ, Heilig E, Kelsey KT. (2002). Alternations of the $p16^{INK4}$ locus in human malignant mesotheial tumors. *Carcinogenesis* 23:1127-30.

Hofmann J, Mintzer D, Warhol MJ. (1994). Malignant mesothelioma following radiation therapy. *American Journal of Medicine* 97:379-82.

Homa DM, Garabrant DH, Gillespie BW. (1994). A meta-analysis of colorectal cancer and asbestos exposure. *American Journal of Epidemiology* 139:1210-22.

Hoskins JA, Lange JH. (2004). A Survey of the Health problems associated with the Production and Use of High Density Chrysotile Products, http://www.chrysotile.com /data/newsletter

Hubbard R. (1997). The aethiology of mesothelioma: are risk factors other than asbestos exposure important? *Thorax* 52: 496-7/

Hughes RS. (2005). Malignant pleural mesothelioma. *American Journal of Medical Science* 329:29-44.

Huncharek M. (2002). Non-asbestos related diffuse malignant mesothelioma. *Tumori* 88: 1-9.

Ilgren EB, Wagner JC. (1991). Background incidence of mesothelioma: animal and human evidence. *Regulatory Toxicology and Pharmacology* 13: 133-149.

Ilgren EB (2001). Health risks from exposure to asbestos, metals, and various chemicals due to collapse of the world trade center: an environmental residential survey with commentary related to ground zero workers. *Indoor and Built Environment* 10:361-83.

Ishikawa Y, Mori T, Machinami R. (1995). Lack of apparent excess of malignant mesothelioma but increased overall malignancies of peritoneal cavity in Japanese autopsies with thorotrast injection into blood vessels. *Journal of Cancer Research Clinical Oncology* 121:567-70.

Jaurand MC, Fleury-Feith J. (2005). Pathogenesis of malignant pleural mesothelioma. *Respirology* 10:2-8.

Kang BC, Lee YS, Lee SK. (2004). Malignant pleural mesothelioma in a wood chuck (*Marmota monax*). *Journal of Veterinary Medicine* 66:1617-9.

Kannerstein M, Churg J. (1980). Mesothelioma in man and experimental animals. *Environmental Health Prospective* 34:31-6.

Kelsey TK, Yano E, Liber HL, Little JB. (1986). The in vitro genetic effects of fibrous erionite and crocidolite asbestos. *British Journal of Cancer* 54:107-114.

Kim DK, Nelson HH, Wiencke JK, Zheng S, Christiani DC, Wain JC, Mark EJ, Kelsey KT. (2001). P16 and histology-specific methylation of CpG island by exposure to tobacco smoke in non-small cell lung cancer. *Cancer Research* 61:3419-24.

Kim Y, Ton TV, Deangelo AB, Morgan K, Devereux TR, Anna C, Collins JB, Paules RS, Crosby LM, Sills RC. (2006). Major carcinogenic pathways identified by gene expression analysis of peritoneal mesotheliomas following chemical treatment in F344 rats. *Toxicological and Applied Pharmacology* Feb 3 [Epub ahead of print].

King JE, Thatcher N, Pickering CA, Hasleton PS. (2006). Sensitivity and specificity of immunohistochemical markers used in the diagnosis of epitheliod mesothelioma: a detailed systemic analysis using published data. *Histopathogy* 48: 223-32.

Kinutani M, Nagai N, Kunhara K, Sakata K, Tanimoto H, Murakami T, Takehara K, Takenka M, Okamoto E, Ohama K. (1994). A case of malignant mesoithelioma arising from uterine seroso after radiation therapy in uterine cervical cancer. *Nippon Sanka Fujinka Gakkai Zasshi* 46:911-4 (Japanese)

Ko LJ and Prives C. (1996). P53: puzzle and paradigm. Genes Development 10:1054-1072.

Kops SP. (2000). Oral polio vaccine and human cancer: a reassessment of SV40 as a contaminant based upon legal documents. *Anticancer Research* 20:4745-50.

Kovalivker M, Motovic A. (1985). Malignant peritoneal mesothelioma on children: description of two cases and review of the literature. *Journal of Pediatrics Surgery* 20:274-5.

Kramer G, Gans S, Rijnders A, Leer J. (2000) Long term survival of a patient with malignant pleural mesothelioma as a late complication of radiotherapy for Hodgkin's disease treated with ^{90}yttrium-silicate. *Lung Cancer* 27:205-8.

Ladero-Quesada JM, Amarillas Sanchez L, Furio Bacete V, Laredo Velasco L. (1991). Peritoneal mesothelioma and complete auricular-ventricular block as late complications in Hodgkin's disease. *Revista Clínica Española.* 189:221-3. (Spanish).

Lange JH, Weyel DA, Rosato LM, Tucker D, Malek DE, Mayernick JA, Ryan L. (1987). Preliminary results of smoking patterns for workers attending an asbestos abatement course. *Scandinavian Journal Work, Environmental, Health* 13:459.

Lange, JH (1992) A survey of cigarette smoking patterns among asbestos abatement workers attending an initial training course. International Journal of Environmental Studies B: *Environmental Science and Technology.* 42:73-79.

Lange, JH. (2001). Has the World Trade Center tragedy established a new standard for asbestos? *Indoor and Built Environment* 10: 346-369.

Lange JH. (2002). How do you interpret regulations through science or agency rules? *Toxicological and Industrial Health* 18:107-8.

Lange JH (2004). Mesothelioma trends in the United States: an update based on surveillance, epidemiology, and end results program data for 1973 through 2003. *American Journal of Epidemiology* 160:823 (letter).

Lange JH (2006). Reduced lung cancer in workers exposed to endotoxin-containing organic dust: experimental evidence and a review of epidemiology. *Current Topics in Toxicology.* (in press).

Lange JH, Hoskins JA. (2004). Asbestos in drinking water does not cause mesothelioma. *International Journal of Gynecological Cancer* 14:1048-9.

Lange JH, Priolo G, Mastrangelo G. (2004). Smoking trend in a high-risk group: asbestos abatement workers. *Journal of Occupational and Environmental Medicine* 46:1195 (letter).

Lanneau GS, McLaughlin D, O'Boyle J, Magann EF, Morrison JC. (2005). Well-differentiated papillary mesothelioma of the uterine serosa identified as cesarean section: a case report. *Journal of Reproductive Medicine* 50:860-2.

Law MR, Ward FG, Hodson ME, Heard BE. (1983). Evidence for longer survival of patients with pleural mesothelioma with asbestos exposure. *Thorax* 38:744-6.

Lee PN. (2001). Relation between exposure to asbestos and smoking jointly and the risk of lung cancer. *Occupational and Environmental Medicine* 58: 145-53.

Le Frere-Belda MA, Gil Diez de Medina S, Daher A, Martin N, Albaud B, Heudes D, Abbou CC, Thiery JP, Zafrani ES, Radvanyi F, Chopin D. (2004). Profiles of the 2 INK4a products of p16 and p14ARF, in human reference urothelium and bladder carcinomas, according to pRb and p53 protein status. *Human Pathology* 35:817-24.

Lerman Y, Learman Y, Schachter P, Herceg E, Lieberman Y, Yellin A. (1991). Radiation associated malignant pleural mesothelioma. *Thorax* 46:463-4.

Lopez-Rios F, Ladanyi M. (2006). *Malignant mesothelioma.* 354:306.

Lopez-Rios F, Chuai S, Flores R, Shimizu S, Ohno T, Wakahara K, Illei PB, Hussain S, Krug L, Zakowski MF, Rusch V, Olshen AB, Ladanvi M. (2006). Global gene expression profiling of pleural mesothelioma overexpression of aurora kinases and P16/CDKN2A detection as prognostic factors and critical evaluation of microarray-based prognostic prediction. *Cancer Research* 15:2970-9.

Lucas DR, Pass HI, Madan SK, Adsay NV, Wali A, Tabaczka P, Lonardo F. (2003). Sarcomatoid mesothelioma and its histological mimics: a comparative immunohistochemical study. *Histopathology* 42:270-9.

Lynch DW, Lewis TR, Moorman WJ, Burg JR, Groth DH, Khan A, Ackerman LJ, Cockrell BY. (1984). Carcinogenic and toxicological effects of inhaled ethylene oxide and propylene oxide in F344 rats. *Toxicological and Applied Pharmacology* 76:69-84.

Maltoni C. (2000). Call for an international ban on asbestos. *Toxicology and Industrial Health* 15:529-31.

Manfredi JJ, Dong J, Liu WJ, Resnick-Silverman L, Oiao R, Chahinian P, Saric M, Gibbs AR, Phillips JI, Murray J, Axten CW, Nolan RP, Aaronson SA. (2005). Evidence against a role for SV40 in human mesothelioma. *Cancer Research* 65:2602-9.

Mark EJ, Yokoi T. (1991). Absence of evidence for a significant background incidence of diffuse malignant mesothelioma apart from asbestos exposure. *Annals of the New York Academy of Science* 643:196-204.

Marsella JM, Liu BL, Vaslet CA, Kane AB. (1997). Susceptibility of p53-deficient mice to induction of mesothelioma by crocidolite asbestos fibers. *Environmental Health Prospective* 105 (Suppl) 5:1069-72.

Marsh CM, Gula MJ, Youk AO, Buchanich JM, Churg A, Colby TV. (2001). Historical cohort study of US man-made vitreous fiber production workers. II mortality from mesothelioma. *Journal of Occupational and Environmental Medicine* 43:757-66.

Mauch PM, Kalish LA, Marcus KC, Coleman CN, Shulman LN, Krill E, Come S, Silver B, Canellos GP, Tarbell NJ. (1996). Second malignancies after treatment for laparotomy staged Ia-IIIB Hodgkin's disease: long-term analysis of risk factors and outcome. *Blood* 87:3625-32.

Maurer R, Egloff B. (1975). Malignant peritoneal mesothelioma after cholangiography with thorotrast. *Cancer* 36:1381-1385.

Mayall PG, Jacobson G, Wilkins R. (1999). Mutations of p53 gene and SV40 sequences in asbestos associated and non-asbestos-associated mesotheliomas. *Journal of Clinical Pathology* 52:291-3.

Mayne ST, Janerich DT, Greenwald P, Chorost S, Tucci C, Zaman MB, Melamed MR, Kiely M, McKneally MF. (1994). Dietary beta carotene and lung cancer risk in US smokers. *Journal of National Cancer institute* 86:33-8.

McDonald JC, Liddell FDK, Dufresne A, McDonald AD. (1993). The 1891-1920 birth cohort of Quebec chrysotile miners and millers: morbidity 1976-1988. *British Journal of Industrial Medicine* 50:1073-81.

McDonald JC, McDonald AD. (1996). The epidemiology of mesothelioma in historical context. *European Respiratory Journal* 9:1932-42.

Melato M. and Rizzardi C. (2001). Malignant pleural mesothelioma following chemotherapy for breast cancer. *Anticancer Research* 21:3094-6.

Mesurolle B, Oanadli SD, Merad M, Mignon F, Baldeyrou P, Tardivon A, Lacombe P, Vanel D. (2000). Unusual radiologic findings in the thorax after radiation therapy. *Radiographics* 20:67-81.

Miller FD, Reed DM, Banta J. (1993). Sugarcane workers: morbidity and mortality. *Hawaii Medical Journal* 52:300-6.

Mishra A, Shet T. (2004). Clear cell mesothelioma of the testis with decuiduioid areas – a case report. *Indian Journal of Pathology and Microbiology* 47:544-6.

Mizuki M, Yukishige K, Abe Y, Tsuda T. (1997). A case of malignant pleural mesothelioma following exposure to atomic radiation in Nagasaki. *Respirology* 2:201-5.

Muscat JE, Huncharek M. (1996). Dietary intake and the risk of malignant mesothelioma. *British Journal of Cancer* 73:1122-1125.

Musti M, Cavone D, Aalto Y, Scattone A, Serio G, Knuutila S. (2002). A cluster of familial malignant mesothelioma with del(9p) as the sole chromosomal anomaly. *Cancer Genetics and Cytogenetics* 138:73-6.

Mutafoglu-Uysal K, Kargi A, Sarialioglu F, Olgun N, Kovanlikaya A. (2002). Malignant pleural mesothelioma in a child: long-term survival with ICE-WAC chemotherapy regimen. *Turkey Journal of Pediatrics* 44:244-7.

Mutsaers SE, Prele CM, Brody AR, Idell S. (2004). Pathogenesis of pleural fibrosis. *Respirology* 9:428-40.

National Toxicology Program. (1999). NTP toxicology and carcinogenesis studies of pentachlorophenol (CAS no. 87-86-5) in F344/N rats (feed study). *National Toxicology Program Technical Report* 483:1-182.

National Toxicology Program. (2000). NTP toxicology and carcinogenesis of methyleugenol (CAS No. 93-15-2) in F344/N rats and B6C3F1 mice (Gavage studies). *National Toxicological Program Technical Service Report.* 491:1-412.

National Toxicology program. (2002). Toxicology and carcinogenesis studies of o-nitrotoluene sulfone (CAS no. 88-72-2) in F344/N rats and B6C3F(1) mice (feed study). *Technical report Service* 504:1-357.

Neuberger M, Vutuc C. (2003). Three decades of pleural cancer and mesothelioma registration in Austria where asbestos cement was invented. *International Archives of Occupational and Environmental Health.* 76:161-166.

Neugut AI, Ahsan H, Antman KH. (1997). Incidence of malignant pleural mesothelioma after thoracic radiotherapy. *Cancer* 80: 948-50.

Newhouse ML, Thompson H. (1965). Mesothelioma of pleura and peritoneum following exposure to asbestos in the London area. *British Journal of Industrial Medicine* 22:261-269.

Newhouse ML, Thompson H. (1965a). Epidemiology of mesothelial tumors in the London area. *Annals of the New York Academy of Science* 132:579-588.

Newman R. (1986). Fine biogenic silica fibers in sugarcane: a possible hazard. *Annals of Occupational Hygiene* 30: 365-70.

Oels HC, Harrison EG, Carr DT, Bernatz PE. (1971). Diffuse malignant mesothelioma of the pleura: a review of 37 cases. *Chest* 60: 564-70.

Okada S, Hamazaki S, Toyokuni S, Midorikawa O. (1989). Induction of mesothelioma by intraperitoneal injections of ferric saccharate in male Wister rats. *British Journal of Cancer* 60:708-11.

Pappo AS, Santan VM, Firman WL, Kun LE, Walter AW, Jemkins JJ, Rao BN, Pratt CB. (1997). Post irritation malignant mesothelioma. *Cancer* 79:192-3.

Park JF, Howard EB, Bair WJ. (1970). Acute toxicity on inhaled 238 PuO_2 in beagles, BNWL-1050. BNLW Report January: 3:6.

Peterson JT, Greenberg SD, Buffler PA. (1984). Non-asbestos-related malignant mesothelioma. *A review. Cancer* 54:951-60.

Picklesimer AH, Zanagnolo V, Niemann TH, Eaton LA, Copeland LJ, (2005). Case report: malignancy peritoneal mesothelioma in two siblings. *Gynecological Oncology* 99: 512-6.

Price B, Ware A. (2004). Mesothelioma trends in the United States: an update based on surveillance, epidemiology, and the end results program data for 1973 through 2003. *American Journal of Epidemiology* 159:107-112.

Priest ND and Giannola SJ. (1980). ^{241}Plutonium deposition and redistribution in the rat rib. *International Journal of Radiation Biology Related Studies in Chemical Medicine* 37:281-98.

Prieto VG, Kenet BJ, Varghese M. (1997). Malignant mesothelioma metastatic to the skin, presenting as inflammatory carcinoma. *American Journal of Dermatopathology* 19:261-5.

Richie JP, Travis LB, Fossa SD, Schonfeld SJ, McMaster ML, Lynch CF, Storm H, Hall P, Holowaty E, Andersen A, Pukkala E, Andersson M, Kaijser M, Gospodarowicz M, Joensuu T, Cohen RJ, Boice JD Jr, Dores GM, Gilbert ES. (2006). Second cancers among 40,576 testicular cancer patients: focus on long-term survivors Division of Cancer Epidemiology and Genetics, National Cancer Institute, National Institutes of Health, Bethesda, MD. *Urologic Oncology* 24:171-2.

Risberg B, Nickels J, Waggermark J. (1980). Familial clustering of malignant mesothelioma. *Cancer* 45:2422-7.

Robinson BW, Musk AW, Lake RA. (2005). Malignant mesothelioma. *Lancet* 366:397-408.

Robinson BWS, Lake RA (2006). Advances in malignant mesothelioma. New England *Journal of Medicine* 353:1591-603.

Rollison DE, Page WE, Crawford H, Gridley G, Wacholder S, Martin J, Miller R, Engels EA. (2004). Case-control study of cancer among US Army veterans exposed to simian virus 40-contaminated adenovirus vaccine. *American Journal of Epidemiology* 160:317-24.

Rom WN. (1983). Asbestos and related fibers. In *Environmental and Occupational Medicine*, Rom WN, editor, Little, Brown and Company, Boston, MA, Pages 157-182.

Ross M, Nolan RP. (2003). History of asbestos discovery and use and asbestos-related disease in context with the occurrence of asbestos within ophiolite complexes. *Geological Society of America, Special Paper* 373. Boulder CO.

Roushdy-Hammady, Siegel J, Emri S, Testa JR, Carbone M. (2001). Genetic susceptibility factor and malignant mesothelioma in the Cappadocian region of Turkey. *Cancer* 357: 444-5.

Rustemeyer P, Micke O, Blasius S, Peters PE. (1997). Radiation-induced malignant mesenchymoma of the chest wall following treatment for breast cancer. *British Journal of radiology* 70:424-6.

Saggia C, Forti G, Biaggi G, Lattuada S, Santagostino A, Angeli G, Pollo MC, Negru MF, Alabiso O. (2004). Two cases of secondary soft tissue sarcomas after radiotherapy and radiochemotherapy. *Tumori* 90: 622-4.

Sanders CL and Jackson TA. (1972). Induction of mesothelioma and sarcomas from "hotspots" of $^{239}PuO_2$ activity. *Health Physics* 22:755-9.

Sanders CL. (1992). Pleural mesothelioma in the rat following exposure to PuO_2. *Health Physics* 63:695-7.

Sato F, Yamazaki H, Ataka K, Mashima I, Suzuki K, Takahashi T, Umezu H, Geiyo F. (2000). Malignant peritoneal mesothelioma associated with deep vein thrombosis following radiotherapy for seminoma of the testis. *Internal Medi*cine 39:920-4.

Sato T, Miyoshi T, Shibuya H, Fujikura J, Koie H, Miyazaka Y. (2005). Peritoneal biphasic mesothelioma in a dog. Journal of the Veterinary Medical, A: *Physiological Pathology Clinical Medicine* 52:22-5.

Schiffman MH, Pickle LW, Fontham E, Zahm SH, Falk KR, Mele J, Correa P, Fraumeni JF. (1988). Case-control study of diet and mesothelioma in Louisiana, *Cancer Research* 48: 2911-5.

Shannon VR, Nesbitt JC, Libshitz HI. (1995). Malignant pleural mesothelioma after radiation therapy for breast cancer. A report of two additional patients. *Cancer* 76:437-41.

Shieh S, Grassi M, Schwartz JK, Cheney RT. (2004). Pleural mesothelioma with cutaneous extension to chest wall scars. *Journal of Cutaneous Pathology* 31:497-501.

Sorahan T, Kinlen LJ, Doll R. (2005). Cancer risks in a historical UK cohort of benzene exposed workers. *Occupational and Environmental Medicine* 62:231-6.

Steineck G, Carstensen J, Wiklund K. (1983). Mesothelioma among sugar refinery workers. *Lancet* 2:1503.

Steinmetz KS, Potter JD. (1991). Vegetables, fruit, and cancer. I. Epidemiology. *Cancer Causes and Control* 2:325-57.

Stock RJ, Fu YS, Carter JR. (1979). Malignant peritoneal mesothelioma following radiotherapy for seminoma of the testis. *Cancer* 44: 914-9.

Taguchi T, Jhanwar SC, Siegfried JM, Keller SM, Testa JR. (1993). Recurrent deletions of specific chromosomal sites in 1p, 3p, 6q, and 9p in human malignant mesothelioma. *Cancer Research* 53:4349-4355.

Tassile D, Roth AD, Kurt AM, Rohner A, Morel P. (1998). Colon cancers and peritoneal mesothelioma occurring 29 years after abdominal radiation for testicular seminoma: a case report and review of the literature. *Oncology* 55:289-92.

Travis LB, Fossa SD, Schonfeld SJ, McMaster ML, Storm H, Hall P. Holowaty E, Anderson A, Pukkala E, Andersson M, Kaiiser M, Gospodarowicz M, Joensuu T, Cohen RJ, Boice JD, Dores GM, Gilbert ES. (2005). Second cancers among 40,576 testicular cancer patients: focus on long-term survivors. *Journal of the National Cancer Institute* 97:1354-65.

Truman KJ, Chilcote RR, Berkow RI, Moohr JW. (1980). Mesothelioma in child with prenatal exposure to isoniazid. *Lancet* 2:362.

Van Cleemput J, Hilde DR, Verschakelen JA, Rombouts J, Lacquet LM, Nemery B. (2001). Surface of localized pleural plaques quantified by computed tomography scanning. *American Journal of Respiratory and Critical Care Medicine* 163:705-10.

Van Kaick G, Dalheimer A, Hornik S, Kaul A, Liebermann D, Luhrs H, Wesch H. (1999). The German thorotrast study: recent results and assessment of risks. *Radiation Research* 152 (Suppl): s64-71.

Van Kesteren P, Bulten J, Schijf C, Boostra H, Massuger L. (2004). Malignant peritoneal mesothelioma in a 76-yesr-old woman with history of asbestos fiber ingestion. *International Journal of Gynecological Cancer* 14:162-5.

Vecker N. (1999). Cancer mortality among arc welders exposed to fumes containing chromium and nickel. Results of a third follow-up:1989-1995. *Journal of Occupational and Environmental Medicine* 41:294-303.

Velissaris TJ, Tang AT, Millward-Sadler GH, Morgan JM, Tsang GM. (2001). Pericardial mesothelioma following mantle field radiotherapy. *Journal of cardiovascular Surgery* (Torino) 42:425-7.

Vilchez RA, Kozinetz CA, Arrington AS, Madden CR, Butel JS. (2003). Simian virus 40 in human cancers. *American Journal of Medicine* 114:675–84.

Vilchez RA, Arrington AS, Butel JS. (2003a). Re: Cancer incidence in Denmark following exposure to poliovirus vaccine contaminated with simian virus 40. *Journal of the National Cancer Institute* 95:1249 (letter).

Vilchez RA, Butel JS. (2004). Emergent human pathogen simian virus 40 and its role in cancer. *Clinical Microbiology Reviews* 17:495-508.

Wagner JC, Steggs CA, Marchand P. (1960) Diffuse pleural mesothelioma and asbestos exposure in the North-West Cape Province. *British Journal of Industrial Medicine* 17:260-71.

Wagner JV, Skidmore JW, Hill RJ, Griffiths DM. (1985). Erionite exposure and mesothelioma in rats. *British Journal of Cancer* 51:727-30.

Warren S, Brown CE, Chute RN, Federman M. (1981). Mesothelioma relative to asbestos, radiation, and methylchoanthrene. *Archives of Pathology and Laboratory Medicine* 105:305-12.

Weill H, Hughes JM, Churg AM. (2004). Changing trends in US mesothelioma incidence. *Occupational and Environmental Medicine* 61:438-41.

Weissmann LB, Corson JM, Neugut AI, Antman KH. (1996). Malignant mesothelioma following treatment for Hodgkin's disease. *Journal of Clinical Oncology* 14:2098-100.

Wong O, Foliart DE. (1993). Epidemiological factors of cancer in Louisiana. *Journal of Environmental Pathology, Toxicology and Oncology* 12:171-83.

Yarborough CM. (2006). Chrysotile as a cause of mesothelioma: an assessment based on epidemiology. *Critical Reviews in Toxicology* 36:165-187.

Yates DH, Corrin B, Stidolph PN, Browne K. (1997). Malignant mesothelioma in south east of England: clinicopathological experience of 272 cases. *Thorax* 52:507-12.

Yeung P, Rogers A, Johnson A. (1999). Distribution of mesothelioma cases in different occupational groups and industries in Australia, 1979-1995. *Applied Occupational and Environmental Hygiene* 14:759-67.

In: Mesothelioma from Bench Side to Clinic
Editor: Alfonso Baldi, pp. 105-116
ISBN: 978-1-60021-789-0

Chapter V

Pathogenesis of Mesothelioma

***Haining Yang*[*], *Harvey I. Pass*[+] *and Michele Carbone*[*]**
[*] Thoracic Oncology Program,
Cancer Research Center of Hawaii, Honolulu, HI
[+] Department of Cardiothoracic Surgery,
New York University, New York, NY

Abstract

Malignant mesothelioma (MM) is a very aggressive tumor that arises from mesothelial cells. About 2,000 to 3,000 people are diagnosed with mesothelioma each year in the US. The prognosis of MM is poor and median survival from diagnosis is about 9-12 months [1]. MM was extremely rare until the second half of the 20th century. The first case report of MM was in 1947[2]. By 1960, the incidence of MM had increased enough for J. C. Wagner to report a MM epidemic among asbestos miners. The continuing increase in the incidence of MM since 1960 has been linked to the widespread use of asbestos in the past century.

Asbestos

In 1960, J.C.Wagner et al first demonstrated a relationship between asbestos exposure and mesothelioma [3]. Since then, a large body of epidemiological data and experimental evidence *in vitro* and in animals associated asbestos exposure to MM. Epidemiological studies found that approximately 80% of patients with MM in the United States have been exposed to asbestos [4]. The latency period between the time of exposure and diagnosis is about 30 to 40 years [5, 6].

Asbestos refers to a group of naturally occurring hydrated mineral silicate fibers including two major forms: serpentine, represented by chrysotile (white asbestos); and amphibole, which includes crocidolite (blue asbestos), amosite (brown asbestos), anthophyllite, actinolite and tremolite [7, 8].

The role of amphibole asbestos in the pathogenesis of MM is well accepted, and crocidolite (blue asbestos) is considered by some experts as the most oncogenic type of asbestos [9]. The long and thin fibers (especially > or = 8 mm in length and < or = 0.25 mm in width) are considered more dangerous since they have longer biopersistance in the pleura [10, 11]. These fibers are able to penetrate the lung and cause repeated damage, tissue repair and local inflammation.

Chrysotile, is the most common type of asbestos and accounts for about 90% of the world's asbestos production. Whether chrysotile causes MM is still controversial [12, 13]. Some scientists believe that chrysotile does not cause MM and that it is the tremolite that often contaminates chrysotile that causes MM [14, 15]. Other scientists believe that chrysotile plays an important role in the pathogenesis of MM, because chrysotile fibers induce DNA damage and chromosome abnormalities in human and rat mesothelial cells *in vitro* [16, 17], and because chrysotile causes MM in animals [18, 19]. Roggli et al suggested that chrysotile may cause MM but at a lower rate compared to amphibole asbestos [20]. Similarly, Hodgson and Darnton suggested that the exposure specific risk of MM is broadly in the ratio of 1:100:500 fro chrysotile, amosite and crocidolite respectively [21]. Instead, Suzuki Y et al analyzed lung and mesothelial tissues taken from 168 cases of MM and found that short, thin, asbestos fibers were the predominant fiber type detected in lung and mesothelial tissues form MM patients. Among these short thin asbestos fibers, chrysotile was the most common asbestos type, and therefore these authors proposed that chrysotile is the main contributor to the causation of MM [22]. We have conducted an extensive review of the literature but found that the data were so dramatically opposite that it was not possible to conclude whether chrysotile does or does not cause MM [23].

The mechanisms of asbestos carcinogenicity are not fully understood. During the long latency period of MM, many pathogenentic events may occur that can contribute to MM pathogenesis.

Compared to other cell types, human mesothelial cells are very susceptible to asbestos cytotoxicity. For example, when exposed to amosite asbestos, mesothelial cells were 10 and 100 times more sensitive to the cytotoxic effects of asbestos than normal human bronchial epithelial or fibroblastic cells [24]. Asbestos fibers induce toxicity in a dose-dependent manner. In tissue culture, doses equal to or higher than 5 micro gram/cm^2 of crocidolite fibers induce 100% cell death in less than a week [25]. The observation raises the issue of how can asbestos cause MM if HM exposed to asbestos die. Recent findings addressed this paradox and demonstrated a critical role for Tumor Necrosis Factor-alpha (TNF-α) and NF-kB signaling in mediating human mesothelial cell responses to asbestos [26]. It was known that *in vivo*, following asbestos exposure there is an inflammatory reaction with a large component of mononuclear phagocytes [27]. Upon differentiation into macrophages, these cells phagocytize asbestos and, in response, release TNF-α. At the same time, asbestos induces HM to express TNF-α receptor TNF-R1 and also stimulates the secretion of TNF-α (both paracrine and autocrine effects). TNF-α binds to its receptor and activates the NF-kB pathway, which increases the percent of HM survive asbestos exposure [27]. HM exposed to asbestos can accumulate DNA damages. Asbestos causes DNA strand breaks mediated by iron-catalyzed free radicals [28]. In addition, by causing the release of reactive oxygen species (ROS) and reactive nitrogen species (RNS), asbestos fibers can indirectly induce genotoxicity including base substitutions, deletions, rearrangements, insertions, sister chromatid exchanges, and chromosomal aberrations which may lead to a broad spectrum of mutations in mammalian cells [29, 30]. The activation of the NF-κB pathway stimulated by TNF-α allows HM with asbestos-induced DNA damage to divide rather than die, and if sufficient genetic damage accumulates to eventually develop into a MM [27] (Figure 1).

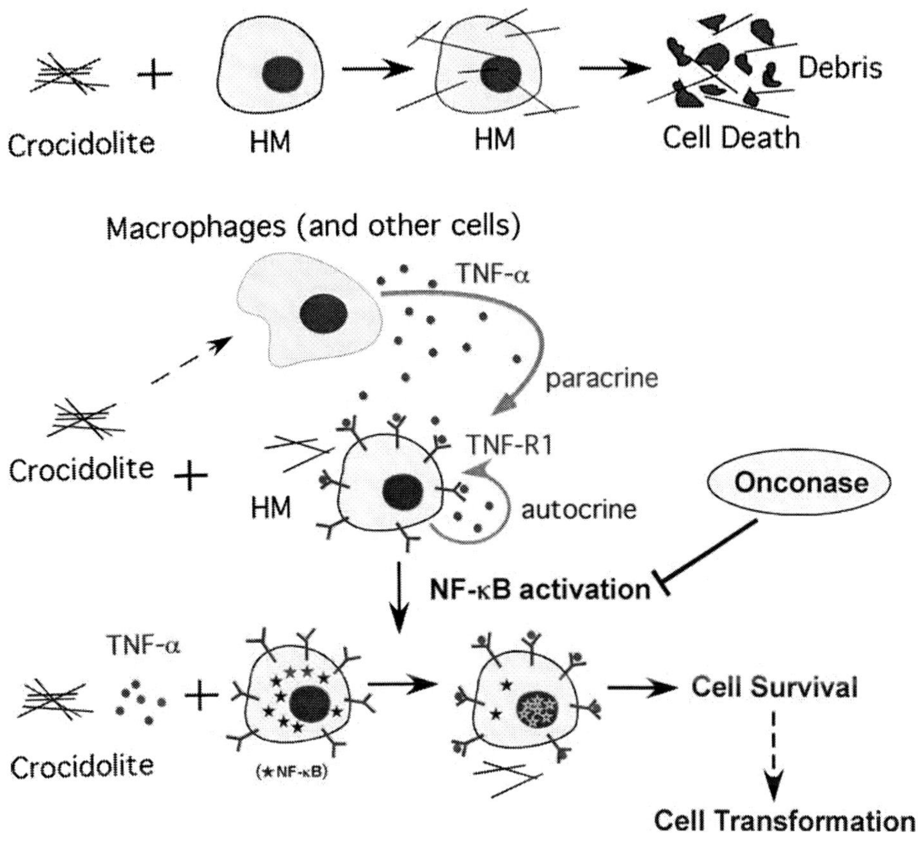

Figure 1. TNF-α inhibits asbestos induced cytotoxicity via a NF-κB dependent pathway: a possible mechanism for asbestos induced oncogenesis. In tissue culture, crocidolite is very cytotoxic to human mesothelial cells (HM), causing extensive cell death. Crocidolite causes accumulation of macrophages in the pleura and lung. These macrophages or some other cells release TNF-α when they encounter asbestos. At the same time, asbestos induces HM to secrete TNF-α (both paracrine and autocrine effects). TNF-α induces translocation of the NF-κB subunit, and the activation of NF-κB increases HM survival. This allows HM with asbestos-induced DNA damage to divide rather than die, and if sufficient genetic damage accumulates to eventually develop into a MM. Moreover, some drugs that specifically target the molecular pathways that lead to MM are already available, such as Onconase can inhibit NF-kB activation, stop cell cycle proliferation, and induce apoptosis.

Karyotypic and comparative genomic hybridization analyses of MMs detected frequent deletions of specific regions within chromosome arms 1p, 3p, 4p, 4q, 6q, 9p, 13q,14q and 22q [31, 32]. Certain tumor suppressor genes (TSGs) located in these areas were also studied, such as p16/CDKN2A at 9p21, p53 at 17p13 and NF2 at 22q12 [33, 34, 35, 36]. Loss and/or inactivation of TSGs may play an important role in development and progression of MM.

In additional to TNF-α, other growth factors and cytokines have been related to asbestos carcinogenesis and their role in pathogenesis is being investigated. These include: Transforming growth factor beta (TGF-b), which might have a role in stimulating tumor growth [37]; platelet-derived growth factor (PDGF), which may act as a regulatory factor in MM cell proliferation [38], Insulin-like growth factor (IGF), which may associate with tumor proliferation and migration [39]; Interleukins (ILs) such as IL-6 and IL-8, which appear responsible for the development of new capillaries and may promote tumor growth [40, 41]; vascular endothelial growth factors (VEGF), which also promotes tumor angiogenesis [42] and hepatocyte growth factor (HGF), which appears to influence mesothelioma cell invasion [43].

After interaction with mesothelial cells, asbestos triggers multiple cell-signaling pathways. Crocidolite fibers can induce autophosphorylation of the epidermal growth factor receptor, which stimulates the extracellular signal regulated kinase (ERK1/2) signaling pathway. This effect in turn increases activator protein (AP)-1 activity, and mitosis of mesothelial cells [44]. Asbestos also activates the NF-kB pathway, which leads to the activation of multiple prosurvival genes that promote tumor development [45].

SV40

Simian virus 40 (SV40) is a DNA monkey virus that has been associated with MM [8]. The most likely route of SV40 transmission from monkey to human was through the SV40 contaminated polio vaccines produced between 1955 and 1978 [46].

Analysis of human mesotheliomas revealed that SV40 sequences are present in tumor cells but not in the normal adjacent tissue [47, 48]. SV40 has been detected in human specimens by using several techniques including Southern blot; immunostaining; polymerase chain reaction (PCR); real-time PCR; RNA in situ hybridization, microdissection and electron microscopy [49]. Animal experiments demonstrated a clear association between SV40 and mesothelioma. 100% of hamsters injected intrapleurally with SV40 and 60% of those injected intracardially developed mesothelioma within 6 months [50].

SV40 produces two proteins that are oncogenic, which are Large T and small t antigens. In human MM biopsies, the large T antigen (Tag) was found to bind and inhibit p53 and the pRb family proteins, thus contributing to MM carcinogenesis [51, 52]. The small t antigen (tag) inhibits cellular phophatase 2A (PP2A), a protein involved in the dephosphorylation of many protein substrates, including components of the MAP-kinase (MAPK) pathway. Through inhibition of PP2A, tag may activate MAPK signaling and induce AP-1 activity [53, 54]. Tissue culture experiments showed that SV40 induces HGF/Met receptor activation [55], telomerase activity [56] and Notch-1 activation in human mesothelial cells [57].

Although over 50 different laboratories have reported a positive association of SV40 with MM, some have not, and this has caused a controversy [58]. The majority of the "negative" reports detected SV40 in only 6% of the specimens tested and conc luded that SV40 was not important in mesothelioma pathogenesis. Moreover, one study had initially found an association of 60% and then determined that most of the positive results were caused by plasmid PCR contamination. Only 6% of the initial 60% positive samples were confirmed to contain SV40 DNA [59].

That SV40 and asbestos might be cocarcinogens was first observed by Bocchetta et al in human mesothelial cells in tissue culture [25]. This hypothesis was confirmed by Kroczynska B et al who demonstrated a strong co-carcinogenesis among asbestos and SV40 [60]: Asbestos and SV40 (SV40 dl883 which does not express the small t antigen, and it does not cause MM in animals) together caused MM in 90% of hamsters, SV40 dl883 alone did not cause MM in any animal, and asbestos alone caused MM in 20% of hamsters. Importantly, significantly lower amounts of asbestos were sufficient to cause MM in animals infected with SV40. Molecular studies showed that asbestos and SV40 in combination had a co-stimulatory effect in inducing ERK1/2 phosphorylation and AP-1 activity in both Syrian hamsters and human primary mesothelial cells. AP-1 activation stimulated the expression and activation of matrix metalloproteases MMP-1 and MMP-9, which in turn led to cell invasion [60]. These findings indicate that mineral fibers and viruses can be co-carcinogens. Moreover, these data suggest that lower amounts of asbestos may be sufficient to cause MM in individuals infected with SV40. These results are important for determining levels of asbestos exposure that are supposedly "safe". Such supposedly safe levels may not be safe at all for the millions of individuals who were exposed to SV40 contaminated polio vaccines.

Erionite

Erionite is another type of mineral fiber that has been linked to the cause of mesothelioma [61]. Erionite has been detected in the lungs of villagers of Cappadocia, Turkey, where 50% or more of deaths are caused by MM [62]. Animal experiments showed that erionite is the most potent fiber in causing MM. Erionite induced pleural mesotheliomas in 40/40 rats compared to 19/40 rats injected with chrysotile) [63]. Inhalation of the erionite fibers induced a similar effect [27/28 rats developed mesotheliomas compared to 11/648 mesotheliomas observed in rats exposed to various types of asbestos) [63, 64].

Genetics

Genetic susceptibility to MM was observed in Cappadocian (Turkey) villages of Tuzkoy, Karain, and "Old" Sarihidir. Although mineralogical studies showed that all the houses contained similar amounts of erionite, MM was prevalent in certain families but not in others. Pedigree studies of the three MM villages showed that MM seemed to be inherited in an autosomal dominant pattern (Figure 2). When high-risk MM family members married into families with no history of it, MM developed in the descendants (Figure 2). The results of mineralogical studies and pedigree analysis indicate that the MM epidemic in Cappadocia is caused by erionite exposure in genetically predisposed individuals. Moreover, it was also found that genetically predisposed family members born and raised outside the MM villages did not seem to develop MM, which supported the observation that genetics and erionite exposure in causing MM [65, 66].

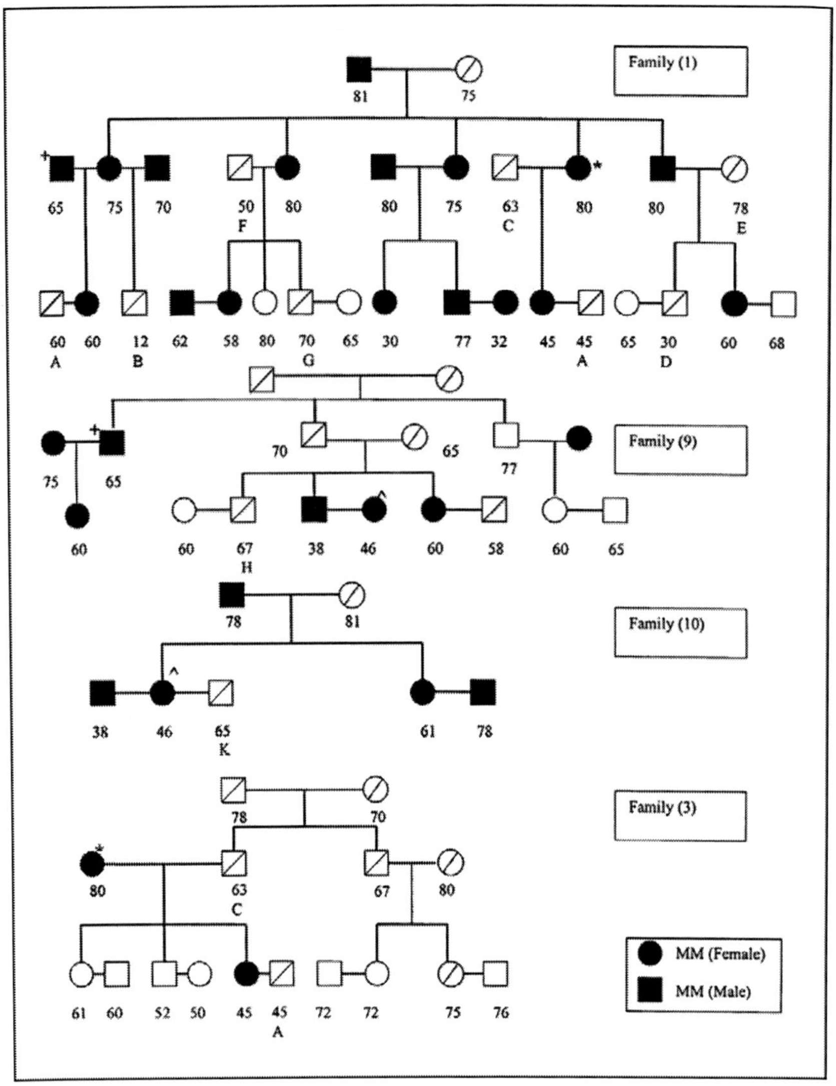

Figure 2. Family 1: Pedigree from the now abandoned village of "Old" Sarihidir showing a family of 30 in which 17 died of malignant mesothelioma (*black symbols*), 4 died of other cancers [osteosarcomas (*B*), leukemia (*D*), prostate cancer (*F*), and pancreatic cancer (*G*)], 4 died of reasons other than cancer [2 traffic accidents (*A*), 1 intestinal occlusion (*C*), 1 congestive hearth failure (*E*), and 1 unknown reason (first generation, female; *F*)], and 4 are alive (*white symbols*). Five malignant mesothelioma developed in individuals who married into the family. They were also from malignant mesothelioma families. *Bottom,* representative examples. Family 9: Pedigree of the family of origin of 65-year-old male (+) marrying into family 1. Seven of the 17 people of this two-generation pedigree died of malignant mesothelioma, 1 of liver cancer (*H*), and 5 unknown. The deaths for malignant mesothelioma include a 46-year-old female (^) who married into family 9. The family of origin of this woman (family 10) has a very high incidence of malignant mesothelioma: 5 of the 7 family members died of malignant mesothelioma and 1 of lung cancer (*K*); the remaining cause of death is unknown. Family 3: When members of family 1 (*) marry into a non–malignant mesothelioma family, malignant mesothelioma appears in the descendents. *A,* traffic accident; *C,* intestinal occlusion; the other causes of death were not cancer related but could not be established with certainty.

Radiation

Several case reports have documented MM in patients who received radiation to the thorax or abdomen [8, 67]. It was reported that the average interval between radiotherapy and MM was 21 years [68]. Animal studies using rats supported the role of radiation as a causative factor of MM [69].

Other Carcinogens and MM

There is no evidence showing an association between mesothelioma with smoking. There are some anecdotal case reports suggesting that chronic inflammation and scaring of the pleura, intrapleural thorium dioxide and some chemicals may cause mesothelioma [70, 71].

Conclusion

MM is a malignancy caused by multiple factors that may work alone or in combination. It is hoped that the recent advances in understanding the mechanisms of MM pathogenesis will lead to novel preventive and therapeutic strategies for MM patients. Importantly, some drugs that specifically target the molecular pathways that lead to MM are already available and can be tested in high-risk cohorts. For example, Onconase (Ranpirnase), which is an RNase that inhibits NF-kB activation (Figure 1), is going to be tested in the near future in some high-risk cohorts in Turkey.

Acknowledgements

The work was supported by the grant from Riviera Country Club in Illinois.

References

[1] Robinson BW, Musk AW, Lake RA. Malignant mesothelioma. *Lancet.* 2005; 366: 397-408.

[2] Case records of the Massachusetts General Hospital (case 33111). *N. Engl. J. med.* 1947; 236: 407-412.

[3] Wagner JC, Sleggs CA, Marchand P. Diffuse pleural mesothelioma and asbestos exposure in the North Western Cape Province. *Br. J. Ind. Med.* 1960, 17: 260-271.

[4] Carbone M, Rdzanek MA. Pathogenesis of Malignant Mesothelioma. *Clin. Lung Cancer. 2004, Suppl* 2, S46-S50.

[5] Mossman B, Kamp D, Weitzman S. Mechanisms of carcinogenesis and clinical features of asbestos-associated cancers. *Cancer Invest.* 1996, 14: 466-480.

[6] Sluis-Cremer GK: Asbestos disease at low exposures after long residence times. *Ann. NY Acad. Sci.* 1991, 643: 182-193.

[7] Mossman B, Bignon J, Corn M, Seaton A, Gee J. Asbestos: Scientific developments and implications for public policy. *Science*. 1990, 247: 294-301.

[8] Carbone M, Kratzke RA, Testa JR. *Semin. Oncol.* 2002, 29: 2-17.

[9] Brown R, Hoskins J, Miller K, Mossman B. Pathogenetic mechanisms of asbestos and other mineral fibers. *Mol. Aspects Med.* 1990,11: 325-349.

[10] Stanton MF, Layard M, Tegeris A, Miller E, May M, Morgan E, Smith A. Relation of particle dimension to carcinogenicity in amphibole asbestoses and other fibrous minerals. *J. Natl. Cancer Inst.* 1981, 67: 965-975.

[11] McDonald JC, Armstrong B, Case B, Doell D, McCaughey WT, McDonald AD, Sebastien P. Mesothelioma and asbestos fiber type. Evidence from lung tissue analyses. *Cancer.* 1989, 63:1544-1547.

[12] Smith AH, Wright CC. Chrysotile asbestos is the main cause of pleural mesothelioma. *Am. J. Ind. Med.* 1996, 30: 252-266.

[13] McDonald JC, McDonald A. Mesothelioma and asbestos exposure, in Pass HI, Vogelzang NJ, Carbone M (eds): *Maliganant Msothelioma.* New York, NY, Springer, 2005: 267-292.

[14] Dunnigan J. Linking chrysotile asbestos with mesothelioma. *Am. J. Ind. Med.* 1988, 14: 205-209.

[15] McDonald JC. Asbestos, in McDonald JC (ed): *Epidemiology of Work Related Diseases.* London, UK, BMJ Books. 2000: 85-108.

[16] Jaurand MC., Kheuang L, Magne L and Bignon J. Chromosomal changes induced by chrysotile fibres or benzo-3,4-pyrene in rat pleural mesothelial cells. *Mutat. Res.* 1986, 169: 141-148.

[17] Dong H, Buard A, Renier A, Levy F, Saint-Etienne L, Jaurand MC. Role of oxygen derivatives in the cytotoxicity and DNA damage produced by asbestos on rat pleural mesothelial cells in vitro. *Carcinogenesis.* 1994, 15: 1251-1255.

[18] Wagner JC, Berry G, Timbrell V. Mesotheliomata in rats after inoculation with asbestos and other materials. *Br. J. Cancer.* 1973, 28:173-185.

[19] Minardi F, Maltoni C. Results of recent experimental research on the carcinogenicity of natural and modified asbestos. *Ann. NY Acad. Sci.* 1988, 534: 754-761.

[20] Roggli VL, Sharma A, Butnor KJ, Sporn T, Vollmer RT. Malignant mesothelioma and occupational exposure to asbestos: a clinicopathological correlation of 1445 cases. *Ultrastruct Pathol.* 2002, 26: 55-65.

[21] Hodgson JT, Darnton A. The quantitative risks of mesothelioma and lung cancer in relation to asbestos exposure. *Ann. Occup. Hyg.* 2000, 44: 565-601.

[22] Suzuki Y, Yuen SR, Ashley R. Short, thin asbestos fibers contribute to the development of human malignant mesothelioma: pathological evidence. *Int. J. Hyg. Environ. Health.* 2005, 208: 201-210.

[23] Powers A, Carbone M: The role of environmental carcinogens, viruses and genetic predisposition in the pathogenesis of mesothelioma. *Cancer Biol. Ther.* 2002, 1: 348-353.

[24] Lechner JF, Tokiwa T, LaVeck M, Benedict WF, Banks-Schlegel S, Yeager H Jr, Banerjee A, Harris CC. Asbestos-associated chromosomal changes in human mesothelial cells. *Proc. Natl. Acad. Sci. USA*. 1985, 82: 3884-3888.

[25] Bocchetta M, Di Resta I, Powers A, Fresco R, Tosolini A, Testa JR, Pass HI, Rizzo P, Carbone M. Human mesothelial cells are unusually susceptible to simian virus 40-mediated transformation and asbestos cocarcinogenicity. *Proc. Natl. Acad. Sci. USA*. 2000, 97: 10214-10219.

[26] Yang H, Bocchetta M, Kroczynska B, Elmishad AG, Chen Y, Liu Z, Bubici C, Mossman BT, Pass HI, Testa JR, Franzoso G, Carbone M. TNF-alpha inhibits asbestos-induced cytotoxicity via a NF-kappaB-dependent pathway, a possible mechanism for asbestos-induced oncogenesis. *Proc. Natl. Acad. Sci. USA*. 2006, 103:10397-402.

[27] Choe N, Tanaka S, Xia W, Hemenway DR, Roggli VL, Kagan E. Pleural macrophage recruitment and activation in asbestos-induced pleural injury. *Environ. Health Perspect*. 1997, Suppl 5:1257-1260.

[28] Kamp DW, Israbian VA, Preusen SE, Zhang CX, Weitzman SA. Asbestos causes DNA strand breaks in cultured pulmonary epithelial cells: rold of iron-catalyzed free radicals. *Am. J. Physiol.* 1995, 268: L471-L480.

[29] Xu A, Zhou H, Yu DZ, Hei TK. Mechanisms of the genotoxicity of crocidolite asbestos in mammalian cells: implication from mutation patterns Induced by reactive oxygen species. *Environ. Health Perspect*. 2002, 110: 1003-1008.

[30] Shukla A, Gulumian M, Hei TK, Kamp D, Rahman Q, Mossman BT. Multiple roles of oxidants in the pathogenesis of asbestos-induced diseases. *Free Radic Biol. Med*. 2003, 34: 1117-1129.

[31] Lee WC, Testa JR. Somatic genetic alterations in human malignant mesothelioma. *Int. J. Oncol.* 1999, 14:181-188.

[32] Krismann M, Muller KM, Jaworska M, Johnen G. Molecular cytogenetic differences between histological subtypes of malignant mesotheliomas: DNA cytometry and comparative genomic hybridization of 90 cases. *J. Pathol.* 2002, 197: 363-371.

[33] Cheng JQ, Jhanwar SC, Klein WM, Bell DW, Lee WC, Altomarc DA, Nobori T, Olopade OI, Buckler AJ, Testa JR. p16 alterations and deletion mapping of 9p21-p22 in malignant mesothelioma. *Cancer Res*. 1994, 54:5547-5551.

[34] Metcalf RA, Welsh JA, Bennett WP, Seddon MB, Lehman TA, Pelin K, Linnainmaa K, Tammilehto L, Mattson K, Gerwin BI, et al. p53 and Kirstein-ras mutations in human mesothelioma cell lines. *Cancer Res.* 1992, 52: 2610-2615.

[35] Sekido Y, Pass HI, Bader S, Mew DJ, Christman MF, Gazdar AF, Minna JD. Neurofibromatosis type 2 (NF2) gene is somatically mutated in mesothelioma but not in lung cancer. *Cancer Res*. 1995, 55:1227-1231.

[36] Bianchi AB, Mitsunaga SI, Cheng JQ, Klein WM, Jhanwar SC, Seizinger B, Kley N, Klein-Szanto AJ, Testa JR. High frequency of inactivating mutations in the neurofibromatosis type 2 gene (NF2) in primary malignant mesotheliomas. *Proc. Natl. Acad. Sci. USA*. 1995, 92:10854-10858.

[37] Fitzpatrick DR, Bielefeldt-Ohmann H, Himbeck RP, Jarnicki AG, Marzo AL, Robinson BW. Transforming growth factor-beta: antisense RNA-mediated inhibition affects

anchorage-independent growth, tumorigenicity and tumor-infiltrating T-cells in malignant mesothelioma. *Growth factors.* 1994, 11: 29-44.

[38] Langerak AW, van der Linden-van Beurden CA, Versnel MA. Regulation of differential expression of platelet-derived growth factor alpha- and beta-receptor mRNA in normal and malignant human mesothelial cell lines. *Biochim. Biophys. Acta* 1996, 1305: 63-70.

[39] Liu Z, Klominek J. Chemotaxis and chemokinesis of malignant mesothelioma cells to multiple growth factors. *Anticancer Res*. 2004, 24: 1625-1630.

[40] Cohen T, Nahari D, Cerem LW, Neufeld G, Levi BZ. Interleukin 6 induces the expression of vascular endothelial growth factor. *J. Biol. Chem*. 1996, 271:736-741.

[41] Galffy G, Mohammed KA, Dowling PA, Nasreen N, Ward MJ, Antony VB. Interleukin 8: an autocrine growth factor for malignant mesothelioma. *Cancer Res.* 1999, 59: 367-71.

[42] Strizzi L, Catalano A, Vianale G, Orecchia S, Casalini A, Tassi G, Puntoni R, Mutti L, Procopio A. Vascular endothelial growth factor is an autocrine growth factor in human malignant mesothelioma. *J. Pathol.* 2001, 193:468-475.

[43] Harvey P, Warn A, Dobbin S, Arakaki N, Daikuhara Y, Jaurand MC, Warn RM. Expression of HGF/SF in mesothelioma cell lines and its effects on cell motility, proliferation and morphology. *Br. J. Cancer.* 1998, 77:1052-1059.

[44] Ramos-Nino ME, Timblin CR, Mossman BT. Mesothelial cell transformation requires increased AP-1 binding activity and ERK-dependent Fra-1 expression. *Cancer Res.* 2002, 62: 6065-6069.

[45] Mossman BT, Faux S, Janssen Y, Jimenez LA, Timblin C, Zanella C, Goldberg J, Walsh E, Barchowsky A, Driscoll K. Cell signaling pathways elicited by asbestos. *Environ. Health Perspect. 1997, 105 Suppl* 5: 1121-1125.

[46] Cutrone R, Lednicky J, Dunn G, Rizzo P, Bocchetta M, Chumakov K, Minor P, Carbone M. Some oral poliovirus vaccines were contaminated with infectious SV40 after 1961. *Cancer Res.* 2005, 65:10273-10279.

[47] Carbone M, Pass HI, Rizzo P, Marinetti M, Di Muzio M, Mew DJ, Levine AS, Procopio A. Simian virus 40-like DNA sequences in human pleural mesothelioma. *Oncogene* 1994, 9: 1781-1790.

[48] Shivapurkar N, Wiethege T, Wistuba II, Salomon E, Milchgrub S, Muller KM, Churg A, Pass H, Gazdar AF. Presence of simian virus 40 sequences in malignant mesotheliomas and mesothelial cell proliferations. *J. Cell Biochem.* 1999, 76: 181-188.

[49] Gazdar AF, Butel JS, Carbone M. SV40 and human tumours: myth, association or causality? *Nat. Rev. Cancer.* 2002, 2: 957-964.

[50] Cicala C, pompetti F, Carbone M. SV40 induces mesotheliomas in hamsters. *Am. J. Pathol.* 1993, 142: 1524-33.

[51] Carbone M, Rizzo P, Grimley PM, Procopio A, Mew DJ, Shridhar V, de Bartolomeis A, Esposito V, Giuliano MT, Steinberg SM, Levine AS, Giordano A, Pass HI. Simian virus-40 large-T antigen binds p53 in human mesotheliomas. *Nat. Med.* 1997, 3: 908-912.

[52] De Luca A, Baldi A, Esposito V, Howard CM, Bagella L, Rizzo P, Caputi M, Pass HI, Giordano GG, Baldi F, Carbone M, Giordano A. The retinoblastoma gene family

pRb/p105, p107, pRb2/p130 and simian virus-40 large T-antigen in human mesotheliomas. *Nat. Med.* 1997, 3: 913-916.

[53] Mungre S, Enderle K, Turk B, Porras A, Wu YQ, Mumby MC, Rundell K. Mutations which affect the inhibition of protein phosphatase 2A by simian virus 40 small-t antigen in vitro decrease viral transformation. *J. Virol.* 1994, 68:1675-1681.

[54] Frost JA, Alberts AS, Sontag E, Guan K, Mumby MC, Feramisco JR. Simian virus 40 small t antigen cooperates with mitogen-activated kinases to stimulate AP-1 activity. *Mol. Cell Biol.* 1994, 14: 6244-6252.

[55] Cacciotti P, Libener R, Betta P, Martini F, Porta C, Procopio A, Strizzi L, Penengo L, Tognon M, Mutti L, Gaudino G. SV40 replication in human mesothelial cells induces HGF/Met receptor activation: a model for viral-related carcinogenesis of human malignant mesothelioma. *Proc. Natl. Acad. Sci. USA.* 2001, 98: 12032-12037.

[56] Foddis R, De Rienzo A, Broccoli D, Bocchetta M, Stekala E, Rizzo P, Tosolini A, Grobelny JV, Jhanwar SC, Pass HI, Testa JR, Carbone M. SV40 infection induces telomerase activity in human mesothelial cells. *Oncogene*, 2002, 21, 1434-1442.

[57] Bocchetta M, Miele L, Pass HI, Carbone M. Notch-1 induction, a novel activity of SV40 required for growth of SV40-transformed human mesothelial cells. *Oncogene*. 2003, 22: 81-89.

[58] Wong M, Pagano JS, Schiller JT, Tevethia SS, Raab-Traub N, Gruber J. New associations of human papillomavirus, Simian virus 40, and Epstein-Barr virus with human cancer. *J. Natl. Cancer Inst.* 2002, 94:1832-1836.

[59] Lopez-Rios F, Illei PB, Rusch V, Ladanyi M. Evidence against a role for SV40 infection in human mesotheliomas and high risk of false-positive PCR results owing to presence of SV40 sequences in common laboratory plasmids. *Lancet.* 2004, 364:1157-1166.

[60] Kroczynska B, Cutrone R, Bocchetta M, Yang H, Elmishad AG, Vacek P, Ramos-Nino M, Mossman BT, Pass HI, Carbone M. Crocidolite asbestos and SV40 are cocarcinogens in human mesothelial cells and in causing mesothelioma in hamsters. *Proc. Natl. Acad. Sci. USA.* 2006, 103: 14128-14133.

[61] Emri S, Demir A, Dogan M, Akay H, Bozkurt B, Carbone M, Baris I. Lung diseases due to environmental exposures to erionite and asbestos in Turkey. Toxicol Lett. 2002, 127:251-257.

[62] Baris YI, Artvinli M, Sahin AA. Environmental mesothelioma in Turkey. *Ann. NY Acad. Sci.* 1979, 330: 423-432.

[63] Wagner JC, Skidmore JW et al, Erionite exposure and mesotheliomas in rats. *Br. J. Cancer.* 1985, 51:727-730.

[64] Saffiotti U: mesothelioma carcinogenesis:in vivo models, in pass HI, Vogelzang NJ, Carbone M (eds): *malignant Mesotehlioma.* New York, NY, Springer, 2005, pp 60-86.

[65] Roushdy-Hammady I, Siegel J, Emri S, Testa JR, Carbone M. Genetic-susceptibility factor and malignant mesothelioma in the Cappadocian region of Turkey. *Lancet.* 2001, 357: 444-445.

[66] Dogan AU, Baris YI, Dogan M, Emri S, Steele I, Elmishad AG, Carbone M. Genetic predisposition to fiber carcinogenesis causes a mesothelioma epidemic in Turkey. *Cancer Res.* 2006, 66: 5063-5068.

[67] Amin AM, Mason C, Rowe P. Diffuse malignant mesothelioma of the peritoneum following abdominal radiotherapy. *Eur. J. Surg. Oncol.* 2001, 27: 214-215.

[68] Cavazza A, Travis LB, Travis WD, Wolfe JT 3rd, Foo ML, Gillespie DJ, Weidner N, Colby TV. Post-irradiation malignant mesothelioma. *Cancer.* 1996, 77:1379-1385.

[69] Sanders CL, Jackson TA. Induction of mesotheliomas and sarcomas from "hot spots" of 239 PuO 2 activity. *Health Phys.*1972, 22: 755-759.

[70] Peterson JT Jr, Greenberg SD, Buffler PA. Non-asbestos-related malignant mesothelioma: A review. *Cancer.* 1984, 54: 951-960.

[71] Comin CE, de Klerk NH, Henderson DW. Malignant mesothelioma: current conundrums over risk estimates and whither electron microscopy for diagnosis? *Untrastruct Pathol.* 1997, 21: 315-320.

In: Mesothelioma from Bench Side to Clinic
Editor: Alfonso Baldi, pp. 117-135

ISBN: 978-1-60021-789-0

Chapter VI

Molecular Pathways Involved in the Pathogenesis of Mesothelioma

Monica Falleni, Solange Romagnoli and Silvano Bosari
Pathology Unit, Department of Medicine, Surgery and Dentistry,
University of Milan School of Medicine

Abstract

Malignant mesothelioma (MM) is a tumour of serosal surfaces with increasing worldwide incidence, likely determined by widespread asbestos exposures. MM patients have poor outcome and surgery, chemotherapy and radiation therapy do not provide satisfactory results. For the most part, current therapeutic approaches have no sound evidence-based foundations and clinical trials are needed. Some molecular alterations that characterize neoplastic transformation of mesothelial cells are now better understood, although we still do not have a comprehensive knowledge of MM, which would be fundamental to develop new molecular-targeted therapies. We will review here some of the data available, whereas the molecular effects of SV40 virus are described elsewhere in the book.

Oncogenes and Growth Factors

The first striking feature regarding the molecular alterations displayed by MM is the difference with most common solid tumours, including lung cancer. It does not appear that MM display any mutation of the most common oncogenes, such as those belonging to the Ras family, that are frequently mutated in solid tumours (Bueno R et al, 2004).

However, altered expression of several growth factors is significant in MM and may possibly be exploited for therapeutic purposes.

Epidermal growth factor receptor (EGFR), a tyrosine kinase receptor linked to cellular proliferation, cell death and angiogenesis, is over-expressed in a significant percentage of MM. The prevalence of EGFR expression, as documented by immunohistochemical analysis, ranges from 55% up to 97% of tumours (Destro A et al, 2006; O'Byrne KJ et al, 2004; Dazzi H et al, 1990; Govindan R et al, 2005). Destro and co-workers documented also increased EGFR mRNA levels by quantitative real time PCR.

Interestingly, in experimental systems asbestos exposure triggers increased expression of EGFR (Faux SP et al, 2000; Pache JC et al, 1998) thus initiating a signalling cascade considered important in mitogenesis and carcinogenesis.

Gefitinib is an inhibitor of EGFR that is used in selected subgroups of lung cancers; of note mutation of the EGFR intracytoplasmic domain are considered the most reliable indicator of tumor sensitivity to Gefitinib (Ono M et al, 2006; Helfrich BA et al, 2006). Although EGFR mutations have not been found in MM (Cortese JF et al, 2006; Destro A et al, 2006), Gefitinib has marked in vitro growth inhibitory effect for mesothelioma cell lines (Janne PA et al, 2002). Given these premises Gefitinib based EGFR inhibition was tested in clinical trial enrolling 43 patients and proved to have no survival benefits (Govindan R et al, 2005). Whether better selection of patients for EGFR inhibition, alone or in combination with other targeted therapies, could improve survival, remain to be established.

Insulin-like Growth Factor (IGF) can stimulate tumor growth and/or growth of adjacent stroma, with stimulatory effects on extracellular matrix development (Syrokou A et al, 1999). It has been documented that IGF is overexpressed in mesothelial cell lines and tumors and this observation has led to the study of the IGF family pathway (Hoang CD et al, 2004). IGF receptors, IGF-R1 and IGF-R2, are present in all mesothelioma cell lines (Liu Z et al, 2003). IGFR adaptor proteins, insulin receptor substrate (IRS)-1 and –2 play a role in MM. Tumors that signal through IRS-1 are associated with increased cellular growth while those that signal through IRS-2 are associated with increased cellular motility, therefore in the former case tumors are expected to be locally invasive while in the latter tumors are more prone to metastasis.

Tumor Suppressors

Mutations in the p53 gene are extremely common in human cancer. However p53 mutations occur rarely, if at all in MM (Mor O et al, 1997; Mayall FG et al, 1999). Conversely, the immunohistochemical finding of p53 reactivity in MM is relatively common, being documented in up to 70 % of cases (Kafiri G et al., 1992). This finding points to a different mechanism, instead of gene mutation, to determine p53 expression. To this end it should be noted that a loss of p14 ^{ARF} can be observed in 70% of tumours (Xio S et al, 1995; Yang CT et al, 2000). This gene maps on 9p21 and p14 bind and degrade MDM2, which inactivate p53. Thus p14 neutralizes the action of MDM2 and stabilizes p53, promoting apoptosis and tumour suppression.

One of the best studied target of p53 activation is p21, a multifunctional CDK inhibitor. p21 expression is detectable in 35% mesotheliomas (Isik R et al, 2001) and interestingly p21 immunoreactivity has been linked with improved patient survival (Baldi A et al, 2002)

One of the most critical transitions in cell cycle progression is the transition at the G1-S point. This checkpoint is guaranteed by the hypophosphorylated pRb that maintains the cell in a quiescent state. Phosphorylation of pRb is mediated by CDK and inhibited by CDK inhibitors. CDK inhibitors encompass p16^{INK4a}, p15^{INK4b}, p18^{INK4c}, p19^{INK4d}, p21, p27. P15 and p16 genes map on 9p21 and in many tumours a direct correlation between wild type pRb and loss of p16^{INK4a} has been noted (Otterson GA et al, 1994; Geradts et al, 1995). This holds true also in mesothelioma where p16 loss is common in tumors and cell lines (Kratke RA et al, 1995; Cheng JQ et al, 1994; Xio S et al, 1995). In MM loss of pRB has not been documented (Kratze RA et al, 1995; Carbone M et al, 2002).

P27 is one of the best characterized among the CDK inhibitors proteins and it is considered a significant prognostic marker in several cancers. Bongiovanni et al. evaluated 27 pleural mesothelioma patients documenting that high levels of p27 expression correlated with better survival (Bongiovanni M et al, 2001). The significance of p27 in MM was further demonstrated by other studies that showed the worse survival of patients with low levels of p27 expression (Beer TW et al, 2001; Beer TW, 2001).

The neurofibromatosis 2 (NF2) tumour suppressor gene, located on 22q, is involved in development of familial and spontaneous tumours of neuroectodermal origin (Bianchi AB et al, 1995). The gene encodes for the protein Merlin which inhibits cell proliferation and cell cycle progression through the repression of cyclin D1 expression (Xiao GH et al, 2005). Loss of chromosome 22 is a frequent event in MM cell lines and primary tumours (Flejter WL et al, 1989), thus prompting the search for the presence of tumour suppressor genes alteration in this location. Indeed high frequency of inactivating mutations of the NF2 gene was documented in MM (Bianchi AB et al, 1995) and mutations are highly correlated to loss of Merlin expression (Cheng JQ et al, 1999). The clinical significance of Merlin loss remains to be established although it has been recently demonstrated that Merlin, via Focal Adhesion Kinase (FAK) regulation, inhibits motility and invasiveness of MM cells (Poulikakos PI et al, 2006)

The Ras-association domain family 1 (RASSF1A) gene is a candidate tumor suppressor gene located in 3p21.3, probably involved in the apoptotic pathway as a negative regulator of Ras (Damman R et al, 2003). RASSF1A inactivation by allelic loss or methylation is frequent in human cancer and associated with features associated with poor prognosis such as high tumour grade and aggressive behaviour (Damman R et al, 2003). RASSF1A silencing by methylation is a frequent event in mesothelioma cells, associated with the presence of SV40 large T-antigen sequences (Toyooka S et al, 2001).

The Wilms tumor susceptibility 1 (WT1) gene was originally described as a tumor suppressor usually inactivated in the kidney Wilms tumor. WT1 expression has been documented in MM and mutations have also been described (Park S et al, 1993, Kumar-Singh S et al, 1997). Indeed expression of WT1 has important diagnostic implications in surgical pathology (Ordonez NG, 2006). The clinical significance for MM patients may depend in the future on the introduction of cancer immunotherapy targeting WT1, which has interesting preliminary results (Sugiyama H, 2005).

Cell Cycle Regulation and Loss of CDKN

Uncontrolled proliferation of neoplastic cells is one of the most important features of all type of cancers: tumour cells regularly acquire defects in the set of genes that positively or negatively regulate the cell cycle (Sherr CJ, 1996).

The G1-S checkpoint is crucial in cell cycle control and is mainly regulated by Rb and p53. CDK inhibitors are involved in the regulation of Rb functional status and p53 expression.

Gene abnormalities at CDKN2A locus, the site encoding two CDK inhibitors, p16INK4a and p14ARF, are a common findings in human mesotheliomas (Whitson BA et al, 2005; Kratzke RA et al, 1995; Wong L et al, 2002; Hirao T et al, 2002; Ladanyi M, 2005). Homozygous deletion of the ARF locus results in loss of p14ARF, in MDM2 increase and in functional inactivation of p53 (Xia C, 2002). P14^{ARF} reintroduction in MM cells results in G1-phase arrest and apoptotic cell death (Yang CT et al, 2000).

P16 ^{INK4a} encodes for a protein inducing cell cycle arrest by inhibition of pRb phosphorylation. Loss of p16^{INK4a}, the most common acquired molecular lesion in MM tumors and cell lines, seems to be the critical target of deletions at 9p21 locus. Loss or inactivation of p16 would thus cause defects in the regulation of the pRb-dependent growth pathway. P16 protein abnormalities have been frequently detected both in MM cell lines and tissues (Kreutzer et al, 1995) Loss of p16 ^{INK4a} are frequently associated to p15 ^{INK4b} and p14ARF (Hirao T et al, 2002; Xio S et al, 1995); this latter alteration leads to p53 destabilization and increased malignant potential of MM cells (Hopkins-Donaldson S et al, 2006). Experimental reintroduction in MM cell lines of p16^{INK4A} and of p14^{ARF} has produced positive results, with decreased phosphorilation of Rb and increased levels of p53 and p21 and increased Rb dephosphorilation, respectively. Adenoviral gene replacement therapy of p14 ^{ARF} and p16 ^{INK4a} in human MM cells has been documented to inhibit cell proliferation and improve response to chemotherapy (Yang CT et al, 2003).

Gene Expression Profiling and Cell Cycle Regulation

The modern analytical gene chip technologies provide the means to evaluate the expression levels all known genes and EST in any type of specimens. Large expression profiling datasets have been collected in MM by different groups in order to identify prognostic markers and therapeutic targets.

Pass et al (Pass HI et al, 2004) identified a 27-gene classifier from 21 MM to classify patients in short-term and long-term survivors.

Further studies were conducted to assess prognostic genes and Gordon et al first identified a 22-gene list (Gordon GJ et al, 2003) and subsequently a non-overlapping 7-gene list (Gordon GJ et al, 2005). The 22-gene list was used to derive a prognostic predictor of 1-year survival based on expression ratios of quantitative RT-PCR and applied to an independent set of 20 short-term (<6.8 months) or long-term (>24.8 months) survivors obtaining an accuracy of 75%. The 7-gene list was used to obtain a second prognostic predictor of 1-year survival based on expression ratios and found an accuracy of 69% in predicting survival in a cohort of 13 short-term (< 5 months) and 13 long-term (>18 months) survivors (Gordon GJ et al, 2005).

Recently Ladanyi's group (Lopez-Rios F et al, 2006) has identified a list of genes predicting survival, although it has a limited overlap with the other previously published datasets. Data were used to develop a microarray-based predictors of 1 year survival achieving a 68% maximum accuracy in cross validation and accuracies ranging from 63 to 67% when applied to other groups' outcome prediction models microarray-based and published recently. The work by Ladanyi et al. reports overexpression in a set of genes , most of which (11 out of 29, 38%) linked directly or indirectly in a network, either by protein-protein or regulatory interactions. This highly significant network is mainly associated with cell cycle regulation and cell death.

Our group (manuscript in preparation) has evaluated by real time quantitative RT-PCR and microfluidic card technology the expression levels of a set of genes involved in cell cycle progression and regulation in a series of MM. We have documented the abnormal expression of several genes of this network, notably: we observed in tumours a significant up-regulation of seven genes compared to normal tissue and down-regulation in two other genes as summarized in Figure 1 and 2 illustrating genes involved (Figure 1) and their functional role in cell cycle regulation (Figure 2).

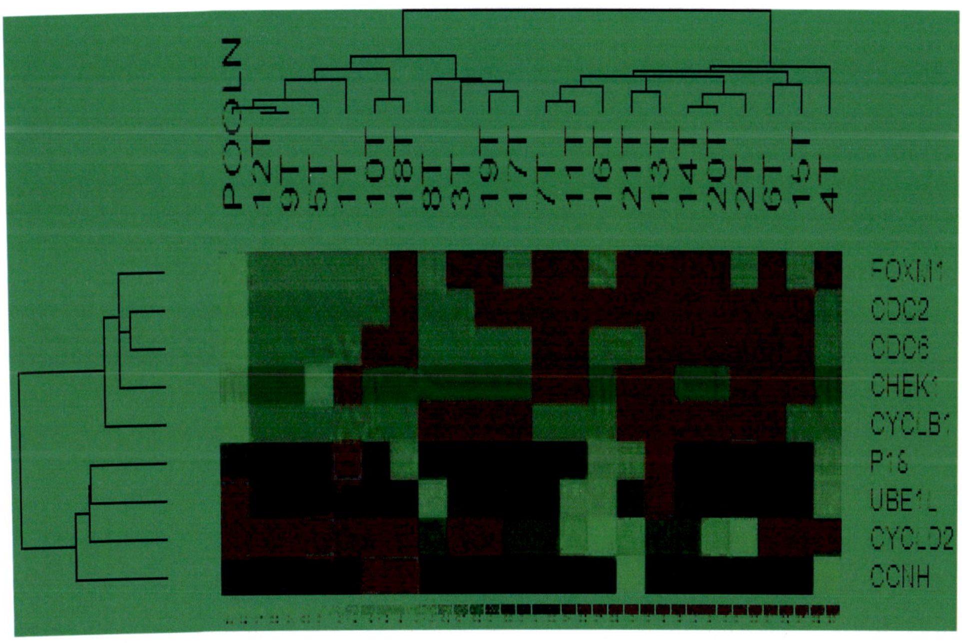

Figure 1. Real time RT-PCR analysis with microfluidic card technology of cell cycle gene expression in a series of mesotheliomas (T) compared to a pool of normal pleural tissues (pool N). Red colours indicate over-expressed genes while green colours correspond to down-regulated genes. FOXM1, CDC2, CDC6, Chek1, CyclB1, p18, CCNH are over-expressed whereas Cyclin D2 and UBE1L are down-regulated.

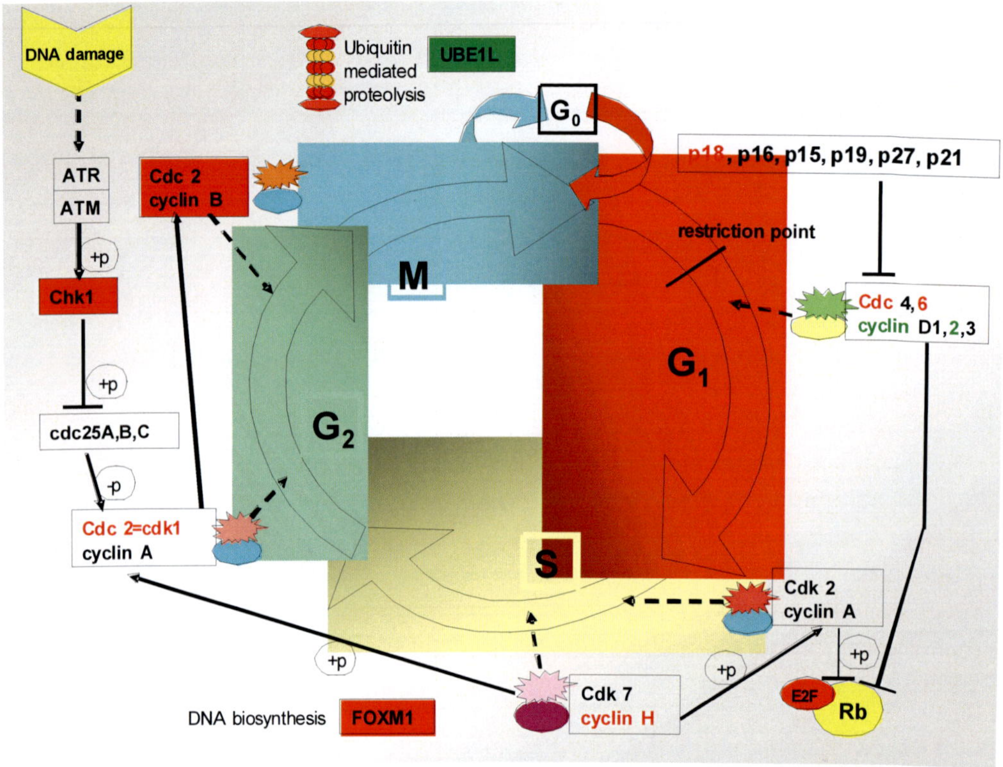

Figure 2. Cartoon of genes involved in cell cycle progression and its regulation, including G1/S and G2/M checkpoints. Degradation by ubiquitination, a mechanisms commonly used to rapidly reduce the concentration of cell-cycle control proteins, is also shown. The G1/S checkpoint controls the progression of eukaryotic cells from the steady-state (G1) into the DNA synthesis phase (S). The complexes formed by the cell cycle kinases CDK4/6 with cyclin D and by CDK2-cyclin E, along with the transcription factors Rb and E2F are crucial in controlling this step. At this checkpoint p18, CDC6, E2F, CCNH (cyclin H), FOXM1 were found to be overexpressed in the majority of MM. The G2/M checkpoint prevents the cell from entering mitosis (M phase) if the DNA is damaged. The main regulatory event in this transition is the activation of Cdc2-cyclin B complex by cdc25, which drives the cell into mitosis. DNA damage activates the DNA-PK/ATM/ATR kinases, initiating the cascade blocking cycle progression. Genes overexpressed at this step are depicted in red (CDC2, Chek1 and CyclinB1). Two down-regulated genes are also observed: CyclinD2 that prevents RB phosphorylation, and UBE1L involved in ubiquitin mediated proteolysis.

Apoptosis

Defects in the programmed cell death pathway affect the balance between cell proliferation and cell death, leading to uncontrolled cell growth.

MM displays drug and radio-resistance that may be related to defects of expression of genes involved in apoptosis and its regulatory mechanisms. Restoring the cell ability to execute apoptosis is now considered an attractive therapeutic strategy to selectively target tumor cells. Apoptosis is induced by two main pathways: the extrinsic receptor pathway activated by members of the TNF family ligands, and the intrinsic or mitochondrial pathway, activated by DNA damage and cellular stress. The two ways converge to activate effector caspases which cleave distinct substrates leading to cell death.

Studies evaluating the functional integrity of the extrinsic pathway still show contrasting results. Recently it has been suggested that tumour cells can take advantage of the FAS system to escape from cytotoxic T cell-induced apoptosis and to evade immune response. Rippo et al (Rippo MR et al, 2004) have recently observed that MM cells are resistant to Fas and TNF-related apoptosis-inducing ligand (TRAIL) induced apoptosis. Furthermore they found that caspase 8/FLICE was not activated and that FLIP (FLICE inhibitory protein) is costitutively expressed. Others observed no defects in the Fas/FasL pathway (Stewart JH 4th et al, 2002), even if FAS receptor downregulation have been observed (Kokturk N et al, 2005). In contrast to the lack of FAS receptor immunostaining, FASL immunoreactivity has been observed in MM; FASL tumor expression is a significant prognostic factor, possibly due to FAS L suppression of tumour growth by induction of inflammatory reactions (Seino K et al, 1997; Arai H et al, 1997; Kayagaki N et al, 1995).

TRAIL binds two proapoptotic receptors, DR4 and DR5, which induce procaspase –8 recruitment and activation (Broaddus VC et al, 2005); TRAIL also binds two receptors lacking death domains with potential anti-apoptotic function, DcR1 and DcR2. Apoptotic synergy between TRAIL signalling and DNA damage induced by etoposide, mediated by Bid activation of mithocondrial apoptotic pathway, is now considered an important strategy in order to treat refractory tumours with combination of differing proapoptotic and sublethal signals (Broaddus VC et al, 2005). Aberrant methylation of DcR1 and DcR2 genes and consequent silencing and loss of gene expression has been documented in up to 63% primary malignant mesotheliomas (Shivapurkar N et al, 2004).

Defects in the IAP and Bcl-2 families which are among the main regulators of the mithocondrial apoptotic pathway, have been documented in MM.

Survivin is a IAP family member which is considered an ideal therapeutic target due to its tissue expression and biological cellular function. In fact it is usually detectable at very low levels in human differentiated tissues, but overexpressed in a large variety of human malignancies, in which it is related to poor prognostic factors and chemoresistance (Altieri DC, 2006). It is a bifunctional protein involved both in cell cycle and in apoptosis regulation. Its antiapoptotic function is exerted by selective inhibition of the intrinsic caspase –9 apoptotic pathway. Survivin is up-regulated at both mRNA and protein levels in MM (Xia C et al, 2002; Falleni M et al, 2005), thus suggesting it may play important roles in MM aggressiveness and resistance to therapies. Furthermore, experimental antisense therapies down-regulating Survivin expression in MM cell lines caused increased caspase-3 activity and tumour cell death in a dose-dependent manner (Xia C et al, 2002).

IAP-1 (Inhibitor of apoptosis protein –1), also known as MIHC/cIAP2, is a protein which directly binds and inhibits caspase–9 proform activation, therefore acting in the mithochondrial intrinsic apoptotic pathway. IAP-1/MIHC/cIAP2 is highly expressed in MMs, both at protein and at mRNA levels. Reduced IAP-1 mRNA by antisense approaches, has been documented to decrease cell viability and increase MM cell sensitivity to cisplatin by nearly 20-fold (Gordon GJ et al, 2002).

Bcl-2 is rarely overexpressed in MM (Hopkins-Donaldson D et al, 2003; Narasimhan SR et al, 1998; Soini Y et al, 1999; Segers K et al, 1994; Cao XX et al, 2001; Chilosi M et al,

1997) but it may nevertheless play a significant role in MM cells survival and chemoresistance (Hopkins-Donaldson D et al, 2003). Unlike Bcl-2, Bax protein overexpression in MM cell lines and tissues is a common event (Narasimhan SR et al 1998; Soini Y et al, 1999; Cao XX et al, 2001), causing low Bcl-2/Bax ratios in MM cell lines (Narasimhan SR et al 1998). Low Bcl-2/Bax ratios, usually associated with tumors with low grade histology and better outcome with good response to chemotherapy, suggest that there must be other mechanisms counteracting Bax proapoptotic function. Possible explanations include the possibility that proapoptotic proteins found to be overexpressed maybe non-functional or not efficient enough to induce apoptosis; otherwise gene expression alterations may involve other apoptotic genes. Bcl-xL is usually overexpressed in MM and its downregulation is the aim of novel experimental therapies (Russo P et al, 2005, Ozvaran KM et al, 2004; Fox SA et al, 2005). The PI3-Akt survival pathway, which is constitutively activated in MM cells by cell membrane receptor tyrosine kinases such as EGFR (Rascoe PA et al, 2005), is involved in defects of apoptosis. In fact this pathway promotes Bcl-xL, XIAP and Survivin trascription (Catalano A et al, 2004; Janne PA et al, 2002), together with inactivation of proapoptotic proteins such as BAD and caspase –9. Recent data suggest that the different morphology of MM may reflect different biological characteristics of tumor cells. Apoptotic gene alterations have been more commonly detected in epithelioid MM, whereas defects in cell cycle progression has been mainly observed in sarcomatoid MM variants. Experimental therapeutic approaches by Sun (Sun X et al, 2006) have shown that epithelioid mesothelioma cells are more sensitive to proteosomal inhibitors than the sarcomatoid ones. These data highlight a novel approach to induce apoptosis in MM.

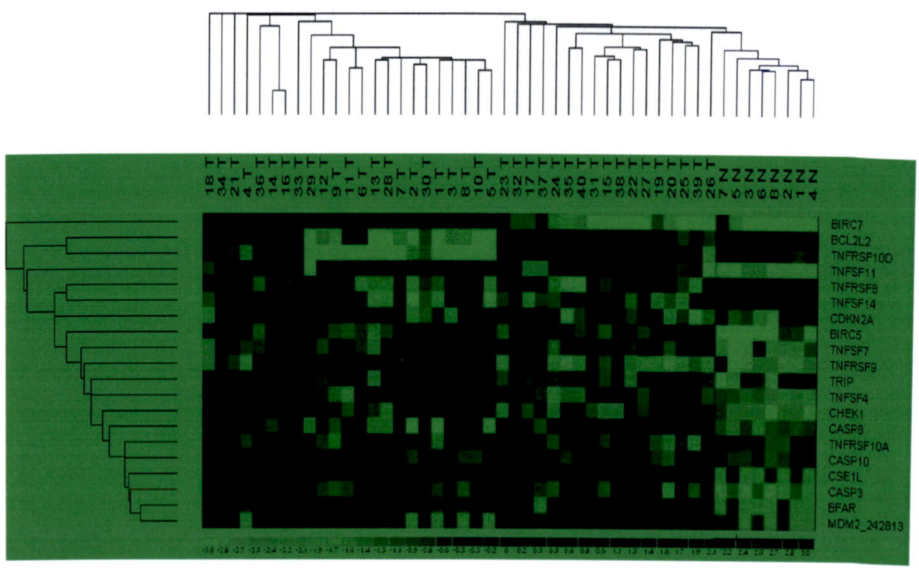

Figure 3. Real time RT-PCR analysis with microfluidic card technology of apoptosis gene expression in a series of mesotheliomas (T) compared to a series of normal pleural tissue (N). Red colour indicates up-regulated genes and green colour down-regulated genes. Up-regulation is observed in genes belonging to IAP family, comprising Survivin and Livin. Other up-regulated genes include members of the caspase family, tumor necrosis factor receptors, ligands and adaptors. Down-regulation is observed for BCL2L2, TNFRSF10D, TNFRSF8 and TNFSF14.

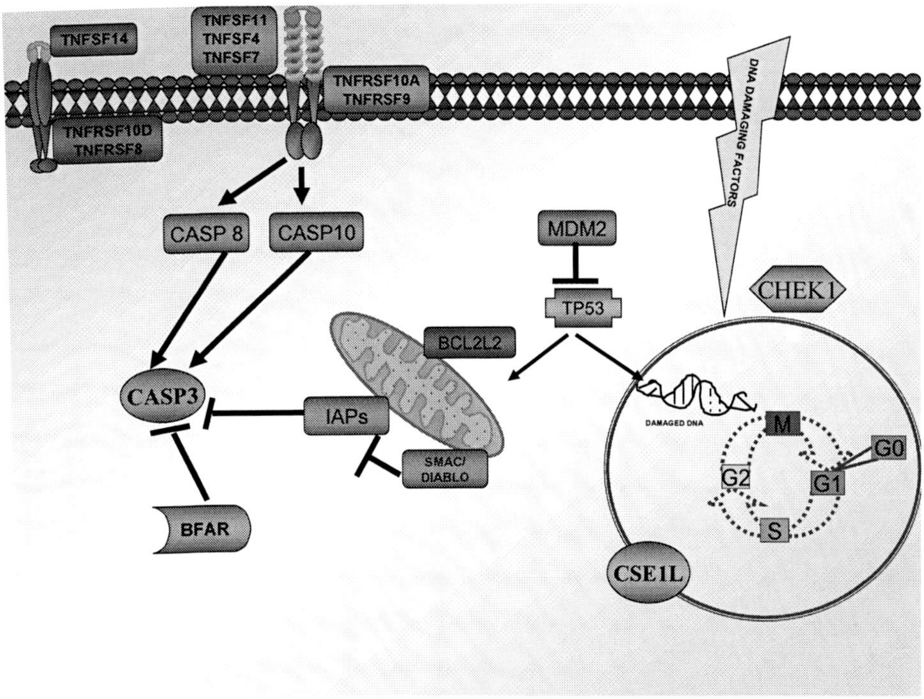

Figure 4. Cartoon of programmed cell death (apoptosis): involvement of genes investigated and their role in intrinsic and extrinsic pathways. The main regulators of the intrinsic pathway are located within the mitochondrial membrane. The release of cytochrome *c* into the cytoplasm is crucial for the formation of the "apoptosome", a complex formed by cytocrome c, apaf-1 and pro-caspase 9. The subsequent proteolysis of initiator caspase 9 drives the cascade of cleavages of effector caspases (caspase3 and 7). Inhibitor of apoptosis proteins (IAPs) block programmed cell death by two means: counteracting the formation of the apoptosome and by directly binding to caspase9 and 3. These proteins are in turn hampered by Smac/DIABLO or by pro-apoptotic Bcl2 family member as BCL2L2. Apoptosis by the extrinsic pathway begins at cellular membrane level where death receptors, as tumor necrosis factor receptor family (TNFRSF) are activated by their ligands (TNFSF). Death receptor ligands initiate signaling via receptor oligomerization, recruitment of specialized adaptor proteins and activation of caspase cascades. The two independent mechanisms, the intrinsic and the extrinsic pathways, merge at caspase 3 level. The genes overexpressed in MM belong to both apoptotic cascades, involving in particular members of IAP and TNF families converging at caspase3 level. An important factor that is down-expressed in mesothelioma tumors is BCL2L2, a fine regulator located at mitochondrial membrane involved in cytochrome *c* release and therefore, in cell fate.

We have quantitatively evaluated mRNA levels of 92 apoptotic genes by microfluidic card technique (manuscript in preparation). Our data document apoptotic defects both in the extrinsic pathway activating apoptotic with disregulation of death receptor and/or ligands, and in the intrinsic mithocondrial pathway with gene expression abnormalities of members belonging to families known as main regulators of the process, the IAPs, and the Bcl-2 family members. Furthermore, defects have been documented in effectors caspases leading to final steps of the apoptotic pathway (see Figure 3, 4).

Angiogenesis

Tumor angiogenesis plays a crucial role in tumor progression and in the metastatic process (Stacker SA et al, 2001; Holmgren L et al, 1995) and this general tenet of cancer biology holds true for MM (O'Birne KJ et al, 2000). Furthermore, accumulating evidence suggests that angiogenesis precedes the overt neoplastic disease, and that it may actually play an important role in the development of cancer in susceptible individuals (Sherr CJ, 2004).

Of particular importance in the understanding of the angiogenetic process is the evaluation of the multiple factors that either promote or inhibit tumor vascularization.

Among factors implicated in this phenomenon, Vascular Endothelial Growth Factor (VEGF), basic Fibroblast Growth Factor (bFGF), the Platelet Derived Growth Factor (PDGF), the Transforming Growth Factor (TGF)-beta, the Epidermal Growth Factor (EGF) and Interleukins -6 and –8 are important in MM since they are over-expressed in MM cell lines and/or tissues (Kumar-Singh S et al, 1999; Tolnay E at al, 1998; Antony VB, et al, 1995).

VEGF binds to VEGF R1 and R2 receptors, expressed by endothelial cells, thus promoting angiogenesis, and VEGF expression is correlated to high microvessel density, a feature associated to poor survival in MM patients (Otha Y et al, 1999; Kumar-Singh S et al, 1997). VEGF itself is an independent prognostic factor in MM and tumor necrosis can stimulate VEGF expression, and both factors appear to be associated with short patients' survival (Demirag F et al, 2005)

Several types of neoplastic cells, including MM cells, also express VEGF receptors. These findings indicate that VEGF role may extend beyond angiogenesis and also act stimulating cancer cells directly through autocrine/paracrine mechanisms. VEGF alterations have been documented in MM cell lines (Ohta Y et al, 1999; Kumar-Singh S et al, 1999) and the role of VEGF as an autocrine growth factor for MM has been documented (Strizzi L et al, 2001), Several factors can stimulate the production of VEGF by tumor cells or by stromal cells, including tumor infiltrating monocytes/macrophages. Among these factors, it is interesting to note that VEGF production can be induced by inflammatory mediators such as interleukin-6 and by 5-lipoxygenase (Romano M et al, 2001). High levels of VEGF in MM cells have been also associated to SV40 infection and linked to the biological effects of SV40 large T antigen (Catalano A et al, 2002).

Furthermore, VEGF has been documented to be involved in cell cycle abnormalities of SV40 infected MM cells with p53 inactivation (Catalano A et al, 2002).

The important roles that VEGF play in MM may represent the basis of future molecular therapies with VEGF inhibitors. In fact in animal models VEGF inhibition has been associated with MM growth reduction (Merritt RE et al, 2004). VEGF antibodies and cisplatinum chemotherapy, documented to induce an inhibitory effect in animal MM models, will be evaluated in MM patients in phase II trials.

PDGF, through its alfa and beta receptors, plays a dual role in tumor biology. PDGF can promote angiogenesis by stimulating endothelial cells proliferation and can induce tumor growth by autocrine stimulation. A striking redistribution of both PDGF A-chain and B-chain, as well as PDGF receptors occurs in MM. In fact MM cell lines express PDGF A-chain and B-chain whereas cultured normal mesothelial cells express low-levels of PDGF A-chain and no PDGF B-chain. Similarly PDGF alfa receptors are detectable in normal mesothelial cells whereas PDGF beta receptors are expressed in MM cells (Versnel MA et al, 1991). Taken together the data suggest that PDGF, with the beta receptors upregulation, acts as an autocrine growth factor for MM (Langerak AW et al, 1996; Strizzi L et al, 2001). An important practical consequence of these findings therefore involves the targeting of PDGF and indeed it has been shown that a hammerhead ribozyme against PDGF-beta mRNA can significantly decrease cell growth of MM cell lines.

Basic fibroblast growth factor (b-FGF) is a potent angiogenic factor promoting growth of endothelial cells growth in vitro and vessel formation in vivo. b-FGF overexpression has been correlated with poor MM patient survival although it poorly correlates with tumour vessel density, thus suggesting a mechanism probably independent of its angiogenic potential (Strizzi et al, 2001).

Invasion and Metastasis

MM has a marked tendency to invade adjacent tissues but can also spread to distant sites (Robinson and Lake, 2005). Genes involved in tissue invasion and metastasis have been investigated by immunohistochemistry and by DNA and tissue microarray. Results have been obtained on neoplastic tissue, cell lines and cytologic specimens and address alterations pertaining several pathways involving cell adhesion, cell migration, and matrix remodelling.

Liu et al (2001) evaluated the expression and activity of matrix metalloproteases (MMPs), as well as the expression of tissue inhibitors of metalloproteases (TIMPs) in several mesothelioma cell lines, documenting the widespread expression of interstitial collagenases (MMP-1), gelatinase A (MMP-2), stromelysin 1 (MMP-3) and gelatinase B (MMP-9). TIMPs 1, 2 and 3 were also commonly detected. A subsequent study (Liu and Klomonik 2003) demonstrated that this increased expression of MMPs could be modulated by several growth factors commonly present in MM, including the epidermal growth factor, transforming growth factor-alpha, stem cell factor, hepatocytes growth factor, and insulin-like growth factor I and II. The alterations of MMP first documented in cell lines have been confirmed in primary human MM, where MMP-2 and 9 activity are both independent poor prognostic factors in multivariate analysis in conjunction with weight loss (Edwards 2003).

Using cDNA and tissue microarrays Kettunen at al (2005) investigated malignant mesotheliomas and compared them to mesothelial cell lines and pleural mesothelium. Genes encoding two adhesion molecules (COL1A2 and integrin β4) and a chemokine (INP10) were up-regulated in MM compared to controls. INP10 has chemotactic and mitogenic activity and modulates the expression of adhesion molecules. INP10, through a novel INP-10 receptor well described in epithelial cell lines, may activate a specific signal transduction pathway and play a role in the metastatic process. Integrin β4 forms a dimer with integrin α6 and functions as an adhesion molecule and also plays a role as a component of the metastatic pathway associated with the HGF-receptor Met (Trusolino et al 2001). Kettunen et al. (2005) also reported a specific gene overexpression in MM histotypes: semaphorin E, integrin β4 and P-cadherin in epithelioid MM, matrix metalloproteinase 9 (MMP9) and tissue-type plasminogen activator (tPA) in sarcomatoid MM, neural cell adhesion molecule L1 (L1CAM) and INP10 in biphasic MM. Semaphorins are implicated in invasive growth and their expression was relatively higher in good-outcome vs poor-outcome MM (Gordon et al., 2003).

Cadherins are transmembrane glycoproteins responsible for calcium dependente cell-cell adhesion. They interact with the same cadherin type on adjacent cells and they are anchored into the cell by cytoplasmic proteins, the catenins, comprising the α, β and γ catenins. The APC protein plays a role in regulating β-catenin since it forms complexes between β-catenin and the serine/threonine kinase GSK-3β, therefore promoting β-catenin degradation (Hinoi et al. 2000).

Abutaily et al. evaluated E-cadherin, N-cadherin, α-catenin, β-catenin and c-terminal and N-terminal APC in MM tissues (Abutaily et al, 2003). Interestingly, E-cadherin expression was observed in 48% of epithelioid mesotheliomas but only in 7% of sarcomatoid mesotheliomas. Abnormal nuclear localization of β-catenin was demonstrated in 19% of mesotheliomas. APC expression was altered in 14 cases, two of which with nuclear staining for β-catenin. The investigators suggested that truncating mutations in APC may explain β-catenin in a subgroup of MM.

An additional gene involved in the metastatic process has been reported by Kratze (Hoang et al, 2004) who identified matriptase overexpression in MM. Matriptase is a type II transmembrane serine protease able to activate hepatocyte growth factor/scatter factor a mesenchymal cell-derived cancer cell growth and motility protein. In addition it is also an in vitro activator of prourokinase plasminogen activator.

The data presented in our review document a wide range of molecular defects currently known in MM: there will be many candidate therapeutic targets in the near future.

Acknowledgments

We thank Valentina Vaira and Ester Fasoli for discussion and editorial assistance.

This work was supported by MIUR, AIRC and CARIPLO.

References

Abutaily AS, Collins JE, Roche WR. Cadherins, catenins and APC in pleural malignant mesothelioma. *J. Pathol.* 2003;201:355-62.

Altieri DC. Targeted therapy by disabling crossroad signalling networks: the surviving paradigm. *Mol. Cancer Ther.* 2006; 5: 478-82.

Antony VB, Hott JW, Godbey SW, Holm K. Angiogenesis in mesotheliomas: role of mesothelial cell derived IL-8. *Human Pathol.* 1995; 26:1196-200.

Arai H, Gordon G, Nabel EG, Nabel GJ. Gene transfer of Fas ligand induces tumor regression in vivo. *Proc. Natl. Acad. Sci.* 1997; 94: 13862-7.

Baldi A, Groeger AM, Esposito V, Cassandro R, Tonini G, Battista T, Di Marino MP, Vincenzi B, Santini M, Angelini A, Rossiello R, Baldi F, Paggi MG. Expression of p21 in SV40 large T antigen positive human pleural mesothelioma: relationship with survival. *Thorax* 2002; 57: 353-356.

Beer TW, Shepherd P, Pullinger NC. P27 immunostaining is related to prognosis in malignant mesothelioma. *Histopathology* 2001; 38: 535-541.

Beer TW. Immunohistochemical MIB-1 and p27 as prognostic factors in pleural mesothelioma. *Pathol. Res. Pract.* 2001;197: 859.

Bianchi AB, Mitsunaga SI, Cheng JQ, Klein WM, Jhanwar SC, Seizinger B, Kley N, Klein-Szanto AJ, Testa JR. High frequency of inactivating mutations in the neurofibromatosis type 2 gene (NF2) in primary malignant mesotheliomas. *Proc. Natl. Acad. Sci.* 1995; 92: 10854-8.

Bongiovanni M, Cassoni P, De Giuli P, Viberti L, Cappia S, Ivaldi C, Chiusa L, Bussolati G. p27(kip1) immunoreactivity correlates with long-term survival in pleural malignant mesothelioma. *Cancer* 2001;92:1245-50.

Broaddus VC, Dansen TB, Abayasiriwardana KS, Wilson SM, Finch AJ, Swigart LB, Hunt AE, Evan GI. Bid mediates apoptotic synergy between tumor necrosis factor-related apoptosis-inducing ligand (TRAIL) and DNA damage. *J. Biol. Chem.* 2005; 280:12486-93.

Bueno R, Gordon GJ. Genetics of malignant pleural mesothelioma: molecular markers and biologic targets. *Thorac. Surg. Clin.* 2004; 14: 461-468.

Cao XX, Mohuiddin I, Ece F, McConkey DJ, Smythe RW: Histone deacetylase inhibitor downregulation of bcl-xl gene expression leads to apoptotic cell death in mesothelioma. *Am. J. Respir. Cell Mol. Biol.* 2001; 5: 562-8.

Carbone M, Kratzke RA, Testa JR. The pathogenesis of mesothelioma. *Semin Oncol.* 2002;29:2-17.

Catalano A, Romano M, Martinotti S, Procopio A. Enhanced expression of vascular endothelial growth factor (VEGF) plays a critical role in the tumor progression potential induced by simian virus 40 large T antigen. *Oncogene* 2002 ;21:2896-900.

Catalano A, Graciotti L, Rinaldi L, Raffaelli G, Rodilossi S, Betta P, Gianni W, Amoroso S, Procopio A. Preclinical evaluation of the nonsteroidal anti-inflammatory agent celecoxib on malignant mesothelioma chemoprevention. *Int. J. Cancer* 2004; 109:322-8.

Cheng JQ, Jhanwar SC, Klein WM, Bell DW, Lee WC, Altomare DA, Nobori T, Olopade OI, Buckler AJ, Testa JR. P16 alterations and deletion mapping of 9p21-p22 in malignant mesothelioma. *Cancer Res.* 1994; 54 : 5547-51.

Cheng JQ, Lee WC, Klein MA, Cheng GZ, Jhanwar SC, Testa JR. Frequent mutations of NF2 and allelic loss from chromosome band 22q12 in malignant mesothelioma evidence for a two hit mechanism of NF2 inactivation. *Genes Chromosomes Cancer* 1999; 24: 238-242.

Chilosi M, Facchetti F, Dei Tos AP, Lestani M, Morassi ML, Martignoni G, Sorio C, Benedetti A, Morelli L, Doglioni C, Barberis M, Menestrina F, Viale G. Bcl-2 expression in pleural and extrapleural solitary fibrous tumours. *J. Pathol.* 1997; 181: 362-367.

Cortese JF, Gowda AL, Wali A, Eliason JF, Pass HI, Everson RB. Common EGFR mutations conferring sensitivity to gefitinib in lung adenocarcinoma are not prevalent in human malignant mesothelioma. *Int. J. Cancer* 2006; 118: 521-522.

Dammann R, Schagdarsurengin U, Liu L, Otto N, Gimm O, Dralle H, Boehm BO, Pfeifer GP, Hoang Vu C. Frequent RASSF1A promoter hypermethylation and K-ras mutations in pancreatic carcinoma. *Oncogene* 2003; 22: 3806-12.

Dazzi H, Hasleton PS, Thatcher N, Wilkes S, Swindell R, Chatterjee AK. Malignant pleural mesothelioma and epidermal growth factor receptor (EGF-R). Relationship of EGF-R with histology and survival using fixed paraffin embedded tissue and the F4 monoclonal antibody. *Br. J. Cancer* 1990; 61: 924-926.

Demirag F, Unsal E, Yilmaz A, Caglar A. Prognostic significance of vascular endothelial growth factor, tumor necrosis, and mitotic activity index in malignant pleural mesothelioma. *Chest* 2005; 128: 3382-7.

Destro A, Ceresoli GL, Falleni M, Zucali PA, Morenghi E, Bianchi P, Pellegrini C, Cordani N, Vaira V, Alloisio M, Rizzi A, Bosari S, Roncalli M. EGFR overexpression in malignant pleural mesothelioma. An immunohistochemical and molecular study with clinico-pathological correlations. *Lung Cancer* 2006; 51: 207-215.

Edwards JG, McLaren J, Jones JL, Waller DA, O'Byrne KJ. Matrix metalloproteinases 2 and 9 (gelatinases A and B) expression in malignant mesothelioma and benign pleura. *Br. J. Cancer* 2003; 88: 1553-9.

Falleni M, Pellegrini C, Marchetti A, Roncalli M, Nosotti M, Palleschi A, Santambrogio L, Coggi G, Bosari S. Quantitative evaluation of the apoptosis regulating genes Survivin, Bcl-2 and Bax in inflammatory and malignant pleural lesions. *Lung Cancer* 2005; 48: 211-6.

Faux SP, Houghton CE, Hubbard A, Patrick G. Increased expression of epidermal growth factor receptor in rat pleural mesothelial cells correlates with carcinogenicity of mineral fibres. *Carcinogenesis* 2000; 21: 2275-2280.

Flejter WL, Li FP, Antman KH, Testa JR. Recurring loss involving chromosome 1, 3 and 22 in malignant mesothelioma: possible sites of tumor suppressor genes. *Genes Chromosomes Cancer* 1989; 1: 148-154.

Fox SA, Kusmiaty, Loh SS, Dharmarajan AM, Garlepp MJ. Cisplatin and TNF-alpha downregulate transription of Bcl-xL in murine malignant mesothelioma cells. *Biochem. Biophys. Res. Commun* 2005;337: 983-91.

Geradts J, Kratzke RA, Niehans GA, Lincoln CE. Immunohistochemical detection of the cyclin-dependent kinase inhibitor 2/multiple tumor suppressor gene 1 (CDKN2/MTS1) product p16INK4A in archival human solid tumors: correlation with retinoblastoma protein expression. *Cancer Res.* 1995;55:6006-11.

Gordon GJ, Appasani K, Parcells JP, Mukhopadhyay NK, Jaklitsch MT, Richards WG, Sugarbaker DJ, Bueno R. Inhibitor of apoptosis protein-1 promotes tumor cell survival in mesothelioma. *Carcinogenesis* 2002; 23: 1017-24.

Gordon GJ, Jensen RV, Hsiao LL, Gullans SR, Blumenstock JE, Richards WG, Jaklitsch MT, Sugarbaker DJ, Bieno R. Using gene expression ratios to predict outcome among patients with mesothelioma. *J. Natl. Cancer Inst.* 2003; 95: 598-605.

Gordon GJ, Rockwell GN, Godfrey PA, Jensen RV, Glickman JN, Yeap BY, Richards WG, Sugarbaker DJ, Bueno R. Validation of genomics-based prognostic tests in malignant pleural mesothelioma. *Clin. Cancer Res.* 2005; 11: 4406-4414.

Govindan R, Kratzke RA, Herndon JE 2nd, Niehans GA, Vollmer R, Watson D, Green MR, Kindler HL, Cancer and Leukemia Group B (CALGB 30101). Gefitinib in patients with malignant mesothelioma: a phase II study by the Cancer and Leukemia Group B. *Clin. Cancer Res.* 2005; 11: 2300-2304.

Helfrich BA, Raben D, Varella-Garcia M, Gustafson D, Chan DC, Bemis L, Coldren C, Baron A, Zeng C, Franklin WA, Hirsch FR, Gazdar A, Minna J, Bunn PA Jr. Antitumor activity of the epidermal growth factor receptor (EGFR) tyrosine kinase inhibitor gefitinib (ZD1839, Iressa) in non-small cell lung cancer cell lines correlates with gene copy number and EGFR mutations but not EGFR protein levels. *Clin. Cancer Res.* 2006; 12: 7117-25.

Hirao T, Bueno R, Chen CJ, Gordon GJ, Heilig E, Kelsey KT. Alteratuions of the p16 (INK4) locus in human malignant mesothelial tumors. *Carcinogenesis* 2002; 23: 1127-1130.

Hoang CD, D'Cunha J, Kratzke MG, Casmey CE, Frizelle SP, Maddaus MA, Kratzke RA. Gene expression profiling identifies matriptase overexpression in malignant mesothelioma. *Chest* 2004;125:1843-52.

Hinoi T, Yamamoto H, Kishida M, Kikuchi A. Complex formation of adenomatous polyposis coli gene product and axin facilitates glycogen synthase kinase-3 beta-dependent phosphorylation of beta-catenin and down-regulates beta-catenin. *J. Biol. Chem.* 275:34399-406.

Hoang CD, Zhang X, Scott PD, Guillaume TJ, Maddaus MA, Yee D, Kratzke RA. Selective activation of insulin receptor substrate 1 and 2 in pleural mesothelioma cells: association with distinct malignant phenotypes. *Cancer Res.* 2004; 64: 7479-85.

Holmgren L, O'Reilly MS, Folkman J. Dormancy of micrometastasis: balanced proliferation and apoptosis in the presence of angiogenesis suppression. *Nat. Med.* 1995; 1: 149-53.

Hopkins-Donaldson D et al. Inductions of apoptosis and chemosensitization of mesothelioma cells by Bcl-2 and Bcl-xL antisense treatment. *Int. J. Cancer* 2003; 106: 160-6.

Hopkins-Donaldson S, Belyanskaya AL, Simões-Wüst AP, Sigrist B, Kurtz S, Zagenmeister-Wittke U, Stahel R. p53-induced apoptosis occurs in the absence of p14(ARF) in malignant pleural mesothelioma. *Neoplasia* 2006;8:551-9.

Isik R, Metintas M, Gibbs AR, Metintas S, Jasani B, Oner U, Harmanci E, Demircan S, Isiksoy S. p53, p21 and metallothionein immunoreactivities in patients with malignant pleural mesothelioma: correlations with the epidemiological features and prognosis of mesotheliomas with environmental asbestos exposure. *Respir Med.* 2001;95:588-93.

Janne PA, Taffaro ML, Salgia R, Johnson BE. Inhibition of epidermal growth factor receptor signaling in malignant pleural mesothelioma. *Cancer Res.* 2002 ;62:5242-7.

Kafiri G, Thomas DM, Shepherd NA, Krausz T, Lane DP, Hall PA. P53 expression is common in malignant mesothelioma. *Histopathology* 1992; 21: 331-4.

Kayagaki N, Kawasaki A, Ebata T, Ohmoto H, Ikeda S, Inoue S, Yoshino K, Okumura K, Yagita H. Metalloproteinase-mediated release of human Fas ligand. *J. Exp. Med.* 1995;182:1777-83.

Kettunen E, Nicholson AG, Nagy B, Wikman H, Seppanene JK, Stjernvall T, Ollikainen T, Kinnula V, Nordling S, Hollmen J, Anttila S, Knuutila S. L1 CAM, INP10, P-cadherin, tPA and ITGB4 over expression in malignant pleural mesotheliomas revealed by combined use of cDNA and tissue microarray. *Carcinogenesis* 2005; 26: 17-25.

Kokturk N, Firat P, Akay H, Kadilar C, Ozturk C, Zorlu F, Gungen Y, Emri S. Prognostic significance of Bax and Fas ligand in erionite and asbestos induced Turkish malignant pleural mesothelioma. *Lung Cancer* 2005; 50: 189-98.

Kratzke RA, Otterson GA, Lincoln CE, Ewing S, Oie H, Geradts J, Kaye FJ. Immunohistochemical analysis of the p16INK4 cyclin-dependent kinase inhibitor in malignant mesothelioma. *J. Natl. Cancer Inst.* 1995;87:1870-5.

Kumar-Singh S, Weyler J, Martin MJ, Vermeulen PB, Van Marck E. Angiogenic cytokines in mesothelioma: a study of VEGF, FGF-1 and -2, and TGF beta expression. *J. Pathol.* 1999; 189:72-8.

Kumar-Singh S, Vermeulen PB, Weyler J, Segers K, Wein B, Van Daele A, Dirix LY, Van Oosterom AT, Van Marck E. Evaluation of tumour angiogenesis as a prognostic marker in malignant mesothelioma. *J. Pathol.* 1997; 182:211-6.

Ladanyi M, Implications of P16/CDKN2A deletion in pleural mesotheliomas. *Lung Cancer* 2005; 49 Suppl 1: S95-98.

Langerak AW, De Laat PA, Van Der Linden-Van Beurden CA, Delahaye M, Van Der Kwast TH, Hoogsteden HC, Benner R, Versnel MA. Expression of platelet-derived growth factor (PDGF) and PDGF receptors in human malignant mesothelioma in vitro and in vivo. *J. Pathol.* 1996; 178: 151-60.

Liu Z, Ivanoff A, Klominek J. Expression and activity of matrix metalloproteases in human malignant mesothelioma cell lines. *Int. J. Cancer* 2001; 91: 638-43.

Liu Z, Klominek J. Inhibition of proliferation, migration, and matrix metalloprotease production in malignant mesothelioma cells by tyrosine kinase inhibitors. *Neoplasia* 2004;6:705-12.

Liu Z, Klominek J. Regulation of matrix metalloprotease activity in malignant mesothelioma cell lines by growth factors. *Thorax* 2003; 58: 198-203.

Lopez-Rios F, Chuai S, Flores R, Shimizu S, Ohno T, Wakahara K, Illei PB, Hussain S, Krug L, Zakowski MF, Rusch V, Olshen AB, Ladanyi M. Global gene expression profiling of pleural mesotheliomas: overexpression of aurora kinases and P16/CDKN2A deletion as prognostic factors and critical evaluation of microarray-based prognostic prediction. *Cancer Res.* 2006 ; 66: 2970-2979.

Mayall FG, Jacobson G, Wilkins R. Mutations of p53 gene and SV40 sequences in asbestos associated and non asbestos-associated mesotheliomas. *J. Clin. Pathol.* 1999; 52: 291-293.

Merritt RE, Yamada RE, Wasif N, Crystal RG, Korst RJ. Effect of inhibition of multiple steps of angiogenesis in syngeneic murine pleural mesothelioma. *Ann. Thorac. Surg.* 2004; 78: 1042-51.

Mor O, Yaron P, Huszar M, yellin A, Jakobovitz O, Brok-Simoni F, Recavi G, Reichert N. Absence of p53 mutations in malignant mesotheliomas. *Am. J. Respir. Cell Mol. Biol.* 1997; 16: 9-13.

Narasimhan SR, Yang L, Gerwin BI, Broaddus VC. Resistence of pleural mesothelioma cell lines to apoptosis: relations to expression of Bcl-2 and Bax. *Am. J. Physiol.* 1998; 275: 5315-20.

O'Byrne KJ, Dalgleish AG, Browning MJ, Steward WP, Harris AL. The relationship between angiogenesis and the immune response in carcinogenesis and the progression of malignant disease. *Eur. J. Cancer* 2000; 36: 151-169.

O'Byrne KJ, Edwards JG, Waller DA. Clinico-pathological and biological prognostic factors in pleural malignant mesothelioma. *Lung Cancer* 2004;45 Suppl 1:S45-8.

Ono M, Kuwano M. Molecular mechanisms of epidermal growth factor receptor (EGFR) activation and response to gefitinib and other EGFR-targeting drugs. *Clin. Cancer Res.* 2006; 12: 7242-51.

Ordonez NG. The diagnostic utility of immunohistochemistry in distinguishing between epithelioid mesotheliomas and squamous carcinomas of the lung: a comparative study. *Mod. Pathol.* 2006; 19: 417-28.

Otha Y, Shridar V, Bright RK, Kalemkerian GP, Du W, Carbone N, Watanabe Y, Pass HI. VEGF and VEGF type C play an important role in angiogenesis and lymphangiogenesis in human malignant mesothelioma tumours. *Br. J. Cancer* 1999;81:54-61.

Otterson GA, Kratzke RA, Coxon A, Kim YW, Kaye FJ. Absence of p16INK4 protein is restricted to the subset of lung cancer lines that retains wildtype RB. *Oncogene* 1994; 11:3375-8.

Ozvaran KM, Cao XX, Miller SD, Monia BA, Hong WK, Smythe WR. Antisense oligonucleotides directed at the bcl-xl gene product augment chemotherapy response in mesothelioma. *Mol. Cancer Ther.* 2004;3:545-50.

Pache JC, Janssen YM, Walsh ES, Quinlan TR, Zanella CL, Low RB, Taatjes DJ, Mossman BT. Increased epidermal growth factor receptor protein in a human mesothelial cell line in response to long asbestos fibers. *Am. J. Pathol.* 1998; 152: 333-340.

Park S, Schalling M, Bernard A, Maheswaran S, Shipley GC, Roberts D, fletcher J, Shipman R, Rheinwald J, Demetri G et al. The Wilms tumour gene WT1 is expressed in murine mesoderm derived tissues and mutated in a human mesothelioma. *Nat. Genet.* 1993; 4: 415-20.

PassHI, Liu Z, Wali A, Bueno R, Land S, Lott D, Siddiq F, Lonardo F, Carbone M, Draghici S. Gene expression profiles predict survival and progression of pleural mesothelioma. *Clin. Canc Res.* 2004;10: 849-859.

Poulikakos PI, Xiao GH, Gallagher R, Jablonski S, Jhanwar SC, Testa JR. Re-expression of the tumor suppressor NF2/merlin inhibits invasiveness in mesothelioma cells and negatively regulates FAK. *Oncogene* 2006; 25: 5960-8.

Rascoe PA, Cao X, Daniel JC, Miller SD, Smythe WR. Receptor tyrosine kinase and phosphoinositide-3 kinase signaling in malignant mesothelioma. *J. Thorac. Cardiovasc. Surg.* 2005;130:393-400.

Rihn BH, Mohr S, McDowell SA, Binet S, Loubinoux J, galateau F, Keith G, Leikauf GD. Differential gene expression in mesothelioma. *FEBS Lett.* 2000;480:95-100.

Rippo MR, Moretti S, Vescovi S, Tomasetti M, Orecchia S, Amici G, Catalano A, Procopio A. FLIP overexpression inhibits death receptor-induced apoptosis in malignant mesothelial cells. *Oncogene* 2004;23:7753-60.

Romano M, Catalano A, Nutini M, D'Urbano E, Crescenzi C, Claria J, Libner R, Davi G, Procopio A. 5-lipoxygenase regulates malignant mesothelial cell survival: involvement of vascular endothelial growth factor. *FASEB J.* 2001;15:2326-36.

Russo P, Catassi A, Malacarne D, Margaritora S, Cesario A, Festi L, Mule A, Ferri L, Granone P. Tumor necrosis factor enhances SN38-mediated apoptosis in mesothelioma cells. *Cancer* 2005; 103: 1503-18.

Segers K, Ramael M, Singh SK, Weyler J, Van Meerbeeck J, Vermeire P, Van Marck E. Immunoreactivity for bcl-2 protein in malignant mesotelioma and non neoplastic mesothelium. *Virchows Arch.* 1994; 424: 631-4.

Seino K, Kayagaki N, Okumura K, Yagita H. Antitumor effect of locally produced CD95 ligand. *Nat. Med.* 1997;3(2):165-70.

Sherr CJ. Cancer cell cycles. *Science* 1996; 274: 1672-7.

Sherr CJ. Principles of tumor suppression. *Cell* 2004; 116: 235-46.

Shivapurkar N, Toyooka S, Toyooka KO, Reddy J, Miyaima K, Suzuki M, Shigematsu H, Takahashi T, Parikh G, Pass HI, Chadhary PM, Gazdar AF. Aberrant methylation of trail decoy receptor genes is frequent in multiple tumor types. *Int. J. Cancer* 2004; 109:786-92.

Syrokou A, Tzanakakis GN, Hjerpe A, Karamanos NK. Proteoglycans in human malignant mesothelioma. Stimulation of their synthesis induced by epidermal, insulin and platelet derived growth factors involves receptors with tyrosine kinase activity. *Biochimie* 1999; 81: 733-744.

Soini Y, Kinnula V, Kaarteenaho-Wiik R, Kurttila E, Linnainmaa K, Paakko P. Apoptosis and expression of apoptosis regulating proteins bcl-2, mcl-1, bcl-X, and bax in malignant mesothelioma. *Clin. Cancer Res.* 1999; 5: 3508-3515.

Stacker SA, Caesar C, Baldwin ME, Thornton GE, Williams RA, Prevo R, Jackson DG, Nishikawa S, Kubo H, Achen MG. VEGF-D promotes the metastatic spread of tumor cells via the lymphatics. *Nat. Med.* 2001; 7: 186-191.

Stewart JH4th, Nguyen DM, Chen GA, Schrump DS. Induction of apoptosis in malignant pleural mesothelioma cells by activation of the Fas (Apo-1/CD95) death-signal pathway. *J. Thorac. Cardiovasc Surg.* 2002;123:295-302.

Strizzi L, Catalano A, Vianale G, Orecchia S, Casalini A, Tassi g, Puntoni R, Mutti L, Procopio A. Vascular endothelial growth factor is an autocrine growth factor in human malignant mesothelioma. *J. Pathol.* 2001;193:468-75.

Sugiyama H. Cancer immunotherapy targeting Wilms' tumor gene WT1 product. *Expert. Rev. Vaccines* 2005; 4: 503-512.

Sun X, Gulyàs M, Hjerpe A, Dobra K. Proteasome inhibitor PSI induces apoptosis in human mesothelioma cells. *Cancer Lett.* 2006;232:161-9.

Tolnay E, Kuhnen C, Wiethege T, Konig JE, Voss B, Muller KM. Hepatocyte growth factor/scatter factor and its receptor c-Met are overexpressed and associated with an increased microvessel density in malignant pleural mesothelioma. *J. Cancer Res. Clin. Oncol.* 1998; 124:291-6.

Toyooka S, Pass HI, Shivapurkar N, Fukuyama Y, Maruyama R, Toyooka KO, Gilcrease M, Farinas A, Minna JD, Gazdar AF. Aberrant methylation and simian virus 40 tag sequences in malignant mesothelioma. *Cancer Res.* 2001; 61: 5727-5730.

Trusolino L, Bertotti A, Comoglio PM. A signaling adapter function for alpha6beta4 integrin in the control of HGF-dependent invasive growth. *Cell* 2001; 107: 643-54.

Versnel MA, Claesson-Welsh L, Hammacher A, .human malignant mesothelioma cell lines express PDGF beta-receptors whereas cultured normal mesothelial cells express predominantly PDGF alpha receptors. *Oncogene* 1991; 6: 2005-11.

Whitson BA, Kratzke RA. Molecular pathways in malignant pleural mesothelioma. *Cancer Letters* 2006; 239: 183-189.

Wong L, Zhou J, Anderson D, Kratzke RA. Inactivation of p16INK4a expression in malignant mesothelioma by methylation. *Lung Cancer* 2002; 38: 131-6.

Xia C, Xu Z, Yuan X, Uematsu K, You L, Li K, Li L, McCormick F, Jablous DM. Induction of apoptosis in mesothelioma cells by antisurvivin oligonucleotides. *Molecular Cancer Therapeutics* 2002; 1: 687-94.

Xiao GH, Gallagher R, Shetler J, Skele K, Altomare DA, Pestell RG, Jhanwar S, Testa JR. The NF2 tumor suppressor gene product, merlin inhibits cell proliferation and cell cycle progression by repressing cyclin D1 expression. *Mol. Cell Biol.* 2005; 25: 2384-94.

Xio S, Li D, Vijg J, Sugarbaker DJ, Corson JM, Fletcher JA. Codeletion of p15 and p16 in primary malignant mesothelioma. *Oncogene* 1995; 11: 511-5.

Yang CT, You L, Lin YC, Lin CT, McCormick F, Jablons DM. A comparison analysis of anti-tumor efficacy of adenoviral gene replacement therapy (p14ARF and p16INK4A) in human mesothelioma cells. *Anticancer Res.* 2003; 23:33-8.

Yang CT, You L, Yet C-C, Chang J W-C, Zhang F, McCormick F, Jablons DM. Adenovirus-mediated p14(ARF) gene transfer in human mesothelioma cells. *J. Natl. Cancer Inst.* 2000; 92:636-41.

In: Mesothelioma from Bench Side to Clinic
Editor: Alfonso Baldi, pp. 137-155

ISBN: 978-1-60021-789-0

Chapter VII

Cell-Cycle Molecules in Mesothelioma

Mara Campioni[1], Vincenzo Ambrogi[2], Anna Severino[3], Tommaso Claudio Mineo[2], Mario Caputi[4], and Alfonso Baldi[1]

[1]Dept. Biochemistry, Sect. Pathology, Second University of Naples, Italy
[2]Dept. Thoracic Surgery, Tor Vergata University, Rome, Italy
[3]Inst. Cardiology, Catholic University, Rome, Italy
[4] Dept. Cardiological, Respiratory and Thoracic Medical Sciences, Second University of Naples, Italy

Abstract

The cell cycle is the cascade of events that allows a growing cell to duplicate all its component and split into two daughter cells. Several studies report the importance of cell cycle proteins in the pathogenesis and the prognosis of mesothelioma. Cell cycle progression is mediated by the activation of a highly conserved family of protein kinases, the cyclin-dependent kinases (CDKs). CDKs are also regulated by related proteins called cdk inhibitors grouped into two families: the INK4 inhibitors (p16, p15, p19 and p18) and the Cip/Kip inhibitors (p21, p27 and p53). This article will review the most recent data from the literature about the expression and the diagnostic and prognostic significance of cell cycle molecules in mesothelioma.

Introduction

Malignant mesothelioma is a rare, highly aggressive tumour, which accounts for less than 1% of all cancer deaths [1]. This neoplasm arises from the surface serosal cells of the pleural (>90% of cases), peritoneal, and pericardial cavities and from the tunica vaginalis of the testis [2]. Although the association between exposure to asbestos and the development of mesothelioma is commonly accepted, the exact mechanism whereby asbestos induces the mesothelioma is unknown [3]. The prognosis is generally poor with a reported median survival of 4–12 months in either untreated or treated (surgery, radiotherapy, or chemotherapy) patients [4]. Moreover, mesothelioma has proved resistant to classical chemotherapeutic and radiation regimes and the natural history has not been influenced by standard therapy [5]. Several studies report the importance of cell cycle proteins in the pathogenesis and the prognosis of this neoplasm [6].

Cell Cycle

The cell cycle is the cascade of events that allows a growing cell to duplicate all its components and split into two daughter cells; it consists of four distinct phases: G1 phase, S phase, G2 phase (collectively known as interphase) and M phase. High fidelity duplication of DNA in each cell during the S phase and the proper migration of the duplicated chromosomes in mitosis are highly regulated processes.

Eukaryotic cells have evolved cell cycle machinery with a series of surveillance pathways, termed cell cycle checkpoints, so the progression through the cell cycle is ensured by intrinsic mechanisms that regulate the dependence of one cell cycle event on another.

Cyclins and *cyclin-dependend kinases (CDKs)* are the two critical classes of molecules involved in the regulation of cell cycle progression. These proteins form an heterodimer in which cyclins are the regulatory subunits and CDKs are the catalytic subunits; when the complex is activated from external signals, CDKs activates or inactivates downstream target proteins to orchestrate coordinated entry into the next phase of the cell cycle [7].

In normal cells, CDKs are expressed throughout all the cycle; however, each cyclin protein has a restricted period of expression, and this limited expression of each cyclin protein is due to cell cycle-dependent regulation of both cyclin gene transcription and protein degradation.

The cyclin/CDK complex is regulated by a number of phosphorylation and dephosphorylation events, resulting either in activation or inhibition of kinase activity [8]: phosphorylation is carried out by *cyclin-activating kinase (CAK),* and dephosphorylation is mediated by members of the *Cell Division Cycle 25 family (Cdc25)* of dual-specificity protein phosphatases. The mammalian Cdc25 family consists of three members: Cdc25A, Cdc25B, and Cdc25C. Cdc25A promotes entry into S phase by acting on cyclin A/CDK2 and cyclin E/CDK2 and is required for DNA replication [9-12]. Cdc25B activation occurs during S phase and peaks during the G2 phase [13, 14]. Both Cdc25B and Cdc25C play roles in the G2/M transition. Cdc25C dephosphorylates cyclin B1/cdc2 and is essential for progression through the G2/M phase of the cell cycle [15].

Decision to enter S phase is made in mid-to-late G1 and is called the *restriction point.* Molecular switch from G1 to S phase and targets of the G1 phase cyclin/CDK complexes are members of the retinoblastoma protein (RB) family: RB, p107 and p130 [16]. RB can function as either a transcriptional repressor or a transcriptional activator depending on its phosphorylation state and the proteins with which it binds: when hypophosphorylated and bound to the E2F family of transcription factors it works as a transcriptional repressor [17]. The E2F family mediates transcription of genes required for DNA synthesis, including cyclin E, cyclin A, cyclin B, dihydrofolate reductase, and thymidine kinase [18]. Sequential phosphorylation of RB by cyclin D/CDK4/6 and cyclinE/CDK2 complexes inhibits the repressor activity of RB, as it results in the dissociation of E2F and RB, and S phase entry. As cells progress into S phase, maintenance of RB hyperphosphorylation is necessary for the successful completion of DNA replication [19]. Mutations that affect the RB signaling pathway have been identified in the majority of human cancers [20].

CDKs are also regulated by a group of functionally related proteins called *CDK inhibitors*. The CDK inhibitors are grouped into two families: the INK4 inhibitors (p16, p15, p19 and p18) and the Cip/Kip inhibitors (p21, p27 and p53). The INK4 family specifically inhibits CDK4 and CDK6 activity during the G1 phase of the cell cycle, while the Cip/Kip family inhibits CDK activity during all phases of the cell cycle. Both families of these inhibitors can arrest cells in the G1 phase of the cell cycle by inhibiting the activities of CDKs and preventing their ability to phosphorylate and inactive RB and other RB-family proteins [7].

The *S phase* of the cell cycle is the stage in which occurs the DNA replication. At the beginning of the S phase, each chromosome is composed of one coiled DNA double helix molecule; at the end of this stage each chromosome has two identical DNA double helix molecules, and therefore is composed of two sister chromatids. During this phase, the centrosome is also duplicated [21,22]. It is proposed that replication origins are in two different states during the cell cycle: one during G1 phase, before DNA replication begins, when a multiprotein pre-replicative complex (*pre-RC*) assembles on the origin. The second state exists from the initiation of S phase to the end of M phase, when a post-replicative complex (*post-RC*) is present at the replication origins.

Initiator proteins required for pre-RC formation include the Origin Recognition Complex (ORC), MCM proteins (that forms the replicative elicase), Cdc6 and Cdt1 (required to load MCM proteins on chromatin)[23-26]. This multiprotein complex is activated at the G1/S transition; subsequently, DNA replicating proteins such as DNA polymerase α and β. are recruited to initiation sites [27]. An increase in CDK2 and hcdc7 activity at the G1/S transition triggers initiation and converts the origin to the post-RC state. The CDK cycle controls the two states at replication origins, couples the initiation of S phase to the completion of M phase, and prevents re-replication events from occurring during a single round of the cell cycle [28, 29].

As cells enter into *G2 phase,* the cyclin B/cdc2 complexes are kept inactive by phosphorylation. At the end of this phase the cells are ready to enter into mitosis, and cyclin B/cdc2 complexes are activated by dephosphorylation [30]. The enzyme that dephosphorylates and activates cdc2 at the end of G2 and initiates mitosis is Cdc25C [31]. This transition point is one of the most important during the progression of cell cycle, and different mechanisms control this stage. Cdc25C is localized in the cytoplasm during interphase and enters the nucleus just before mitosis. Also cyclin B1 is in the cytoplasm during S phase and G2 phase and is translocated to the nucleus at the beginning of mitosis [32]. It is thought that the precise regulation of cyclin B1 localization prevents premature mitosis during interphase, while allowing regulated access of cyclin B1/cdc2 complexes to their nuclear substrates at the onset of mitosis. Although less well understood, Cdc25B and A/Cdc2 also play a role at the mitotic transition.

As cells enter *mitosis,* phosphorylation of key components causes significant changes in the architecture of the cell and this phosphorylation is due mainly to cyclin B/cdc2 activity [33]. This complex induces changes in the microtubule network, in the actin microfilaments, and in the nuclear lamina [34]. Other cyclin B/cdc2 substrates include histone H1 and microtubule-associated proteins such as MAP4, MAP2, and stathmin [35]. The family of polo-like protein kinases (Plks) also plays a critical role in several mitotic events [36]. They are critical for the formation of a bipolar spindle. It is proposed that Plks initiate the onset of mitosis by activating Cdc25C. Plks are also important regulators of mitotic exit.

Mitotic exit requires sister chromatid separation, spindle disassembly, and cytokinesis. The initiation and coordination of these processes are controlled by degradation of key regulatory proteins. The mediator of this protein destruction is a multisubunit protein called the *anaphase-promoting complex (APC)* or cyclosome [37]. Key APC substrates are the mitotic A- and B-type cyclins. Cyclin A is degraded in metaphase, whereas B-type cyclins are degraded when cells enter anaphase [38]. Cyclin B1 destruction starts as soon as the last chromosomes are aligned on the metaphase plate and is complete by the end of metaphase [39]. Another group of APC substrates are proteins that function as anaphase inhibitors. During G2, sister chromatids are held together by proteins called cohesins, which require inactivation by APC for anaphase initiation [40]. Overall, the APC regulates two different steps in mitosis. First, sister chromatid separation is triggered by destruction of the anaphase inhibitors, after which spindle disassembly and mitotic exit are initiated by the degradation of mitotic cyclins. These two steps allow the cell to couple the exit from mitosis to the prior completion of anaphase.

Cell Cycle Checkpoint

Cell cycle checkpoints are signal transduction pathways monitoring the successful completion of events in one phase of the cell cycle before proceeding to the next phase. Cell cycle checkpoints contain sensor proteins that scan chromatin for partially replicated DNA, DNA breaks, or other abnormalities. Sensor proteins are thought to translate DNA-derived stimuli into biochemical signals that modulate specific downstream target proteins and activate signaling pathways involved in DNA repair and cell cycle arrest [41]. Further, when cellular damage is irreparable, checkpoint signaling could eliminate potentially hazardous cells by permanent cell cycle arrest or apoptosis.

The physiological relevance of these signaling pathways is supported by their evolutionary conservation and the finding that the major consequence of their alteration in humans is tumorigenesis [41]; in fact, the loss of cell cycle checkpoints is a universal alteration identified in human cancer. Although numerous genetic alterations can result in loss of normal checkpoints, the hope is that common strategies will be developed against a wide variety of cancers.

G1/S Phase Checkpoint

The G1 cell cycle checkpoint prevents damaged DNA from being replicated and is the best understood checkpoint in mammalian cells. Progression of cells through early G1, across the restriction point into late G1 and then into S phase requires the coordinated regulation of multiple positive and negative factors [42]. Cyclin D-CDK4/6 complexes promote early G1 progression, but cyclin E (or cyclin A)-CDK2 (or CDK1) activity is required to inactive RB by hyperphosphorylation to transit the restriction point into late G1 phase [43]. RB inactivation results in release of E2F transcription factors and induction of late-G1-specific genes, including dihydrofolatereductase (DHFR), Emi1, and cyclin A [44]. Cyclin A-associated kinase activity is required to initiate DNA synthesis, prevent rereplication, and enter mitosis.

Although cyclin A is transcriptionally induced by E2Fs at the restriction point, cyclin A protein does not accumulate until the late G1/S phase transition due to ubiquitination by the anaphase promoting complex (APC) and subsequent proteolysis by the 26S proteasome. APC is active throughout G1 phase by association with Cdh1 (APCCdh1), an activator that confers substrate specificity [45]. Prior to initiation of S phase, APCCdh1 is inactivated by the binding of Emi1 to Cdh1, resulting in stabilization of cyclin A, activation of cyclin A-associated kinase activity, and subsequent inactivation of Cdh1 by phosphorylation [46]. Thus, tight regulation of cyclin E- and A-associated kinase activity results in a coordinated G1 cell cycle progression [47].

If DNA is damaged the G1/S checkpoint prevent transition of cells into S phase. Due to its essential and rate-limiting role in G1/S transition, cyclin E/CDK2 is a key target for the DNA damage checkpoint [12]. Damage to DNA inhibits the action of CDK2 thus stopping the progression of the cell cycle until the damage can be repaired. If the damage is so severe that it cannot be repaired, the cell self-destructs by apoptosis. It is proposed that after exposure of cells to UV or IR, the level of Cdc25A phosphatase rapidly decreases [12]. Cdc25A removes the inhibitory phosphorylation on CDK2 that is required for G1/S transition. After IR or UV exposure, Cdc25A is rapidly phosphorylated by Chk2 and Chk1, respectively. Chk-mediated phosphorylation triggers accelerated turnover of Cdc25A and thus inhibition of CDK2 [48]. An endpoint of this checkpoint signaling is inhibition of CDK2-dependent loading of Cdc45 onto the DNA prereplication complexes and thus inhibition of S phase [49].

Another important target for checkpoint signaling in cells that are in G1/S transition before the restriction point is the p53 tumor suppressor protein [50]. In normal, non stressed cells, p53 protein has short half-life as result of the rapid MDM2-mediated degradation of the protein after synthesis [51, 52].

After exposure of cells to stress p53 phosphorylation changes and protein levels increase significantly [50]. Transducers that are required for p53-mediated maintenance of G1 checkpoint arrest are the same as those required for activation of the checkpoint, namely the ATM/ATR and Chk2/Chk1kinases. Among the genes regulated by p53, the CDK-inhibitor p21WAF1/Cip1 plays a central role in G1 checkpoint by inhibiting CDKs that are essential for entry into S phase [53-55]. Thus, although ATM/ATR-mediated signaling can phosphorylate key targets Cdc25A and p53 within minutes after DNA damage, the impact of the signaling pathways regulated by Cdc25A and p53 on CDK2 activity and G1/S blockage are separated in time, due to the dependence of p53 signaling on transcription and protein synthesis.

Human cells also have evolved additional mechanisms to prolong a G1 cell cycle checkpoint arrest. For example, after exposure of keratinocytes and melanocytes to physiological doses of UV radiation, there is an increase of the CDK-inhibitor p16INK4a [56]. This factor acts as tumor suppressor which inhibits the activities of cyclin D-dependent kinases, CDK4 and CDK6, and regulates the activities of RB [57]. Given the direct role that CDK-inhibitors play in regulation of the G1/S transition, it is not surprising that CDK-inhibitor function is often compromised in human tumors. The p16INK4A gene is the frequent target of mutations that ablate its function, including point mutations, promoter methylation, or homozygous deletions [58]. Likewise, many human breast cancers have reduced p27Kip1 protein expression or aberrant sub-cellular localization of the protein that has been correlated with more aggressive tumors [59,60].

S Phase Checkpoint

The S-phase checkpoint monitors cell cycle progression and decreases the rate of DNA synthesis following DNA damage. The responses of cells that are already in S phase at the time of the DNA damage will be critical for optimal outcome of the cell. These cells must respond virtually instantaneously to halt initiation of new replication forks throughout S phase, and the first action to prevent wrong DNA synthesis is the activation of the ATM (ataxia telangiectasia mutated) and/or ATR (ATM and Rad3-related) protein kinase [54]. Both of these proteins belong to a structurally unique family of serine-threonine kinases, but they generally respond to distinct types of DNA damage.

ATM is the primary mediator of the response to DNA double strand breaks (DSBs) that can arise by exposure to ionizing radiation (IR). [61]. For responses to other types of DNA damage, such as base damage caused by exposure to ultraviolet light or alkylating agents, the ATR kinase appears to be important for initiating the relevant signal transduction pathways [62].

Once ATM or ATR has been activated by the introduction of DNA damage, these protein kinases begin to phosphorylate substrates to help the cell arrest cell cycle progression or repair DNA. As discussed previously, the phosphorylation of p53, MDM2, and Chk2 by ATM following DNA damage contributes to the arrest of cells in G1 before the restriction point. Among the proteins phosphorylated by ATM that contribute to arrest of cells in S phase are Nbs1, Brca1, SMC1, and FAncD2 [63-66]. The importance of this process in cancer formation in humans is suggested by the fact that many of these genes are mutated in familial cancer syndromes. For example, the cancer susceptibility syndromes Ataxia-telangiectasia, Nijmegen breakage syndrome, Fanconi's anemia, and familial breast/ovarian carcinoma syndrome are caused by inherited mutations in ATM, Nbs1, FAncD2, and Brca1, respectively.

G2 Checkpoint

In addition to activation of the G1/S and S phase checkpoints, DNA damage also activates checkpoint arrest in G2 to prevent the passage of DNA lesions to two daughter cells during mitosis. At this stage entry into mitosis is controlled by the activity of the cyclin dependent kinase Cdc2. Maintenance of the inhibitory phosphorylations on Cdc2 is essential for G2 checkpoint activation. ATM and ATR indirectly modulate the phosphorylation status of these sites in response to DNA damage. These DNA damage checkpoint pathways all share common upstream signaling pathways made up of the ATM/ATR transducer and Chk2/Chk1 effector kinases [67].

Activation of the G2 checkpoint after genotoxic stress involves ATM-mediated phosphorylation and activation of the Chk1 and Chk2 kinases [68,69]. It is proposed that direct inhibition of Cdc25 activity by Chk1 is sufficient for proficient checkpoint regulation of Cdc25 and that Cdc25C might be inhibited by another upstream kinase, Plk1 [70]. The activity of Plk1 is inhibited in the G2 phase of human tumor cells exposed to ionizing radiation, camptothecin, and doxorubicin. Further, expression of a mutant Plk1 in which residues necessary for Plk1 activation are altered, prevents Plk1 inactivation and leads to G2 override in cells treated with doxorubicin [71].

In addition to a role in G1/S checkpoint function, p53-mediated signaling plays an integral role in maintenance of the G2 checkpoint delay after activation of the checkpoint. p53 is believed to exert G2 checkpoint responses through transcriptional up-regulation of the downstream target genes p21, 14-3-3, and GADD45. Similar to its regulation of the cyclin D1/cdk4,6 or cyclin E/cdk2 complexes at the G1/S checkpoint, p21 can bind to and inhibit the cyclin B1/cdc2 complex and inhibit cyclin-activated kinase-mediated cdc2 activation [72]. The p53-dependent increase in 14-3-ȝmodulates the sub-cellular localization of the cyclin B1/Cdc2 complex, as the binding of 14-3-ȝto cdc2 results in retention of the kinase in the cytoplasm [73]. The p53-mediated GADD45-dependent G2 arrest is induced only after specific types of DNA damage, as lymphocytes from GADD45 knockout mice failed to arrest after exposure to UV radiation but retained the G2 checkpoint initiated by ionizing radiation [74].

Spindle Checkpoint

The mitotic spindle checkpoint monitors spindle microtubule structure, chromosome alignment on the spindle, and chromosome attachment to kinetochores during mitosis [75]. The spindle checkpoint delays the onset of chromosome segregation during anaphase until any defects in the mitotic spindle are corrected. Unattached kinetochores are thought to be the source of the checkpoint signal, and mechanical tension at the kinetochore dictates whether the checkpoint is initiated or not [76]. Activation of the spindle checkpoint prevents mitotic progression through inhibition of the anaphase-promoting complex activator, Cdc20 [76]. Mediators of the spindle checkpoint pathway include the Mad2, Bub1, and Bub3 proteins [75]. Mad2 localizes to the kinetochores during prometaphase until alignment of the chromosomes occurs in metaphase and regulates mitotic exit by interaction with components of the APC machinery (such as Cdc20) that mediate anaphase entry. Bub1 and Bub3 also localize to kinetochores and regulate chromosome/kinetochore interactions, and both are required for cell cycle arrest after disruption of microtubule dynamics during mitosis [35]. Inactivating mutations in Bub1 have been identified in human colon carcinoma cell lines, suggesting that disruption of the spindle checkpoint could occur during tumor progression.

Integral to cell cycle regulation is the proper coordination of mitotic exit and subsequent S phase entry. After DNA synthesis, cells have a tetraploid (4N) DNA content that is reduced to a diploid (2N) DNA content in each daughter cell after successful completion of mitosis. Intact checkpoint pathways are needed to prevent the S phase entry of cells that have failed to properly segregate their chromosomes during mitosis. Cells with defective spindle checkpoint function can exit from mitosis with a 4N DNA content [35]. These cells can inappropriately continue to the next cell cycle division and, in the absence of a functional G1/S checkpoint, enter S phase with a 4N DNA content; this process is known as endoreduplication. Endoreduplication results in the generation of polyploid cells—that is, cells with a 4N or greater DNA content after mitotic exit. Cells that are RB-, p53-, p21-, or p16-deficient can endoreduplicate after microtubule inhibitor treatment [77, 78].

The G1 cell cycle regulators, however, do not directly regulate the mitotic arrest induced by microtubule inhibitors; rather, absence of these proteins allows deregulated CDK2 activity, the precise control of which is required for normal cells to maintain proper coupling of mitotic exit and S-phase entry [78, 79].

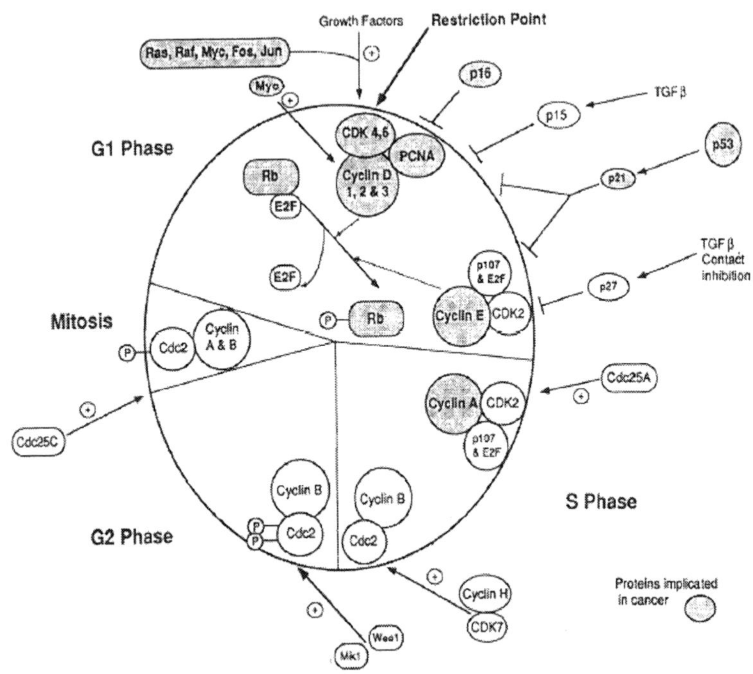

Figure 1. cell cycle and cancer.

Thus, in addition to playing a role in checkpoint function after DNA damage, proteins that mediate the G1/S checkpoint through regulation of cdk2 activity also prevent inappropriate S-phase entry after an abnormal mitotic exit and are critical to proper coordination of S-phase and mitosis.

In figure 1 the most important cell cycle molecules involved in cancer pathogenesis and progression, are depicted.

Cell Cycle Genes in Mesothelioma

First studies about cell cycle protein interference in mesothelioma dated 1998. In that period Beer et al [80] investigated the expression of the Ki-67 nuclear antigen detected by MIB-1 immunoreactivity as an indicator of cell proliferation and survival in pleural malignant mesotheliomas. Ki-67 is a well known nuclear antigen highly expressed in proliferating cells, routinely used as a prognostic factor in the assessment of tumour behaviour [81]. Beer and coll. showed that patients with a MIB-1 proliferation index less than 30% had a significantly longer survival than patients with a proliferation index exceeding that value. Similar observations were confirmed by Comin et al in 2000 [82].

A low mitotic count and a low apoptotic index defined by in situ end-labeling were also found to be associated with a significant survival advantage. The proliferation index, the mitotic count, and the apoptotic index, therefore, were proposed as useful prognostic markers in pleural malignant mesotheliomas [83].

In 2001 Bongiovanni and colleagues [84] provided the first evidence of a role of p27kip1 in predicting survival in a large series of long-term survival patients. As described previously, p27kip1 acts as inhibitor during the cell cycle progression from G1-phase to the S-phase; than this protein is defined a cell cycle regulator and a putative tumor suppressor gene [85,86]. In this paper the authors described as p27kip1 positively correlated to the length of survival: all patients presenting with length of survival exceeding 24 months had high p27kip1 values. They also found that the MIB-1/Ki-67 positivity, instead, was inversely correlated to the survival. In the same work they reported also that the combined evaluation of Ki-67 and p27kip1 together allowed a gain of additional reliability in the prediction of survival with a 100% specificity and sensitivity. Nuclear staining intensity of p27kip1 was found to be associated with survival: the higher the intensity, the longer the survival. The cytoplasmic localization of p27kip1 immunoreactivity was instead of little significance. Gunther et al, however, showed such localization to be a common event in rectal carcinoma and proved it to be the best prognostic factor of disease free survival in such neoplasms [87]. Moreover, in this study patients with intensive cytoplasmic p27kip1 expression showed a significantly poorer outcome, irrespective of their nuclear staining. Further investigations are needed to explain whether the nuclear and cytoplasmic distribution reflect two different biologic activities or two different regulative mechanism of p27kip1.

Histologic subtyping was considered one of the more useful criteria to recognize lesions with a favourable prognosis: epithelioid type usually is considered less aggressive than the biphasic and pure sarcomatoid types. However, the definite identification of the subtype could be difficult on small biopsy specimens especially for recognizing the mixed lesions.

Johansson and collegues showed that p27kip1 immunoreactivity was significantly higher in pure epithelioid compared with biphasic ones and they found also that Ki-67 had opposite expression in the two histotypes. This observation could provide a possible biologic counterpart to the usual, although not univocally recognized, better prognosis of epithelioid mesothelioma [88].

Several studies have investigated the potential prognostic value of other Cip/Kip inhibitors, as p53 and p21, and the role of the SV40 large T antigen (L-Tag) in malignant mesotheliomas.

It has been proposed that malignant transformation of human mesothelioma cells does not require inactivation of p53 by point mutations in the conserved regions of the gene [89]. Moreover, there are observation that p53 overexpression did not correlate in a statistical manner with survival, but its overexpression is a frequent feature of pleural mesothelioma and is useful for routine differentiating between malignant and non-neoplastic mesothelial alterations [90].

In 2001 Yang et al. [91] proposed that p53 is inactive in malignant pleural mesothelioma cells as a result of $p14^{ARF}$ deficiency. Homozygous deletions of INK4a/ARF locus have been shown to be the predominant events which occur at a frequency of >70% in this malignancy [92,93]. The INK4a/ARF locus [94] on human chromosome 9p21 plays an important role in both the pRB and p53 tumor suppressor pathways by encoding two distinct proteins translated from alternatively spliced mRNAs: $p16^{INK4a}$ regulates pRB phosphorylation and induces cell cycle arrest in G1 phase [95]; $p14^{ARF}$ plays a role as a negative regulator of MDM2, interfering with MDM2-mediated shuttling and degradation of p53 [96-98]. A single mutational event at the INK4a/ARF locus therefore has the potential to disrupt both pRB and p53 tumor suppressor pathways.

In a recent study, Hopkins-Donaldson et al [99] investigated the status of p53 in malignant pleural mesothelioma cells lacking $p14^{ARF}$. In contrast with the precedent observations, their findings suggest that p53 is functional in malignant pleural mesothelioma in the absence of $p14^{ARF}$; they found that p53 is activated by DNA damage, and in this way it contributes to the apoptotic response induced by cisplatin (CDDP). Moreover, Hopkins-Donaldson and collegues also demonstrates that removal of downstream inhibitors such as survivin can enhance this response more successfully than the disruption of p53–MDM2 interaction by $p14^{ARF}$.

In regard to the role of SV40 protein, De Luca et collegues found the presence of SV40-like sequences in 86% of 35 archival specimens of mesothelioma. They demonstrated that SV40 Tag, isolated from frozen biopsies of human mesothelioma, binds each of the retinoblastoma family proteins, pRb, p107 and pRb2/p130. They proposed that the tumorigenic potential of SV40 Tag in some human mesotheliomas may arise from its ability to interact with and thereby inactivate several tumor and/or growth suppressive proteins [100].

Baldi et al have investigated the expression of p21 in a group of mesothelioma specimens already characterized for the expression of p53 and for the presence of SV40 sequences [101]. In this study they did not found relationship between p21 expression and histological type in the mesothelioma specimens, but they showed that there was a significant positive relationship between p21 expression level and the overall survival of the patients, which suggests that the p21 pathway is involved in the pathogenesis of mesothelioma. This could occur by silencing p21 through p53 inactivation by SV40 proteins and/or the weaker activation of p21 by alternative pathways. A greater reduction in p21 expression will cause greater aggression and result in a poorer prognosis.

In a different work, Baldi et al analyzed the potential prognostic value of the immunohistochemical expression of cyclooxygenase-2 (COX-2) and p27 in 29 malignant mesotheliomas already screened for the expression of p21 and p53 [102]. COX-2 has been implicated in carcinogenesis of several neoplasms and it over-expression has been noted in many solid tumours and has been correlated with a worse prognosis in colorectal cancer, non-small cell lung cancer, and gastric cancer [88,103]. A recent study showed that COX-2 expression is a strong prognostic factor in human mesothelioma, which contributes independently to the other clinical and histopathological factors in determining a short survival [104]. It has been also proposed that COX-2 exerts its influence on mesangial cell proliferation in vitro by a novel mechanism involving the tumour suppressor p53 and the cell cycle inhibitors p21 and p27 [105]. In this work Baldi et al did not find any relationship between the levels of expression of the COX-2, p27, p21 and p53 and the histological types in their patients, but they observed that a high level of COX-2 expression and low p21 and p27 expression were associated with a statistically significant decrease in survival (Figure 2). These data agree with the lack of correlation reported by others between COX-2, p21 and p53 and type of mesothelioma [106, 107], but other groups have found a significant correlation between p27 expression and epithelioid histotype [108,109]. The data suggest that COX-2 expression may be a useful prognostic parameter and thus support further investigations into the clinical usefulness of COX-2 inhibitors in the treatment of malignant mesotheliomas.

In a recent study by Vivo et al [110] it has been investigated the anti-tumoral activity of recombinant human interferon gamma (r-hu-IFNgamma) on nine different human malignant mesothelioma cell lines. The authors showed that r-hu-IFNgamma produced an arrest in the G1 and G2-M phases of the cell cycle, associated with a reduction in both cyclin A and cyclin dependent kinase inhibitors (CDKIs) expression. Moreover cyclin B1/cdc2 activity was decreased. The cell cycle arrest induced by r-hu-IFNgamma seems to depend on cyclin regulation through p21(WAF1/CIP1)- and p27(Kip1)-independent mechanisms and is not directly related to the induced DNA damage.

Another interesting study by Mukohara et al [111] investigated a potential therapeutic role for the Met receptor in malignant pleural mesothelioma. Expression of the Met receptor and its ligand, hepatocyte growth factor (HGF), has been observed in 74% to 100% and 40% to 85% of malignant pleural mesothelioma specimens, respectively [112,113]. HGF stimulation has been shown to enhance malignant pleural mesothelioma cell proliferation, migration, cell scattering, and invasiveness [114]. The authors provided evidence supporting the possibility of therapeutic targeting HGF/Met signaling in malignant pleural mesothelioma. Disrupting HGF/Met signaling is potentially attractive as it may not only inhibit malignant pleural mesothelioma growth but also alter the rate of migration and invasion in a disease that is clinically characterized by local extension. However, the effects of Met receptor inhibition are limited to a minority of malignant pleural mesothelioma cell lines, those that also produce HGF. This study would predict that clinical trials of Met inhibitors, such as PHA-665752, in malignant pleural mesothelioma would be most effective in patients whose tumors express both Met and HGF.

Finally, a recent work by Adusumilli and collegues analyzed the effects of a potential oncolytic viral therapy in the treatment of malignant pleural mesothelioma [115]. The authors showed that cisplatin induces GADD34 (Growth Arrest and DNA Damage-Inducible Protein) expression in ten human malignant pleural mesothelioma cell lines, and that this up-regulation selectively enhanced the cytotoxicity of the gamma134.5-deficient oncolytic virus, NV1066. This provides a cellular basis for combination therapy with cisplatin and NV1066 to treat malignant pleural mesothelioma and achieve synergistic efficacy, while minimizing dosage and toxicity.

Conclusion

In conclusion, all the works mentioned here would provide useful information on the prognosis of newly diagnosed cases and would allow researchers to recognize a subgroup of patients with significantly improved survival, in which it could be possible to achieve better response to therapy. Nevertheless, targeting multiple checkpoint proteins may represent a good therapeutic strategy for the development of new molecular treatments for pleural mesothelioma. The data presented in this chapter support this hypothesis and strongly suggest further works aimed at investigating the simultaneous expression of numerous cell cycle regulators in mesotheliomas.

References

[1] Peto J, DeCarli A, La Vecchia C, et al. The European mesothelioma epidemic. *Br. J. Cancer* 1999; 79: 666–72.

[2] Attanos RI, Gibbs AR. Pathology of malignant mesothelioma. *Histopathology* 1997; 30: 403–18.

[3] Hughes JM, Weill H. Asbestos exposure: quantitative assessment of risk. *Am. Rev. Respir. Dis.* 1986; 133: 5–13.

[4] Sugarbaker DJ, Flores RM, Jaklitsch MT, et al. Resection margins, extrapleural nodal status, and cell type determine postoperative longterm survival in trimodality therapy of malignant pleural mesothelioma: results in 183 patients. *J. Thorac. Cardiovasc. Surg.* 1999; 117: 54–63.

[5] Pass HI, Robinson BW, Testa JR, et al. Emerging translational therapies for mesothelioma. *Chest* 1999;116:455–60S.

[6] Carbone M, Fisher S, Powers A, et al. New molecular and epidemiological issues in mesothelioma: role of SV40. *J. Cell Physiol.* 1999; 180: 167–72.

[7] Matsushime H, Ewen ME, Strom DK, et al: Identification and properties of an atypical catalytic subunit (p34*PSK-J3*/cdk4) for mammalian D type G1 cyclins. *Cell* 1992;71:323–334.

[8] Sherr CJ, Roberts JM: CDK inhibitors: Positive and negative regulators of G1-phase progression. *Genes Dev.* 1999;13:1501–1512.

[9] Jinno S, Suto K, Nagata A, et al: Cdc25A is a novel phosphatase functioning early in the cell cycle. *Embo J.* 1994;13:1549–1556.

[10] Saha P, Eichbaum Q, Silberman ED,Mayer BJ,Dutta A: p21CIP1 and Cdc25A: Competition between an inhibitor and an activator of cyclin-dependent kinases. *Mol. Cell Biol.* 1997;14:4338–4345.

[11] Hoffmann I, Draetta G, Karsenti E:Activation of the phosphatase activity of human cdc25A by a cdk2-cyclin E dependent phosphorylation at the G1/S transition. *Embo J.* 1994;13:4302–4310.

[12] Blomberg I, Hoffmann I: Ectopic expression of Cdc25A accelerates the G1/S transition and leads to premature activation of cyclin E and cyclin A-dependent kinases. *Mol. Cell Biol.* 1999;19:6183–6194.

[13] Lammer C,Wagerer S, Saffrich R, Mertens D,Ansorge W, Hoffmann I:The cdc25B phosphatase is essential for the G2/M phase transition in human cells. *J. Cell Sci.* 1998;111:2445–2453.

[14] Garner-Hamrick PA, Fisher C:Antisense phosphorothioate oligonucleotides specifically down-regulate cdc25B causing S-phase delay and persistent antiproliferative effects. *Int. J. Cancer* 1998;76:720–728.

[15] Strausfeld U, Fernandez A, Capony JP, et al:Activation of p34cdc2 protein kinase by microinjection of human cdc25C into mammalian cells. Requirement for prior phosphorylation of cdc25C by p34cdc2 on sites phosphorylated at mitosis. *J. Biol. Chem.* 1994;269:5989–6000.

[16] Adams PD: Regulation of the retinoblastoma tumor suppressor protein by cyclin/cdks. *Biochim. Biophys. Acta* 2001;1471:M123–M133.

[17] Sellers WR, Kaelin WG: pRB as a modulator of transcription. *Biochim. Biophys. A*cta 1996;1288:M1–M5.

[18] Sladek TL: E2F transcription factor action, regulation, and possibile role in human cancer. *Cell Prolif.* 1997;30:97–105.

[19] Knudsen ES, Buckmaster C, Chen TT, Feramisco JR,Wang JYJ: Inhibition of DNA synthesis by RB: Effects on G1/S transition and S-phase progression. *Genes Dev.* 1998;12:2278–2292.

[20] Sellers WR, Kaelin WGJ: Role of the retinoblastoma protein in the pathogenesis of human cancer. *J. Clin. Oncol.* 1997;15:3301–3312.

[21] Diffley JF: Eukaryotic DNA replication. *Curr. Opin. Cell Biol.* 1994;6:368–372.

[22] Rowley A, Dowell SJ, Diffley JF: Recent developments in the initiation of chromosomal DNA replication: a complex picture emerges. *Biochim. Biophys. Acta* 1994;1217:239–256.

[23] Bell SP, Stillman B:ATP-dependent recognition of eukaryotic origins of DNA replication by a multiprotein complex. *Nature* 1992;357:128–134.

[24] Stillman B, Bell SP,Dutta A, Marahrens Y:DNA replication and the cell cycle. *Ciba Found Symp.* 1992;170:147–156; discussion 156–160.

[25] Dutta A, Bell SP: Initiation of DNA replication in eukaryotic cells. *Annu. Rev. Cell Dev. Biol.* 1997;13:293–332.

[26] Maine GT, Sinha P,Tye BK: Mutants of S. cerevisiae defective in the maintenance of minichromosomes. *Genetics* 1984;106:365–385.
[27] Takisawa H, Mimura S,Kubota Y: Eukaryotic DNA replication: from pre-replication complex to initiation complex. *Curr. Opin. Cell Biol.* 2000;12:690–696.
[28] Wuarin J, Nurse P: Regulating S phase: CDKs, licensing and proteolysis. *Cell* 1996;85:785–787.
[29] Stillman B: Cell cycle control of DNA replication. *Science* 1996;274:1659–1664.
[30] Krek W, Nigg EA: Differential phosphorylation of vertebrate p34cdc2 kinase at the G1/S and G2/M transitions of the cell cycle: Identification of major phosphorylation sites. *Embo J.* 1991;10:305–316.
[31] Coleman TR, Dunphy WG: Cdc2 regulatory factors. *Curr. Opin. Cell Biol.* 1994;6:877–882.
[32] Hagting A, Karlsson C, Clute P, Jackman M, Pines J: MPF localization is controlled by nuclear export. *Embo J.* 1998;17:4127–4138.
[33] Nigg EA:Targets of cyclin-dependent protein kinases. *Curr. Opin. Cell Biol.* 1993;5:187–193.
[34] Blangy A, Lane HA, d'Herin P, Harper M, Kress M, Nigg EA: Phosphorylation by p34cdc2 regulates spindle association of human Eg5, a kinesin-related motor essential for bipolar spindle formation in vivo. *Cell* 1995;83:1159–1169.
[35] Sorger PK, Dobles M,Tournebize R, Hyman AA: Coupling cell division and cell death to microtubule dynamics. *Curr. Opin. Cell Biol.* 1997;9:807–814.
[36] Llamazares S, Moreira A,Tavares A, et al: Polo encodes a protein kinase homolog required for mitosis in Drosophila. *Genes Dev.* 1991;5:2153–2165.
[37] Morgan DO: Regulation of the APC and the exit from mitosis. *Nat. Cell Biol.* 1999;1:E47–E53.
[38] Gallant P, Nigg EA: Cyclin B2 undergoes cell cycle-dependent nuclear translocation and, when expressed as a non-destructible mutant, causes mitotic arrest in HeLa cells. *J. Cell Biol.* 1992;117:213–224.
[39] Clute P, Pines J:Temporal and spatial control of cyclin B1 destruction in metaphase. *Nat. Cell Biol.* 1999;1:82–87.
[40] Funabiki H,Yamano H,Kumada K, Nagao K, Hunt T,Yanagida M: Cut2 proteolysis required for sister-chromatid seperation in fission yeast. *Nature* 1996;381:438–441.
[41] Boddy MN, Russell P:DNA replication checkpoint. Curr Biol 2001;11:R953–R956.
[42] Ho, A., and S. F. Dowdy. Regulation of G1 cell-cycle progression by oncogenes and tumor suppressor genes. *Curr. Opin. Genet. Dev.* 2002;12:47-52.
[43] Aleem, E., H. Kiyokawa, and P. Kaldis. Cdc2-cyclin E complexes regulate the G1/S phase transition. *Nat. Cell Biol*. 2005; 7:831-836.
[44] Ezhevsky, S. A., A. Ho, M. Becker-Hapak, P. K. Davis, and S. F. Dowdy. Differential regulation of retinoblastoma tumor suppressor protein by G1 cyclin-dependent kinase complexes in vivo. *Mol. Cell. Biol.* 2001; 21:4773-4784.
[45] Fang, G., H. Yu, and M. W. Kirschner. Direct binding of CDC20 protein family members activates the anaphase-promoting complex in mitosis and G1. *Mol. Cell.* 1998;2:163-171.

[46] Hsu, J. Y., J. D. Reimann, C. S. Sorensen, J. Lukas, and P. K. Jackson. E2F-dependent accumulation of hEmi1 regulates S phase entry by inhibiting APC(Cdh1). *Nat. Cell Biol.* 2002; 4:358-366.

[47] Lukas, C., C. S. Sorensen, E. Kramer, E. Santoni-Rugiu, C. Lindeneg, J. M. Peters, J. Bartek, and J. Lukas. Accumulation of cyclin B1 requires E2F and cyclin-A-dependent rearrangement of the anaphase-promoting complex. *Nature*, 1999; 401:815-818.

[48] Falck J, Mailand N, Syljuåsen RG, Bartek J, Lukas J:The ATM-Chk2-Cdc25A checkpoint pathway guards against radioresistant DNA synthesis. *Nature* 2001;410:842–847.

[49] Costanzo V, Robertson K,Ying CY, et al: Reconstitution of an ATM-dependent checkpoint that inhibits chromosomal DNA replication following DNA damage. *Mol. Cell* 2000; 6: 649–659.

[50] Kastan MB, Onyekwere O, Sidransky D,Vogelstein B, Craig RW: Participation of p53 protein in the cellular response to DNA damage. *Cancer Res.* 1991;51:6304–6311.

[51] Reich NC, Levine AJ: Growth regulation of a cellular tumour antigen, p53, in nontransformed cells. *Nature* 1984;308:199–201.

[52] Reihsaus E,Kohler M, Kraiss S, Oren M, Montenarh M: Regulation of the level of the oncoprotein p53 in non-transformed and transformed cells. *Oncogene* 1990;5:137–145.

[53] Harper JW,Adami GR,Wei N,Keyomarsi K, Elledge SJ:The p21 Cdk-interacting protein Cip1 is a potent inhibitor of G1 cyclindependent kinases. *Cell* 1993;75:805–816.

[54] Deng CX, Zhang PM, Harper JW, Elledge SJ, Leder P: Mice lacking p21CIP1/WAF1 undergo normal development, but are defective in G1 checkpoint control. *Cell* 1995;82:675–684.

[55] Waldman T, Kinzler KW,Vogelstein B: p21 is necessary for the p53-mediated G1 arrest in human cancer cells. *Cancer Res.* 1995;55:5187–5190.

[56] Pavey S, Conroy S, Russell T, Gabrielli B: Ultraviolet radiation induces p16CDKN2A expression in human skin. *Cancer Res.* 1999;59:4185–4189.

[57] Quelle DE, Zindy F,Ashmun RA, Sherr CJ:Alternative reading frames of the INK4a tumor suppressor gene encode two unrelated proteins capable of inducing cell cycle arrest. *Cell* 1995;83:993–1000.

[58] Sharpless NE, DePinho RA:The INK4A/ARF locus and its two gene products. *Curr. Opin Gen.* 1999;9:22–30.

[59] Porter PL, Malone KE, Heagerty PJ, et al: Expression of cell-cycle regulators p27Kip1 and cyclin E, alone and in combination, correlate with survival in young breast cancer patients. *Nature Med.* 1997;3:222–225.

[60] Viglietto G, Motti ML, Bruni P, et al: Cytoplasmic relocalization and inhibition of the cyclin-dependent kinase inhibitor p27Kip1 by PKB/Akt-mediated phosphorylation in breast cancer. *Nat. Med.* 2002;8:1136–1144.

[61] Bakkenist CJ, Kastan MB:DNA damage activates ATM through intermolecular autophosphorylation and dimer dissociation. *Nature* 2003;421:499–506.

[62] Shiloh Y, Kastan MB:ATM: genome stability, neuronal development, and cancer cross paths. *Adv. Cancer Res.* 2001;83:209–254.

[63] Lim DS, Kim ST, Xu B, et al:ATM phosphorylates p95/nbs1 in an S-phase checkpoint pathway. *Nature* 2000;404:613–614.

[64] Taniguchi T, Garcia-Higuera I, Xu B, et al: Convergence of the fanconi anemia and ataxia telangiectasia signaling pathways. *Cell* 2002;109:459–472.

[65] Yazdi PT,Wang Y, Zhao S, Patel N, Lee EY, Qin J: SMC1 is a downstream effector in the ATM/NBS1 branch of the human S-phase checkpoint. *Genes Dev.* 2002;16:571–582.

[66] Xu B, O'Donnell AH, Kim ST, Kastan MB: Phosphorylation of serine 1387 in Brca1 is specifically required for the Atm-mediated S-phase checkpoint after ionizing irradiation. *Cancer Res.* 2002;62:4588–4591.

[67] Hwang A, Muschell RJ: Radiation and the G2 phase of the cell cycle. *Radiat Res.* 1998;150:S52–S59.

[68] Sanchez Y,Wong S,Thoma RS, et al: Conservation of the Chk1 checkpoint pathway in mammals: Linkage of DNA damage to Cdk regulation through Cdc25C. *Science* 1997;277:1497–1501.

[69] Furnari B, Rhind N, Russell P: Cdc25C mitotic inducer targeted by Chk1 DNA damage checkpoint kinase. *Science* 1997;277:1495–1497.

[70] Smits VAJ, Medema RH: Checking out the G2/M transition. *Biochim. Biophys Acta Gene Struct Expr.* 2001;1519:1–12.

[71] Smits VAJ, Klompmaker R,Arnaud L, Rijksen G, Nigg EA, Medema RH: Polo-like kinase-1 is a target of the DNA damage checkpoint. *Nat. Cell Biol.* 2000;2:672–676.

[72] Innocente SA,Abrahamson JLA, Cogswell JP, Lee JM: p53 regulates a G2 checkpoint through cyclin B1. *Proc. Natl. Acad. Sci. USA* 1999;96:2147–2152.

[73] Chan TA,Hermeking H, Lengauer C, Kinzler KW,Vogelstein B: 14-3-3Sigma is required to prevent mitotic catastrophe after DNA damage. *Nature* 1999;401:616–620.

[74] Wang XW, Zhan QM, Coursen JD, et al: GADD45 induction of a G2/M cell cycle checkpoint. *Proc. Natl. Acad. Sci. USA* 1999;96:3706–3711.

[75] Burke DJ: Complexity in the spindle checkpoint. Curr Opin Genet Dev 2000;10:26–31.

[76] Gorbsky GJ:The mitotic spindle checkpoint. *Curr. Biol.* 2001;11:R1001–R1004.

[77] Khan SH,Wahl GM: p53 and pRb prevent rereplication in response to microtubule inhibitors by mediating a reversible G1 arrest. *Cancer Res.* 1998;58:396–401.

[78] Stewart ZA, Leach SD, Pietenpol JA: p21Waf1/Cip1 inhibition of cyclin E/Cdk2 activity prevents endoreduplication after mitotic spindle disruption. *Mol. Cell Biol.* 1999;19:205–215.

[79] Lanni JS, Jacks TS: Characterization of the p53-dependent postmitotic checkpoint following spindle disruption. *Mol. Cell Biol.* 1998;18:1055–1064.

[80] Beer TW, Buchanan R, Matthews AW, Stradling R, Pullinger N, Pethybridge RJ. Prognosis in malignant mesothelioma related to MIB 1 proliferation index and histological subtype. *Hum. Pathol.* 1998; 29: 246-51.

[81] Brown DC, Gatter KC. Monoclonal antibody Ki-67: its use in histopathology. *Histopathology* 1990; 17: 489-503.

[82] Comin CE, Anichini C, Boddi V, Novelli L, Dini S. MIB-1 proliferation index correlates with survival in pleural malignant mesothelioma. *Histopathology* 2000; 36: 26-31.

[83] Beer TW, Carr NJ, Whittaker MA, Pullinger N. Mitotic and in situ end-labeling apoptotic indices as prognostic markers in malignant mesothelioma. *Ann. Diagn. Pathol.* 2000; 4: 143-8.

[84] Bongiovanni M, Cassoni P, De Giuli P, Viberti L, Cappia S, Ivaldi C, Chiusa L, Bussolati G. p27kip1 immunoreactivity correlates with long-term survival in pleural malignant mesothelioma. *Cancer* 2001; 92: 1245-50.

[85] Sgambato A, Cittadini A, Faraglia B, Weinstein IB. Multiple functions of p27kip1 and its alteration in tumor cells: a review. J Cell Physiol 2000; 183: 18-27. Slingerland J, Pagano M. Regulation of the Cdk inhibitor p27 and its deregulation in cancer. *J. Cell* Physiol. 2000; 183: 10-7.

[86] Tallini G, Garcia-Rostan G, Herrero A, Zelterman D, Viale G, Bosari S, et al. Downregulation of p27kip1 and Ki67/Mib1 labeling index support the classification of thyroid carcinoma into prognostically relevant categories. *Am. J. Surg. Pathol.* 1999; 23: 678-85.

[87] Gunther K, Jung A, Volker U, Meyer M, Brabletz T, Matzel KE, et al. p27(kip1) expression in rectal cancer correlates with disease-free survival. *J. Surg. Res.* 2000; 92: 78-84.

[88] Johansson L, Linden CJ. Aspects of histopathologic subtype as a prognostic factor in 85 pleural mesotheliomas. *Chest* 1996; 109: 109-14.

[89] Mor O, Yaron P, Huszar M, et al. Absence of p53 mutations in malignant mesotheliomas. *Am. J. Respir. Cell Mol Biol.* 1997;16:9–13.

[90] Esposito V, Baldi A, De Luca A, et al. p53 immunostaining in differential diagnosis of pleural mesothelial proliferations. *Anticancer Res.* 1997;17:733–6.

[91] Yang CT, You L, Uematsu K, Yeh CC, McCormick F, and Jablons DM. p14^{ARF} modulates the cytolytic effect of ONYX-015 in mesotheliomacells with wild-type p53. *Cancer Res.* 2001; 61, 5959 – 5963.

[92] Cheng J. Q., Jhanwar S. C., Klein W. M., Bell D. W., Lee W. C., Altomare D. A., Nobori T., Olopade O. I., Buckler A. J., Testa J. R. p16 alterations and deletion mapping of 9p21–p22 in malignant mesothelioma. *Cancer Res.* 1994; *54:* 5547-5551.

[93] Prins J. B., Williamson K. A., Kamp M. M., Van Hezik E. J., Van der Kwast T. H., Hagemeijer A., Versnel M. A. The gene for the cyclin-dependent-kinase-4 inhibitor, CDKN2A, is preferentially deleted in malignant mesothelioma. *Int. J. Cancer*, 1998; *75:* 649-653.

[94] Chin L, Pomerantz J., DePinho R. A. The INK4a/ARF tumor suppressor: one gene–two products–two pathways. *Trends Biochem. Sci.*1998; *23:* 291-296.

[95] Craig C., Kim M., Ohri E., Wersto R., Katayose D., Li Z., Choi Y. H., Mudahar B., Srivastava S., Seth P., Cowan K. Effects of adenovirus-mediated p16INK4A expression on cell cycle arrest are determined by endogenous p16 and Rb status in human cancer cells. *Oncogene,* 1998; *16:* 265-272.

[96] Pomerantz J., Schreiber-Agus N., Liegeois N. J., Silverman A., Alland L., Chin L., Potes J., Chen K., Orlow I., Lee H. W., Cordon-Cardo C., DePinho R. A. The Ink4a tumor suppressor gene product, p19Arf, interacts with MDM2 and neutralizes MDM2's inhibition of p53. *Cell,* 1998; *92:* 713-723.

[97] Zhang Y., Xiong Y., Yarbrough W. G. ARF promotes MDM2 degradation and stabilizes p53: ARF-INK4a locus deletion impairs both the Rb and p53 tumor suppression pathways. *Cell,* 1998; *92:* 725-734.

[98] Piette J., Neel H., Marechal V. Mdm2: keeping p53 under control. *Oncogene*, 1997; *15:* 1001-1010.

[99] Sally Hopkins-Donaldson, Larisa L Belyanskaya, Ana Paula Simões-Wüst, Brigitte Sigrist, Stefanie Kurtz, Uwe Zangemeister-Wittke, and Rolf Stahel. p53 Induced Apoptosis Occurs in the Absence of p14ARF in *Malignant Pleural Mesothelioma. Neoplasia.* 2006 July; *8(7)*: 551–559.

[100] De Luca A, Baldi A, Esposito V, et al. The retinoblastoma gene family pRb/p105, p107, pRb2/p130 and simian virus-40 large T-antigen in human mesotheliomas. *Nature Med.* 1997;3:913–6.

[101] Baldi A, Groeger AM, Esposito V, Cassandro R, Tonini G, Battista T, Di Marino MP, Vincenzi B, Santini M, Angelini A, Rossiello R, Baldi F, Paggi MG. Expression of p21 in SV40 large T antigen positive human pleural mesothelioma: relationship with survival. *Thorax* 2002; 57: 353-6.

[102] Baldi A, Santini D, Vasaturo F, Santini M, Vicidomini G, Di Marino MP, Esposito V, Groeger AM, Liuzzi G, Vincenzi B, Tonini G, Piccoli M, Baldi F, Scarpa S. Prognostic significance of cyclooxygenase-2 (COX-2) and expression of cell cycle inhibitors p21 and p27 in human pleural malignant mesothelioma. *Thorax* 2004; 59; 428-433.

[103] Rusch VW, Venkatraman ES. Important prognostic factors in patients with malignant pleural mesothelioma, managed surgically. *Ann. Thorac. Surg.* 1999;68:1799–804.134.

[104] Grosch S, Tegeder I, Niederberger E, et al. COX-2 independent induction of cell cycle arrest and apoptosis in colon cancer cells by the selective COX-2 inhibitor celecoxib. *FASEB J.* 2001;15:2742–4.

[105] Zahner G, Wolf G, Ayoub M, et al. Cyclooxygenase-2 overexpression inhibits platelet-derived growth factor-induced mesangial cell proliferation through induction of the tumour suppressor gene p53 and the cyclin-dependent kinase inhibitors $p21^{waf-1/cip-1}$ and $p27^{kip-1}$. *J. Biol. Chem.* 2002; 277:9763–71.

[106] Baer AN, Green FA. Cyclooxygenase activity of cultured human mesothelial cells. *Prostaglandins* 1993;46:37–49.

[107] Marrogi A, Pass HI, Khan M, et al. Human mesothelioma samples overexpress both cyclooxygenase-2 (COX-2) and inducible nitric oxide synthase (NOS2): in vitro antiproliferative effects of a COX-2 inhibitor. *Cancer Res.* 2000; 60:3696–700.

[108] Sheehan KM, Sheahan K, O'Donoghue DP, et al. The relationship between cyclooxygenase-2 expression and colorectal cancer. *JAMA* 1999; 282:1254–7.

[109] Hida T, Yatabe Y, Achiwa H, et al. Increased expression of cyclooxygenase-2 occurs frequently in human lung cancers, specifically in adenocarcinomas. *Cancer Res.* 1998; 58:3761–4.

[110] C Vivo, F Lévy, Y Pilatte, J Fleury-Feith, P Chrétien, I Monnet, L Kheuang and M C Jaurand. Control of cell cycle progression in human mesothelioma cells treated with gamma interferon. *Oncogene.* 2001 Mar 1;20(9):1085-93.

[111] Toru Mukohara, Gabriel Civiello, Ian J. Davis, Michele L. Taffaro, James Christensen, David E. Fisher, Bruce E. Johnson and Pasi A. Jänne. Inhibition of the Met Receptor in Mesothelioma. *Clin .Cancer Res.* 2005 Nov 15;11(22):8122-3.

[112] Jeffers M, Fiscella M, Webb CP, et al. The mutationally activated Met receptor mediates motility and metastasis. *Proc. Natl. Acad. Sci. USA* 1998; 95:14417–22.

[113] Danilkovitch-Miagkova A, Zbar B. Dysregulation of Met receptor tyrosine kinase activity in invasive tumors. *J. Clin. Invest.* 2002; 109:863–7.

[114] Klominek J, Robert KH, Sundqvist KG. Chemotaxis and haptotaxis of human malignant mesothelioma cells: effects of fibronectin, laminin, type IV collagen, and an autocrine motility factor-like substance. *Cancer Res.* 1993;53:4376–82.

[115] Prasad S. Adusumilli, M.D., Mei-Ki Chan, B.S., Yun Shin Chun, M.D., Michael Hezel, B.S., Ting-Chao Chou, Ph.D., Valerie W. Rusch, M.D., and Yuman Fong, M.D. Cisplatin-Induced GADD34 Upregulation Potentiates Oncolytic Viral Therapy in the Treatment of Malignant Pleural Mesothelioma. *Cancer Biol. Ther.* 2006 January; 5(1): 48–53.

In: Mesothelioma from Bench Side to Clinic
Editor: Alfonso Baldi, pp. 157-182

ISBN: 978-1-60021-789-0

Chapter VIII

Oxidative Stress and Activation of Survival Pathways as a Basis for Mesothelioma Pathogenesis: New Perspectives for Experimental Therapy

Michele Caraglia[*], *Alfonso Catalano*[°^], *Monica Marra*[*], *Alfredo Budillon*[*] and *Antonio Procopio*[°^]
[*]Experimental Pharmacology Unit, Experimental Oncology Department, National Institute of Tumours, Via Semmola, 80131, Naples, Italy
[°]Department of Molecular Pathology and Innovative Therapies, Polytechnic University of Marche and
[^]Center of Cytology, Department of Gerontological Research, Italian National Research Centers on Aging (INRCA-IRCCS), Ancona, Italy

Abstract

Asbestos, a group of natural hydrated silicates, is considered as a complete carcinogen, which is able to cause malignant transformation. Occupational exposure to asbestos increases the risk of development of mesotheliomas and lung cancers. It was proposed that carcinogenic effects of asbestos are determined both by direct interaction of target cells with asbestos fibers and by generation, in response to asbestos, of an inflammatory environment containing strong proliferative signals as well as reactive oxygen and nitrogen species (ROS/RNS) causing fibroproliferative diseases of the lung and pleura. The activation of AP-1 as well as NF-kB by asbestos in rat lung fibroblasts can be reduced by treatment with vitamin E derivatives. Moreover, ERK1/2 as well as p38 mitogen-activated protein kinases (MAPKs) activation induced by asbestos is

[*] E-mail: michele.caraglia@fondazionepascale.it

diminished by the addition of the anti-oxidant N-acetyl-l-cysteine. These data indicate an involvement of ROS production in asbestos induced effects. This chapter discusses the pathways of oxidant generation induced by asbestos fibers, which may initiate and perpetuate inflammation, cytokine release and proliferative responses to asbestos. Moreover, we will illustrate the signal transduction pathways activated by stress giving relevance to the terminal enzymes NH2 terminal Jun kinase 1 and 2. Once initiated, these pathways can lead to promotion of gene expression critical to cellular injury, proliferation and inflammation-events leading to the development of cancer of the lung and pleura. Another pathway that is specifically activated is that one dependent from Erk. It has been demonstrated that asbestos can activate Erk-5 through the stimulation of Src and independently from epidermal growth factor receptor (EGF-R) in human lung epithelial cells. These effects are associated to cell proliferation and transformation. It has been also reported that asbestos can induce apoptosis through the prolonged and sustained activation of Erk 1 and 2 associated to apoptosis in the absence of EGF in human lung epithelial cells. The concomitant presence of asbestos and EGF induced, on the other hand, proliferation. These studies indicate that the presence of other micro-environmental factors, such as EGF, could be essential for the carcinogenic effect induced by asbestos in mesothelial and epithelial cells. Moreover, these findings open a new scenario of investigation on the correlation between asbestos and the activation of survival and anti-apoptotic pathways. The elucidation and relevance of critical signalling cascades to lung injury or repair following asbestos exposure could aid in developing strategies to prevent or treat asbestos-associated lung and pleural diseases, including lung carcinoma and malignant mesothelioma.

1. Introduction

1.1. General Notions on Mesothelioma

Mesothelioma is a cancer arising from the peritoneal and parietal pleural epithelium or subepithelium. Three main histological patterns are now recognized: epithelial, desmoplastic (a variant is sarcomatoid), and biphasic (mixed). Although there have been case reports with pathological descriptions consistent with the diagnosis since 1870, mesothelioma was not generally considered a distinct cancer entity until the 1960s (Jones, 2001).

There are some known and suspected causes of mesothelioma (Peterson et al., 1984; Pelnar, 1988; Ilgren and Wagner, 1991; Hillerdal, 1999; Sato et al., 2000; Sporn and Roggli, 2004; Sterman, 2004; Lange, 2004). For example, epidemiological evidence indicates that some geologic minerals (e.g., the fibrous silicates erionite–zeolite) are associated with an elevated risk of mesothelioma. In the aftermath of the World Trade Center collapse on September 11, 2001, where widespread exposures to mainly chrysotile asbestos are reported, the long-running debate on the potency of chrysotile fibers of whatever physical dimensions to cause mesothelioma (and other health outcomes, which are beyond the scope of this chapter) hampers unambiguous risk communications (Landrigan et al., 2004; Lange, 2004; Greenberg, 2005; Nolan et al., 2005).

1.2. Asbestos and Mesothelioma

Asbestos is a family of six chemically and physically distinct fibers that are classified, based upon morphology, as serpentine (chrysotile) or amphibole including crocidolite, amosite (both having industrial applications), anthophyllite, actinolite and tremolite (non-commercial fibres). (Guthrie and Mossman, 1993). Chrysotile has been used most often in industry historically, and since this is the type mined in Canada and parts of the US, as well as the most common type of asbestos worldwide, it is studied most often in experimental models. Chrysotile can break down into smaller fibrils in tissue and is cleared more rapidly from the lung and pleura (Churg, 1994; Hume and Rimstidt, 1992), properties that have been attributed to its decreased pathogenicity in the causation of mesothelioma. In addition, size, geometry, chemical composition, and surface charge of various asbestos types play important roles in interactions with cells that lead to cell injury and disease (Guthrie and Mossman, 1993; Kamp and Weitzman, 1999).

Each asbestos type has a distinct chemical formula. Asbestos occurs both as asbestiform (fibrous) and nonasbestiform (massive) structures in nature, and each type retains its chemical composition in either form. Chrysotile is a sheet silicate that rolls into nano-sized tubular structures possessing a hollow core, whereas amphiboles are chain silicates.

Both fibrous and non-fibrous particles have been associated with malignant lung diseases. The most extensively studied of these particulates are asbestos fibres, crystalline silica and more recently ambient particulate matter (PM). Based on epidemiological and mechanistic studies, asbestos and quartz have been classified as carcinogens caused by massive occupational exposure. Particle-induced tumours mainly arise in the lung and pleura. A major fraction of the particles are deposited onto the fragile epithelial structures of the gas exchange region. Most dosimetry models and calculations assume a uniform deposition at the bronchial airway surfaces and therefore a similar target dose for all epithelial cells within the respiratory tract. However, analysis of particles in human lung tissue shows that a rather large particle deposition occurs independently of the particle size at the bronchial airway bifurcations. Moreover, major differences in particle deposition can be found between lung lobes. In particular, cells located in the vicinity of the dividing spur may receive local doses that are a several hundred times higher than the average dose for the total airway. For lung cancer, neoplasia is suggested to originate from bronchiolar non-ciliated epithelial cells (i.e. Clara cells) and alveolar type II pneumocytes in these hot-spot area's. Clara cells and alveolar type II cells are described as progenitor cells of the bronchiolar or the alveolar epithelium, respectively. The high proliferative capacity of these cell types explains their sensitivity for induction of proliferation due to xenobiotics, such as particles. As a second target tissue for particle-induced proliferative or neoplastic effects, the mesothelium must also be considered. Fibrous particles are well known to penetrate the lung tissue and accumulate in the pleura and, less frequently, in the peritoneum. In the mesothelial cell layer, in addition to other pathological effects, such as plaques, tumours are induced. In humans, clinical mesothelioma only occurs after a long period of latency. In this target tissue, as compared with the lung, clearance mechanisms are of minor importance. Therefore, fibrous dust may persist for a very long time and induce pathological reactions. Inhalable fibrous particles can differ in their potency to induce neoplastic changes. Several characteristics have been described as critical in determining the pathological alteration due to inhalation of natural and man made mineral fibres (MMVF).

Asbestos is a group of fibrous, naturally occurring mineral silicates that become problematic to human health when they are inhaled at high airborne concentrations in the workplace or during product usage (Mossman et al., 1990; Mossman and Gee, 1989). Asbestos fibers, defined as having a greater than 3–1 length to diameter ratio, when in a submicron size, can penetrate into the deep lung and cause a number of respiratory and pleural diseases including pulmonary (asbestosis) and pleural fibrosis, lung cancers and mesotheliomas (Mossman et al., 1996). Therefore, understanding how asbestos fibers interact with target cells of disease, i.e. epithelial, mesothelial and fibroblastic cells, and how these events contribute to the pathogenesis of asbestos-associated fibroproliferative and malignant diseases are critical to designing preventive and therapeutic approaches to lung and pleural disorders.

This chapter focuses on key pathways in cell signaling by asbestos that are likely to play a role in cell injury, survival, proliferation, and inflammation in target cells of asbestos-induced diseases of the lung and pleura.

1.3. Cellular and Molecular Responses to Asbestos

After initial contact with cells, asbestos fibers can produce injury at high concentrations and proliferation at low concentrations. Both lytic cell death and apoptosis have been described in response to asbestos fibers in a number of cell types (Mossman and Churg, 1998). These events may result in compensatory proliferation of epithelial cells or mesothelial cells analogous to wounding responses after scraping of cell monolayers (Goldberg et al., 1997). An imbalance in tissue homeostasis maintained by proliferation and apoptosis maybe induced by asbestos fibers such that cell growth predominates and neoplastic growth occurs. In this context, the tissue-specific responsiveness to apoptosis as a reaction to the relevant compounds, is of interest. Viral infections, polycyclic aromatic hydrocarbons (PAH), hyperoxia, but also endogenous substances like ROS/RNS have all been found to shift the balance between apoptosis and proliferation in mesothelium.

Similar responses (i.e apoptosis and proliferation) are seen in epithelial cells after inhalation or intratracheal injection of asbestos fibers in animal models. For example, increased proliferation of terminal bronchiolar epithelial cells, particularly at the alveolar duct junction, is noted shortly after inhalation of asbestos, and this may be in direct response to asbestos fibers that are deposited preferentially at this site after inhalation (BeruBe et al., 1996; Dixon et al., 1995; Donaldson et al., 1995; Robledo et al., 2000). In addition, growth factors and ROS elaborated by alveolar macrophages after endo-cytosis of asbestos fibers may be important not only for inflammatory response, but also for mitogenesis of mesothelial cells. In fact, inflammation occurs rapidly after administration of asbestos fibers *in vivo*, and putative by-products of inflammatory cells also may contribute to cell signaling, injury and proliferation and, in turn, to cancer development.

2. Cell Signaling Pathways and Transcription Factors Activated by Asbestos

Recently, cell injury and S-phase alterations by asbestos have been linked to phosphorylation of the epidermal growth factor receptor (EGFR) and the protracted activation of the extracellular signal-regulated (ERK1/2) pathway (Zanella et al., 1996, 1999; Jimenez et al., 1997; Buder-Hoffmann et al., 2001) or of other intracellular signalling molecules. In fact, mitogen-activated protein kinase (MAPK) signal transduction pathways, including the extracellular signal regulated protein kinases (ERKs 1/2), c-Jun N-terminal kinases (JNKs), p38 and big mitogen kinase 1 (BMK1/ERK5), are activated in response to various agents such as growth factors, tumor promoters and oxidants. Interestingly, ERK5, a more recently characterized member of the ERK family (Lee et al., 1995; Zhou et al., 1995), is strongly activated by EGF as well as other receptor tyrosine kinases (Kamakura et al., 1999; Kato et al., 1998), and is required for cell proliferation and progression through the cell cycle (Kamakura et al., 1999; Kato et al., 1998). Downstream targets of the ERK5 pathway include the MAD-box transcription factor, MEF2C, which acts on the protooncogene c-jun promoter, and the SRE on the c-fos promoter.

Considering that phagocytosis of fibers and the high concentration of iron on the surface of crocidolite fibers may catalyse the formation of reactive oxygen species (ROS) that can interact with EGFR and mediate cell proliferation and toxicity, it was hypothesized that ERK5, a redox-sensitive kinase (Abe et al., 1999) could be an MAPK pathway contributing to asbestos-induced cell signaling in pulmonary epithelial cells.

All the above mentioned cell signaling cascades may lead to activation of transcription factors and alterations in gene expression. The most studied transcription factors after asbestos exposures are activator protein-1 (AP-1) and nuclear factor-kappa B (NF-κB). Moreover, asbestos has other effects, such as modulation of intracellular ROS production and activation of isoforms of protein kinase C (PKC). Therefore, we provide an overview of regulation of different signaling events by asbestos fibers.

2.1. Mitogen-Activated Protein Kinases (MAPK)

The mitogen-activated protein kinase (MAPK) cascade is characterized by a sequential series of phosphorylation events catalyzed by three pathways: extracellular signal-regulated kinases (ERK), c-jun NH2-terminal kinases (JNK) or stress-activated protein kinases (SAPK), and p38 kinases (Karin, 1995). The MAPK module (cascade) is composed by an upstream serine threonine kinase that is called MAPK kinase kinase (i.e Raf-1 is the upstream kinase that leads to the final activation of Erk1 and 2), by an intermediate dual kinase called MAPK kinase (i.e. Mek-1 leads to the phosphorylation of Erk-1 and 2 in both threonine and tyrosine) and finally by MAPK (i.e. Erk 1 and 2). MAPK, after the phosphorylation and consequent activation, migrates from the cytoplasm to the nucleus where they phosphoprylate their substrate that are transcription factors responsible for the synthesis of genes involved in the control of cell proliferation and survival. For the activation of the upstream MAPK kinase kinase is required the interaction of the latter with signaling molecules that are intimately associated to the cell membranes such as the small GTP binding proteins including molecules behaving to the ras family. These proteins, in turn, are activated by cell surface signals such as transmembrane receptors that receive extracellular stimuli (for a summary see Figure 1). On the basis of these considerations, these MAPK pathways are induced by a number of cell surface stimuli and act in the transactivation of multiple nuclear transcription factors, such as AP-1, to mediate gene expression by asbestos. These events promote cellular responses, such as proliferation, apoptosis or inflammation (Ramos-Ninos et al., 2002a, Caraglia et al., 2005).

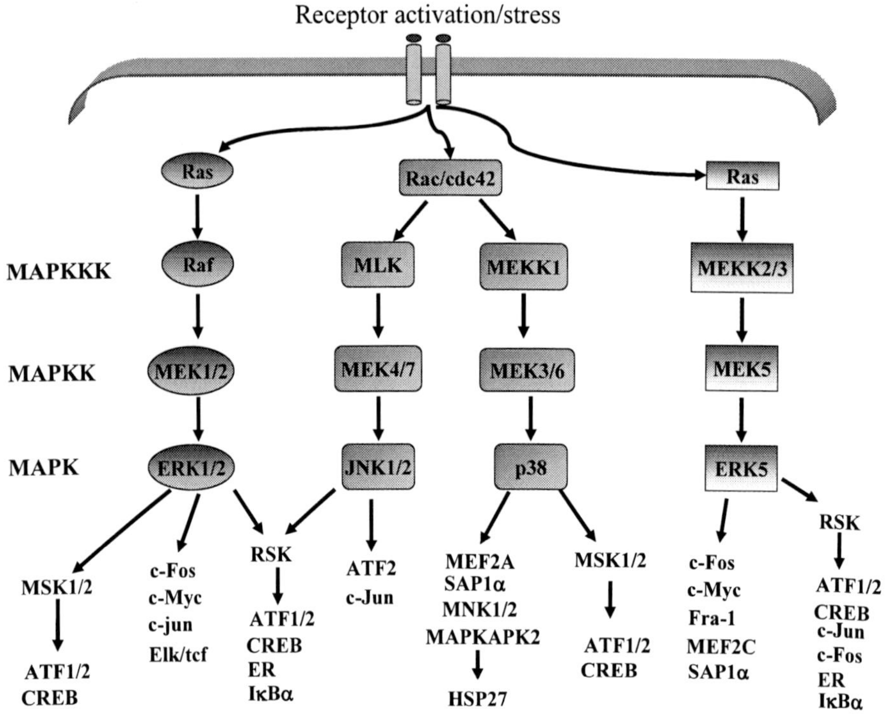

Figure 1. Model for signal transduction pathways regulating MAP kinases. The mitogen-activated protein kinase (MAPK) family is an evolutionarily conserved class of proline-directed serine/threonine kinases. The four major groupings are the Erk, JNK or SAPK, p38 and the Big MAPK or ERK5 cascades. Each of the MAPK modules operates as a three-tier system. The MAPK, a serine/threonine kinase, is activated by a MAPK kinase (MAPKK), which is a 'dual-specific' kinase that phosphorylates at both Ser/Thr and Tyr sites. In turn, the MAPKK is activated by a MAPKK kinase (MAPKKK) that receives signals from stimulus-activated receptors on the cell surface or through interactions with GTP-binding proteins and/or other kinases. The MAPKs at the end of these signaling cascades phosphorylate their target proteins, many of which are nuclear proteins such as transcription factors. The ERK module responds primarily to growth factors and mitogens and stimulates transcriptional responses in the nucleus. ERK1 and 2 are activated by MAPK/ERK kinase (MEK) 1 and 2. The MEKs, in turn, are activated by Raf, the MAPKKK of this signaling pathway, that is in turn regulated by growth factor receptors and tyrosine kinases activating through Ras. Upon translocation to the nucleus, ERKs are responsible for the phosphorylation of multiple substrates, depending on the initial stimulus. These include activators of transcription including RSK kinase. RSK or 90 kDa ribosomal S6 kinases (also known as p90rsk or MAPK-activated protein kinase-1, MAPKAP-K1) regulates gene expression via association and phosphorylation of transcriptional regulators including c-Fos, estrogen receptor (ER), NFκB/IκBα, cAMP-response element-binding protein (CREB) and CREB-binding protein. A family of RSK-related kinases, named mitogen- and stress-activated protein kinases (MSK), are also activated by

ERK as well as p38 MAPK. JNKs respond to a variety of stress signals including heat shock, osmotic stress, pro-inflammatory cytokines, ischemia and UV. The JNKs are activated by dual phosphorylation by MEK 4 and MEK7. Upstream of the MEKs are their MAPKKKs, which include a member of the mixed-lineage kinases (MLK). In turn, these are activated by GTP-binding proteins of the Rho family (Rac, Rho, Cdc42). JNKs were originally identified as the major kinases responsible for the phosphorylation of c-Jun, leading to increased activity of the AP-1 (activator protein-1) transcription factor; other nuclear transcription factors are also now known to be targets including ATF-2. JNKs are responsible for the phosphorylation of activators of transcription including RSK kinase. Activation of the JNK signaling cascade generally results in apoptosis, although it has also been shown to promote cell survival under certain conditions. Enzymes in the p38 MAPK module are subject to dual phosphorylation and are generally activated by environmental stresses. The upstream kinases acting on p38 include MEK 3 and 6. These upstream kinases are in turn activated by MEKK1. GTPases are responsible for the transmission of stress stimuli to the MAPKKKs of this pathway, including Rac, Rho and Cdc42. The five p38 isoforms defined to date (p38a, p38b, p38g, p38d and p38-2) vary, based on their substrate specificity. They are responsible for the activation of HSP27 by Sap-1α, myocyte enhancer factor-2A (MEF-2A), MNK1/2 and MAPK-activated protein kinase-2 (MAPKAPK2) originally identified as a substrate for ERKs but now recognized as a physiological substrate for p38. Other targets including ATF1/2 and Ca^{+2}/cAMP response element binding protein (CREB) are produced through the activation of MSK1. Similarly to ERK1/2, ERK5 [also known as Big MAP kinase (Bmk1)] is activated by serum, growth factors and G protein coupled receptors. Upstream components of the ERK5 pathway include Ras, MEKK2 and 3, MEK5. ERK5 translocates into the nucleus and phosphorylates the kinase RSK, which phosphorylates transcriptional regulators including c-Fos, estrogen receptor (EP), NΦκB/IκBα, cAMP-response element-binding protein (CREB). Other downstream targets of the ERK5 pathway include MEF2C, Fra-1, c-myc, c-Fos.

The ERK1/2 Pathway

For asbestos, the ERK1/2 pathway was demonstrated to be the predominant MAPK pathway relevant for the induction of apoptosis and proliferation in mesothelial cells (Goldberg et al., 1997; Jimenez et al., 1997; Zanella et al., 1996). The initiation of the ERK cascade in mesothelial cells by asbestos is due to autophosphorylation of the EGF receptor (EGFR) (Zanella et al., 1996). In these studies, the specific activation of EGFR and ERK1/2 by asbestos but not by non-pathogenic particles was also demonstrated. Aggregation of the EGFR by long crocidolite fibers may initiate cell signaling cascades important for asbestos-induced mitogenesis and mesothelioma (Pache et al., 1998). However, diverse ERK stimuli like H_2O_2, EGF and asbestos cause different time patterns of accumulation of activated, i.e. phosphorylated ERK1/2, which then mediate cell-cycle alterations during the development of epithelial cell apoptosis or proliferation (Buder-Hoffmann et al., 2001). Inhalation studies have also shown a striking increase in ERK phosphorylation within pulmonary epithelial cells at sites of developing fibrotic lesions after 14–20 days of chrysotile asbestos inhalation by mice (Robledo et al., 2000). PDGF-A and TGF-α gene expression by amosite asbestos in tracheal explants are also ERK-dependent (Dai and Churg, 2001). Two phases of the C10 cell cycle appear particularly sensitive to environmental insults: transition from G0 to G1 as assessed by expression of cyclin D1 (Yuan et al. 2003 and 2004, Burch et al., 2004) and progression through the S phase.

Yuan et al indicated expression of cyclin D1 as a reliable marker for serum-stimulated cells that are destined to enter the S phase, whereas migration of AIF into the cell nucleus represents a marker for cells destined to die of apoptosis. The expression of both of these markers correlated with the subcellular localization of phospho-ERK1/2 over time, supporting the notion that the duration of ERK1/2 signaling in the nucleus is intimately connected to cell fate (Yuan et al. 2004).

These data suggest that termination of nuclear ERK1/2 signaling is required to exit G0. However, once cells exit G0 and express cyclin D1, they are destined to continue through G1, phosphorylate pRB, and enter into the S phase.

In some models of cell stress, inhibition of caspases does not prevent cell death (Penninger and Kroemer 2003). AIF is a mitochondrial intermembrane flavoprotein that induces nuclear fragmentation when added directly to nuclei *in vitro* (Susin et al., 1999) and therefore may be responsible for some aspects of cell death that occur under conditions in which caspases have been inhibited. Necrosis and apoptosis also may share features in common when ATP levels are low (Susin et al., 2000). The migration of AIF from mitochondria to the nucleus provided a dose-dependent marker of cell fate in response to persistent nuclear phospho-ERK1/2. Nearly all of the cells that expressed nuclear phospho-ERK1/2 8 hours after serum stimulation in the presence of any dose of asbestos also stained positive for nuclear AIF. Previous work indicates that AIF is released from mitochondria slightly before cytochrome *c*, supporting the interpretation that it represents an early marker for the induction of apoptosis and, under some conditions, necrosis (Susin et al., 2000). Therefore, analysis of those signaling events that correlate with migration of AIF into the nucleus represents a useful approach to examine the responses of individual cells to environmental agents.

Cell fate in response to asbestos, either entry into the S phase or induction of apoptosis, was strongly correlated with the trafficking of ERK1/2 over time. In response to serum, phosphorylated ERK1/2 entered the nucleus by 15 minutes, and by 2 hours most of the phosphorylated kinase was observed in the cell periphery. It is not known whether nuclear ERK1/2 relocates to the cell periphery under these conditions or whether control of kinase activity in these locations occurs independently. However, sequestration of p42/p44 mitogen-activated protein kinase (*i.e.,* ERK1/2) in the cytoplasm by expression of a catalytically inactive form of a cytoplasmic mitogen activated protein kinase phosphatase does not prevent phosphorylation of cytoplasmic substrates (Brunet et al., 1999).

Cells expressing nuclear phospho-ERK1/2 at 8 hours in response to asbestos often showed high levels of phospho-ERK1/2 in the cytoplasm and the nucleus, indicating that mechanisms that regulate the kinases in these two locations may be independent of one another.

The p38 Kinase Pathway

A recent study investigating the induction of the p38 pathway in mesothelial cells after treatment with crocidolite asbestos convincingly showed a dose-dependent phosphorylation of this protein (Swain et al., 2004). The relevance of this signalling pathway was demonstrated by its correlation with the asbestos induced AP-1 binding activity which can be blocked by an inhibitor of p38. In addition to ERK, p38 kinase also is activated by asbestos in normal alveolar macrophages (Geist et al., 2000).

The JNK Pathway

As another MAPK pathway, JNK has been investigated for its inducibility by particles. Both DEP and crystalline silica are able to induce JNK activation in mouse lung epithelial cells, resulting in an upregulation of mRNA coding for AP-1 proteins. In the same cell system, crocidolite asbestos induced a moderate activation of JNK and AP-1 mRNA (Shukla et al., 2001). In earlier studies using mesothelial cells, however, crocidolite asbestos failed to induce JNK (Jimenez et al., 1997). The relative importance of each of the three MAP-kinase pathways as well as their contribution to AP-1 activation and the induction of the endpoints apoptosis and proliferation are still an open question. Moreover, the interference of these pathways between each other as well as with other pathways induced by growth factors or particle associated compounds remains to be clarified.

The ERK5 Pathway

The ERK family consists of at least seven isoforms, and little is known about their regulation and function. Scapoli et al (2004) showed for the first time that asbestos, but not glass beads or the nonfibrous, chemically similar analog, riebeckite, causes protracted activation of ERK5, a redox-sensitive kinase known to mediate c-jun proto-oncogene expression and critically related to proliferation in other cell systems (Kato et al., 1998; Esparis-Ogando et al., 2002), is activated by asbestos. Inducible ERK5 phosphorylation is observed in C10 epithelial cells in a time- and dose-dependent manner after exposure to EGF, H_2O_2 or crocidolite asbestos. This observation supports the concept that frustrated phagocytosis of asbestos fibers (Mossman et al., 1996) is a source of oxidant production relevant to ERK5 activation. ERK5 activation by asbestos is Src-dependent as demonstrated using transfection of a dominant-negative Src (dnSrc) construct into C10 cells. In fact, the cells transfected with an empty vector (controls) showed an increase in ERK5 phosphorylation after asbestos exposure, while the dnSrc-transfected cells did not. The protracted responses in ERK5 phosphorylation by asbestos resemble those observed for ERK1/2 (Buder-Hoffmann et al., 2001), and may be due to the fact that asbestos fibers slowly settle on cells and are phagocytized or cycled between cells over time. The use of small molecule inhibitors suggests that ERK5 activation by asbestos is similar to that of H_2O_2. The blockage of EGFR or MEK1/2 phosphorylation does not reduce ERK5 activation by asbestos or H_2O_2, implying an EGFR-independent pathway of activation. In contrast, ERK1/2 phosphorylation by asbestos, but not H_2O_2, is dependent on phosphorylation of the EGFR.

Src involvement has been implicated in signalling from many receptors, including EGFR, although the interactions between Src and the EGFR are multidimensional and poorly understood (Abram and Courtneidge, 2000). It has been suggested that Src binds directly to the EGFR, leading to the activation of Src and Src phosphorylation of the EGFR at sites that hyperactivate the kinase activity of the EGFR (Abram and Courtneidge, 2000). Scapoli et al showed that phosphorylation of Src occurs prior to phosphorylation of the EGFR, and these observations are consistent with the hypothesis that Src phosphorylates the EGFR, a requirement for ERK1/2 phosphorylation (Scapoli et al., 2004). Alternatively, Src activation of ERK5 could be downstream of the EGFR and mediated by other kinases. Src, ERK1/2 and ERK5 are all important in asbestos-induced proliferation and this may be the result of increases in the mRNA levels of AP-1 family members as shown in Figure 2.

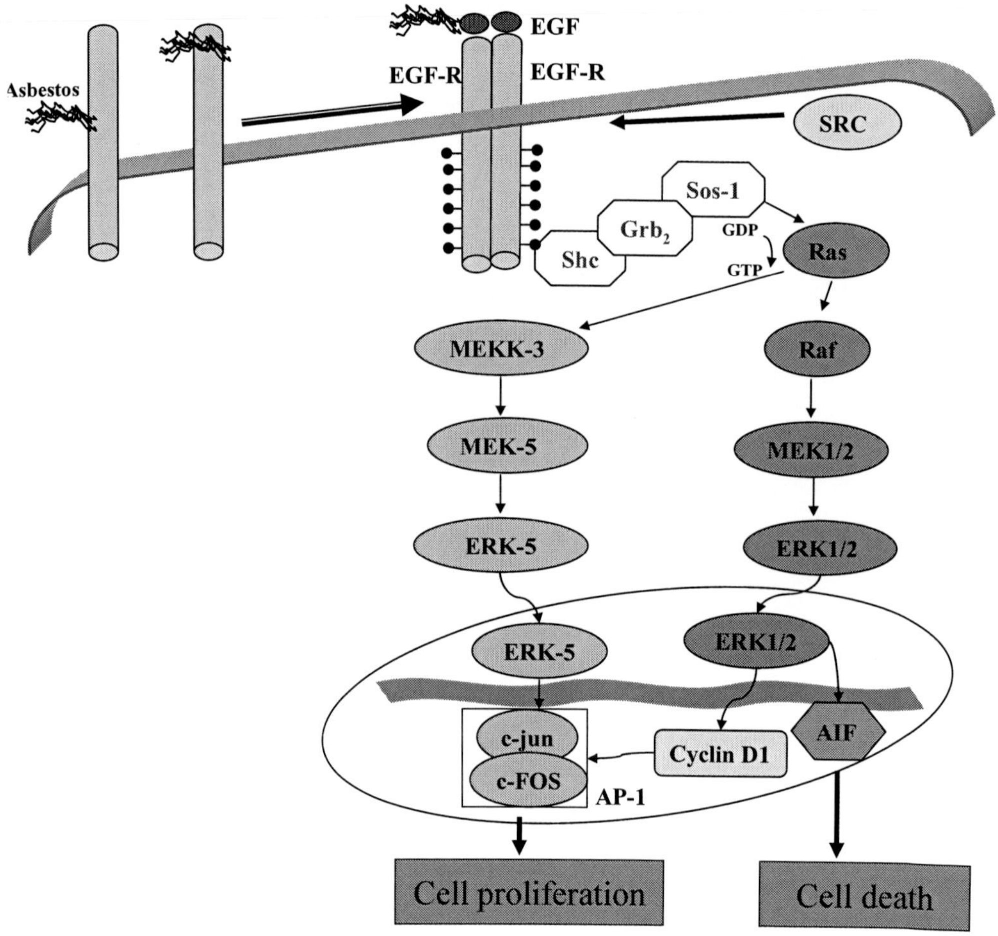

Figure 2. Cell signaling pathways elicited by asbestos fibers. Asbestos fibers cause aggregation of the EGFR, a phenomenon leading to phosphorylation of the EGFR which is critical to ERK1/2 activation. ERK1/2 activated through an EGFR-dependent pathway, enters the nucleus. In absence of asbestos signaling by ERK1/2 in the nucleus decrease and expression of cyclin D1 ensues, thereby driving cells through G1 and into the S phase. In presence of asbestos, signaling by ERK1/2 in the nucleus is prolonged, AIF relocates to the nucleus, and cell death ensues. Src activation by asbestos may lead to phosphorylation of the EGFR and/or downstream events linked to ERK5 phosphorylation. AP-1 member protooncogenes most importantly, ERK1/2- and ERK5-dependent, c-fos, c-jun, and fra-1, are observed. The possible synergy between Src- and EGFR-dependent signaling are critical to cell proliferation.

The ERK5 pathway may contribute selectively to the regulation of c-jun, whereas both the Src and ERK1/2 pathways may regulate c-fos, fra-1 and c-jun. Moreover, it has been recently linked ERK1/2-dependent fra-1 expression on mesothelial cell transformed by asbestos (Ramos-Nino et al., 2002, 2003) to the protracted expression of this gene that may be a result of initial increases in c-fos and c-jun (Shukla et al., 2001; Ramos-Nino et al., 2002, 2003).

2.2. Transcription Factor AP-1

AP-1 is a family of transcription factors comprised of homo- and heterodimers of the Jun and Fos early response oncogenes. It is a redox-sensitive transcription factor classically associated with the development of cell proliferation and tumor promotion (Su and Karin, 1996). These proteins are phosphorylated and activated by MAPK signaling cascades (Seger and Krebs, 1995). Strikingly persistent and dose-dependent increases in c-fos and c-jun mRNA by crocidolite asbestos were originally reported in rat pleural mesothelial cells (Heintz et al., 1993). AP-1 activation after asbestos exposure in vivo was then demonstrated in transgenic mice bearing AP-1-luciferase reporter sequences (Ding et al., 1999). Crocidolite increased AP-1 activity in these animals in a dose and time dependent manner. This suggests a model of asbestos-induced mesothelioma involving chronic stimulation of cell proliferation via an activation of the early response gene pathway. The induction of AP-1 by asbestos is cell type specific. For example, in hamster tracheal epithelial cells, increased c-jun expression after asbestos exposure was not accompanied by elevations in c-fos expression (Heintz et al., 1993). The increased expression of c-jun in hamster tracheal epithelial cell by asbestos led to increased proliferation and enhanced ability of these cells to grow in soft agar, an indication of cellular transformation (Timblin et al., 1995). The asbestos-induced overexpression of c-fos in rat mesothelial cells is mediated via phosphorylation of EGFR (Zanella et al., 1999). Thus, the ability to block asbestos-induced elevations in c-fos mRNA levels and apoptosis by small molecule inhibitors of EGFR phosphorylation may have therapeutic implications in asbestos-related disease (Zanella et al., 1999).

The fos-family member Fra-1 (fos related antigen-1) was also demonstrated to be upregulated in pretumorous tissues from crocidolite treated animals as well as in mesothelioma induced by this fibre sample. In vitro assays revealed that, comparable to other members of the jun and fos families, fra-1 is induced as an early response gene in a fibre-specific manner by natural and man made fibres but not by granulous control particles (Ramos-Ninos et al., 2003). Expression of fra-1 is ERK-dependent and related directly to growth in soft agar and conversion of cells to a fibroblastic-like phenotype.

Furthermore, crocidolite asbestos increases expression of redox factor-1 (Ref-1 or APE) in mesothelial cells (Fung et al., 1997) and in alveolar macrophages. This is accompanied by an oxidant stimulus-mediated increase in AP-1 DNA binding activity (Flaherty et al., 2002). These findings indicate that high airborne concentrations of asbestos cause molecular changes in pleural spaces that also may be related to upregulation of antioxidant defenses and triggering of cell proliferation.

2.3. Transcription Factor NF kappa B (NF-κB)

Although the direct effects of particles may influence proliferation and apoptosis, important signaling pathways can also be activated by the release of growth factors and cytokines consequent to inflammatory response. This protein secretion may lead to the induction of autocrine growth loops. On the other hand, cytokine release is followed by the recruitment of inflammatory cells, which may also influence initiation and tumour promotion.

Nuclear factor-kappa B (NF-κB) is a redox sensitive transcription factor that also regulates expression of genes intrinsic to inflammation and cell proliferation (Janssen-Heininger et al., 2000). The NF-κB family consists of five different family members including NF-κB1 (p50/p105), NF-κB2 (p52/p100), RelA (p65), RelB and c-Rel. The highly conserved Rel proteins are responsible for DNA-binding, dimerization and interaction with IκB the intracellular inhibitor of NFκB. A wide range of stimuli, which typically includes cytokines, mitogens, environmental and occupational particles, toxic metals, intracellular stress, viral and bacterial products, and UV light, induce expression of early response genes through the NFκB family of transcription factors. Moreover, since inflammation and proliferation are associated with the development of asbestos-associated diseases, this family of transcription factors has been studied extensively both in vitro and in vivo after asbestos exposures.

Crocidolite asbestos was first discovered to cause protracted and dose-responsive increase in NF-κB binding proteins in hamster tracheal epithelial cells (Janssen et al., 1995). Asbestos-induced redox changes and phosphorylation events in vitro activate nuclear proteins recognizing the NF-κB/NF-IL-6 binding sites of the IL-8 promoter and contribute to the regulation of IL-8 gene expression, a major chemo-attractant in lung (Luster and Simeonova, 1998; Simeonova and Luster, 1996). Using rat inhalation models of crocidolite- and chrysotile-induced inflammation and asbestosis, it was observed striking immunolocalization of RelA in bronchiolar and alveolar epithelial cells at 5 days after inhalation which persisted at sites of lesion development for 20 days (Janssen et al., 1997). Asbestos fibers stimulate IL-6 expression and secretion in pulmonary type II-like epithelial A549 cells as well as in normal human bronchial epithelial cells (Simeonova et al., 1997). This may be relevant to the development of asbestosis as elevated IL-6 levels are found in bronchoalveolar lavage fluids from patients diagnosed with fibrosis or having work-related histories of long-term asbestos exposure (Simeonova et al., 1997).

Activation of NFκB in cells which are mainly important in the inflammatory response, i.e. alveolar macrophages, has been demonstrated in several studies following particle exposure. Exposure of human alveolar macrophages to indoor air pollutants like chrysotile B induce transcription and production of pro-inflammatory cytokines via NF-κB, suggesting an important role in the pathogenesis of airway disease and lung parenchymal injury (Drumm et al, 1999; Drumm et al., 1998; Oettinger et al., 1999). Since alveolar macrophages are located adjacent to bronchial and bronchiolar epithelial cells, an interaction between these cells may be conducive to the process of inflammation. For example, in an in vitro model of co-cultured blood monocytes and epithelial cells in a transwell system, exposure of monocytes to chrysotile increases the level of NF-κB and cytokine genes in epithelial cells (Drumm et al., 1999). In addition, urokinase type plasminogen activator and its receptor mRNA levels are increased in human bronchial epithelial cells and endothelial cells exposed to chrysotile fibers, and this is associated with increased nuclear levels of NF-κB (Barchowsky et al., 1998).

Like several other pro-inflammatory cytokines, tumor necrosis factor-alpha (TNF-α) is a critical mediator of the pathogenic responses of asbestosis (Liu et al., 1998). Asbestos-induced TNF-α gene expression in alveolar macrophages is mediated through a process that involves NF-κB activation and a free radical process (Cheng et al., 1999). A work of Xie et al. (2000) suggests that mineral fibers may cause pathological lesions via an autocrine-like process in which the response evoked by particles, for example, TNF-α production acts to enhance subsequent interaction of particles with tissue. In these studies, TNF-α released from alveolar macrophages after phagocytosis of asbestos fibers increased epithelial binding of fibers by a NF- κB-dependent mechanism. Although EGFR phosphorylation has been linked to alterations of NF-κB activity in some models, EGFR phosphorylation is not essential for NF-κB activation by asbestos (Ramos-Ninos et al., 2002). In addition, several studies have also described the involvement of NFκB in cell cycle regulation, apoptosis as well as tumourigenic processes (Chen et al., 2002). The authors described NFκB as a pivotal transcription factor in silica-induced diseases. The understanding of how silica induces NFκB activation as well as which signalling pathways are involved has been emphasized as important for new information regarding aetiology and potential treatment of silica-related lung diseases.

On the other hand, other transcription factors may be involved. The nuclear factor of activated T cells (NFAT) is a transcription factor that is expressed only in activated but not in resting T cells (Rincon and Flavell, 1997). The induction of this factor in T cells requires a calcium-activated signaling pathway and may play an important role in cancer development (Jiang et al., 1993). In mouse embryo fibroblasts, asbestos induces NFAT activation through a H_2O_2-dependent and cyclosporine A-sensitive pathway, an observation which may be relevant to asbestos-induced inflammation and cancers (Li et al., 2002).

2.4. Protein Kinase C (PKC)

Another signalling pathway responding to various extracellular stimuli and possibly involved in regulation of proliferation and apoptosis is the protein kinase C (PKC) pathway. This family of proteins has been shown to exhibit effects on several endpoints such as growth, differentiation and apoptosis. A feature of tumor promoters, such as phorbol esters, i.e. 12-O-tetradecanoylphorbol-13-acetate (TPA) is their ability to stimulate PKC activity. Phorbol esters, such as TPA resembles diacylglycerol in structure, thus activate PKC directly. In contrast, asbestos is an insoluble fiber that increases hydrolysis of inositol phospholipids and amounts of diacylglycerol in respiratory epithelial cells in vitro (Sesko et al., 1990). These signaling events may be linked to asbestos-induced stimulation of MAPK pathways, activation of fos/jun early response genes, and outcomes, such as injury and/or proliferation of epithelial cells. Like other tumor promoters, both chrysotile and crocidolite forms of asbestos have been shown to induce the activity of ornithine decarboxylase (ODC) and DNA synthesis in a hamster tracheal epithelial cell line (Landesman and Mossman, 1982). Use of protein kinase C inhibitors blocked the ODC activity in a dose-dependent manner, showing the involvement of PKC in the asbestos-induced mitogenic response (Marsh and Mossman, 1988). Asbestos increases the activity of PKC in hamster tracheal epithelial cells using a histone phosphorylation assay (Perderiset et al., 1991). However, the mechanism seems to be different from TPA. Whereas TPA causes redistribution of almost all the PKC activity from the cytosol to membrane fraction, the majority of activity is still associated with the cytosolic fraction at various time periods after exposure to asbestos (Perderiset et al., 1991). Asbestos-stimulated TNF-α release from alveolar macrophages is dependent on fiber length and opsonization and can be blocked using PKC inhibitors, thus indicating a role of PKCs in asbestos-induced TNF release (Donaldson et al., 1992). Using a specific inhibitor for protein kinase C, Ro 31-7549, other studies suggest that PKC may have also an important role in the activation of neutrophils and their production of ROS after exposure to particulate or soluble stimuli (Ruotsalainen and Savolainen, 1995).

There are several isoforms of PKC that may act differentially in asbestos-induced signaling events. Using specific inhibitors and down-modulation of PKC, it was showed that inhibition of PKC-δ blocked asbestos-induced c-fos/c-jun expression in rat mesothelial cells (Fung et al., 1998). PKC may be involved in oxygen radical generation from different asbestos fibers as the protein kinase C inhibitors, sphingosine and staurosporine, suppressed ROS generation by asbestos in alveolar macrophages (Lim et al., 1997). Using a pulmonary epithelial cell line (C10), enhanced immunoreactivity of PKC- δ was observed in epithelial cells expressing proliferating cell nuclear antigen (PCNA) after mechanical wounding or exposure to asbestos fibers, indicating an involvement of PKC- δ in asbestos-induced proliferation (Lounsbury et al., 2002).

2.5. Reactive Oxygen and Nitrogen Species (ROS/RNS)

Asbestos fibers, which contain transition metals or which have reactive surface characteristics, are able to induce signaling pathways via the generation of reactive oxygen species (ROS) (Fubini et al., 1997). Reduction or blocking of this ROS generation demonstrated that ROS are involved in asbestos-induced cellular effects (Shukla et al., 2003). The activation of AP-1 as well as NFκB by crocidolite asbestos in rat lung fibroblasts can be reduced by treatment with vitamin E (α-tocopherol). These data indicate an involvement of ROS generated via lipid peroxidation in asbestos induced effects (Faux et al., 1997). ERK1/2 as well as p38 activation by crocidolite asbestos could be diminished by the addition of N-acetyl-l-cysteine, a general anti-oxidant, and furthermore, the involvement of hydrogen peroxide was demonstrated using catalase as blocking substance (Swain et al., 2004). The generation of hydrogen peroxide may be explained by the presence of intrinsic iron in the asbestos sample which may serve as the transition metal involved in Fenton chemistry. The ROS activation of the JNK pathway was studied in mouse lung epithelial cells treated with crystalline silica. In these experiments, JNK-activity as well as Fra-1 mRNA levels were reduced by the addition of tetramethylthiourea (TMTU), a specific intracellular scavenger of hydroxyl radicals (Shukla et al., 2001). Moreover, cell proliferation, as well as activation of ERK1/2, was reduced by TMTU.

In addition to ROS, other signaling may be triggered by reactive nitrogen species (RNS) like nitric oxide (NO•) or peroxynitrite (ONOO−). There are some indications that asbestos is able to induce nitric oxide synthase (iNOS) in rat lung as well as in rat pleural mesothelial cells (Choe et al., 1998). In vivo, RNS can be produced by macrophages activated during particle-induced inflammation. In rats treated by asbestos both the activation of iNOS in lung macrophages as well as the immunoreactivity for nitrotyrosine in the target cells of lung epithelium and mesothelium have been observed (Tanaka et al., 1998). Studying MAPK signaling in asbestos treated rat lung, it was shown that nitrotyrosine immunoreactivity and

ERK1/2 phosphorylation co-localise in the same target tissues suggesting a role for ONOO– in ERK signaling (Iwagaki et al., 2003). However, contrasting data come from in vitro studies investigating the role of RNS on lung epithelial cells using donor substances for NO• and ONOO–. While NO• was able to induce c-fos and c-jun expression and AP-1 binding, ONOO– failed to exhibit these effects (Janssen et al., 1997b). Although the development of asbestos-related diseases is complex, a number of studies suggest that ROS mediate asbestos-induced pathogenesis. In an environment of increased oxidative stress as the one found in the pleura, mesothelial cells might develop particular defenses against the oxidative environment leading to the development of mesothelioma. This particular conditioning environment could be one of the causes of the resistance of mesothelioma to ROS produced by the most part of anticancer drugs.

2.6. Membrane Receptors

Possible targets of particle-cell interaction as well as of exogenous ROS or RNS are cell surface receptors. The epidermal growth factor receptor (EGFR) is the best studied receptor involved in MAPK activation, which is discussed as a possible target for ROS and RNS (Klotz et al., 2002). However, the molecular mechanisms by which these radicals may induce autophosphorylation of EGFR are not understood. For asbestos, an involvement of EGF-R autophosphorylation in the signalling pathways via ERK1/2 and AP-1 activation associated with apoptosis has been demonstrated convincingly. Using the specific EGF-R inhibitor Tyrphostin AG-1478, the fibre effects could be blocked (Zanella et al., 1999). In experiments with transgenic mice expressing dominant-negative EGF-R in lung tissue, the asbestos induced expression of genes of the fos and jun family could be linked to this receptor (Manning et al., 2002).

In further studies, a synergism between oxidants and TNFα in the activation of NFκB was shown, supported by the observation of TNFα-induced IκB degradation in contrast to ROS/RNS. In addition, by using dominant-negative Ras-constructs, the requirement of Ras only in ROS-induced NFκB activation is shown. In both (ROS/RNS, TNFα) downstream events, the MEKK1-JNK pathway seems to play a key role in NFκB activation, whereas the MEK-ERK pathway negatively regulates NFκB (Janssen et al., 1999). EGF-R may be the critical protein governing particle-cell-interaction. In co-localisation studies with asbestos fibres and EGF-R-specific antibodies, differences due to physical characteristics were observed. In these studies only cells which came into contact with very long fibres showed increased protein levels of EGF-R (Pache et al., 1998; Faux et al., 2000). Since the same cells expressed proliferating cell nuclear antigen (PCNA) this may be associated with EGF-R clustering and subsequent induction of the MAPK and AP-1 signaling pathway.

The fibrous effect of asbestos was first tested in vitro in lung epithelial cells cultured in a stretching chamber mimicking cyclic cell motion during breathing (Tsuda et al., 1999). Fibre treatment during cyclic stretch resulted in an increased release of the pro-inflammatory cytokine IL-8. Interestingly, fibres coated with fibronectin, a protein of the extracellular matrix (ECM), increased this mechanically induced effect. The involvement of integrins as cell surface receptors was indicated by the abolishment of IL-8 release in cells pre-treated with an excess of integrin blocking peptides. Therefore, the extracellular matrix, cell surface receptors, and the cell membrane itself must be considered as target compartments of the cell with a pivotal role for signal transduction.

The very first target for interaction with the particle may be the ECM proteins of the cell which are directly linked to integrins by protein–protein interaction (Dedhar et al., 2001). Integrins are transmembrane proteins consisting of an extracellular domain which is in contact with the ECM, a transmembrane domain, and an intracellular domain linked to the focal contacts. Alterations in the structure of the ECM which may be induced by physical or chemical reactions are perceived by integrins and this information is relayed into the cell (Aplin et al., 1998). Signal transduction proteins, such as focal adhesion kinase (FAK) or integrin linked kinase (Ilk) are located in focal contacts and can be activated by integrins. Further indications for the involvement of ECM proteins and integrins come from mesothelial cells, treated with crocidolite or chrysotile asbestos (Wu et al., 2000). Coating of fibres with vitronectin led to increased phagocytosis, resulting in enhanced levels of intracellular oxidative stress and apoptosis. Again, these effects could be blocked by integrin-ligand blockade with the respective arginine–glycine–aspartic acid (RGD) peptides. In these assays, endpoints like oxidative DNA-damage as well as apoptosis appeared to be linked to phagocytosis.

Indications for the in vivo relevance of integrins in fibre-cell interaction come from mRNA expression analysis during asbestos induced mesothelioma carcinogenesis. In these assays three genes that are directly linked to integrin mediated signal transduction, have been demonstrated to be upregulated. Apart from zyxin, a shuttle protein of the focal contact, and the ECM protein osteopontin, integrin linked kinase as a cytoplasmic integrin binding partner was identified (Liu et al., 1997). Ilk is described to activate protein kinase B (AKT), as well as glycogensynthase kinase 3 (GSK-3) and therefore may play a key role in cell cycle regulation (Persad et al., 2001). Based on these in vivo observations, a series of experiments investigating the induction of integrin mediated signal transduction in response to fibrous particles has been performed in mesothelial cells. As a relevant endpoint, particle-induced apoptosis was demonstrated to be influenced by integrins. Similar results were obtained for fibre-induced cell proliferation which occurs in parallel to apoptosis.

Recently, it was observed that fibre-induced activation of ERK1/2 is strongly linked to ß1-integrins (Berken et al., 2003). Moreover, protein kinase B (AKT) was activated in parallel to ERK1/2 with similar kinetics and integrin linkage. The results are the first demonstration of particle-induced AKT activation, a pathway that allows cells to escape from apoptosis and instead undergo proliferation.

3. Conclusion

The ability of asbestos fibers to stimulate multiple cell signaling pathways suggest the involvement of a myriad of transcription factors and their cross-talk in asbestos-induced gene expression. A hypothetical schema showing the plausible interactions between these signaling cascades is presented in Figure 3.

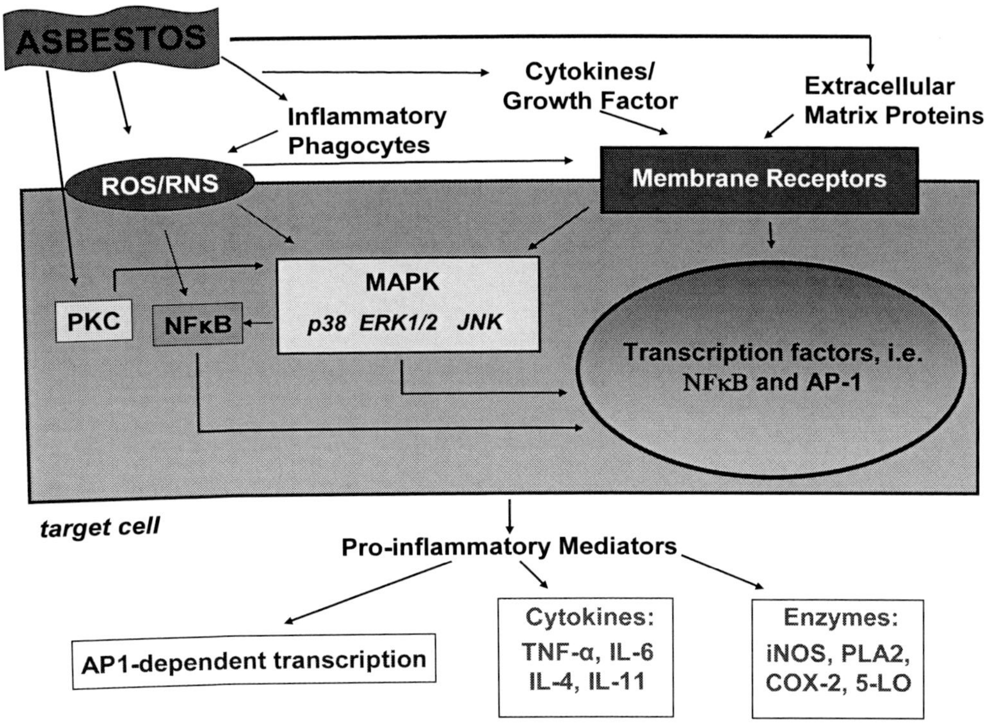

Figure 3. Hypothetical representation showing the interactions of various cell signaling pathways elicited by asbestos fibers and their relationships to activation of transcription factors and gene expression (see the text).

Although the relationships between NF-κB and AP-1 dependent gene expression are undoubtedly complex, both are regulated by redox changes and inhibited by antioxidants (Meyer et al., 1994; Pinkus, et al., 1996). Moreover, these transcription factors act in concert in the induction of neoplastic transformation (Li et al., 1997). The demonstration that inhibitors of NF-κB (Baichwal and Baeuerle, 1997) and ERK phosphorylation (Sebolt-Leopold et al., 1999) block survival responses and proliferation of tumor cells suggest novel preventive and therapeutic approaches to asbestos-associated tumors and fibrosis.

The selective inhibition of a suspected target of these multiple cell signaling pathways could be an interesting strategy in the chemoprevention of mesothelioma. In this view, different single-target agent was been studied: the specific EGF-R-associated kinase inhibitors Gefitinib (ZD1839 [IRESSA]), already used in phase II/III clinical trials in the therapy of lung epidermoid cancer, and Erlotinib are coupled to complete inhibition of ras and erk activity. Moreover, the selective inhibition of ras with gene transfer therapeutic strategies based on the delivery of dominant negative forms of ras such as RASN17 or with agents that block ras farnesylation such as the farnesyltransferase inhibitors (FTI) could be also considered new molecular-targeted therapies. Raf-1, MEK-1 and consequently the activation of ERK-1/2 could be also evaluated as additional target through the use of selective inhibitors such as Sorafenib or U0126 (Figure 4).

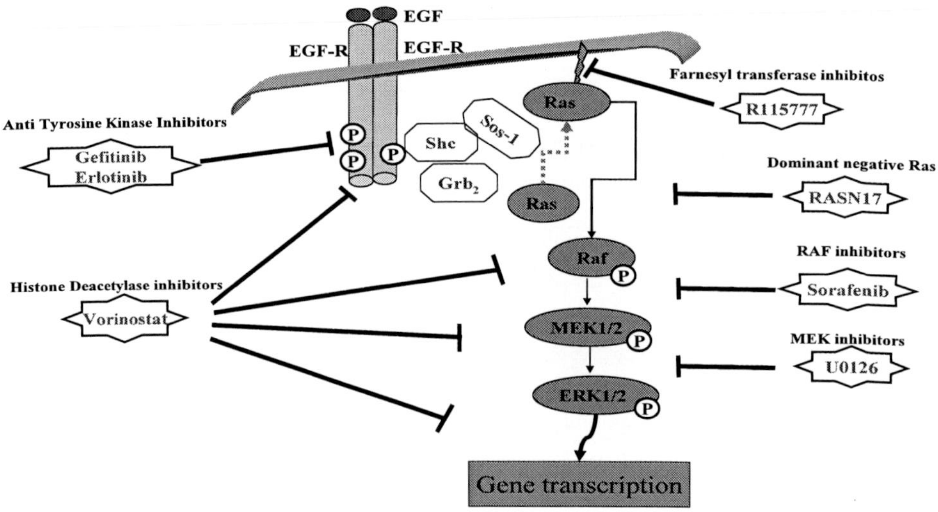

Figure 4. Signal transduction pathways inhibited by single- and multi-target agents. The inhibition of EGF-ras dependent pathway through the use of single-target agents, the EGF-R-associated tyrosine kinase inhibitor Gefitinib or Erlotinib or the dominant negative ras RASN17 or FTI R115777 or the Raf-1 inhibitor Sorafenib or the MEK-1 inhibitor U0126 and of multi-target agents, the HDAC inhibitor Vorinostat, induces the release of this anti-apoptotic pathway.

Inhibitors of histone deacetylase (HDAC), such as suberoylanilide hydroxamic acid (SAHA, vorinostat), represent a novel class of multi-target agents entered recently in clinical studies that target histones and other proteins involved in the regulation of gene expression and cell cycle progression (Budillon et al., 2005) (Figure 4). Phase I trials of intravenous and oral formulations of vorinostat, have shown that it is safe and tolerable, that it inhibits histone deacetylation in peripheral blood mononuclear cells, and that it has a broad range of antitumor activity and partial clinical activity in some tumors subtype including mesothelioma (Kelly et al., 2005). In particular, among thirteen patients with mesothelioma, previously treated with chemotherapy and included in a phase I trial of oral vorinostat, four patients completed at least 6 cycles of therapy and two patients demonstrated a partial response (Krug et al. 2006). Given the dearth of treatment options for patients with advanced mesothelioma who have progressed after first-line chemotherapy, these results are encouraging. A placebo-controlled, randomized phase III study of oral SAHA is now open for patients with mesothelioma in whom treatment with pemetrexed has failed (Krug et al. 2006).

Together with the newer drugs, rapidly emerging from the laboratory to be applied in the clinic, we have the hope of making further advances in the effort against this rare disease.

Acknowledgements

This work was supported in part by grants from AIRC, FIRC, MIUR and Ministero della Sanità, Rome, Italy (FSN2005).

References

Abe M, Kuo W-L, MB H and Rosner M. Extracellular signal-regulated kinase 7 (ERK7), a novel ERK with a C-terminal domain that regulates its activity, its cellular localization, and cell growth. *Mol. Cell. Biol.* 1999, 19, 1301–1312.

Abram CL, Courtneidge SA. Src family tyrosine kinases and growth factor signaling. *Exp. Cell Res.* 2000, 254(1):1-13.

Aplin AE, Howe A, Alahari SK, Juliano RL. Signal transduction and signal modulation by cell adhesion receptors: the role of integrins, cadherins, immunoglobulin-cell adhesion molecules, and selectins, *Pharmacol. Rev.* 1998, 50, 197–263.

Baichwal V and Baeuerle P. Activate NF-kappa B or die? *Current Biology* 1997, 7, R94–R96.

Barchowsky A, Roussel R, Krieser R, Mossman B and Treadwell M. Expression and activity of urokinase and its receptor in endothelial and pulmonary epithelial cells exposed to asbestos. *Toxicology and Applied Pharmacology* 1998, 152, 388–396.

Berken A, Abel J, Unfried K. β1-Integrin mediates asbestos induced activation of Akt and Erk1/2 in a rat pleural mesothelial cell line. *Oncogene* 2003, 22, 8524–8528.

BeruBe K, Quinlan T, Fung H, Magae J, Vacek P, Taatjes D and Mossman B. Apoptosis is observed in mesothelial cells after exposure to crocidolite asbestos. *American Journal of Respiratory Cell and Molecular Biology* 1996a, 15, 141–147.

Brunet A, Roux D, Lenormand P, Dowd S, Keyse S, Pouyssegur J. Nuclear translocation of p42/p44 mitogen-activated protein kinase is required for growth factor induced gene expression and cell cycle entry. *EMBO J.* 1999;18:664–74.

Buder-Hoffmann S, Palmer C, Vacek P, Taatjes D and Mossman B. Different accumulation of activated extracellular signal-regulated kinases (ERK 1/2) and role in cell-cycle alterations by epidermal growth factor, hydrogen peroxide, or asbestos in pulmonary epithelial cells. *American Journal of Respiratory Cell and Molecular Biology* 2001, 24, 405–413.

Budillon A, Bruzzese F, Di Gennaro E, Caraglia M. Multiple-target drugs: inhibitors of heat shock protein 90 and of histone deacetylase. *Curr. Drug Targets* 2005, 6(3):337-51.

Burch PM, Yuan Z, Loonen A, Heintz NH. An extracellular signal-regulated kinase 1- and 2-dependent program of chromatin trafficking of c-Fos and Fra-1 is required for cyclin D1 expression during cell cycle reentry. *Mol. Cell Biol.* 2004;24:4696–709.

Caraglia M, Budillon A, Tagliaferri P, Marra M, Abbruzzese A, Caponigro F. Isoprenylation of intracellular proteins as a new target for the therapy of human neoplasms: preclinical and clinical implications. *Curr. Drug Targets* 2005, 6(3):301-23.

Chen F, Shi X. NF-kappaB, a pivotal transcription factor in silica-induced diseases. *Mol. Cell Biochem.* 2002, 34-235(1-2):169-76.

Cheng N, Shi X, Ye J, Castranova V, Chen F, Leonard S, Vallyathan V and Rojanasakul Y. Role of transcription factor NF-kappaB in asbestos-induced TNF-alpha response from macrophages. *Experimental and Molecular Pathology* 1999, 66, 201–210.

Choe N, Tanaka S, Kagan E. Asbestos fibers and interleukin-1 upregulate the formation of reactive nitrogen species in rat pleural mesothelial cells. *Am. J. Respir. Cell Mol. Biol.* 1998, 19(2):226-36.

Churg A. Deposition and clearance of chrysotile asbestos. *Annals of Occupational Hygiene* 1994, 38, 625–633.

Dai J and Churg A. Relationship of fiber surface iron and reactive oxygen species to expression of procollagen, PDGF-A, and TGF-beta(1) in tracheal explants exposed to amosite asbestos. *American Journal of Respiratory Cell and Molecular Biology* 2001, 24, 427–435.

Dedhar S, Hannigan GE. Integrin cytoplasmic interactions and bidirectional transmembrane signalling, *Curr. Opin. Cell Biol.* 2001, 24, 405–413.

Dixon D, Bowser A, Badgett A, Haseman J and Brody A. Incorporation of bromodeoxyuridine (BrdU) in the bronchiolar-alveolar regions of the lungs following two inhalation exposures to chrysotile asbestos in strain A/J mice. *Journal of Environmental Pathology, Toxicology and Oncology* 1995, 14, 205–213.

Donaldson K, Brown D, Miller B and Brody A. Bromo-deoxyuridine (BrdU) uptake in the lungs of rats inhaling amosite asbestos or vitreous fibres at equal airborne fibre concentrations. *Experimental and Toxicologic Pathology* 1995, 47, 207–211.

Donaldson K, Li X, Dogra S, Miller B and Brown G. Asbestos-stimulated tumour necrosis factor release from alveolar macrophages depends on fibre length and opsonization. *Journal of Pathology* 1992, 168, 243–248.

Drumm K, Messner C and Kienast K. Reactive oxygen intermediate-release of fibre-exposed monocytes increases inflammatory cytokine-mRNA level, protein tyrosine kinase and NF-kappaB activity in co-cultured bronchial epithelial cells (BEAS-2B). *European Journal of Medicinal Research* 1999, 4, 257–263.

Drumm K, Oettinger R, Smolarski R, Bay M and Kienast K. In vitro study of human alveolar macrophages inflammatory mediator transcriptions and releases induced by soot FR 101, Printex 90, titandioxide and Chrysotile B. *European Journal of Medicinal Research* 1998, 3, 432–438.

Esparis-Ogando A, Diaz-Rodriguez E, Montero JC, Yuste L, Crespo P, Pandiella A. Erk5 participates in neuregulin signal transduction and is constitutively active in breast cancer cells overexpressing ErbB2. *Mol. Cell Biol.* 2002, 22(1):270-85.

Faux S and Howden P. Possible role of lipid peroxidation in the induction of NF-κB and AP-1 in RFL-6 cells by crocidolite asbestos: Evidence following protection by Vitamin E. *Environmental Health Perspectives* 1997, 105, 1127–1130.

Faux S, Houghton C, Hubbard A and Patrick G.. Increased expression of epidermal growth factor receptor in rat pleural mesothelial cells correlates with carcinogenicity of mineral fibres. *Carcinogenesis* 2000, 21, 2275–2280.

Flaherty D, Monick M, Carter A, Peterson M and Hunninghake G. Oxidant-mediated increases in redox factor-1 nuclear protein and activator protein-1 DNA binding in asbestos-treated macrophages. *Journal of Immunology* 2002, 168, 5675–5681.

Fubini B. Surface reactivity in the pathogenic response to particulates. *Environ. Health Perspect.* 1997 105(Suppl 5): 1013–1020.

Fung H, Kow Y, Van Houten B, Taatjes D, Hatahet Z, Janssen Y, Vacek P, Faux S and Mossman B. Asbestos increases mammalian major AP-endonuclease (APE) gene expression, protein levels and enzyme activity in rat pleural mesothelial cells. *Cancer Research* 1998, 58, 189–194.

Fung H, Quinlan TR, Janssen YM, Timblin CR, Marsh JP, Heintz NH, Taatjes DJ, Vacek P, Jaken S and Mossman BT. Inhibition of protein kinase C prevents asbestos-induced c-fos and c-jun proto-oncogene expression in mesothelial cells. *Cancer Research* 1997, 57, 3101–3105.

Geist L, Powers L, Monick M and Hunninghake G. Asbestos stimulation triggers differential cytokine release from human monocytes and alveolar macrophages. *Experimental Lung Research* 2000, 26, 41–56.

Goldberg J, Zanella C, Janssen Y, Timblin C, Jimenez L, Taatjes D and Mossman B. Novel cell imaging approaches show induction of apoptosis and proliferation in mesothelial cells by asbestos. *American Journal of Respiratory Cell and Molecular Biology* 1997, 17, 265–271.

Greenberg M. The art of perpetuating a public health hazard. *J. Occup. Environ. Med.* 2005, 47:137–144.

Guthrie G and Mossman B. (Eds.). *Health Effects of Mineral Dusts* 1993 (Vol. 28, pp. 1–584). Washington, DC: Mineralogical Society of America.

Heintz N, Janssen Y and Mossman B. Persistent induction of c-fos and c-jun expression by asbestos. *Proceedings of the National Academy of Sciences of the United States of America,* 1993, 90, 3299–3303.

Hillerdal G. Mesothelioma: Cases associated with nonoccupational and lowdose exposures. *Occup. Environ. Med.* 1999, 56:505–513.

Hume L and Rimstidt J. The biodurability of chrysotile asbestos. *American Mineralogist* 1992, 77, 1125–1128.

Ilgren EB and Wagner JC. Background incidence of mesothelioma: Animal and human evidence. *Regul. Toxicol. Pharmacol.* 1991, 13:133–149.

Iwagaki A, Choe N, Li Y, Hemenway DR, Kagan E. Asbestos inhalation induces tyrosine nitration associated with extracellular signal-regulated kinase 1/2 activation in the rat lung. *Am. J. Respir Cell Mol. Biol.* 2003, 28(1):51-60.

Janssen YM, Matalon S, Mossman BT. Differential induction of c-fos, c-jun, and apoptosis in lung epithelial cells exposed to ROS or RNS. *Am. J. Physiol.* 1997a, 273(4 Pt 1):L789-96.

Janssen Y, Driscoll K, Howard B, Quinlan T, Treadwell M, Barchowsky A and Mossman B. Asbestos causes translocation of p65 protein and increases NF-kappa B DNA binding activity in rat lung epithelial and pleural mesothelial cells. *American Journal of Pathology*, 1997b, 151, 389–401.

Janssen Y, Heintz N and Mossman B. Induction of c-fos and c-jun proto-oncogene expression by asbestos is emeliorated by N-acetyl-l-cysteine in mesothelial cells. *Cancer Research*, 1995, 55, 2085–2089.

Janssen YMW, Macara I, Mossman BT. Cooperativity between oxidants and tumor necrosis factor in the activation of nuclear factor (NF)-κB, *Am. J. Respir. Cell Mol. Biol.* 1999, 20, 942–952.

Janssen-Heininger Y, Poynter M and Baeuerle P. Recent advances towards understanding redox mechanisms in the activation of nuclear factor kappaB. *Free Radical Biology and Medicine* 2000, 28, 1317–1327.

Jiang H, Yamamoto S, Nishikawa K and Kato R. Anti-tumor-promoting action of FK506, a potent immunosuppressive agent. *Carcinogenesis* 1993, 14, 67–71.

Jimenez L, Zanella C, Fung H, Janssen Y, Vacek P, Charland C, Goldberg J and Mossman B. Role of extracellular signal-regulated protein kinases in apoptosis by asbestos and H_2O_2. *American Journal of Physiology* (Lung Cellular and Molecular Physiology) 1997, 273, L1029–L1035.

Jones JS. The pleura in health and disease. *Lung* 2001, 179:397–413.

Kamakura S, Moriguchi T and Nishida EJ. Activation of the protein kinase ERK5/BMK1 by receptor tyrosine kinases. Identification and characterization of a signaling pathway to the nucleus. *Biol. Chem.* 1999, 274, 26563–26571.

Kamp D and Weitzman S. The molecular basis of asbestos induced lung injury. *Thorax* 1999, 54, 638–652.

Karin M. The regulation of AP-1 activity by mitogenactivated protein kinases. *Journal of Biological Chemistry* 1995, 270, 16483–16486.

Kato Y, Tapping RI, Huang S, Watson MH, Ulevitch RJ, Lee JD. Bmk1/Erk5 is required for cell proliferation induced by epidermal growth factor. *Nature* 1998, 395(6703):713-6.

Kelly WK, O'Connor OA, Krug LM, Chiao JH, Heaney M, Curley T, MacGregore-Cortelli B, Tong W, Secrist JP, Schwartz L, Richardson S, Chu E, Olgac S, Marks PA, Scher H, Richon VM. Phase I study of an oral histone deacetylase inhibitor, suberoylanilide hydroxamic acid, in patients with advanced cancer. *J. Clin. Oncol.* 2005, 23(17):3923-31.

Klotz LO, Schroeder P, Sies H. Peroxynitrite signaling: receptor tyrosine kinases and activation of stress-resposive pathways, *Free Radic. Biol. Med.* 2002, 33, 737–747.

Krug LM, Curley T, Schwartz L, Richardson S, Marks P, Chiao J, Kelly WK. Potential role of histone deacetylase inhibitors in mesothelioma: clinical experience with suberoylanilide hydroxamic acid. *Clin. Lung Cancer*. 2006, 7(4):257-61.

Landesman, JM and Mossman BT. Induction of ornithine decarboxylase in hamster tracheal epithelial cells exposed to asbestos and 12-O-tetradecanoylphorbol-13-acetate. *Cancer Research* 1982, 42, 3669–3675.

Landrigan PL, Lioy PJ, Thurston G, et al. Health and environmental consequences of the World Trade Center disaster. *Environ. Health Perspect.* 2004, 112:731–739.

Lange JH. Letter to the editor—Re: “Mesothelioma trends in the United States: An update based on surveillance, epidemiology, and end results program data for 1973 through 2003.” *Am. J. Epidemiol.* 2004, 160:823.

Lee J, Ulevitch R and Han J. Primary structure of BMK1: a new mammalian map kinase. *Biochem. Biophys. Res. Commun.* 1995, 213, 715–724.

Li J, Huang B, Shi X, Castranova V, Vallyathan V and Huang C. Involvement of hydrogen peroxide in asbestos-induced NFAT activation. *Molecular and Cellular Biochemistry* 2002, 234–235, 161–168.

Li J, Westergaard C, Ghosh P and Colburn, N. Inhibitors of both nuclear factor-kappaB and activator protein-1 activation block the neoplastic transformation response. *Cancer Research* 1997, 57, 3569–3576.

Lim Y, Kim S, Kim K, Oh M, Lee K. Involvement of protein kinase C, phospholipase C, and protein tyrosine kinase pathways in oxygen radical generation by asbestos-stimulated alveolar macrophage. *Environmental Health Perspectives* 1997, 105, 1325–1327.

Liu J, Brass D, Hoyle G and Brody A. TNF-alpha receptor knockout mice are protected from the fibroproliferative effects of inhaled asbestos fibers. *American Journal of Pathology* 1998, 153, 1839–1847.

Liu YK, Uemura T, Nemoto A, Yabe T, Fujii N, Ushida T, Tateishi T. Osteopontin involvement in integrin-mediated cell signaling and regulation of expression of alkaline phosphatase during early differentiation of UMR cells, *FEBS Lett.* 420 (1997) 112–116.

Lounsbury KM, Stern M, Taatjes D, Jaken S and Mossman B. T. Increased localization and substrate activation of protein kinase C delta in lung epithelial cells following exposure to asbestos. *American Journal of Pathology* 2002, 160, 1991–2000.

Luster M and Simeonova P. Asbestos induces inflammatory cytokines in the lung through redox sensitive transcription factors. *Toxicology Letters* 1998, 102–103, 271–275.

Manning CB, Cummins AB, Jung MW, Berlanger I, Timblin CR, Palmer C, Taatjes DJ, Hemenway D, Vacek P, Mossman BT. A mutant epidermal growth factor receptor targeted to lung epithelium inhibits asbestos-induced proliferation and proto-oncogene expression, *Cancer Res.* 2002, 624169–4175.

Marsh JP and Mossman BT. Mechanisms of induction of ornithine decarboxylase activity in tracheal epithelial cells by asbestiform minerals. *Cancer Research* 1988, 48, 709–714.

Meyer M, Pahl H and Baeuerle P. Regulation of the transcription factors NF-kappa B and AP-1 by redox changes. *Chemico-Biological Interactions* 1994, 91, 91–100.

Mossman B and Churg A. State-of-the-art: Mechanisms in the pathogenesis of asbestosis and silicosis. *American Journal of Respiratory and Critical Care Medicine* 1998, 157, 1666–1680.

Mossman B and Gee J. Asbestos related disease. *New England Journal of Medicine* 1989, 320, 1721–1730.

Mossman B, Bignon J, Corn M, Seaton A and Gee J. Asbestos: Scientific developments and implications for public policy. *Science* 1990, 247, 294–301.

Mossman B, Kamp D and Weitzman S. Mechanisms of carcinogenesis and clinical features of asbestos-associated cancers. *Cancer Investigation* 1996, 14, 466–480.

Nolan RP, Ross M, Nord GL, Axten CW, Osleeb JP, Domnin SG, Price B and Wilson R. Risk assessment for asbestosrelated cancer from the 9/11 attack on the World Trade Center. *J. Occup. Environ. Med.* 2005, 47:817–825.

Oettinger R, Drumm K, Knorst M, Krinyak P, Smolarski R and Kienast K. Production of reactive oxygen intermediates by human macrophages exposed to soot particles and asbestos fibers and increase in NF-kappa B p50/p105 mRNA. *Lung* 1999, 177, 343–354.

Pache, J., Janssen, Y., Walsh, E., Quinlan, T., Zanella, C., Low, R., Taatjes, D., and Mossman, B. Increased epidermal growth factor-receptor (EGF-R) protein in a human mesothelial cell line in response to long asbestos fibers. *American Journal of Pathology* 1998, 152, 333–340.

Pelnar PV. Further evidence of nonasbestos-related mesothelioma. *A review of the literature. Scand. J. Work Environ. Health* 1988, 14:141–144.

Penninger JM, Kroemer G. Mitochondria, AIF and caspases--rivaling for cell death execution. *Nat. Cell Biol.* 2003, 5(2):97-9.

Perderiset M, Marsh JP and Mossman BT. Activation of protein kinase C by crocidolite asbestos in hamster tracheal epithelial cells. *Carcinogenesis* 1991, 12, 1499–1502.

Persad S, Attwell S, Gray V, Mawji N, Deng JT, Leung D, Yan J, Sanhera J, Walsh MP, Dedhar S. Regulation of protein kinase B /Akt-serine 473 phosphorylation by integrin-linked kinase, *J. Biol. Chem* 2001 276, 27462–27469.

Peterson JT Jr., Greenberg SD and Buffler PA. Nonasbestos-related malignant mesothelioma.Areview. *Cancer* 1984, 54:951–960.

Pinkus R, Weiner L and Daniel V. Role of oxidants and antioxidants in the induction of AP-1s, NF-kappaB, and glutathione S-transferase gene expression. *Journal of Biological Chemistry* 1996, 271, 13422–13429.

Ramos-Ninos M, Haegens A, Shukla A and Mossman B. Role of mitogen-activated protein kinases (MAPK) in cell injury and proliferation by environmental particulates. *Molecular and Cellular Biochemistry* 2002, 234–235, 111–118.

Ramos-Ninos M, Scapoli L, Martinelli M, Land S and Mossman B. Microarray analysis and RNA silencing link fra-1 to cd44 and c-met expression in mesothelioma. *Cancer Research* 2003, 63, 3539–3545.

Ramos-Ninos M, Timblin C and Mossman B. Mesothelial cell transformation requires increased AP-1 binding activity and ERK-dependent Fra-1 expression. *Cancer Research* 2002, 62(21):6065-9.

Rincon M and Flavell R. Transcription mediated by NFAT is highly inducible in effector CD4+ T helper 2 (Th2) cells but not in Th1 cells. *Molecular and Cellular Biology* 1997, 17, 1522–1534.

Robledo R, Buder-Hoffmann S, Cummins A, Walsh E, Taatjes D and Mossman B. Increased phosphorylated ERK immunoreactivity associated with proliferative and morphologic lung alterations following chrysotile asbestos inhalation in mice. *American Journal of Pathology* 2000, 156, 1307–1316.

Ruotsalainen M and Savolainen K. Effects of a protein kinase C inhibitor, Ro 31-7549, on the activation of human leukocytes by particulate stimuli. *Human Experimental Toxicology* 1995, 14, 266–272.

Sato F, Yamazaki H, Ataka K, Mashima I, Suzuki K, Takahashi T, et al. Malignant peritoneal mesothelioma associated with deep vein thrombosis following radiotherapy for seminoma of the testis. *Intern. Med.* 2000, 39:920–924.

Scapoli L, Ramos-Nino ME, Martinelli M and Mossman BT. Src-dependent ERK5 and Src/EGFR-dependent ERK1/2 activation is required for cell proliferation by asbestos. *Oncogene* 2004, 23, 805–813.

Sebolt-Leopold J, Dudley D, Herrera R, Van Becelaere K, Wiland A, Gowan R, Tecle H, Barrett S, Bridges A, Przybranowski S, Leopold W and Saltiel A. Blockade of the MAP kinase pathway suppresses growth of colon tumors in vivo. *Nature Medicine* 1999, 5, 810–816.

Seger R and Krebs E. The MAPK signaling cascade. *FASEB Journal* 1995, 9, 726–735.

Sesko A, Cabot M and Mossman B. Hydrolysis of inositol phospholipids precedes cellular proliferation in asbestos-stimulated tracheobronchial epithelial cells. *Proceedings of the National Academy of Sciences of the United States of America*, 1990, 87, 7385–7389.

Shukla A, Gulumian M, Hei TK, Kamp D, Rahman Q, Mossman BT. Multiple roles of oxidants in the pathogenesis of asbestos-induced diseases. *Free Radic Biol. Med.* 2003, 34(9):1117-29.

Shukla A, Timblin C, Hubbard A, Bravman J and Mossman B. Silica-induced activation of c-Jun-NH2-terminal amino kinases, protracted expression of the activator protein-1 proto-oncogene, fra-1, and S-phase alterations are mediated via oxidative stress. *Cancer Research* 2001, 61, 1791–1795.

Simeonova P and Luster M. Asbestos induction of nuclear transcription factors and interleukin 8 gene regulation. *American Journal of Respiratory Cell and Molecular Biology* 1996, 15, 787–795.

Simeonova P, Toriumi W, Kommineni C, Erkan M, Munson A, Rom W and Luster M. Molecular regulation of IL-6 activation by asbestos in lung epithelial cells: Role of reactive oxygen species. *Journal of Immunology* 1997, 159, 3921–3928.

Sporn TA and Roggli VL. Mesothelioma. In: *Pathology of Asbestos-Associated Diseases* 2004, 2nd ed., Roggli, V.L., Oury, T.D., and Sporn, T.A., eds., chapter 5 New York: Springer.

Sterman DH, Litzky LA, Kaiser LR and Albelda SM. Epidemiology and pathology of malignant mesothelioma. 2004 In: Rose, B.D., ed., *UpToDate*. Wellesley, MA: UpToDate.

Su B and Karin M. Mitogen-activated protein kinase cascades and regulation of gene expression. *Current Opinion in Immunology* 1996, 8, 402–411.

Susin SA, Daugas E, Ravagnan L, et al. Two distinct pathways leading to nuclear apoptosis. *J. Exp. Med.* 2000, 192:571–80.

Susin SA, Lorenzo HK, Zamzami N, et al. Molecular characterization of mitochondrial apoptosis-inducing factor. *Nature* 1999, 397:441–6.

Swain WA, O'Byrne KJ, Faux SP. Activation of p38 MAP kinase by asbestos in rat mesothelial cells is mediated by oxidative stress. *Am. J. Physiol. Lung Cell Mol. Physiol.* 2004 286(4):L859-65.

Tanaka S, Choe N, Hemenway DR, *et al.* Asbestos inhalation induces reactive nitrogen species and nitrotyrosine formation in the lungs and pleura of the rat. J Clin Invest 1998; 102:445-454

Timblin C, Janssen Y and Mossman B. Transcriptional activation of the protooncogene c-jun by asbestos and H_2O_2 is directly related to increased proliferation and transformation of tracheal epithelial cells. *Cancer Research* 1995, 55, 2723–2726.

Tsuda A, Stringer BK, Mijailovich SM, Rogers RA, Hamada K, Gray ML. Alveolar cell streching in the presence of fibrous particles induces interleukin-8 responses, *Am. J. Respir. Cell Mol. Biol.* 1999, 21, 455–462.

Wu J, Liu W, Koenig K, Idell S, Broaddus VC. Vitronectin adsorption to chrysotyle asbestos increases fiber phagocytosis and toxicity for mesothelial cells. *Am. J. Physiol. Lung Cell Mol. Physiol.* 2000, 279, L916–L923.

Xie C, Reusse A, Dai J, Zay K, Harnett J and Churg A. TNF-alpha increases tracheal epithelial asbestos and fiberglass binding via a NF-kappaB-dependent mechanism. *American Journal of Physiology* (Lung Cellular and Molecular Physiology), 2000, 279, L608–L614.

Yuan Z, Schellekens H, Warner L, Janssen-Heininger Y, Burch P, Heintz NH. Reactive nitrogen species block cell cycle re-entry through sustained production of hydrogen peroxide. *Am. J. Respir. Cell Mol. Biol.* 2003, 28:705–12.

Yuan Z, Taatjes DJ, Mossman BT, Heintz NH The duration of nuclear extracellular signal-regulated kinase 1 and 2 signaling during cell cycle reentry distinguishes proliferation from apoptosis in response to asbestos. *Cancer Research* 2004, 64, 6530–6536.

Zanella C, Posada J, Tritton T and Mossman B. Asbestos causes stimulation of the ERK-1 mitogen-activated protein kinase cascade after phosphorylation of the epidermal growth factor receptor. *Cancer Research* 1996, 56, 5334–5338.

Zanella C, Timblin C, Cummins A, Jung M, Goldberg J, Raabe R, Tritton T and BT M. Asbestos-induced phosphorylation of epidermal growth factor receptor is linked to c-fos expression and apoptosis. *American Journal of Physiology* (Lung Cellular and Molecular Physiology) 1999, 277, L684–L693.

Zhou G, Bao Z and Dixon J. Components of a new human protein kinase signal transduction pathway. *J. Biol. Chem.* 1995, 270, 12665–12669.

In: Mesothelioma from Bench Side to Clinic
Editor: Alfonso Baldi, pp. 183-205

ISBN: 978-1-60021-789-0

Chapter IX

Functional Genomic Applications in Understanding Molecular Basis of the Mesothelioma Progression: Use of Transcriptomics and Proteomics Technologies

Stefania Crispi[1] and Raffaele Calogero[2]
[1] Gene Expression Core - Human Molecular Genetics Laboratory, Institute of Genetics and Biophysics "A. Buzzati-Traverso" CNR via P. Castellino, 111, 80125 Naples
[2] Bioinformatics and Genomics Unit Dipartimento di Scienze Cliniche e Biologiche c/o Az. Ospedaliera S. Luigi, Regione Gonzole 10, 10043 OrbassanoTorino

Abstract

Malignant mesothelioma is a fatal cancer of the pleural and peritoneal spaces whose incidence is mainly related to the asbestos exposure.

To date the molecular basis that induce carcinogenesis are still unknown, and there are different problems related to a precise diagnosis with non-invasive techniques that often requires a thoracoscopic or pleural biopsy.

The application of the new post genomic technologies could represent a good challenge to identify specific gene and protein changes in malignant mesothelial cells.

Functional genomic starts after the completion of the sequence of the human genome when it begins the so-called “post-genomic era”. The aim of the functional genomic is to understand gene and protein functions and it is adverse to the structural genomic that analyses the gene and protein sequences.

Functional genomic is based on two main technologies that recently have contributed to shed light in understanding the molecular basis of cancer progression: the DNA microarrays and the protein microarrays.

A cancer peculiarity is the heterogeneity that involves difference in gene and protein expression. The DNA microarrays technique, through the simultaneous analysis of the expression of thousands of genes, permits to classify human tumors into homogeneous groups and the data obtained can be used to predict clinical behavior study by detecting similarities and differences among tumors. This analysis is broadly known as "expression profiling". A DNA microarray contains many DNA sequences (cDNA or oligonucleotides) corresponding to a gene positioned on a solid support. Multiple sequences correspond to each gene. The binding between the probe positioned on the array and the target that corresponds to the mRNAs present in the sample analyzed is based on complementarities. The target is labeled with fluorescent dyes that can be analyzed by a laser scanner.

The protein microarrays technique is helpful to distinguish among the proteins expressed in a specific behavior and even this approach can be used in cancer studies. It is possible to analyze a particular biological sample - as a tumor biopsy - performing a proteomic analysis and potentially to measure the abundance, modification, activity, localization and interaction of all the proteins in a sample. This experiment is the protein equivalent of expression profiling and it is known as 'protein profiling'. The protein microarrays technology is based on combination of two-dimensional gel electrophoresis and mass spectrometry, and its development is related to the immunoassays technique improvment. A protein-detecting microarray contains many antibodies arrayed at high spatial density on a solid support. Each antibody recognizes and binds its target protein present in serum or cell lysate, and the captured proteins are subsequently detected and quantified.

Microarray and proteomic analysis of mesothelioma and normal pleural samples could be of a great relevance to identify genes or proteins involved in the pathophysiology of mesothelioma, or that might serve as diagnostic markers to improve the accuracy of tumor classification.

The application of these technologies will help the development of new therapeutic target and the definition of clinical trials tumor-specific.

Introduction

Cell biology studies were completely transformed after the complete sequencing of the human genome that gave rise to the birth of a new biological era containing different *-omics* disciplines.

"*Omics*" is a term referred to the analysis of a specific compartment in a biological system. Different "*omics*" approach were minted for specific cellular compartments like *glicomics* for the total list of carbohydrates in an organism, *lipidomics* for the totality of lipids, *spliceomics* for the totality of the alternative splicing and so on.

Genomics is the discipline that analyses the DNA structure and function through the analysis of individual polimorphisms present in the genome (SNPs, Single Nucleotide Polymorphisms) that are potentially involved in disease development or in disease predisposition, yielding changes in protein function. The development of these studies was obtained thanks to the automation of the sequencing procedures. (Prober et al., 1987).

The term *Transcriptomics* indicates the global analysis of gene expression in a cell and it is usually referred as microarray analysis, a technology that enables measurement of thousands of genes in a single RNA sample. Using this technology the understanding of cell biology and the molecular mechanisms underlying normal and pathological biological processes were totally revisited.

Proteomics is a large-scale systematic study of the proteic complement with the aim to analyse its structure and function in an organism o cell. This approach relies on the quantitative measurements of the global proteic levels by two-dimensional polyacrylamide gel electrophoresis (2-DE analysis, O'Farrell, 1975). The initial studies of protein expression profiling became more specific and sensitive with the application of mass spectrometry (MS) technologies that allows to analyse post-translation modifications and protein-protein interactions.

The publication of the draft sequence of the human genome (Venter et al., 2001) revealed that it contained about 30,000 open reading frames (ORFs) encoding over 100,000 functional proteins, showing that one gene can addresses for different proteins. The discrepancies existing between mRNA and amount of the corresponding functional protein lead to the birth of proteomics.

Both genomic and proteomic cancer profiling studies aim to identify clinical biomarkers. A biomarker include any pattern changes correlate with the characteristics of a disease (SNPs, DNA methylation, protein amount) and it was recently defined as: 'A characteristic that can be measured and evaluated as an indicator of normal biologic processes, pathologic processes or pharmacological responses to therapeutic intervention' (Biomarkers Definitions Working Group, 2001). Any alteration in gene transcription and translation or in a protein product can potentially serve as specific biomarkers for disease (Srinivas et al., 2001). Because transcriptome studies decode the gene expression patterns disease-related without no indication of the related and biologically active proteic complement, it is though that direct measurement of protein expression could more accurately indicate cellular dysfunction underlying the development of disease because they represent the majority of active molecules responsible for most cellular functions.

Recently is emerging the importance of analyze the whole results coming from transcriptomics and proteomics analyses. The new exploration of the biological systems will elucidate our understanding of the phenotypes of both normal and diseased cells and it will undoubtedly help in the discovery of new therapeutics.

Basic Understanding of Microarrays

The DNA microarray technology is a high-throughput method for gaining information on gene function. A microarray is an orderly arrangement of samples where matching of known and unknown DNA samples is done based on base pairing rules. Thousands of spotted samples known as probes (with known identity) are immobilized on a solid support. The spots can be DNA, cDNA, or oligonucleotides. These are used to determine complementary binding of the unknown sequences thus allowing parallel analysis for gene expression and gene discovery. An experiment with a single DNA chip can provide information on thousands of genes simultaneously. An orderly arrangement of the probes on the support is important as the location of each spot on the array is used for the identification of a gene.

Microarray can be a valuable tool to define transcriptional signatures bound to a pathological condition or to rule out molecular mechanisms tightly bound to transcription. However, because our current knowledge of gene function in high eukaryotes is quite incomplete, microarray analysis frequently does not imply a final answer to a biological question, but allows the discovery of new research paths for its exploration from a different perspective (Saviozzi et al., 2004).

Many microarray platforms are actually available. We can distinguish microarrays in two main groups:

- Double channel microarrays
- Single channel microarray

Double channel microarray represents the first approach used to query the expression level of multiple transcripts at the same time (Shalon et al., 1996). This method is based on the use of cDNA or oligonucleotides spotted on a solid surface and hybridized at the same time with two different samples. The samples can be mixed and hybridized to one single microarray that is then scanned, allowing the visualization of up-regulated and down-regulated genes in one go. Relative expression of the two samples can be detected since they are labeled with different fluorofores. The downside of this is that the absolute levels of gene expression cannot be observed.

Single channel technology instead is based on spotted or "in situ" synthesized oligonucleotides on a solid surface. In this case each specimen is hybridized on a single array. Affymetrix GeneChips® represent the most used worldwide single channel microarray technology. GeneChips® have been developed by photolithographic oligonucleotide synthesis (www.affymetrix.com). In GeneChips® multiple short oligonucleotides are used to detect the expression level of each transcript. GeneChips® have the advantages to allow a very high density of oligonucleotide synthesis. In the most recent GeneChips® releases more than 4,000,000 probes can be accommodated on a 1.28. x 1.28 cm surface.

Wet approaches for the use of microarrays are well consolidated and especially for Affymetrix GeneChips® there are commercial kits available for this. A different story regards the analysis of the data generated by microarrays and the paragraph below will focus on the basic handling approaches for GeneChips® data analysis.

1. Oligonucleotide Arrays: An Introduction to Data Analysis

Computational tools are essential in microarray data analysis and mining to extract information knowledge from the experimental results. In this section we present some of the basic steps in the data analysis pipe-line (Figure 1). All approaches described in this section can be applied to the single channel arrays platform produced by Affymetrix (Santa Clara, CA).

In GeneChips® a probe set is composed of a different number of probes (4-20) due to the specific release of the GeneChip®. Probes belonging to the same probe set are distributed in various locations on the chip.

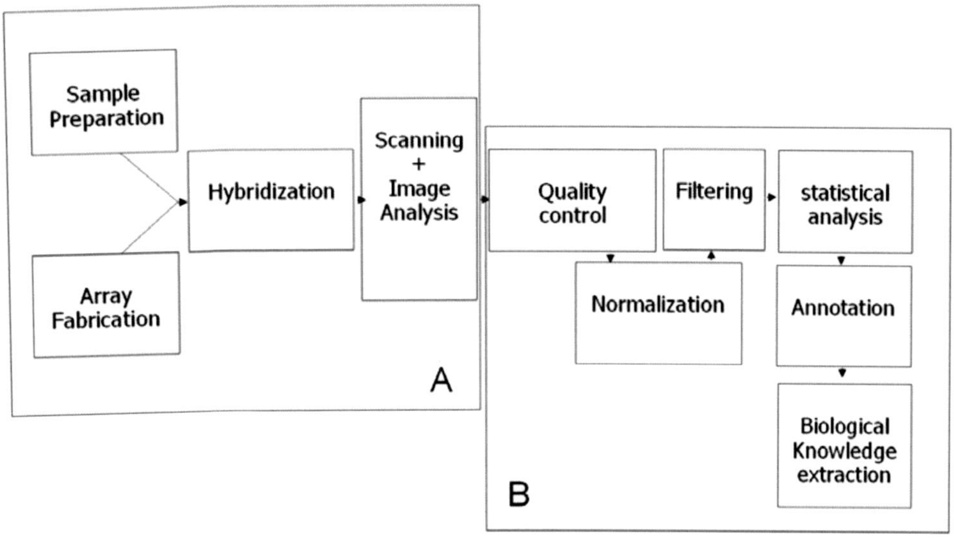

Figure 1. Microarray flowchart. Microanalysis data analysis pipe-line is part of the Microarray flowchart. The flowchart can be organized in two big blocks: the first one, which is dependent on the microarray platform in use (A) and the second which represent the basic steps necessary in a microarray analysis (B). The steps of the analysis pipe-line are clearly defined, but there is not a globally accepted unique method to be applied for each step of the pipe-line, since computational methods are rapidly improving and new analysis approaches are constantly coming out.

In GeneChips® designed to investigate the expression level of transcripts using the most 3' end of the transcripts, each probe, also called perfect match (PM), is associated with a "negative control" oligonucleotide, called mismatch (MM), whose sequence is equal to that of PM apart from a single central mismatch that greatly strongly destabilizes hybridization of the target molecule: PM/MM is called the probe pair. The definition of the probe set intensity summary might be calculated, depending on the chosen algorithm, using the PM only or the probe pair, where MM is used as the measure of nonspecific hybridization (Irizarry et al., 2003a, b).

2. Microarray Data Analysis

The main steps in a microarray data analysis are:

- Hybridization/construction artifacts identification and probe intensity distribution evaluation.
- Replicates quality evaluation.
- Data normalization.
- Data filtering.
- Statistical validation.
- Data annotation.

2.1. Hybridization/Construction Artifacts Identification and Probe Intensity Distribution Evaluation

A useful tool to identify hybridization/washing artifacts for Affymetrix GeneChips® is the "fitPLM" function implemented in the "affyPLM" Bioconductor package (www.bioconductor.org). This function produces probe level models by fitting a linear model to the probe data, and enables a model to be fitted with probe level and chip level parameters for each probe set. It produces chip pseudo-images which are very useful for detecting artifacts on arrays that could cause potential quality problems. Local artifacts have limited impact on probe set intensity calculation, since probe pairs of the same probe set are scattered over the array. However, if artifacts affect a vast part of an array, it should be discarded (Figure 2A). Another quality control parameter is the distribution of probe intensities. This is evaluated with "hist" function implemented in the "affy" Bioconductor package (Gautier et al., 2004). The distribution of probe intensities should have a log-normal shape and be spread over more than two logs (Figure 2B, black arrow). If the distribution is too narrow, as typically happens if the cRNA amount used for the hybridization is over-estimated (Figure 2B, dashed and dotted lines), many PM signals will be below the instrumental sensitivity. The probe set intensity will be under-estimated and information will be lost.

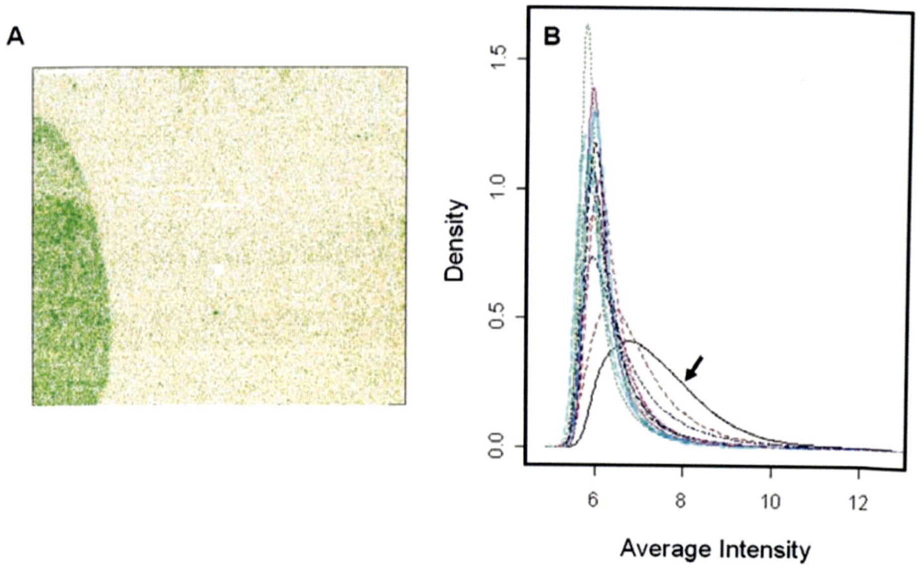

Figure 2. A) Pseudo-image generated by the fitPLM function (affyPLM Bioconductor package). The weight plot in the affyPLM package shows how well the model is fitted over all probes of a probe set, strong colours represent strong deviation from the calculated probe set model. In this plot probe outliers are represented by their weight in the definition of the modeled intensity of the probe set; low weights are represented by greener dots. B) PMs density distribution plots. PM distribution should log-normal over a large interval of log2(intensities) (black arrow). If the amount of cRNA used in the hybridization is over-estimated the overall distribution of the PM signals is very narrow (dashed and dotted curves).

2.2. Replicates Quality Evaluation

An important issue in microarray analysis is the quality of replicates. To perform statistical validation analysis, each experimental point should be replicated a few times to estimate the technical and experimental variability associated with the experiment. Replicates are of two types: technical and biological. Technical replicates are used to estimate the variability associated with instrumental and methodological effects (e.g. different lots of array, cRNA synthesis, etc.). They are generated by dividing a sample of total RNA into two/three aliquots and converting them into cRNA to be hybridized on different chips. The recent improvement in GeneChips® technology has made technical replicates inessential, whereas biological replicates are essential, because the main source of variation is related to the biological issue under study. An efficient way to evaluate homogeneity has been introduced by Irizarry (Irizarry et al., 2005). It is based on the use of a reference array against which biological replicates are compared. The homogeneity within replicates is then evaluated at the level of absolute expression fold change variation of each probe set with respect to the reference. Each biological replicate is described as the sorted list (fold change variation descending order) of all probe sets. Homogeneous replicates must have at the top rank positions (e.g. 100-1000) a concordance in probe set composition of at least 40%, corresponding to a r-squared between replicates greater than 0.8 (Irizarry et al., 2005).

2.3. Data Normalization

This is an important issue in microarray since it ensures that differences in intensities are indeed due to differential expression, and not to technical artifacts, and it is also required prior to any analysis that involves between-array comparisons of intensities. Affymetrix has proposed that intensities should be scaled so that each array has the same average value (constant normalization, in affy Bioconductor package). This approach, however, is less effective in the case of non-linear relationships between arrays, which are efficiently dealt with by the approaches of Bolstad (2003).

Bolstad proposes two methods. Both are implemented in the affy Bioconductor package:

- Cyclic loess. This approach stems from the M versus A plot, where M is the difference in log expression values and A is the average of those (Dudoit et al., 2002). A normalization curve is fitted to this M versus A plot by using loess, which is a method of local regression (Cleveland and Devlin, 1988). The fits based on the normalization curve are subsequently subtracted from the M values. However, rather than being applied to two-color channels on the same array, as is done in the cDNA case, normalization is applied to probe intensities from two arrays at a time. An M versus A plot for normalized data should show a point cloud scattered about the M = 0 axis. To deal with more than two arrays, the method is extended to look at all distinct array pairwise combinations.
- Quantile normalization. The goal of the quantile method is to make the distribution of probe intensities for each of a set of arrays the same. The idea behind the method

is that a quantile-quantile plot shows that the distribution of two data vectors is the same if the plot is a straight diagonal line, but not if it is other than a diagonal. This concept can be extended to "n" dimensions if more then two arrays are available. This suggests that an n set of data can be made to have the same distribution by projecting the points of the n dimensional quantile plot onto the diagonal. This normalization can be easily done by organizing the arrays to be normalized in a matrix, where columns represent the arrays and the rows gene-specific PMs. Each column is then sorted in a descending order. The means across rows are taken and assigned to each element of the rows. Columns are then reordered as the original matrix to generate the normalized set.

In our hands, cyclic-loess normalization performs better than the quantile method although it si more slow.

2.4. Data Filtering

The premise of this important step in microarray data analysis is removal of genes deemed to be not expressed according to some specific criterion under the control of the user (von Heydebreck et al., 2004). It can also be used to eliminate genes that do not show sufficient variation in expression across all samples, since their little discriminatory power. There are various approaches for data filtering:

- Removing probe sets with an intensity below a user-defined threshold (von Heydebreck et al. 2004).
- Removing probe sets that do not vary in function of the experimental conditions (von Heydebreck et al., 2004).
- Removing probe sets that do not belong to a specific functional class (e.g. transcription factors).

2.5. Statistical Validation

Statistical validation is an important issue for the identification of differentially expressed genes. Optimization of validation tools for microarray data has been sought since microarray experiments are generally conducted on a very limited number of replicates (biological replicates) and involve many parallel tests (genes to be evaluated for differential expression). This situation, of course, is the exact opposite of the ideal definition of a statistical test case: many replicates for few parallel tests.

It is not true that new statistical tests have been excogitated for microarray analysis. Instead known tests (e.g. t-test, ANOVA, linear model analysis, etc.) have been subjected to sophisticated optimization to secure a good estimate of inter/intra sample variance despite to the limited number of replicates. All methods for statistical validation start from the assumption that the transcription expression level of one gene is independent from that of the others.

The best way of identifying differentially expressed genes cannot be determined. Each method will catch only a part of the biologically meaningful differential expressions (Hosack et al., 2003) (Figure 3). Results obtained with multiple statistical methods have in common a core of very robust differentially expressed genes which are always identified (Figure 3).

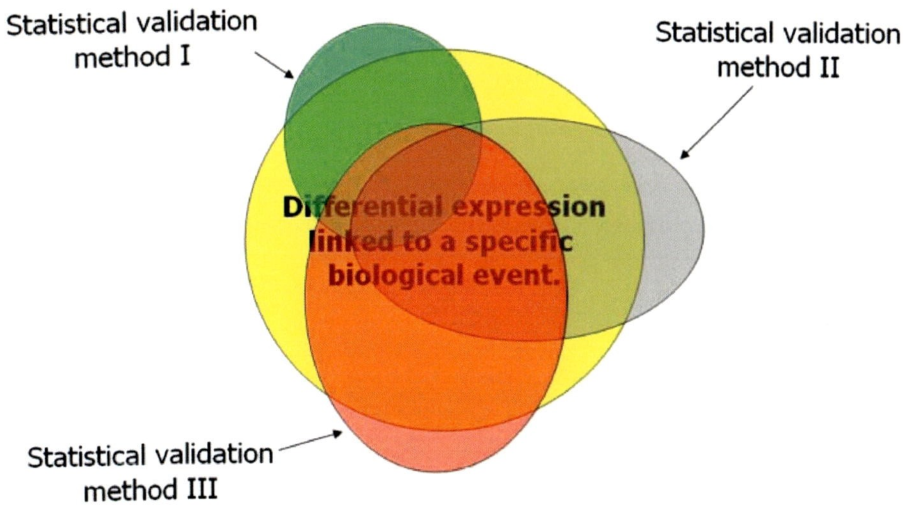

Figure 3. Ability of different statistical methods to catch differential expression. In yellow is shown the unknown set of differential expressed genes generated by a biological experiment. Different statistical approaches will catch only a part of the biologically meaningful differential expressions and each of them will be also characterized by a certain level of false positives (i.e. genes that are not differentially expressed but are detected within the pool of differential expressed genes).

In microarray analysis, identification of differentially expressed genes requires methods that can deal with multiple testing problems (i.e. when performing multiple statistical tests two types of errors are possible: Type I error or false positive, a gene is identified as differentially expressed when it is not; Type II error or false negative, failure to identify a truly differentially expressed gene). The Bioconductor package multitest implements widely applicable resampling based single-step and stepwise multiple testing procedures (MTP) for controlling a broad class of Type I error rates, in testing problems involving general data generating distributions (with arbitrary dependence structures among variables), null hypotheses, and test statistics (Dudoit, 2004). A key feature of these MTPs is the test statistics null distribution (rather than data generating null distribution) used to derive rejection regions (i.e., cut-offs) for the test statistics and the resulting adjusted p-values.

2.6. Data Annotation

Another important issue in microarray data analysis is the specific association of probe set identifiers with genome annotated transcripts. A critical point in annotation is the way in which the association between probe sets and genes is produced. When a GeneChips® is designed, probes are defined from the transcript sequences in the most recent Unigene release (www.ncbi.nlm.nih.gov/entrez/query.fcgi?db=unigene). Unigene is the major repository of sequences belonging to transcriptomes for all known organisms and a system for automatically partitioning GenBank sequences into a non-redundant set of gene-oriented clusters. Each cluster contains sequences that represent a single gene, as well as related information such as the tissue types in which gene has been expressed and its map location (Wheeler et al., 2003).

Probe sets are not simply designed to secure good recognition of the target, but also to reduce as much as possible unwanted cross-hybridization with other clusters. However, since new sequences are constantly being added to Unigene, gene-oriented clusters are rebuilt and this process may change the transcript structure (e.g. a transcribed sequence changes cluster or two or more clusters are joined in a single one).

GeneChip® probes are not updated at every Unigene rebuild, but only when a new GeneChip® version becomes available. After a few Unigene releases, therefore, a set that initially mapped all probes to a specific transcript may map only some of them to the target sequence. Therefore, the lack of synchronization between Unigene and GeneChips® probes may reduce the specificity of a probe set in target recognition (Mecham et al., 2004), while the addition of new sequences to the Unigene database may mean that unwanted cross-mapping to other transcripts occurs for some probes. All this information is available on the GeneChip®-specific annotation files at the Affymetrix web site (www.affymetrix.com/support/technical/index.affx), and on their on-line annotation tool, Netaffx (www.affymetrix.com/analysis/netaffx/index.affx). Both are updated quarterly.

When the first GeneChip® appeared, the only annotation tool was that provided by Affymetrix. Today three other public tools (www.bioconductor.org/packages/data/annotation /stable/src/contrib/html/; www.tigr.org/tigr-scripts/magic/r1.pl; www.ensembl.org/Multi/martview) are available on the net. These repositories use different approaches to associate a probe set with a specific gene.

Bioconductor uses a specific annotation library, AnnBuilder, to create Bioconductor annotation libraries or XML annotation files starting from the association "probe set identifier"/"GeneBank accession number" (i.e. the primary target for probes design).

The relationships captured in the RESOURCERER (Tsai et al., 2001), the annotation tool at TIGR center (www.tigr.org), are elaborated from EST and gene sequences stored in the TGI databases (www.tigr.org/tdb/tgi.shtml). They provide an analysis of publicly available EST and gene sequence data for the identification of transcripts and their placement in a genomic context, and the identification of orthologs and paralogs wherever possible.

Neither Bioconductor nor TIGR methods operate at the probe level, nor do they consider the limited reliability of some sets due to probe cross-hybridization or erroneous probe/transcript annotation.

Annotation with the Ensembl tool is built by direct matching of Affymetrix probes over the Ensembl sequence database. Its weak point is that matching of only 50% of the probes of a specific set to an Ensembl gene is needed for a true association definition "probe set identifier"/"Ensembl gene identifier". Once again, the presence of unwanted cross-mapping is not taken into account. Furthermore, since these resources are not synchronized and their annotation methods differ, some discrepancy between their results is inevitable.

Recently Dai (2005) demonstrated that the original Affymetrix probe set definitions could be inaccurate in some cases. Therefore, these Authors reorganized probes on GeneChips® into gene-, transcript- and exon-specific probe sets in light of up-to-date genome and cDNA/EST clustering information (i.e. custom probe sets). For example generation of custom probe sets to search for RefSeq records (Pruit et al., 2005) is done identifying all perfect match probes on a GeneChip® to the corresponding RefSeq records, removing probes with more than one perfect hit on the corresponding genomic sequence. This remapping of probes to RefSeq or other genes/transcript identifiers also removes the problem to handle multiple probe set mapping to the same genes which is a characteristics of Affymetrix annotation. In our hands, RefSeq remapping works better than Entrez Genes (EG, Maglott et al., 2005) remapping since some qPCR validated probe sets based on Affy probe sets are lost using the EG based Dai's annotation. Furthermore, comparing fold changes between the same subset of genes identified using Affy probesets or EG based probesets a generalized reduction of fold change range is observed.

Basic Understanding in Proteomics

The idea of mapping the human complement of expressed protein was firstly suggested with the development of the 2D polyacrylamide gel electrophoresis (2-DE; O'Farrell, 1975) a technique that allows the simultaneous separation of large numbers of proteins. Only after ten years was defined "proteome" the protein complement of a genome (Wasinger et al., 1995).

Proteomics studies are based on Mass spectrometry (MS) a methodology made possible after the discovery of protein ionization for which the 2002 Nobel Prize in chemistry was conferred (Cho and Normile, 2002).

A proteomic analysis (Figure 4) can be performed following different steps starting with a peptide gel-based separation followed by a spectrometric analysis that generate information-rich ion mass spectra from peptide fragments (peptide mass fingerprinting). Then it is possible to proceed in order to obtain the primary proteic structure. Once a protein data set has been generated, it is important to use bioinformatics integration for a systematic assembling of the data.

MS works analysing ionized molecules in a gas phase. These molecules, previously positive or negative charged, can be affected by the effect of an electric or a magnetic field. Wide ranges of analyses are possible using different types of mass spectrometers and different techniques of sample introduction. The MS provides information about the molecular weight of the compound and its chemical structure. MS can be utilised for quantitative and qualitative analysis of different molecules ranging from inorganic molecules to proteins or nucleic acids with a molecular weight of few or million of Dalton.

1. Protein separation and visualization

The starting point of a proteomics experiment is the sample separation realized by the two-dimensional gel electrophoresis or 2-DE, the currently used technique. 2- DE is a high-resolution method that allows to identify protein processing or modification. The separation method is applied after the sample solubilization, a procedure that separates proteic aggregates in individual polypeptides and eliminates molecules that can interfere with the separation itself (nucleic acids, lipids or polysaccharides).

2-DE separates the proteins in two dimensions, the first is made in denaturing conditions according to the isoelectric point while the second, a SDS-PAGE, is made according to the relative molecular mass (M*r*) (Figure 5).

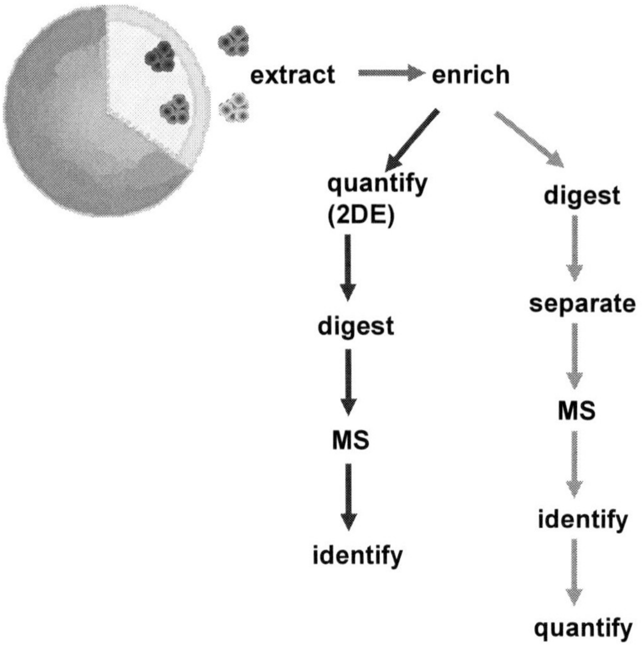

Figure 4. Flow chart of a proteomic analysis.

With 2-DE simultaneously thousands of proteins are analyzed and is possible to identify changes in protein expression level, or post-translational modifications that result in alterations in protein pI or M*r*. It is possible to perform expression profiling of large sets of complex protein mixtures such as whole cell lysates, resolve up to 5000 proteins in a single assay and detect up to 1 ng of protein per spot.

An alternative to 2-DE is the protein fractionation, a method in which proteins can be divided into fractions and digested separately with the enzyme trypsin in order to obtain less complex peptide mixtures. The resulting peptide fragments are then separated by SDS-PAGE followed by liquid-chromatography to reduce the complexity of peptide fractions. The fractions are then introduced in a mass spectrometer for sequence-based identification (liquid-chromatography–MS or LC–MS). This method has been applied to develop the "MudPIT" approach used for detection of 1500 yeast proteins in a single analysis (multidimensional protein identification technology), combining multidimensional LC, tandem MS, and database searching (Washburn et al., 2001).

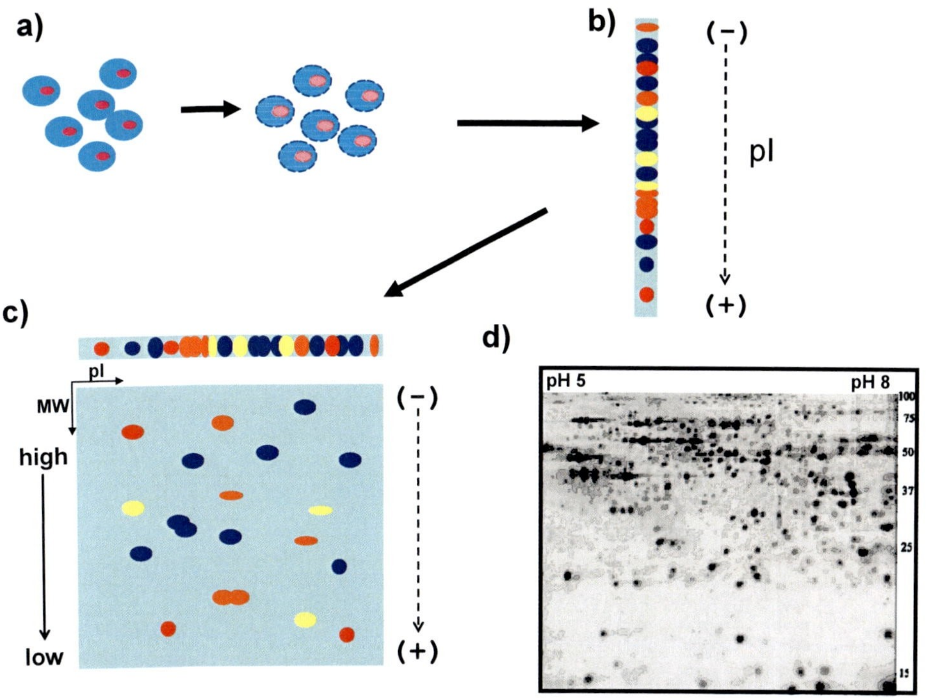

Figure 5. Two dimensional gel electrophoresis: a) solubilization of protein from cells; b) first dimension separation by isoelectrofocusing; c) second dimension separation by SDS-PAGE; d) 2DE image analysis.

After separation, proteins can be visualized by means of high sensitivity methods. The silver staining method (resolution = 0.1 ng protein) was recently replaced by detection methods based on fluorescent dyes to label protein (2D- DIGE, differential in-gel electrophoresis). Fluorescent dyes generally show a linear response to variation in protein concentration over five orders of magnitude (sub-nanogram sensitivity), and are compatible with MS analysis. The standard method is based on separate labeling of protein samples with Cy3 and Cy5 derivatives before their separation on the same 2-DE gel (Karp et al., 2004). Up to three protein extracts, for example one control and two treated, can be labelled with different fluorescent dyes (Cy2, Cy3 and/or Cy5), then combined and separated on the same 2-DE gel. The resulting 2-DE gel is then scanned to acquire the Cy3 and Cy5 images separately. This technique provides increased sensitivity for expression profiling studies of samples as laser-microdissected clinical specimens (Greengauz-Roberts et al., 2005). Other new fluorescent dyes have been introduced for 2-DE gels staining of specific proteins such as phosphorylated/hyper-phosphorylated or glycosylated ones: the Pro-Q Diamond dye for the detection of phosphoserine-, phosphothreonine- and phosphotyrosine containing proteins (Martin et al., 2003), and the Pro-Q Emerald 300 fluorescent stain for the detection of glycoproteins (Steinberg et al., 2001). Both detections are done directly in SDS–polyacrylamide and 2-DE gels.

Finally two new labelling methods have been developed, based on the incorporation of stable isotopes into biological samples (Figure 6). Labelling of cells or tissues with a isotopic variants (e.g., ^{12}C vs.^{13}C) will give rise to "light" and "heavy" populations from different samples that can be mixed at equal amounts (light:heavy) providing a single sample containing peptides from both cellular conditions. The two methods that represent an accurate way to perform quantitative analysis are: the isotope-coded affinity tags (ICAT) and the stable isotope labelling with amino acids in cell culture (SILAC).

The ICAT, relies on the quantification of peptides resulting from the selective isotopic labelling of cysteine residues *in vitro*; an ICAT tag utilizes three elements, an iodoacetamide group to react with cysteine, a linker region substituted with either nine ^{13}C (heavy tag) or ^{12}C (light tag) atoms, and biotin tag to selectively isolate the ICAT-labelled peptides prior to MS. Only cysteine-containing peptides are retained than there will be a significant reduction in mixture complexity. The strength of this technique lies in its ability to allow quantification and identification within a single analysis. (Hansen et al., 2003).

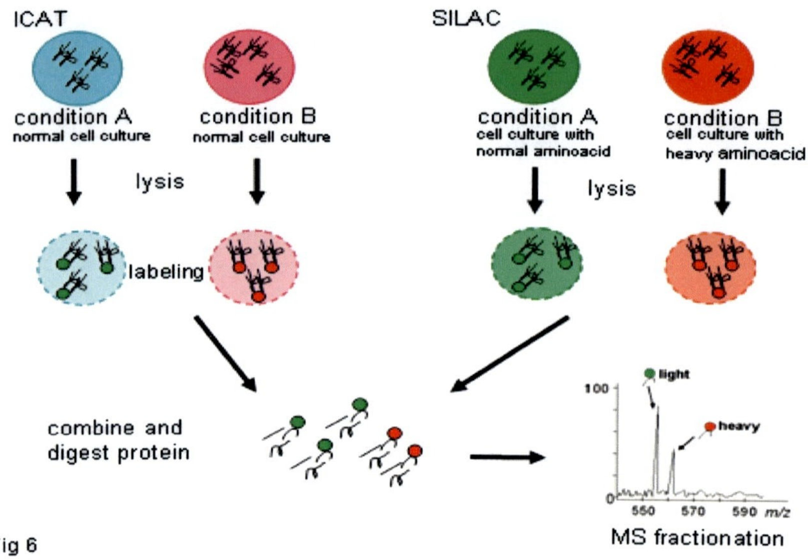

Fig 6

Figure 6. The ICAT and SILAC techniques for proteins labelling with different isotopes.

SILAC differs from ICAT because cells are cultured in the presence of either ^{12}C - or ^{13}C -containing amino acids. Following protein collection, samples are combined, digested, and analysed by MS. The advantage of this metabolic incorporation is the lack of chemical labelling that increases the sensitivity (Ong et al., 2002).

ICAT and SILAC have recently been applied in cancer proteomic applications (Meehan and Sadar, 2004; Everley et al., 2004).

2. Mass Spectrometry Based Proteomics

Following the protein separation each molecule can be analysed within the MS. A mass spectrometer consists of a ion source were the analytes are ionized, a mass analyzer that separates ionized molecules according to the mass to charge ratio (m/z) and a detector that registers the number of ions at each *m/z* value.

All the ionisation, analyser and detector sources are under high vacuum to allow unhindered movement of ions.

Different ionization processes can be used depending on the property of molecule that is being studied but all processes allow to a fast addition of energy to the analytes with production of stable ionic of species in a gas phase. Two methods are mainly used for proteomic studies:

- ESI (Electrospray Ionisation) that gives multiply charged ions by spraying the surface of the analyte (Fenn et al., 1989) (Figure 7).
- MALDI (Matrix Assisted Laser Desorption Ionisation) in which the ions are generated by a laser through a crystalline matrix that transfers energy to the sample ionizing it (Karas and Hillenkamp, 1988).

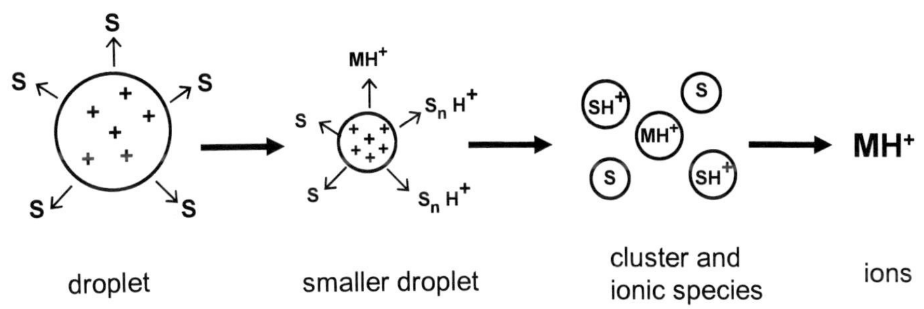

Figure 7. ESI ionization process. The mixture of peptides to analyse is electrostatically dispersed with generation of highly charged droplets (usually positive for the excess of protons), than the solvent evaporation decreases their size and increases their charge density. The electrospray plume is generated at atmospheric pressure in close proximity to the entrance of the mass spectrometer.

For example ESI is preferred for the analysis of complex samples because ionizes the analytes out of a solution and can easily coupled to liquid-based separations (ESI-MS LC-MS) (Zhang et al., 2006; Chen et al., 2005).

The ionized molecules produced are then forced into the mass analyzer where the separation takes place; they are accelerated by manipulation of the charged particles through the mass spectrometer (Figure 8). Four main types of mass analyzer are currently used in proteomics research: the *quadrupole*, the *quadrupole ion trap*, the *time-of-flight* (TOF) and *Fourier transform ion cyclotron resonance* (FT-MS) which differ in the way of determining the mass-to-charge (m/z) ratios of the peptides. For example the *quadrupole* MS uses positive and negative voltage to control the path of the ions; ions travel down the path based on their mass to charge ratio (m/z) and the detector works producing an electronic signal when struck by an ion. Timing mechanisms, which integrate those signals with the scanning voltages, allow the instrument to report which m/z strikes the detector. Then the mass analyzer sorts the ions according to m/z and the detector records the abundance of each m/z.

Another MS-based approach is the SELDI-TOF (SELDI: surface-enhanced laser desorption/ionization; Villanueva et al., 2004) used for diagnostic profiling purposes as serum profiling applied to the early detection of cancer (Petricoin and Liotta, 2004). SELDI TOF-MS combines retention chromatography with TOF-MS. The SELDI surface utilizes a retention chromatography chip (protein chip) to capture specific families of proteins from a biological sample. In fact the surface enhancement facilitates fractionation of samples allowing the detection of specific classes of proteins. Protein chip arrays can have chemically (anionic, cationic, hydrophobic, hydrophilic, metal affinity capture, etc.) or biochemically (immobilized antibody, receptor, DNA, enzyme, etc.) active surface (Figure 9). Chemical surfaces are used to retain particular groups of proteins, whereas surfaces coated with a biochemical reagent are designed to interact with a specific target protein.

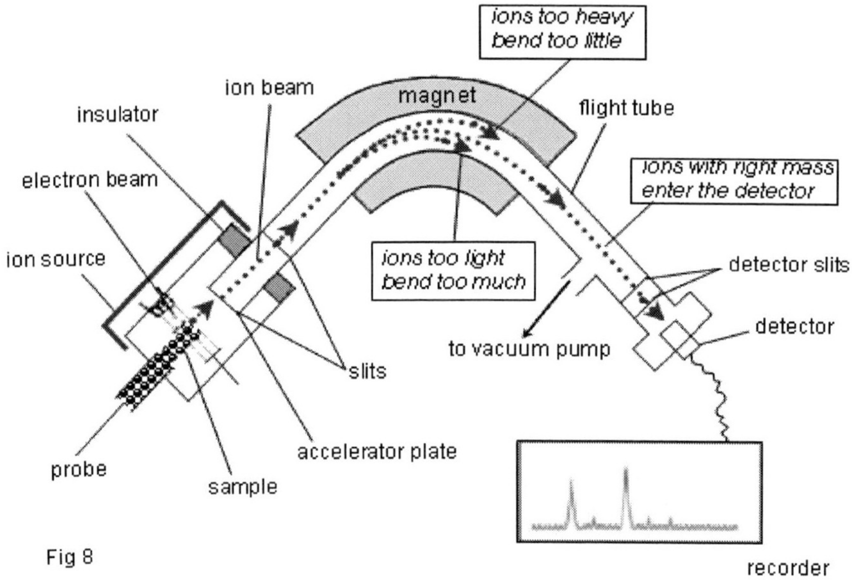

Fig 8

Figure 8. Mass spectrometer components. Particles are ionized, accelerated through magnetic field and their quantity is recorded for the different mass to charge ratio (m/z).

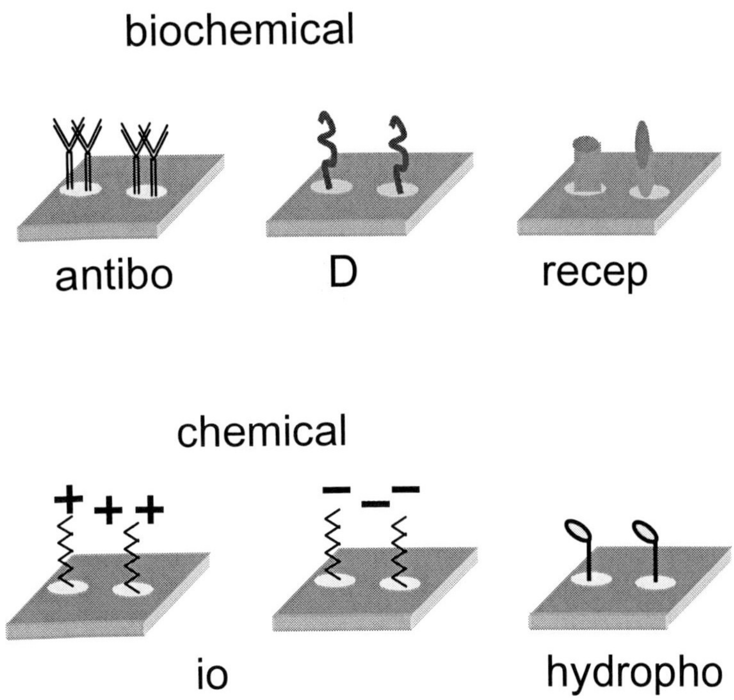

Figure 9. Active surface in protein chip arrays.

The final filtered spectrum generated by MS analysis is called peptide mass fingerprinting (PMF). A MALDI mass spectra usually contain specific peaks corresponding to some ions cluster that mark the relevant features in that mass spectrum. The shape of the peaks is related to the peptides composition while the intensity of peaks is related to their concentration. A complete LC-MALDI measurement shows individual characteristics for each peptide, thus it is possible to have characteristic dose response curve that differs from peptide to peptide. Furthermore the intensities of certain features in one spectrum can be highly correlated with each other; if there is a high correlation the features are not truly independent, and this is very important for the statistical methods applied in data interpretation.

After having determined the spectrum of all molecules it is possible to proceed to obtain primary structure by tandem MS (MS/MS or MS2), that couples two stages of MS. MS/MS takes advantage of two-stage MS instruments (MALDI–MS with postsource decay, MALDI–TOF -MS/MS, or electrospray ionization ESI-MS/MS triple-quadropole, ion-trap, or Q-TOF machines) to induce fragmentation of peptide bonds. It is possible to generate a short partial sequence or "tag," that provide significant additional information when used in combination with the mass of the intact parent peptide ion (Liska et al., 2005). In alternative it is possible to use a database-searching algorithm to match experimental MS/MS spectra with predicted fragment patterns generated *in silico* in protein and nucleotide databases to for the homology search (Kapp et al., 2005) (Figure 10).

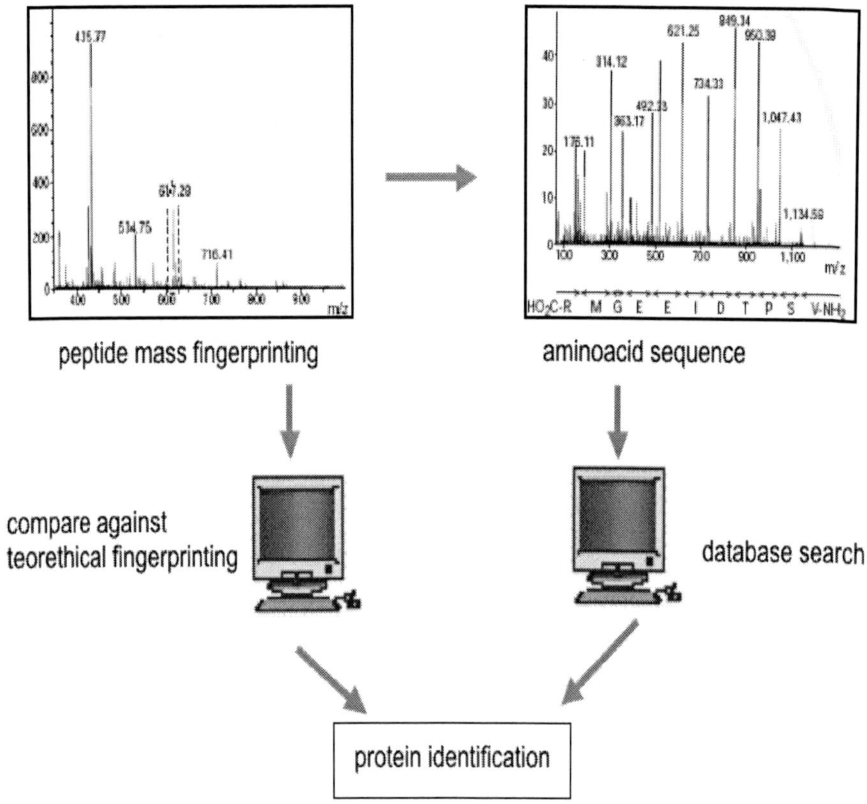

Figure 10. Mass spectrum and methods for protein identification.

Briefly in a tandem MS, molecules resulting from the first MS are selected and further fragmented at a peptide bond producing N-terminal (a-, b-, or c-ions) or C-terminal fragments (x-, y-, or z-ions). These are then analysed by the second MS producing the peptide fragment mass fingerprints (PFMF). MS/MS principally allows to detection of previously unknown peptide sequences and the direct interpretation of PFMFs is also called *de novo* sequencing (Cagney and Emili, 2002).

3. Mass Spectrum Data Analysis

Data acquisition, performed before data analysis, is realized through a high-speed transient recorder that yields thousands of sampling points per spectrum. A mass spectrum is a histogram of a probability density function describing molecules that approach to the mass spectrometric detector simultaneously within subsequent time intervals (bins). Statistical computations and data mining follow different preprocessing steps, starting with the mass calibration of the spectra, that transforms the time based coordinate system into a mass to charge (m/z) ratio based coordinate system. Subsequent steps usually address the alignment of the spectra or the intensity scaling to obtain a valuable data set (Carlson et al., 2005).

The PMF represents the basis to protein identification that can be done searching the measured PMF in a database of *in silico* predicted PMFs. Different bioinformatics tools are available to perform PMF prediction and searching, that vary in the method of generating the theoretical PMFs (FindPept: www.expasy.org/tools/findpept.html; MultiIdent: www.expasy.org/tools/multiident/; *Pep*MAPPER: http://wolf.bms.umist.ac.uk/mapper/). All possible peptides originated from a given database are then used to generate theoretical PFMFs and different searching procedure can be used to find the best match to a given measured PFMF (ProteinProspector: http://prospector.ucsf.edu/ucsfhtml4.0/mshomology.html; SEQUEST: http:// fields.scripps.edu/sequest/).

Protein identification by PMFs is suitable for completely sequenced genomes but there are difficulties for incomplete gene models, or for biological events difficult to model as mRNA splicing. For these reasons identification methods were extended to MS/ MS data and the main goal of bioinformatics tools is just (right) the correct interpretation of the resulting PFMF in order to find all y-ions (see below).

To understand the function of biological processes, it is possible, with specific tools, to assembly proteins in functionally active domains, usually conserved in evolutionarily related proteins, while sequences outside of domains diverge faster during evolution (BLAST, PSI- or PHI-BLAST: www.ncbi.nlm.nih.gov/BLAST/). As mentioned before a limitation of database searching is that large-scale proteomic experiments should only be carried out using organisms that have had their genome sequenced, so that all the possible peptides are known (Liska and Shevchenko, 2003). If a genome is not completely sequenced, it is helpful to search for homologous gene models in related organisms (MS-BLAST: http://dove.embl-heidelberg.de/Blast2/msblast.html; Shevchenko et al., 2001). Finally since cellular functions are realized by a whole set of different interacting proteins (functional modules) conserved among different species, the definition and characterization of the functional modules is one of the most challenging tasks in bioinformatics (Snel et al., 2002). Moreover several *in silico* methods can provide clues of possible network interaction partners.

The term data mining indicates an analytic process designed to explore usually large amounts of data in order to search consistent patterns and/or systematic relationships between variables, and then validate the findings by applying the detected patterns to new subsets of data. Data mining methods suitable for mass spectrometry based profiling data can be found in the same application area of microarrays data. The majority of these tools are available at public web site as Bioconductor (www.bioconductor.org), that is repository for the statistical R-language (www.r-project.org).

The general aim of data mining is to analyse how the mass spectrometric samples are related to each other, to identify relationships between the peptides that are highly correlated with each other and to generate models for the description of relationships between features and objects to be used to make predictions or diagnoses (Lamerz Jet al., 2005).

Peptide-mass mapping by methodologies as MALDI-TOF and peptide sequencing by ESI-MS/MS have become highly efficient for identification of gel-separated proteins.

The comprehension of the huge amount of data produced by the two technologies is possible with advances in bioinformatics. Bioinformatics integration of the data set produced by these new approaches will be useful as atlas of protein properties and functions.

References

Biomarkers Definitions Working Group. "Biomarkers and surrogate endpoints: Preferred definitions and conceptual framework." *Clin. Pharm. Ther.* 2001, 69: 89-95.

Bolstad, B.M., Irizarry, R.A., Astrand, M., Speed, T.P. A comparison of normalization methods for high density oligonucleotide array data based on variance and bias. *Bioinformatics* 2003, 19: 185–193.

Cagney G, Emili A. De novo peptide sequencing and quantitative profiling of complex protein mixtures using mass-coded abundance tagging. *Nat. Biotechnol.* 2002, 20:163-70.

Carlson SM, Najmi A, Whitin JC, Cohen HJ. Improving feature detection and analysis of surface-enhanced laser desorption/ionization-time of flight mass spectra. *Proteomics* 2005, 5: 2778-88.

Chen HS, Rejtar T, Andreev V, Moskovets E, Karger BL. Enhanced characterization of complex proteomic samples using LC-MALDI MS/MS: exclusion of redundant peptides from MS/MS analysis in replicate runs. *Anal. Chem.* 2005, 77: 7816-25.

Cho A, Normile D. Nobel Prize in Chemistry. Mastering macromolecules. *Science* 2002, 298: 527-8.

Cleveland, W.S. Devlin, S.J. Locally-weighted regression: an approach to regression analysis by local fitting. *J. Am. Stat. Assoc.* 1998, 83: 596–610.

Dai M, Wang P, Boyd AD, Kostov G, Athey B, Jones EG, Bunney WE, Myers RM, Speed TP, Akil H, Watson SJ, Meng F: Evolving gene/transcript definitions significantly alter the interpretation of GeneChip data. *Nucleic Acids Res.* 2005, 33: e175.

Dudoit, S., Yang, Y.H., Callow, M.J., Speed, T.P. Statistical methods for identifying genes with differential expression in replicated cDNA microarray experiments. *Stat. Sin.* 2002, 12: 111–139.

Dudoit, S., van der Laan, M.J., Pollard, K.S. Multiple testing. Part I. Single-step procedures for control of general Type I error rates. *Statistical Applications in Genetics and Molecular Biology* 2004 3, Article 13. URL www.bepress.com/sagmb/vol3/iss1/art13.

Everley PA, Krijgsveld J, Zetter BR, Gygi SP. Quantitative cancer proteomics: stable isotope labeling with amino acids in cell culture (SILAC) as a tool for prostate cancer research. *Mol. Cell Proteomics* 2004, 3: 729-35.

Fenn JB, Mann M, Meng CK, Wong SF, Whitehouse CM. Electrospray ionization for mass spectrometry of large biomolecules. *Science* 1989, 246: 64-71.

Greengauz-Roberts O, Stoppler H, Nomura S, Yamaguchi H, Goldenring JR, Podolsky RH, Lee JR, Dynan WS. Saturation labeling with cysteine-reactive cyanine fluorescent dyes provides increased sensitivity for protein expression profiling of laser-microdissected clinical specimens. *Proteomics* 2005, 5: 1746-57.

Gygi SP, Rist B, Gerber SA, Turecek F, Gelb MH, Aebersold R. Quantitative analysis of complex protein mixtures using isotope-coded affinity tags. *Nat. Biotechnol.* 1999, 17: 994-9.

Hansen KC, Schmitt-Ulms G, Chalkley RJ, Hirsch J, Baldwin MA, Burlingame AL. Mass spectrometric analysis of protein mixtures at low levels using cleavable 13C-isotope-coded affinity tag and multidimensional chromatography. *Mol. Cell Proteomics* 2003, 2: 299-314

Hosack DA, Dennis G Jr, Sherman BT, Lane HC, Lempicki RA. Identifying biological themes within lists of genes with EASE. *Genome Biol.* 2003 4: R70.

Irizarry, R.A., Hobbs, B., Collin, F., Beazer-Barclay, Y.D., Antonellis, K.J., Scherf, U., Speed, T.P. Exploration, normalization, and summaries of high density oligonucleotide array probe level data. *Biostatistics* 2003 (a) 4: 249-264.

Irizarry, R.A., Bolstad, B.M., Collin, F., Cope, L.M., Hobbs, B., Speed, T.P. Summaries of Affymetrix GeneChip probe level data. *Nucleic Acids Res.* 2003 (b) 31: e15.

Irizarry, R.A., Warren, D., Spencer, F., Kim, I.F., Biswal S., Frank, B.C., Gabrielson, E, Garcia, J.G., Geoghegan, J., Germino, G., Griffin, C., Hilmer, S.C., Hoffman, E., Jedlicka, A.E., Kawasaki, E., Martinez-Murillo, F., Morsberger, L., Lee, H., Petersen, D., Quackenbush, J., Scott, A., Wilson, M., Yang, Y., Ye, S.Q., Yu, W. Multiple-laboratory comparison of microarray platforms. Nat Methods 2005 2: 345-350. *Erratum in: Nat. Methods* 2005, 2: 477.

Kapp EA, Schutz F, Connolly LM, Chakel JA, Meza JE, Miller CA, Fenyo D, Eng JK, Adkins JN, Omenn GS, Simpson RJ. An evaluation, comparison, and accurate benchmarking of several publicly available MS/MS search algorithms: sensitivity and specificity analysis. *Proteomics* 2005, 5: 3475-90.

Karas M, Hillenkamp F. Laser desorption ionization of proteins with molecular masses exceeding 10,000 daltons. *Anal. Chem.* 1988, 60: 2299-301.

Karp NA, Kreil DP, Lilley KS. Determining a significant change in protein expression with DeCyder during a pair-wise comparison using two-dimensional difference gel electrophoresis. *Proteomics* 2004, 4: 1421-32.

Lamerz J, Selle H, Scapozza L, Crameri R, Schulz-Knappe P, Mohring T, Kellmann M, Khamenia V, Zucht HD. Correlation-associated peptide networks of human cerebrospinal fluid. *Proteomics* 2005, 5: 2789-98.

Liska AJ, Shevchenko A. Expanding the organismal scope of proteomics: cross-species protein identification by mass spectrometry and its implications. *Proteomics* 2003, 3: 19-28.

Liska AJ, Sunyaev S, Shilov IN, Schaeffer DA, Shevchenko. A Error-tolerant EST database searches by tandem mass spectrometry and multiTag software. Proteomics. 2005, 5: 4118-22

Maglott D, Ostell J, Pruitt KD, Tatusova T. Entrez Gene: gene-centered information at NCBI. *Nucleic Acids Res.* 2005, 33(Database issue): D54-8.

Martin K, Steinberg TH, Goodman T, Schulenberg B, Kilgore JA, Gee KR, Beechem JM, Patton WF. Strategies and solid-phase formats for the analysis of protein and peptide phosphorylation employing a novel fluorescent phosphorylation sensor dye *Comb. Chem. High Throughput Screen.* 2003 6: 331-9.

Mecham, B.H., Wetmore, D.Z., Szallasi, Z., Sadovsky, Y., Kohane, I., Mariani, T.J. Increased measurement accuracy for sequence-verified microarray probes. *Physiol. Genomics* 2004, 18: 308-315.

Meehan KL, Sadar MD Quantitative profiling of LNCaP prostate cancer cells using isotope-coded affinity tags and mass spectrometry. *Proteomics* 2004, 4: 1116-34.

O'Farrell PH. High resolution two-dimensional electrophoresis of proteins. *J. Biol. Chem.* 1975, 250: 4007-21.

Ong SE, Blagoev B, Kratchmarova I, Kristensen DB, Steen H, Pandey A, Mann M. Stable isotope labeling by amino acids in cell culture, SILAC, as a simple and accurate approach to expression proteomics. *Mol. Cell Proteomics* 2002, 1: 376-86.

Petricoin EF, Liotta LA. SELDI-TOF-based serum proteomic pattern diagnostics for early detection of cancer. *Curr. Opin. Biotechnol.* 2004, 15: 24-30.

Prober JM, Trainor GL, Dam RJ, Hobbs FW, Robertson CW, Zagursky RJ, Cocuzza AJ, Jensen MA, Baumeister K. A system for rapid DNA sequencing with fluorescent chain-terminating dideoxynucleotides. *Science* 1987, 238: 336-41.

Pruitt KD, Tatusova T, Maglott DR: NCBI Reference Sequence (RefSeq): a curated non-redundant sequence database of genomes, transcripts and proteins. *Nucleic Acids Res.* 2005, 33 (Database issue): D501-4.

Saviozzi, S., Iazzetti, G., Caserta, E., Guffanti, A., Calogero, R.A. Microarray data analysis and mining. *Methods Mol. Med.* 2004 94: 67-90.

Shalon D, Smith SJ, Brown PO. A DNA microarray system for analyzing complex DNA samples using two-color fluorescent probe hybridization. *Genome Res.* 1996, 6: 639-45.

Shevchenko A, Sunyaev S, Loboda A, Shevchenko A, Bork P, Ens W, Standing KG. Charting the proteomes of organisms with unsequenced genomes by MALDI-quadrupole time-of-flight mass spectrometry and BLAST homology searching. *Anal. Chem.* 2001, 73: 1917-26.

Snel B, Bork P, Huynen MA. The identification of functional modules from the genomic association of genes. *Proc. Natl. Acad. Sci. USA*. 2002, 99: 5890-5.

Srinivas PR, Kramer BS, Srivastava S. Trends in biomarker research for cancer detection. *Lancet Oncol.* 2001, 2: 698-704.

Steinberg TH, Pretty On Top, Berggren KN, Kemper C, Jones L, Diwu Z, Haugland RP, Patton WF. Rapid and simple single nanogram detection of glycoproteins in polyacrylamide gels and on electroblots. *Proteomics* 2001, 1: 841-55.

Tsai, J., Sultana, R., Lee, Y., Pertea, G., Karamycheva, S., Antonescu, V., Cho, J., Parvizi, B., Cheung, F., Quackenbush, J. RESOURCERER: a database for annotating and linking microarray resources within and across species. *Genome Biol.* 2001 2, SOFTWARE0002.1 - 0002.4.

Venter JC, Adams MD, Myers EW, Li PW, Mural RJ, Sutton GG, Smith HO, Yandell M, Evans CA, Holt RA, et al. The sequence of the human genome. Science 2001, 291: 1304-51. *Erratum in: Science* 2001, 292: 1838.

Villanueva J, Philip J, Entenberg D, Chaparro CA, Tanwar MK, Holland EC, Tempst P. Serum peptide profiling by magnetic particle-assisted, automated sample processing and MALDI-TOF mass spectrometry. *Anal. Chem.* 2004, 76: 1560-70.

von Heydebreck, Huber W., Gentleman R. "Differential Expression with the Bioconductor Project". 2004 *Bioconductor Project Working Papers*. Working Paper 7, http://www.bepress.com/bioconductor/paper7.

Washburn, M. P., Wolters, D. and Yates, J. R. 3rd. Large-scale analysis of the yeast proteome by multidimensional protein identification technology. *Nat. Biotechnol.* 2001, 19: 242-7.

Wasinger VC, Cordwell SJ, Cerpa-Poljak A, Yan JX, Gooley AA, Wilkins MR, Duncan MW, Harris R, Williams KL, Humphery-Smith I. Progress with gene-product mapping of the Mollicutes: Mycoplasma genitalium. *Electrophoresis* 1995, 16:1090-4.

Wheeler, DL, et al. Database Resources of the National Center for Biotechnology. *Nucl. Acids Res.* 2003, 31: 28-33.

Zhang X, Scalf M, Berggren TW, Westphall MS, Smith LM. Identification of Mammalian Cell Lines Using MALDI-TOF and LC-ESI-MS/MS Mass Spectrometry. *J. Am. Soc. Mass Spectrom.* 2006, 17: 490-9.

In: Mesothelioma from Bench Side to Clinic
Editor: Alfonso Baldi, pp. 207-220

ISBN: 978-1-60021-789-0

Chapter X

Transcriptional Profiling of Malignant Pleural Mesothelioma Using Microarrays

Gautam Maulik, Lingsheng Dong and Gavin J. Gordon*
The Thoracic Surgery Oncology Laboratory and the Division of Thoracic Surgery, Brigham and Women's Hospital, Harvard Medical School, Boston, Massachusetts USA

Abstract

Malignant pleural mesothelioma (MPM) is a highly lethal, poorly understood asbestos-related neoplasm of the thoracic pleura for which effective therapy is limited. The diagnosis of MPM can be difficult in some cases and multiple non-interconvertible staging schemas frequently hinder accurate patient prognosis. Large-scale transcriptional profiling using microarrays is frequently a part of studies to explore gene expression patterns in cancer and other diseases and has the potential to overcome these issues. In general, microarray based experiments can facilitate the identification of tumor molecular markers, provide clues relating to mechanisms of carcinogenesis, and aid in the discovery of candidate targets for therapy. Relatively few studies of this sort have been attempted for MPM, likely due to its relatively rare incidence and by extension the difficulty in acquiring suitable tissues for analysis. Microarray analysis of MPM will likely lead to a better understanding of a highly lethal malignancy and result in the identification of potential therapeutic targets to ultimately affect better treatment options and patient clinical outcome. Here we will address the general issues pertaining to all expression profiling experiments and summarize similar published studies that have been attempted for MPM.

---

* *Correspondence should be addressed to:* Gavin J. Gordon, Ph.D. Brigham and Women's Hospital Division of Thoracic Surgery, 75 Francis Street, Boston, MA 02115, Phone: (617) 732-6526. Fax: (617) 582-6085. Email: ggordon@partners.org

1. Introduction

Malignant pleural mesothelioma (MPM) is an asbestos related, highly lethal neoplasm of the pleura for which current therapy is limited [1]. Approximately 3,000 patients are diagnosed with MPM in the US annually and the incidence worldwide is projected to rise substantially in the next two decades [2-6]. Treatment options are few and the most patients die within two years of diagnosis. Without any treatment, the expected median survival of patients presenting with MPM is between 4 and 12 months [1, 4]. Aggressive cytoreductive therapy including surgery (i.e., extrapleural pneumonectomy, EPP) followed by combination chemotherapy and radiation therapy (trimodality therapy) has been shown to prolong survival in selected patients with early MPM [7-10]. However, most patients do not undergo trimodality therapy due to insufficient cardiopulmonary reserve, advanced disease, or lack of access to specialized centers.

MPM is exceedingly resistant to most chemotherapy regimens examined to date [11, 12] and radiation therapy is generally ineffective as a primary treatment as well [13]. Targeted therapies, such as anti-angiogenic drugs [14] and inhibitors of epidermal growth factor receptor (EGFR) tyrosine kinase [15], have proved equally ineffective at prolonging MPM patient survival despite substantial overexpression of the relevant molecular targets in MPM tumors. Pemetrexed (Alimta) and cisplatin combination chemotherapy was recently shown in a prospective randomized trial to be the best chemotherapy regimen for MPM [16]. However, this therapy only increased median survival from 9 to 12.4 months and the response rate lower than 50% [16]. New therapies for MPM are desperately needed but the process of designing new drugs is costly and time consuming. Emerging molecular targeted therapy (e.g., receptor tyrosine kinase c-Met [17] and others), or gene therapy-based treatment [18], may eventually prove superior in MPM but are not yet ready for clinical implementation.

The pathological diagnosis of MPM is often complex and requires immunohistochemical staining with a panel of antibodies. There are three distinct histologic subtypes of MPM based on the microscopic appearance of the major malignant elements: epithelial, sarcomatoid, mixed. The majority of MPMs are epithelial (50%) and patients with this subtype are generally thought to experience a somewhat longer survival than do patients with the other subtypes [10, 19]. However, clinicians have long noticed a certain degree of variability in patient survival and response to therapy that is not explained solely by the stage or histological appearance and may therefore be due to more subtle biological variability among tumors. However, there are no predictive factors, prognostic molecular markers, or genetic abnormalities other than histological subtype to preoperatively identify these (or other) long-term survivors. In addition, established methods to predict outcome in mesothelioma based on histological appearance are somewhat subjective, prone to human error, and are ineffective for small patient cohorts or in extreme cases for individual patients [19-23].

Large-scale transcriptional studies using microarrays have been reported in multiple cancers. Current bioinformatics tools recently applied to microarray data have shown utility in predicting both cancer diagnosis [24] and outcome [25]. Though highly accurate, their widespread clinical relevance and applicability are unresolved. The minimum number of predictor genes is not known, and the discrimination function can vary (for the same genes) based on the location and protocol used for sample preparation [24]. To date, relatively few gene expression profiling studies using microarrays have been attempted for MPM (compared to other cancers), and most of these published reports have used relatively small numbers of tissues and/or cell lines [26-28]. This is likely the consequence of the relatively low incidence of MPM and by extension, the difficulty of acquiring large numbers of MPM pathological specimens. Expression profiling studies have been attempted in MPM for three primary purposes: i) to discover new diagnostic, prognostic, and histological subtype-specific molecular markers [20, 21, 29-33] ii) to identify genes that may play a role in MPM carcinogenesis [26, 27, 33-35] and iii) to identify genes associated with specific traits of MPM tumors such as drug resistance and invasiveness [27, 35, 36]. Although multiple techniques have been employed in these combined analyses, all of them have in common some measure to identify meaningful up- and down-regulated genes in normal and tumor tissues and/or cell lines. It is not possible in this space to comprehensively address all of the genes and associated molecular pathways discovered in this manner. Therefore, the reminder of this summary will highlight select observations and seminal studies pertaining to microarray analysis in MPM as well as detail some of the technical issues that are important to expression profiling studies in general and in particular for MPM.

2. Technical Aspects of Microarray Studies

Microarrays are typically constructed by arraying oligonucleotides, PCR amplified cDNA clones or full-length genes at high density on derivatized glass slides [37]. For high-density oligonucleotide arrays, total RNA isolated from samples after quality control checks is converted to double-stranded cDNA followed by *in vitro* transcription to produce biotinylated cRNA. The tethered nucleic acids (or "probes") are hybridized to a mixture of labeled "target" nucleic acids and specific interactions can be measured as a detectable signal relating intensity to expression level for any given gene. These devices are routinely used for the simultaneous measurement of the expression levels of as many as 40,000 genes in human cancers (and disease in general). Despite recent design improvements, microarrays continue to remain susceptible to technical issues under routine circumstances that can lead to excessive variability and a lack of reproducibility [38]. When a large number of data points are generated, this can lead to a high number of false-positives when identifying differentially expressed genes, even when measures of statistical significance (i.e., *P* values) are seemingly robust. For example, multiple hypothesis testing dictates that if one uses 12,000 gene microarrays to examine differences in average gene expression levels between 2 tissue types, a significance cut-off of P=0.05 will theoretically result in up to 600 genes falsely called statistically significant. This is frequently overcome using specialized software (e.g., Significance Analysis of Microarrays or SAM, [39] and/or by applying filtering criteria secondary to *P* value (e.g. ratio fold-change). Nevertheless, the currently accepted gold standard is confirmation of microarray data using another technique such as quantitative RT-PCR.

3. Usage of Microarray Data

Another issue common to these types of studies is what to do with the large number of data-points generated after a list of differentially expressed genes is identified. (For example, in a recent analysis in our laboratory we have profiled 40 MPM tumors using microarrays containing approximately 22,000 genes resulting in approximately 800,000 discrete data points.) One common approach is to classify genes with similar distributions and samples with similar gene expression levels using complex bioinformatics tools (i.e., software). However, there are multiple different clustering algorithms available and which are appropriate to use in microarray studies is subject to interpretation [40]. Also, the results of cluster analysis should generally be validated in other ways to determine if the resulting classification scheme is stable. Finally, even robust results should be interpreted carefully to see if the resulting classification has any biological relevance.

There are two major types of clustering used in microarray analysis: hierarchical and non-hierarchical. Hierarchical clustering is essentially an agglomerative process in which single member clusters are fused into larger and larger clusters. The results are visualized using a dendrogram (i.e., classification tree) that contains an increasing number of sub-branches in which samples that are tightly clustered on a single sub-branch have similar gene expression patterns. The same technique can also be used to cluster genes with a similar distribution across all samples. Comprehensive statistical packages (such as S-PLUS [41] are capable of most types of (non-)hierarchical cluster analysis, although Eisen and colleagues have generated two user-friendly programs (i.e., CLUSTER and TREEVIEW) that are in wide use that easily accomplish this task for the non-statistician [42]. Non-hierarchical clustering includes iterative partitioning algorithms (such as *k*-means) that assign samples to a cluster, the center of which is continually adjusted by reassigning genes such that the sum of distances of genes in each cluster to the center is minimized. These techniques necessitate defining the number of expected clusters up-front, and generally are most useful when a known number of groups are expected.

One final aspect common to all clustering algorithms is how to choose which genes to include in the analysis. How genes are chosen directly relates to the question being asked. For example, for sub-class discovery, genes are typically chosen based only on their level of variation across all samples (i.e., unsupervised clustering). Sometimes it is useful to choose genes based on a known hypothesis (i.e., supervised clustering). For example, a set of cancer prognostic genes could be examined for general relevance by using them to cluster a cohort of samples then determining if statistically significant survival differences result for different predicted groups.

4. Microarray Analysis in MPM

Most efforts to transcriptionally profile MPM have used cell lines and/or small numbers of human tumor specimens. The first published report in which MPM was transcriptionally profiled using microarrays appeared in 2000. Rihn and colleagues compared global gene expression patterns between an SV40-immortalized (non-tumorigenic) mesothelial cell line and a malignant mesothelioma cell line using a filter array containing approximately 6,500 genes and discovered genes that may play a role in MPM adhesion (multiple integrins), invasion (PAI-2), and drug resistance (glutathione *S*-transferase) [27]. In a follow-up study, these investigators added microarray data from 2 human MPM specimens to their previous data [27] and have generated an extensive list of differentially expressed genes in MPM tissues and cell lines [36]. In a similar study Kettunen et al. profiled a total of 4 MPM cells lines and 2 primary mesothelial cell cultures using an array containing 588 cancer-related genes [26]. In this study, up- and down-regulated MPM genes included those implicated in a number of diverse processes such as cell cycle (multiple cyclins), cellular growth (FGF3), intracellular signaling (JNK1, NIK, ERK5, PAK1, TRAF2), and drug resistance (Ku80). The most comprehensive published study of this type was conducted by Hoang and colleagues who discovered novel mesothelioma-associated genes (and genes that distinguish between MPM histological subtypes) by profiling 10 MPM cell lines and 4 human MPM tumor specimens using microarrays containing almost 5,000 genes [34].

The studies above primarily utilized established human MPM cell lines, and like similar studies were purely descriptive. In contrast, other investigators have used microarray analysis to explore mechanisms of asbestos-induced carcinogenesis in a rat model of MPM [35]. In this study, Ramos-Nino and colleagues discovered up-and down-regulated genes in rat mesothelial cells after acute exposure to asbestos using a microarray containing nearly 9,000 genes. In a follow-up experiment in the same publication, these investigators used RNA interference (RNAi) technology to abrogate expression of one of the genes found to be upregulated after asbestos exposure (fra-1). They found that mRNA expression levels of CD44 and c-met, genes that encode receptors linked to tumor migration and invasiveness, were substantially lower in fra-1 knockdown cell lines.

Despite the difficulty in acquiring large numbers of human MPM tumor specimens, at least 5 reports have used a substantial number of human MPM tumor specimens for expression profiling analysis. Singhal and colleagues profiled 16 MPM patient tumors and 4 normal pleura tissues using microarray filters containing approximately 4,000 genes [28]. These investigators discovered a number of differentially expressed genes in MPM tumors relating to glucose metabolism, mRNA translation, and cytoskeletal remodeling. In a recent study, Pass and colleagues profiled 21 MPM patient tumors using 12,000 gene microarrays and created a 27-gene neural network classifier that could predict clinical outcome with moderate accuracy [30]. Additionally, our laboratory has profiled 31 MPM tumors (also using 12,000 gene microarrays) to develop and validate diagnostic [29] and prognostic [20] genomics-based tests for MPM using a relatively small number of genes. In more recent efforts [33], we have performed transcriptional profiling of an additional 40 independent MPM tumors, as well as normal lung and pleural tissues (n=9), and tumor-derived and non-tumorigenic cell lines (n=5) using high density oligonucleotide microarrays containing approximately 22,000 genes to better characterize the molecular pathways involved in the pathogenesis of MPM and to further validate MPM prognostic genes and tests. In global expression analysis using unsupervised clustering techniques, we found two potential subclasses of mesothelioma that correlated loosely with tumor histology. We also identified sets of genes with expression levels that distinguish between multiple tumor subclasses, normal and tumor tissues, and tumors with different morphologies. Microarray gene expression data were confirmed using quantitative reverse transcriptase-polymerase chain reaction and protein analysis for three novel candidate oncogenes (NME2, CRI1, and PDGFC) and one candidate tumor suppressor (GSN). Finally, we used bioinformatics tools to create and explore complex physiological pathways. Combined, all of these data may advance our understanding of mesothelioma tumorigenesis, pathobiology, or both.

Although analyses using human and non-human cell lines to discover differentially expressed genes in microarray studies of human malignancies are generally useful, one should realize that there are inherent differences between species, and within species between cell lines and actual tumor specimens, particularly for MPM. This caveat should be kept in mind especially when considering the biological relevance of differentially expressed genes discovered in cell lines that have not yet been examined (or have conflicting expression level patterns) in human tumor specimens. For example, c-fos mRNA levels are elevated in rat mesothelial cells exposed to asbestos but not rat mesothelioma cell lines [35]. Consistent with these findings, we have also observed relatively low (or absent) mRNA levels of c-fos in human MPM cell lines profiled with microarrays in our laboratory [29, 33]. However, we found that c-fos mRNA levels are highly expressed in human MPM specimens profiled in the same study [29]. Another example is the finding of insulin-like growth factor binding protein 5 to be down-regulated in MPM cell lines [34] yet highly expressed in MPM tumor specimens [33]. At least some of these differences may be due in part to the choice of control tissue. There is no standard and universally accepted normal control tissue or cell line for MPM. The result is that genes differentially expressed in mesothelioma have been expressed relative to short-term mesothelial cell cultures, SV40-immortalized (non-tumorigenic) mesothelial cell lines, and normal pleura tissue by multiple of investigators.

In the most recent and comprehensive transcriptional profiling of MPM tumors, Lopez-Rios and colleagues analyzed 99 MPM tumors using a 22,000-gene microarray [43]. They found that the overexpression of Aurora kinases and deletion of p16/CDKN2A were prognostic factors. In a separate analysis within the same publication these investigators developed an independent multi-gene prognostic model for MPM. Finally, Lopez-Rios et al. performed differential gene expression analysis between epithelial and sarcomatoid histological subtypes of MPM and unexpectedly observed that the epithelial subtype overexpressed uroplakins as well as kallikrein11 at the mRNA and protein level.

More recently, gene expression profiling has been used to create a molecular diagnostic test to aid in the distinction of MPM and lung cancer using material obtained from pleural effusions [44]. In other animal model studies, Kim et al. used 20,000-gene microarrays to identify insulin-like growth factor 1 (IGF-1], p38 MAPkinase, Wnt/beta-catenin, and integrin signaling pathways as important in peritoneal mesothelioma carcinogenesis in a rat model [45]. Examination of microarray data for 16 selected genes using Ingenuity Pathway Analysis software demonstrated that peritoneal mesotheliomas in these rats were similar to some degree to mesotheliomas in humans.

5. Translation of Microarray Data into Clinically Relevant Diagnostic and Prognostic Tests in MPM

To overcome the many limitations in the direct clinical application of gene profiling data from microarrays, we have developed and tested a new predictive metric based on ratios of gene expression levels. This method requires an initial gene expression profiling and comparison of two groups of tissues that differ by a single clinical parameter (histology, outcome, etc.) using standard statistical methods. The genes that are found to differ most significantly are identified, selected and used to construct a set of ratios that singly or in combination predict the correct parameter in the training set. The numerical value of gene ratios can be compared to a rationally chosen threshold and used to identify the desired clinical parameter in future samples. The gene expression ratio method, by virtue of the fact that it is a ratio (i) negates the need for a third reference gene when determining expression levels, (ii) is independent of platform used for data acquisition, (iii) requires only small quantities of RNA, (iv) does not require the coupling of transcription to translation for chosen genes, and (v) permits analysis of individual samples without reference additional "training samples" whose data was acquired on the same platform. We have used this technique to discover MPM diagnostic tests [29] and prognostic tests [20, 21] and for the diagnosis of prostate cancer [46], the diagnosis of lung cancer [47] and the prognosis of lung cancer [48]. Other investigators have used this technique to aid in lung cancer detection [49]. We propose that utilizing gene expression ratios is an accurate and inexpensive technique with direct clinical applicability for distinguishing among different tissue types in cancer and other diseases with a basis in differentially expressed genes.

6. Pathway Discovery in MPM Using Microarray Data

What is the next step in microarray studies after cluster analysis and discovering differentially expressed genes? Interpreting the data in a biologically meaningful context is frequently accomplished by considering which molecular pathways are regulated by differentially expressed genes, which has been done in some form for all of the studies cited here for MPM. The challenge is to link the published scientific literature with microarray experiments in such a way as to discover relevant pathways that may not be immediately clear simply by visually scanning a long list of genes and performing standard literature searches on each one. Although a number of free web-based tools are available for this purpose (e.g., GenMAPP, Pubgene), all of them have drawbacks and limitations and work best when their usage is combined. One new commercially developed tool for this purpose is Pathway Analysis from Ingenuity Systems. We have used this software to discover molecular pathways that may be relevant in MPM, identify drugs that are known to act on key differentially expressed genes, and determine the physiological, biochemical, and functional role of key genes in addition to their subcellular localization. Nevertheless, these tools are simply used to generate hypotheses and are not a replacement for "wet lab" molecular biology based studies.

We analyzed tumor molecular markers and computer assisted pathway analysis to create multiple biological networks to define and begin testing hypothesis regarding the pathophysiology of MPM [33]. The combined network consisted of 210 genes, approximately half of which (46%, 97/210) were MPM up-regulated genes. Of these genes, SP1 and SPARC were not previously reported in MPM in the published literature. The SP1 transcription factor has multiple functions and can drive the expression of many cancer-related genes such as VEGF. SPARC, a matrix-associated protein that plays role in cell shape, cell-cycle progression, and influence the synthesis of extra cellular matrix. Pathway analysis revealed that the SPARC/VTN (vitronectin) interaction could also modulate adhesion and spreading of endothelial cells, which may function in angiogenesis in the context of MPM tumorigenesis.

Although MPM tumors and cell lines contained low, but reliably detectable levels of MYCN mRNA by microarray analysis, this gene may be physiologically relevant during MPM tumorigenesis since MYCN protein has been detected in some MPM tumors, [50] and not all neuroblastoma tumors or cell lines have MYCN genomic amplification yet still contain detectable mRNA and protein [51]. Alternatively, genes regulated by multiple *myc* family members could be transcriptionally activated primarily by MYC in MPM. Genes in pathway analysis include well-studied transcription factors regulating proliferation and apoptosis (E2F1, E2F4, FOS, MYC), cell cycle regulators (RB1), and growth factors (VEGF). Several genes have been previously described in MPM and/or are consistent with current knowledge. For example, the up-regulation of genes transcriptionally regulated by TP53 and RB1 tumor suppressors is consistent with the lack of mutations in these genes in MPM [52-54]. Similarly, VEGF and MYC have been previously described as potential proto-oncogenes in MPM [55]. Curiously, we found high levels of the *FMR1* gene in MPM tumors. Mutations in this gene are responsible for X-linked mental retardation (i.e. fragile X syndrome) and the role of this gene (if any) in cancer is unknown. This mRNA binding protein has not previously been described in MPM and forms a node with other genes that have mRNA to which it is capable of binding. These genes (e.g. GNAS, SPP1, CDK4, HINT1, COLL11A1, CDH11, CBX3) are themselves up regulated in MPM. Although the exact functional relevance of these results is unknown at present, at least one of these genes is in a pathway with direct cancer relevance (e.g., *SPP1*, which interacts with the anti-apoptotic protein IGFBP2, also expressed at high mRNA levels in MPM).

In other studies, AP-1 transcription factor family members FOS and FOSL1 were found to associate with MPM tumorigenesis, consistent with our pathway analysis showing that multiple MPM upregulated gene. In these analyses, FOSL1 mRNA levels were found to be elevated in both rat mesothelioma cell lines and rat mesothelial cells exposed to asbestos, but FOS mRNA levels were up-regulated only in the latter [35, 56-58]. This finding prompted these investigators to suggest that FOSL1 may substitute for FOS in AP-1 complexes during human MPM tumorigenesis [35]. Consistent with these findings, we have also observed relatively low (or absent) mRNA levels of FOS and substantially higher mRNA levels of FOSL1 in human MPM cell lines [29, 33]. However, we observed FOS mRNA levels that are 8-fold to 56-fold higher than those of FOSL1 in human MPM specimens [29, 33].

7. Inhibitor of Apoptosis Proteins (IAP) in Mesothelioma

Inhibitor of Apoptosis Proteins (IAP) comprise a family of structurally similar proteins, five of which are widely studied in the context of cancer: IAP-1/MIHC/cIAP2, IAP-2/MIHB/cIAP1, livin/ML-IAP/KIAP, survivin, and XIAP/MIHA/hILP. IAPs are overexpressed by most neoplasms, promote tumor cell survival after a wide variety of apoptotic stimuli, and frequently have gene and/or protein expression patterns associated with a relatively poor prognosis. However, normal tissues also express many IAPs, can facilitate apoptotic cell death, and have expression patterns associated with a relatively favorable prognosis in some cases. The result is that the precise role(s) of IAPs in human tumors is not exactly known. Given the high homology of IAP family members, it is likely that other IAPs will be important in MPM. In our recent work [59] we have determined the gene and protein expression patterns of IAP-1, IAP-2, survivin, livin, and XIAP in MPM cell lines (n=9) and a large number of MPM tumors using high-density oligonucleotide microarrays (n=40) and a MPM tissue array (n=66). Human tumors were linked to clinical data and we discovered that IAP-1 and survivin mRNA expression patterns were associated with relatively shorter patient survival while those of XIAP and livin were associated with a relatively longer patient survival. We also detected abundant protein for all IAPs in MPM tumors, which were expressed primarily in the cytoplasm. Only IAP-1 protein was expressed exclusively in the nucleus of MPM tumors. Using antisense targeting strategies, we demonstrated that attenuation of IAP-1 gene expression in cell lines results in reduced baseline cell viability and heightened sensitivity to cisplatin-induced cytotoxicity [60]. Our results strongly suggest that IAP-1 plays an important role in mediating MPM carcinogenesis and contributes to the inherent resistance of MPM to cisplatin. These combined results provide the rational for additional study of this gene family in MPM and cancer in general.

8. Conclusion

The body of knowledge concerning global gene expression in MPM has benefited greatly from expression profiling studies using microarrays. Since MPM remains a highly lethal and poorly understood neoplasm that is resistant to most types of standard therapy, these studies will drive gene discovery and likely positively impact patient survival by elucidating novel molecular markers and pathways involved in MPM carcinogenesis and/or pathobiology as well as identifying potential new targets for therapy.

References

[1] Pass, H. Malignant pleural mesothelioma: Surgical roles and novel therapies. *Clinical Lung Cancer*, *3:* 102-117, 2001.

[2] Peto, J., Decarli, A., La Vecchia, C., Levi, F., and Negri, E. The European mesothelioma epidemic. *British Journal of Cancer*, *79:* 666-672, 1999.

[3] Peto, J., Hodgson, J. T., Matthews, F. E., and Jones, J. R. Continuing increase in mesothelioma mortality in Britain. *Lancet, 345:* 535-539, 1995.

[4] Sugarbaker, D. J. and Liptay, M. J. Therapeutic approaches in malignant mesothelioma. *In:* J. Aisner, R. Arriagada, M. R. Green, N. Martini, and M. C. Perry (eds.), *Comprehensive Textbook of Thoracic Oncology*, pp. 786-798. Baltimore: Williams and Wilkins, 1996.

[5] Aisner, J. Diagnosis, staging, and natural history of pleural mesothelioma. *In:* J. Aisner, R. Arriagada, M. R. Green, N. Martini, and M. C. Perry (eds.), *Comprehensive Textbook of Thoracic Oncology,* pp. 799-785. Baltimore: Williams and Wilkins, 1996.

[6] Britton, M. The Epidemiology of Mesothelioma. *Seminars in Surgical Oncology*, *29:* 18-25, 2002.

[7] Chang, M. Y. and Sugarbaker, D. J. Extrapleural pneumonectomy for diffuse malignant pleural mesothelioma: Techniques and complications. *Thoracic Surgery Clinics*, *14:* 523-530, 2004.

[8] Richards, W. G., Zellos, L., Bueno, R., Jaklitsch, M. T., Janne, P. A., Chirieac, L. R., Yeap, B. Y., Dekkers, R. J., Hartigan, P. M., Capalbo, L., and Sugarbaker, D. J. Phase I to II study of pleurectomy/decortication and intraoperative intracavitary hyperthermic cisplatin lavage for mesothelioma. *Journal of Clinical Oncology*, *24:* 1561-1567, 2006.

[9] Sugarbaker, D. J., Flores, R. M., Jaklitsch, M. T., Richards, W. G., Strauss, G. M., Corson, J. M., DeCamp, M. M., Jr, Swanson, S. J., Bueno, R., Lukanich, J. M., Baldini, E. H., and Mentzer, S. J. Resection margins, extrapleural nodal status, and cell type determine postoperative long-term survival in trimodality therapy of malignant pleural mesothelioma: results in 183 patients. *Journal of Thoracic and Cardiovascular Surgery*, *117:* 54-65, 1999.

[10] Sugarbaker, D. J., Garcia, J. P., Richards, W. G., Harpole, D. H., Jr., Healy-Baldini, E., DeCamp, M. M., Jr., Mentzer, S. J., Liptay, M. J., Strauss, G. M., and Swanson, S. J. Extrapleural pneumonectomy in the multimodality therapy of malignant pleural mesothelioma. Results in 120 consecutive patients. *Annals of Surgery*, *224:* 288-294, 1996.

[11] Goudar, R. K. New therapeutic options for mesothelioma. *Current Oncology Reports*, *7:* 260-265, 2005.

[12] Krug, L. M. An overview of chemotherapy for mesothelioma. *Hematology and Oncology Clinics of North America*, *19:* 1117-1136, 2005.

[13] Sugarbaker, D. J., Norberto, J. J., and Bueno, R. Current therapy for mesothelioma. *Cancer Control*, *4:* 326-334, 1997.

[14] Dowell, J. E. and Kindler, H. L. Antiangiogenic therapies for mesothelioma. *Hematology and Oncology Clinics of North America*, *19:* 1137-1145, 2005.

[15] Govindan, R., Kratzke, R. A., Herndon, J. E., Niehans, G. A., Vollmer, R., Watson, D., Green, M. R., Kindler, H. L., and 30101), C. a. L. G. B. C. Gefitinib in patients with malignant mesothelioma: a phase II study by the Cancer and Leukemia Group B. *Clinical Cancer Research*, *11:* 2300-2304, 2005.

[16] Vogelzang, N. J., Rusthoven, J. J., Symanowski, J., Denham, C., Kaukel, E., Ruffie, P., Gatzemeier, U., Boyer, M., Emri, S., Manegold, C., Niyikiza, C., and Paoletti , P. Phase III study of pemetrexed in combination with cisplatin versus cisplatin alone in patients with malignant pleural mesothelioma. *Journal of Clinical Oncology, 21:* 2636-2644, 2003.

[17] Jagadeeswaran, R., Ma, P. C., Seiwert, T. Y., Jagadeeswaran, S., Zumba, O., Nallasura, V., Ahmed, S., Filiberti, R., Paganuzzi, M., Puntoni, R., Kratzke, R. A., Gordon, G. J., D.J., S., Bueno, R., Janamanchi, V., Bindokas, V. P., Kindler, H. L., and Salgia, R. Functional analysis of c-Met/hepatocyte growth factor pathway in malignant pleural mesothelioma. *Cancer Research, 66:* 352-361, 2006.

[18] Sterman, D. H. Gene therapy for malignant pleural mesothelioma. *Hematology and Oncology Clinics of North America, 19:* 1147-1173, 2005.

[19] Corson, J. M. and Renshaw, A. A. Pathology of mesothelioma. *In:* J. Aisner, R. Arriagada, M. R. Green, N. Martini, and M. C. Perry (eds.), *Comprehensive Textbook of Thoracic Oncology*, pp. 757-758. Baltimore: Williams and Wilkins, 1996.

[20] Gordon, G. J., Jensen, R. V., Hsiao, L. L., Gullans, S. R., Blumenstock, J. E., Richards, W. G., Jaklitsch, M. T., Sugarbaker, D. J., and Bueno, R. Using gene expression ratios to predict outcome among patients with mesothelioma. *Journal of the National Cancer Institute, 95:* 598-605, 2003.

[21] Gordon, G. J., Rockwell, G. N., Godfrey, P. A., Jensen, R. V., Glickman, J. N., Yeap, B. W., Richards, W. G., Sugarbaker, D. J., and Bueno, R. Validation of genomics-based prognostic tests in malignant pleural mesothelioma. *Clinical Cancer Research, 11:* 4406-4414, 2005.

[22] Ong, S.-T. and Vogelsang, N. J. Current therapeutic approaches to unresectable (primary and recurrent) disease. *In:* J. Aisner, R. Arriagada, M. R. Green, N. Martini, and M. C. Perry (eds.), *Comprehensive Textbook of Thoracic Oncology*, pp. 799-814. Baltimore: Williams and Wilkins, 1996.

[23] Ordonez, N. G. The value of antibodies 44-36A, SM3, HBME-1, and thrombomodulin in differentiating epithelial pleural mesothelioma from lung adenocarcinoma. *American Journal of Surgical Pathology, 21:* 1399-1408, 1997.

[24] Golub, T. R., Slonim, D. K., Tamayo, P., Huard, C., Gaasenbeek, M., Mesirov, J. P., Coller, H., Loh, M. L., Downing, J. R., Caligiuri, M. A., Bloomfield, C. D., and Landers, E. S. Molecular classification of cancer: class discovery and class prediction by gene expression monitoring. *Science, 286:* 531-537, 1999.

[25] Pomeroy, S. L., Tamayo, P., Gaasenbeek, M., Sturla, L. M., Angelo, M., McLaughlin, M. E., Kim, J. Y. H., Goumnerova, L. C., Black, P. M., Lau, C., Allen, J. C., Zagzag, D., Olson, J. M., Curran, T., Wetmore, C., Biegel, J. A., Poggio, T., Mukherjee, S., Rifkin, R., Califano, A., Stolovitzky, G., Louis, D. N., Mesirov, J. P., Lander, E. S., and Golub, T. R. Prediction of central nervous system embryonal tumor outcome based on gene expression. *Nature, 415:* 436-442, 2002.

[26] Kettunen, E., Nissen, A. M., Ollikainen, T., Taavitsainen, M., Tapper, J., Mattson, K., Linnainmaa, K., Knuutila, S., and El-Rifai, W. Gene expression profiling of malignant mesothelioma cell lines: cDNA array study. *International Journal of Cancer, 91:* 492-496, 2001.

[27] Rihn, B. H., Mohr, S., McDowell, S. A., Binet, S., Loubinoux, J., Galateau, F., Keith, G., and Leikauf, G. D. Differential gene expression in mesothelioma. *FEBS Letters, 480:* 95-100, 2000.

[28] Singhal, S., Wiewrodt, R., Malden, L. D., Amin, K. M., Matzie, K., Friedberg, J., Kucharczuk, J. C., Litzky, L. A., Johnson, S. W., Kaiser, L. R., and Albelda, S. M. Gene expression profiling of malignant mesothelioma. *Clinical Cancer Research, 9:* 3080-3097, 2003.

[29] Gordon, G. J., Jensen, R. V., Hsiao, L. L., Gullans, S. R., Blumenstock, J. E., Ramaswamy, S., Richards, W. G., Sugarbaker, D. J., and Bueno, R. Translation of microarray data into clinically relevant cancer diagnostic tests using gene expression ratios in lung cancer and mesothelioma. *Cancer Research, 62:* 4963-4967, 2002.

[30] Pass, H. I., Liu, Z., Wali, A., Bueno, R., Land, S., Lott, D., Siddiq, F., Lonardo, F., Carbone, M., and Draghici, S. Gene expression profiles predict survival and progression of pleural mesothelioma. *Clinical Cancer Research, 10:* 849-859, 2004.

[31] Mohr, S. and Rihn, B. Gene expression profiling in human mesothelioma cells using DNA microarray and high-density filter array technologies. *Bulletin du Cancer, 88:* 305-313, 2001.

[32] Mohr, S., Bottin, M.-C., Lannes, B., Neuville, A., Bellocq, J.-P., Keith, G., and Bertrand, H. R. Microdissection, mRNA amplification, and microarray: a study of pleural mesothelial and malignant mesothelioma cells. *Biochimie, 86:* 13-19, 2004.

[33] Gordon, G. J., Rockwell, G. N., Jensen, R. V., Rheinwald, J. G., Glickman, J. N., Aronson, J. P., Pottorf, B. J., Nitz, M. D., Richards, W. G., Sugarbaker, D. J., and Bueno, R. Identification of novel candidate oncogenes and tumor suppressors in malignant pleural mesothelioma using large-scale transcriptional profiling. *American Journal of Pathology, 166:* 1827-1840, 2005.

[34] Hoang, C. D., D'Cunha, J., Kratzke, M. G., Casmey, C. E., Frizelle, S. P., Maddaus, M. A., and Kratzke, R. A. Gene expression profiling identifies matriptase overexpression in malignant mesothelioma. *Chest, 125:* 1843-1852, 2004.

[35] Ramos-Nino, M. E., Scapoli, L., Matrtinelli, M., Land, S., and Mossman, B. T. Microarray analysis and RNA silencing link fra-1 to cd44 and c-met expression in mesothelioma. *Cancer Research, 63:* 3539-3545, 2003.

[36] Mohr, S., Keith, G., Galateau-Salle, F., Icard, P., and Rihn, B. H. Cell protection, resistance and invasiveness of two malignant mesotheliomas as assessed by 10K-microarray. *Biochimica et Biophysica Acta, 1688:* 43-60, 2004.

[37] The Chipping Forecast. Nature Genetics, *21:* 1-60, 1999.

[38] Gullans, S. R. Of microarrays and meandering data points. *Nature Genetics, 26:* 4-5, 2000.

[39] Tusher, V. G., Tibshirani, R., and Chu, G. Significance analysis of microarrays applied to the ionizing radiation response. *Proceedings of the National Academy of Science,* USA, *98:* 5116-5121, 2001.

[40] Quackenbush, J. Computational analysis of microarray data. *Nature Reviews Genetics, 2:* 418-427, 2001.

[41] Venables, W. N. and Riley, B. D. *Modern Applied Statistics with S-Plus.* New York: Springer, 1997.

[42] Eisen, M. B., Spellman, P. T., Brown, P. O., and Botstein, D. Cluster analysis and display of genome-wide expression patterns. *Proceedings of the National Academy of Science, USA, 95:* 14863-14868, 1998.

[43] Lopez-Rios, F., Chuai, S., Flores, R., Shimizu, S., Ohno, T., Wakahara, K., Illei, P. B., Hussain, S., Krug, L., Zakowski, M. F., Rusch, V., Olshen, A. B., and Ladanyi, M. Global gene expression profiling of pleural mesotheliomas: overexpression of aurora kinases and P16/CDKN2A deletion as prognostic factors and critical evaluation of microarray-based prognostic prediction. *Cancer Res., 66:* 2970-2979, 2006.

[44] Holloway, A. J., Diyagama, D. S., Opeskin, K., Creaney, J., Robinson, B. W., Lake, R. A., and Bowtell, D. D. A molecular diagnostic test for distinguishing lung adenocarcinoma from malignant mesothelioma using cells collected from pleural effusions. *Clin. Cancer Res., 12:* 5129-5135, 2006.

[45] Kim, Y., Ton, T. V., DeAngelo, A. B., Morgan, K., Devereux, T. R., Anna, C., Collins, J. B., Paules, R. S., Crosby, L. M., and Sills, R. C. Major carcinogenic pathways identified by gene expression analysis of peritoneal mesotheliomas following chemical treatment in F344 rats. *Toxicol. Appl. Pharmacol., 214:* 144-151, 2006.

[46] Bueno, R., Loughlin, K. R., Powell, M. H., and Gordon, G. J. A diagnostic test for prostate cancer from gene expression profiling data. *Journal of Urology, 171:* 903-906, 2004.

[47] Gordon, G. J., Deters, L. A., Nitz, M. D., Lieberman, B. C., Yeap, B. Y., and Bueno, R. Differential diagnosis of solitary lung nodules using gene expression ratios. *Journal of Thoracic and Cardiovascular Surgery, 132:* 621-627, 2006.

[48] Gordon, G. J., Richards, W. G., Sugarbaker, D. J., Jaklitsch, M. T., and Bueno, R. A prognostic test for adenocarcinoma of the lung from gene expression profiling data. *Cancer Epidemiol. Biomarkers Prev., 12:* 905-910, 2003.

[49] Hofmann, H.-S., Hansen, G., Burdach, S., Bartling, B., Silber, R.-E., and Simm, A. Discrimination of human lung neoplasm from normal lung by two target genes. *American Journal of Respiratory and Critical Care Medicine, 170:* 516-519, 2004.

[50] Kishimoto, T. The distribution of various type of oncogenes products in the tumor tissue of malignant mesothelioma. *Nihon Kyobu Shikkan Gakkai Zasshi, 29:* 1168-1173, 1991.

[51] Tsuchida, Y., Hemmi, H., Inoue, A., Obana, K., Yang, H. W., Hayashi, Y., Kanda, N., and Shimatake, H. Genetic clinical markers of human neuroblastoma with special reference to N-myc oncogene: amplified or not amplified? *Tumour Biology, 17:* 65-74, 1996.

[52] Metcalf, R. A., Welsh, J. A., Bennet, W. P., Seddon, M. B., Lehman, T. A., Pelin, K., Linnainmaa, K., Tammilehto, L., Mattson, K., Gerwin, B. I., and Harris, C. C. p53 and Kirsten-*ras* mutations in human mesothelioma cell lines. *Cancer Research, 52:* 2610-2615, 1992.

[53] Mor, O., Yaron, P., Huszar, M., Yellin, A., Kakobovitz, O., Brok-Simoni, F., Rechavi, G., and Reichart, N. Absence of p53 mutations in malignant mesotheliomas. *American Journal of Respiratory Cell and Molecular Biology, 16:* 9-13, 1997.

[54] Van der Meeren, A., Seddon, M. B., Kispert, J., Harris, C. C., and Gerwin, B. I. Lack of expression of the retinoblastoma gene is not frequently involved in the genesis of human mesothelioma. *European Respiratory Reviews*, *3:* 177-179, 1993.

[55] Lechner, J. F., Tesfaigzi, J., and Gerwin, B. I. Oncogenes and tumor-suppressor genes in mesothelioma--a synopsis. *Environmental Health Perspectives, 105:* 1061-1067, 1997.

[56] Ramos-Nino, M. E., Timblin, C. R., and Mossman, B. T. Mesothelial cell transformation requires increased AP-1 binding activity and ERK-dependent Fra-1 expression. *Cancer Research, 62:* 6065-6069, 2002.

[57] Heintz, N., Janssen, Y., and Mossman, B. T. Persistent induction of c-fos and c-jun expression by asbestos. *Proceedings of the National Academy of Science*, USA, *90:* 3299-3303, 1993.

[58] Janssen, Y., Heintz, N., Marsh, J., Borm, P., and Mossman, B. T. Induction of c-fos and c-jun protooncogenes in target cells of the lung and pleura by carcinogenic fibers. *American Journal of Respiratory Cell and Molecular Biology, 11:* 522-530, 1994.

[59] Gordon, G. J., Mani, M., Mukhopadhyay, L., Dong, L., Glickman, J. N., Yeap, B. W., Sugarbaker, D. J., and Bueno, R. Expression patterns of inhibitor of apoptosis proteins in malignant pleural mesothelioma. *Journal of Pathology, In Press.*, 2007.

[60] Gordon, G. J., Chen, C.-J., Mukhopadhyay, N. K., Jaklitsch, M., Richards, W. G., Sugarbaker, D. J., and Bueno, R. Inhibitor of apoptosis protein-1 promotes tumor cell survival in mesothelioma. *Carcinogenesis, 23:* 1017-1024, 2002.

In: Mesothelioma from Bench Side to Clinic
Editor: Alfonso Baldi, pp. 221-242
ISBN: 978-1-60021-789-0

Chapter XI

Cyclooxygenase Enzymes: Structure, Function and Involvement in Mesothelioma

***Alessandra Verdina*[*]*, Irene Cardillo*[*]*, Rossella Galati*[*] *and Alfonso Baldi*[**]**

[*] Laboratory D, Dept. for Development of Therapeutic Programs,
Center for Experimental Research,
Regina Elena Cancer Institute, Rome, Italy
[**]Department of Biochemistry, Section of Pathology,
Second University of Naples, Naples, Italy

Abstract

Cyclooxygenases catalyze the rate limiting step in the production of prostanoids. Accumulating data demonstrate that over-expression of these enzymes, and in particular of cyclooxygenase-2, promotes multiple events involved in tumorigenesis; in addition, numerous studies show that inhibition of cyclooxygenase-2 can delay or prevent certain forms of cancer. Moreover, cyclooxygenase-2 has been recently recognized as an important adverse prognostic factor in mesothelioma. Hence, there is an increasing interest in the development of new treatments based on cyclooxygenase-2 inhibitors, to prolong survival and even potentially cure this neoplasia.

This chapter critically reviews the most recent data about the role of COX molecules in mesothelioma pathogenesis and progression. Moreover, the possible clinical implications in the treatment of mesothelioma of these findings are discussed.

COX Enzymes

The cyclooxygenase (COXs) enzymes, also known as prostaglandin endoperoxide H synthases (PGH synthases), catalyze the first step in the biosynthesis of all prostaglandins through the conversion of arachidonic acid to the common intermediate prostaglandin H_2 (PGH_2) [Cardillo I. et al., 2005; Marnett L.J. et al., 1999; Smith W.L. et al., 2000; Smith W.L. et al., 1996] (Figure 1). The first step in PGs synthesis is hydrolysis of membrane phospholipids to produce free arachidonic acid. This reaction is catalyzed by phospholipase A_2. Next COXs catalyze the conversion of arachidonic acid in PGH_2, through two different activities: a cyclooxygenase (bis-oxygenase) one which converts arachidonic acid into an unstable intermediate, PGG_2, and a peroxidase one which reduce PGG_2 to form PGH_2. Specific isomerases then convert PGH_2 to several PGs and thromboxane A_2 [Miyamoto T. et al., 1976; Van der Ouderaa F.J. et al., 1977].

The COX enzymes are glycosylated integral membrane proteins found in the luminal surface of the endoplasmic reticulum and on the outer membrane of the nuclear envelope [Smith W.L. et al., 1996], although they have also been detected in other structures, such as lipid bodies and mitochondria [Bozza P.T. et al., 1997; Coffey R.J. et al., 1997; Liou J.Y. et al., 2000; Liou J.Y. et al., 2001] (Figure 2).

The better known isoforms of PGH synthase in mammals are two: PGH synthase-1 (COX-1) and PGH synthase-2 (COX-2), although a COX-1 variant, COX-3, has been recently demonstrated. COX-1 is the constitutively expressed isoform, while COX-2 is inducible.

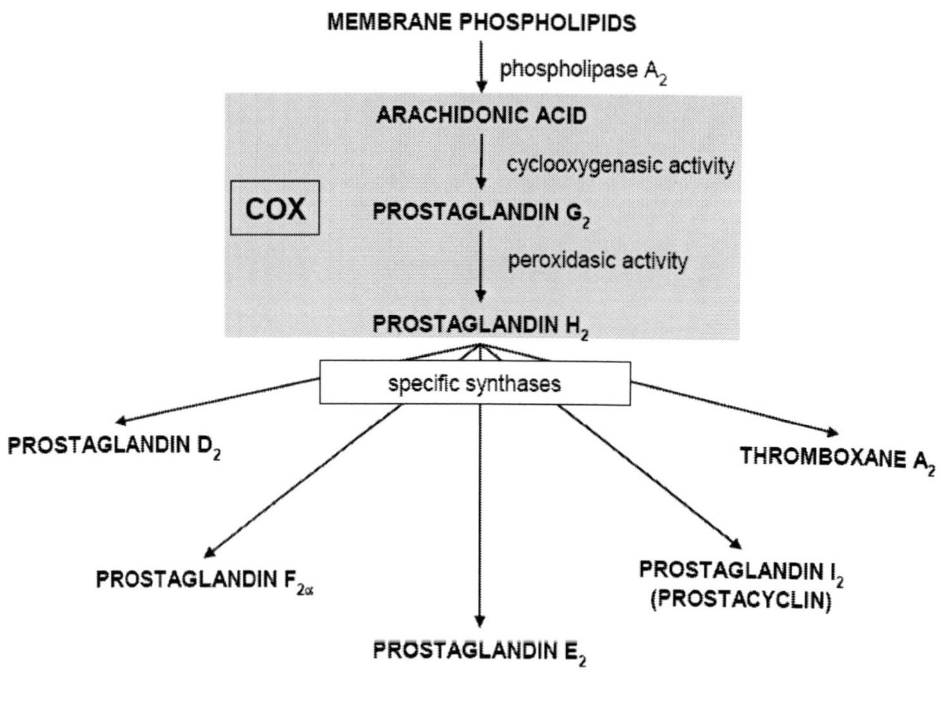

Figure 1. Production of prostaglandins by COXs. The two reactions performed by cyclooxygenases: the conversion of arachidonic acid to PGG_2 by the cyclooxygenase activity and the conversion of PGG_2 to PGH_2 by the peroxidase activity. The conversion of PGH_2 to the five principal prostaglandins by cell specific synthases.

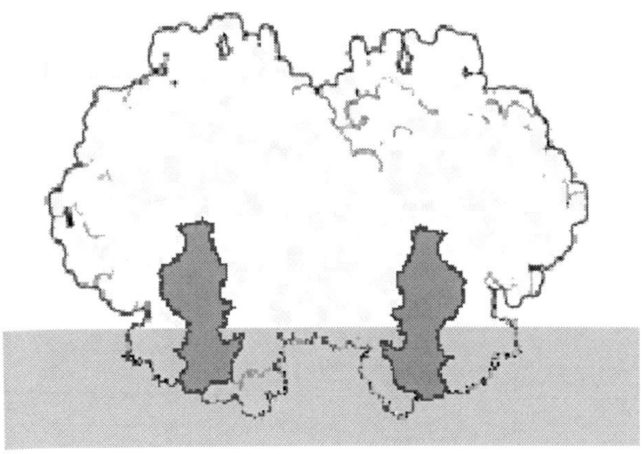

Figure 2. Cyclooxygenase-2. The enzyme is a dimer of two identical subunits, and each subunit contains two separate active sites, which perform the first reactions in prostaglandin synthesis. The active sites are found deep within a pocket that opens into the membrane (yellow in the illustration), allowing easy access to idrofobic arachidonic acid (modified from Goodsell D.S., 2000).

Although encoded by different genes, the two COX isozymes share a relatively conserved primary structure, similar structural topology, and an identical catalytic mechanism [Picot D. et al., 1994; Kurumbail R.G. et al., 1996; Luong C. et al., 1996; Garavito R.M. et al., 2002; Kulmacz R.J. et al., 2003]. However, the patterns of gene expression and regulation differ greatly, pointing to distinct biological roles [Vane J.R. et al., 1998; Hla T. et al., 1999].

COX Isozymes: Gene Structure and Expression

COX isozymes are encoded by separate single copy genes that map to distint chromosomes [Marnett L.J. et al., 1999; Tanabe T. and Tohnai N., 2002], indicating that these genes are not genetically linked; in particular, the localization is 9q32-q33.3 for cox-1 [Funk C.D. et al., 1991] and 1q25.2-q25.3 for cox-2 [Tay A., 1994]. The human gene for COX-1 (cox-1) is about 22 kb in length with 11 exons and is transcribed as 2.8- and 5.2-kb mRNAs variants [Yokoyama C. and Tanabe T., 1989]. The gene for COX-2 (cox-2) is about 8.3 kb long with 10 exons and it is transcribed as 2,8- and 4.6-kb mRNA variants [Appleby S. B. et al., 1994; Kosaka T. et al., 1994; Tazawa R. et al., 1994; Hla T. and Neilson K., 1992; Hla T. et al., 1999]. The genes for both COX-1 and -2 are highly regulated: cox-1 is generally induced by cell quiescence and differentiation whereas cox-2 is an immediate-early gene induced by a variety of stimuli including hormones, growth factors, cytokines and shear stress [Hla T. et al., 1993].

The gene structures of cox-1 and cox-2 demonstrate remarkable conservation of exon/intron junctions [Kraemer S.A. et al., 1992; Xie W. et al., 1993; Boerboom D. and Sirois J., 1998]. The main differences between cox-1 and cox-2 consist of different intron lengths and one missing intron in cox-2 (Figure 3).

In cox-1 there are several putative transcriptional regulatory elements in the promoter region, including two Sp1 motifs, two AP-2 sites, an NF-IL6 motif, and a GATA. The 5'-

flanking region of cox-1 has multiple transcription start sites, it does not possess a canonical TATA or CAAT box, and it is GC-rich (Figure 3).

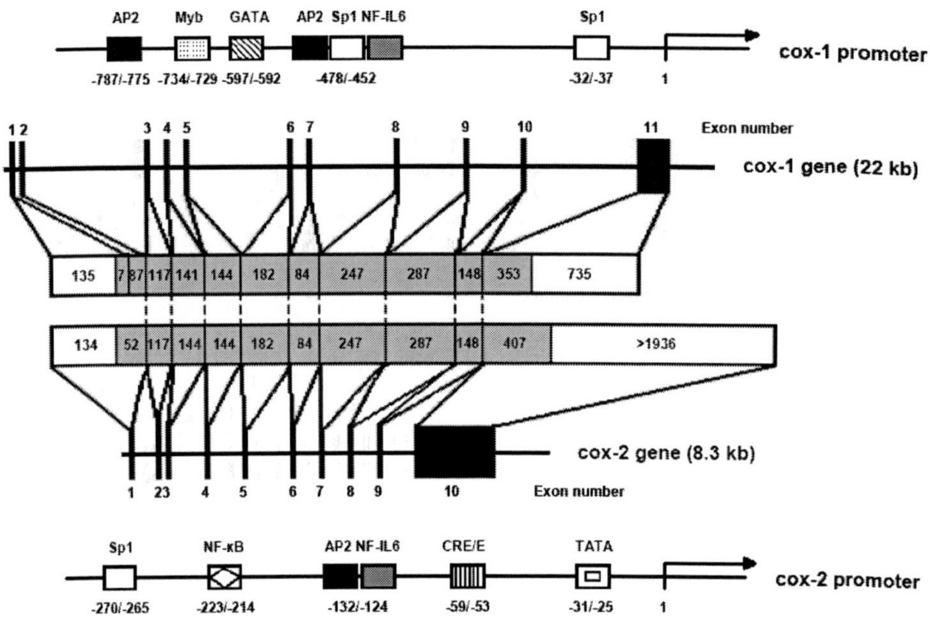

Figure 3. Promoter and Gene structures of human cox-1 and cox-2. The exon-intron structures of human cox-1 and cox-2 genes. Italicized numbers indicate the number of nucleotides comprising the exon. Modified from Kosaka T et al., 1994. Regulatory elements in human cox-1 and cox-2 promoters. Modified from Inoue H. et al., 1995.

These features are consistent with those of a housekeeping gene. Sp1 has been shown to contribute to constitutive expression of cox-1 [Xu X.M. et al., 1997]: mutation of either Sp1 binding site significantly reduce the promoter activity to 40-50% that of the wild type. When both sites are mutated, the basal activity is reduced to 29%. This indicates that the two Sp-1 *cis*-elements constitutively regulate expression of the cox-1 gene by *trans*-acting and maintaining the basal level of transduction.

In cox-2 the largest exon encodes the entire 3'-untraslated region (3'-UTR), containing 23 copies of the 'ATTTA' RNA instability element. Sequence analysis of the 5'-flanking region has shown several potential transcription regulatory elements, including a TATA box, two NF-IL6 motif, two AP-2 sites, three Sp1 sites, two NF-κB sites, a CRE motif and an E-box. ATF/CRE is one of the most important regulatory elements in the cox-2 promoter region: in fact, mutations of this element attenuate the expression of cox-2 in many cases, whereas a destruction of both ATF/CRE and NF-IL6 regulatory elements markedly reduce cox-2 expression (about 75%) in human endothelial cells, although destruction of only the NF-IL6 or the CRE motif caused 40 and 10% reductions, respectively [Inoue H. et al., 1995].

Two NF-IL6 motifs are present in the cox-2 promoter region of most animal species and the expression of cox-2 requires the presence of at least one NF-IL6 motif [Wadleigh D.J. et al., 2000]. In fact, mutation of either NF-IL6 motifs causes only a moderate reduction of cox-2 induction, but mutations of both of them greatly reduce the induction.

NF-κB comprises a family of inducible transcription factors that serve as important regulators of immune and inflammatory responses. Sequencing of the cox-2 promoter region has revealed the presence of two NF-κB consensus sites. Studies on cox-2 expression have implicated NF-κB in signalling [Tanabe T. and Tohnai N., 2002].

E-box element of cox-2 is the binding site for the transcriptional regulatory protein USF-1 in rat granulosa cells [Morris J.K. and Richards J.S., 1996]; the rat E-box element does not show the ATF/CRE activity found in the human and mouse cox-2 promoter, where the E-box and ATF/CRE are overlapping. In rat, as consequence of LH or GnRH induction, the E-box site interacts with other *cis*-acting elements located proximal to the NF-IL6 motifs and *trans*-activates the induction. On the other hand E-box is not involved in the regulation of cox-2 expression in mouse fibroblasts and human epithelial cells [Xie W. and Herschman H.R., 1996; Reddy S.T. et al., 2000], but regulates expression of cox-2 in LPS-treated mouse macrophages [Mestre J.R., Rivadeneira D.E. et al., 2001].

Both the CRE and E-box can individually mediate cox-2 transcription in response to LPS through the binding of c-jun and CREB to the CRE and of USF-1 to the E-box. However, the CRE synergizes with other promoter elements (i.e. NF-κB and NF-IL6) [Mestre J.R., Mackrell P.J. et al., 2001] to induce cox-2 transcription to a greater extent than the E-box, indicating that the complex binding to the CRE is transcriptionally more active.

On the other hand, transcriptional activation through individual CRE or E-box elements is greater than through the overlapping CRE/E-box, suggesting that CRE and E-box binding transcription factors may interfere with the binding of one another to the cox-2 promoter thereby decreasing transcription [Rourke I.J. et al., 1999].

COX Isozymes: Protein Structure

The primary structures of COX-1 and COX-2 shows that nascent proteins are processed into mature enzyme forms containing 576 amino acids and 587 aminoacids, respectively, by removal of signal peptides.

By convention, the residues of COX are often numbered to correspond to the ovine or murine COX-1 sequence [Smith W.L. and DeWitt D.L., 1996] in order to aid convenience of structural and functional comparison across species. The numbering of amino acids begins at the N-terminal methionine of the signal sequence which is removed in the mature protein [Smith W.L. and DeWitt D.L., 1996].

The sequence homology between COX-1 and -2 is high: the two isozymes from the same species display 60-65% sequence identity [Smith W.L. and DeWitt D.L., 1996; Xie W. et al., 1991; Kujubu D.A. et al., 1991; DeWitt D.L. et al., 1990], while sequence identity among different species varies from 85-90% [Smith W.L. and DeWitt D.L., 1996]; in particular, amino acid residues required for the activity of COX-1 are conserved in COX-2.

However, despite a high level of sequence homology between COX isoforms, major differences in primary structure occur in four distint areas of the sequence.

First, both isoforms have distinctly different signal peptides in terms of length and amino acid composition, in particular, COX-2 lacks the large hydrophobic signal peptide of COX-1, containing instead a short, cleaved signal sequence [DeWitt D.L. et al., 1990; Yokoyama C. and Tanabe T., 1989; Simmons D.L. et al., 1991; Sirois J. and Richards J.S., 1992].

Second, substantial sequence differences are found in the membrane binding domains between the two isoforms, although no explanation for this phenomenon is known [Otto J. and Smith W., 1996; Spencer A.G. et al., 1999].

Third, there is an 18-aminoacid cassette located near the carboxyl terminus of COX-2 that is absent from COX-1. This COOH-terminal region of COX-2 contains two additional consensus sequences for N-glycosylation which, in the case of murine COX-2 are located at Asn^{580} and Asn^{592} [Xie W. et al., 1991; Hla T. and Neilson K., 1992]. The function of this insert in COX-2 is not known, but mutations and sequence alterations at C terminus can markedly affect the expression of active protein [Guo Q. and Kulmacz R.J., 2000; Song I. and Smith W.L., 1996]. It may be possible that this insertion is a "signal domain" for controlling protein turnover or subcellular trafficking.

Fourth, COX-1 appears to be uniformly glycosylated at three sites (Asn68, Asn144, and Asn410) and appears as a single band on SDS-PAGE with a molecular weight of about 67 KDa. Native COX-2, on the other hand, is more heterogeneously glycosylated at an additional site (Asn588), and multiple molecular species of COX-2 can be readily observed with SDS-PAGE with a molecular weight of 68-72 KDa.

Due to the high degree of sequence homology between COX-1 and COX-2, it was not surprising that the tertiary and quaternary structures of the COX isozymes are virtually identical [Kurumbail R.G. et al., 1996; Luong C. et al., 1996].

Three crystal structures of COX have been published: ovine COX-1 [Picot D. et al., 1994; Garavito R.M. et al., 1994], recombinant human COX-2 [Luong C. et al., 1996] and recombinant mouse COX-2 [Kurumbail R.G. et al., 1996]. All the crystal structures reveal that COXs are dimers of identical subunits, so there are two cyclooxygenase and two peroxidase sites for each complex: after detergent solubilization, COX-1 and COX-2 appear as homodimers in solution and as 67-72 kDa monomers on SDS-PAGE, depending on isoform and heterogenicity of glycosylation. N-glycosylation may play a role in the maturation of COXs [Otto J. et al., 1993], in particular it seems to be required for enzyme folding and it is required for enzyme activity.

The COX monomer reveals a unique structure comprised of three structural domains, (Figure 4): an N-terminal epidermal growth factor (EGF)-like module, a membrane-binding domain (MBD) and a C-terminal globular catalytic domain.

The *EGF domain*, a domain of about 48 amino acids in length, create a substantial portion of the dimer interface and occurs at a position N-terminal in the primary sequence, such that it always occur on the extracytoplasmic face of the membrane. The functional significance of EGF domain is unclear: however, it was supposed play a role in the insertion of COX into lipid bilayer [Campbell I.D. and Bork P., 1993].

The *MBD* consists of a spiral of four short, consecutive, amphipathic helices; three of them lie in roughly the same plane while last helix merges upwards into catalytic domain. From the helices hydrophobic and aromatic residues protrude in order to create an hydrophobic surface that would interact with only one leaflet of the lipid bilayer and therefore represents an example of monotopic integral membrane protein [Picot D. et al., 1994].

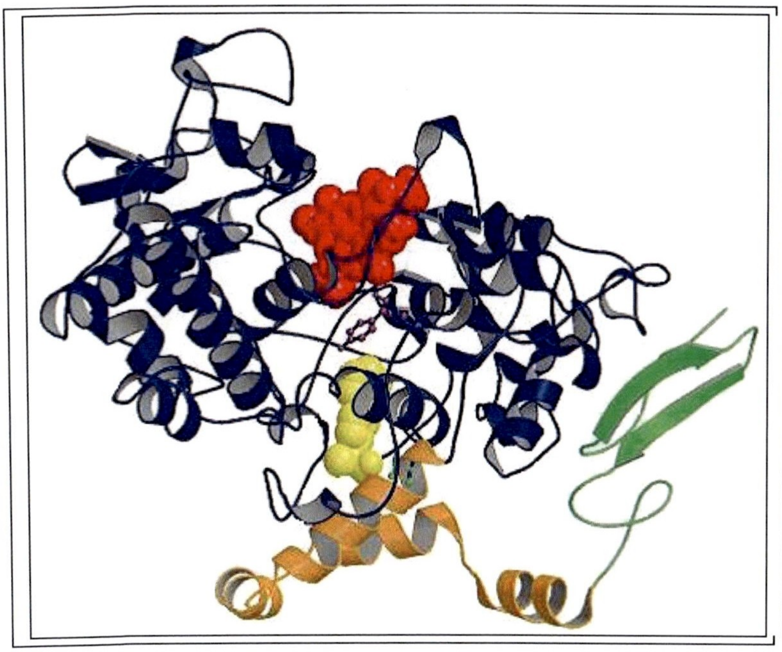

Figure 4. COX monomer structure. A schematic representation of ovine COX-1 monomer (modified from Garavito R.M. et al., 1994). In red is represented the peroxidase site; in green EGF domain; in yellow COX active site and in orange the membrane binding domain.

The *catalytic domain*, that contains the cyclooxygenase and peroxidase active sites and the heme binding site, comprises the bulk of the COX monomer and is almost entirely composed of α-helical secondary structure. The tertiary structure of the catalytic domain bears striking homology with myeloperoxidase and other mammalian peroxidases [Picot D. et al., 1994; Garavito R.M. et al., 1994; Zeng J. and Fenna R.E., 1992]. This suggest that the COX enzymes arose from an ancestral soluble peroxidase which had acquired a membrane binding capability [Picot D. et al., 1994; Garavito R.M. et al., 1994].

The COXs bind 1 mole of ferric-protoporphyrin IX per mole monomer for full activity, as expected for a heme-dependent peroxidase. However, native ovine COX-1 often loses much of the bound heme during detergent solubilization and purification. For recombinant COX-2, detergent solubilization and subsequent purification tends to yield apo-enzyme, suggesting that its affinity for heme is lower than that exhibited by COX-1. Although the heme can be readily removed, active COX-1 and -2 can be easily reconstituted by the addition of hematin to the sample. This behavior makes the COXs rather unusual among the known heme-dependent peroxidases.

The Role of COXs

Recently, there has been considerable interest in the question of which roles the two COX isoforms might play. The results of different studies suggest that there are process in which each isozyme is uniquely involved and others in which both isozymes function co-ordinately. For example COX-1 is the only isoform responsible in platelet aggregation, whereas COX-2 in ovulation. In process such as inflammation, gastric ulceration, carcinogenesis both isoforms are involved.

An interesting model suggests that COX-1 synthesizes prostaglandins that serve noble purposes in housekeeping, such as protecting the stomach from ulcers [Robert A., 1983] and regulating renal blood flow [Whelton A., 1999]. COX-2, on the other hand, is the rogue that synthesizes the excessive amounts of prostaglandins associated with pain and fever [DeWitt D. and Smith W.L., 1995]. In general, COX-1 is constitutively expressed to fulfill its beneficial housekeeping roles. COX-2 is not constitutively expressed in appreciable amounts by most normal tissues, but it is rapidly induced by certain inflammatory cytokines, tumour promoters, growth factors and oncogenes.

Amongst all the actions mediated by COXs, the one currently most investigated is the involvement in tumorigenesis, since several reports indicate that NSAIDs (non steroidal anti-inflammatory drugs), which are COXs inhibitors, can prevent the development of various human tumors including colon [Suh O. et al., 1993; Thun M.J. et al., 1993; Muscat J.E. et al., 1994], breast [Harris R.E. et al., 1996; Harris R.E. et al., 1999], lung [Schreinemachers D.M. and Everson R.B., 1994] and gastric [Thun M.J., 1996; Farrow D.C. et al., 1998] neoplasias. Indeed, to date, most studies have implicated COX-2, rather than COX-1, in multiple events throughout the tumorigenic process [Smith W.L. and Langenbach R., 2001]. For example, in colon carcinogenesis three separate sources of evidence, epidemiology, animal pharmacology, and *in vitro* pharmacology, indicate that COX-2 is a rate-limiting step. Regard to the question of where does COX-2 fit in tumorigenesis and how does it exert its effects, many studies have been done. Some of them suggest that an initiating event, such as the mutation of a "gate-keeper" gene [Kinzler K.W. and Vogelstein B.W., 1996; Prescott S.M. and White R.L., 1996] can result in the induction of COX-2. This appears to occur mainly through increased transcription of the COX-2 gene [Kutchera W. et al., 1996], but it may also occur via translational regulation. This latter possibility is attractive because COX-2 has multiple elements in the 3'-UTR [Jones D.A. et al., 1993] that are known to regulate the stability of messenger RNA and, perhaps, the efficiency of translation [Ristimaki A. et al., 1994].

Once COX-2 is induced and catalyzes the oxidation of arachidonic acid, it produces prostaglandins and highly reactive products that may accelerate the carcinogenesis process. However, the precise mechanism by which COX-2 expression and catalysis results in tumour formation is not understood. A possibility is that COX-2 catalysis removes a protective agent and generates one or more oncogenic agents. This theory has experimental support. Several groups have shown that high concentrations of free arachidonic acid can promote apoptosis, regardless of prostaglandin formation [Surette M.E. et al., 1996; Surette M.E. et al., 1999; Chan T.A. et al., 1998, Longo W.E. et al., 1999]. It is possible that the increased levels of COX-2 serve to lower the intracellular level of free arachidonic acid and thereby prevent apoptosis. In other words, COX-2 catalysis is simply a process that depletes an apoptotic signal. The second possibility is that products formed by the enzymatic action of COX-2, presumably one of the prostaglandins, alter cell growth, apoptosis, angiogenesis or other steps that lead to cancer. A variety of studies have investigated this possibility and it is well established that prostaglandins modulate most cellular process that govern cell growth and differentiation, by working through cell surface receptors or through nuclear receptors. For instance, induction of COX-2 in intestinal epithelial cells increased their adhesion and simultaneously decreased their response to certain apoptotic stimuli [Tsujii M. and DuBois R.N., 1995]. The same group reported that COX-2 and COX-1 cooperate to induce angiogenesis [Tsujii M. et al., 1998] and that PGE_2 inhibits programmed cell death by inducing expression of the Bcl-2 protooncogene [Sheng H. et al., 1998]. Excessive local synthesis of prostaglandins has also been shown to disrupt immune surveillance that may otherwise suppress tumour growth [Stolina M. et al., 2000; Huang M. et al., 1996]. In addition, the direct product of COX-2, PGH_2, can isomerize by both enzymatic and non-enzymatic reactions to form the potent mutagen malondialdehyde, which can induce frame shifts and base pair substitutions [Marnett L.J., 1992]. Moreover, PGE_2 and other prostaglandins often elevate intracellular cyclic AMP concentrations, which can suppress apoptosis [Orlov S.N. et al., 1999].

In addition to the possibility that just prostaglandins mediate the downstream effects of increased COX-2, it may be that there are other products with deleterious effects. COX-2 is an oxygenase and the intermediates are highly reactive. It is possible that these intermediates or other products derivative macromolecules, such as DNA, and facilitate tumour formation. In addition, the second step catalyzed by COX-2 is a reduction for which a cofactor is required and many compounds can be co-oxidized to serve as this cofactor [Smith B. et al., 1991; Marnett L.J., 1990]. For example, this reaction can oxidize estrogen [Degen G.H., 1990] to a carcinogenic by-product.

On the ground of these considerations, we can understand the mechanism through which COX inhibitors exert their preventive and therapeutic action in any forms of cancer. Inhibition of COX-2 by NSAIDs selective for this isoenzyme suppressed the growth of the tumours that had high levels of COX-2 but had no effect on tumours that lacked COX-2 in experiments involving transplantation of human colon cancer cell lines into mice [Sheng H. et al., 1997].

COX-2 potential role in cancer has been evidenced in many tumours: colon [Sheng H. et al., 1997; Fujita T. et al., 1998], breast [Subbaramaiah K. et al., 1996; Egan K.M. et al., 1996], head and neck [Chan G. et al., 1999], lung [Wolff H. et al., 1998; Hida T. et al., 1998], pancreatic [Tucker O.N. et al., 1999], and gastric cancers [Ristimaki A. et al., 1997] and several reports suggest that beneficial effects of NSAIDs extend to these cancer types [Harris R.E. et al., 1996; Farrow D.C. et al., 1998].

Since COX-2 is involved both in inflammation and in cancer induction, it may represent a link between these two processes. For several types of tumours has been evidenced that chronic inflammatory disorders increase the risk of developing cancer: for example, patients with persistent ulcerative colitis have an incidence of colon cancer 5-7-fold higher than expected [Ekbom A. et al., 1990] and colitis persisting for 35-40 years carries an absolute risk of colon cancer ranging from 20 to 35% [Ekbom A. et al., 1990; Lashner B.A., 1994]. Studies on cancer incidence in asthmatic patients are also informative. A study on 78000 patients with asthma reported a significant increase of lung cancer risk in both men and women, consistent with a contribution from local, chronic inflammation [Vesterinen E. et al., 1993]. Another example is represented from chronic pancreatitis that has been demonstrated a risk factor for pancreatic cancer [Bansal P. and Sonnenberg A., 1995; Cylwik B. et al., 1998].

Mesothelioma and COX-2

As we said previously for other types of tumours, one of the risk factor for malignant pleuric mesothelioma (MPM) is chronic inflammation that, in this case, is induced by deposition of insoluble amphibole fibers [Mossman B.T. and Churg A., 1998; Kamp D.W. and Weitzman S.A., 1999]. Asbestos causes chronic inflammation that maintains a high level of COX-2 and consequently it causes the release of PGE_2 from alveolar macrophages and inhibition of mesothelial cell-mediated cytotoxicity [Bissonnette E. et al., 1990; Leikauf G.D. et al., 1995; Prescott S.M. and Fitzpatrick F.A., 2000]. Recent studies highlight a COX-2 overexpression in MPM samples collected during palliative surgery or at diagnostic surgical biopsy and consider this expression a novel prognostic factor in mesothelioma [Edwards J.G. et al., 2002; Baldi A. et al., 2004]. In these studies COX-2 expression was evaluated by immunohistochemistry, western blotting and PGE_2 detection. With western blot technique, COX-2 M_r 72,000 and/or M_r 74,000 was detected, indicating different glycosylation states. In the study of O'Kane et al. [O'Kane S.L. et al., 2005] COX-2 overexpression was identified by immunohistochemistry in 73% of epithelial tumors but in only 37% of sarcomatoid tumours. Marrogi and collegues [Marrogi A. et al., 2000], using the same technique, reported a strong COX-2 expression in 30/30 flash-frozen, paraffin embedded cases (23 epithelial, 4 biphasic and 3 sarcomatoid). Baldi et al. [Baldi A. et al., 2004] reported high COX-2 expression in 66% of sections obtained from 29 formalin-fixed, paraffin-embedded mesothelioma samples consisting of 16 epithelial, 7 biphasic and 6 sarcomatoid tumours. In addition, in the study of Edwards et al. [Edwards J.G. et al., 2002], COX-2 level correlates with a worse prognosis in univariate and multivariate analyses.

A number of growth factors, which play important roles in the pathogenesis of MPM, have been shown to induce COX-2 expression. These include hepatocyte growth factor/scatter factor [Harvey P. et al., 2000; Shimada T et al., 2000], transforming growth factor β [Marzo A.L. et al., 1997; Sheng H. et al., 2000], platelet-derived growth factor [Langerak A.W. et al., 1996], and epidermal growth factor receptor. An over-expression of COX-2 has been shown also in some mesothelioma cell lines and cyclooxygenase activity has been correlated with increased proliferative and invasive potential [Marrogi A. et al., 1996; Catalano A. et al., 2004].

Possible Role of Cox Inhibitors in Malignant Mesothelioma Therapy

Until now, there isn't an effective treatment for malignant mesothelioma and for this reason a lot of studies are addressed toward the search of new therapeutic solutions for this tumour. COX-2 over-expression in tumours, in particular in mesothelioma, has provided the rationale for the development of a new class of drugs, the selective COX-2 inhibitors (coxibs).

The classical non selective nonsteroidal antiinflammatory drugs (NSAIDs) bind to COX-1 and COX-2, interacting with the hydrophobic channel of the COX isoenzymes, and inhibiting prostaglandin synthesis. NSAIDs block COX-1 about halfway down the channel:

this block occurs by hydrogen binding to the polar arginine at position 120 [Picot D. et al., 1994]. Arginine 120 is also present in COX-2. Aspirin, unlike other NSAIDs, irreversibly acetylates a serine residue in both COX-1 and COX-2 to prevent binding of arachidonic acid. Other non selective NSAIDs compete directly for arachidonic acid, inhibiting cyclooxygenase activity in a rapid but reversible manner [Smith W.L. et al., 2000]. Although nonselective NSAIDs bind both COX-1 and COX-2, each isoform is inhibited to different degrees. Coxibs, the COX-2 selective inhibitors, preferentially bind to and inhibit COX-2. Coxibs are selective agents because they bind COX-1 poorly and in a rapidly reversible manner, whereas they bind COX-2 more tightly. This binding occurs in two stages and, in particular, it is tight in the second stage, with dissociation occurring only slowly. Preferential inhibition of COX-2 is thought to be due to the additional space in the COX-2 hydrophobic channel, as well as to the presence of a side pocket in the channel. This side pocket can discriminate the coxibs from nonselective agents based on the different overall structures of these agents, in particular, by the presence in coxibs of specific side chains [Hawkey C.J., 1999]. In particular, the difference of a single aminoacid positioned near Arginine 120 in COXs is the responsible for selectivity of many drugs. In fact, at position 523 of COX-1 there is an isoleucine residue, while in COX-2 there is a valine, smaller by a single methyl group. The smaller valine in COX-2 leaves a gap in the wall of the channel, giving access to a side-pocket, which is thought to be the site of binding of many selective drugs. The bulkier isoleucine at 523 in COX-1 is large enough to block access to the side-pocket. In confirmation of this, targeted single aminoacid substitution of COX-1 isoleucine with valine is sufficient to turn COX-1 into an enzyme that can be inhibited by COX-2 selective agents [Luong C. et al., 1996; Gierse J. et al., 1996] (Figure 5).

Another difference between COXs isozymes is in their inhibition kinetics. COX-1 inhibition is instantaneous and competitively reversible, as would be expected from a process based on hydrogen bond, instead COX-2 inhibition is time-dependent, with selectivity developing over 15–30 minutes and is thereafter essentially irreversible.

Selective COX-2 inhibitors are as effective as nonselective nonsteroidal antiinflammatory drugs in relieving pain and inflammation but are associated with significantly fewer gastric, duodenal, and intestinal ulcers and ulcer complications. This has been the reason for developing new anti-inflammatory agents specific for COX-2. Really, only a few drugs have a COX-1/COX-2 ratio suggesting that limited inhibition of COX-1 would occur. For example, three drugs that have been used in the past, meloxicam, nimesulide and diclofenac, have a COX-1/COX-2 ratio in the range of 10 to 30 and, while preferentially inhibiting COX-2, have considerable COX-1 inhibitory activity. Two drugs approved by the US Food and Drug Administration, rofecoxib and celecoxib, have been shown to have the greatest selectivity for COX-2. In fact these coxibs have COX-1/COX-2 ratios that are 10- to 100-fold greater than existing nonselective NSAIDs [Hawkey C.J., 1999; Patrono C. et al., 2001; Chan C.C. et al., 1999].

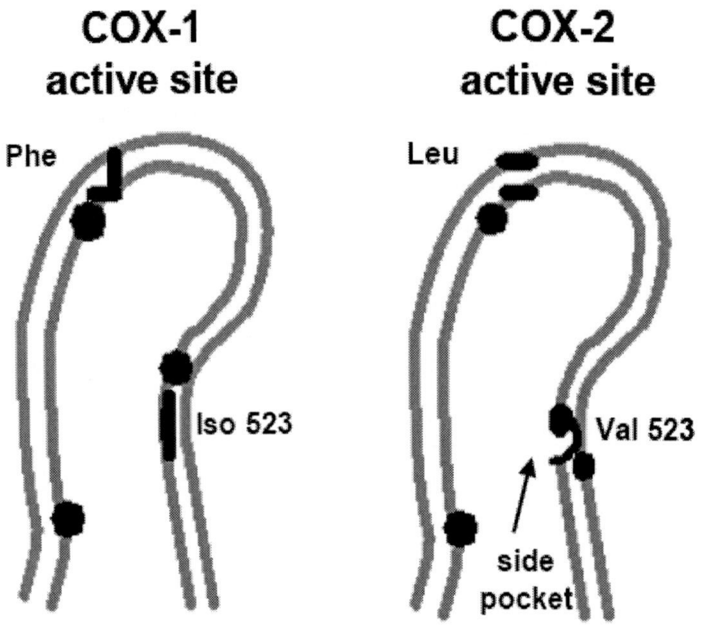

Figure 5. COX-1 and COX-2 are different. Differences between COX-1 and COX-2 active site: at position 523 there is an isoleucine molecule in COX-1 and a valine in COX-2. The smaller valine molecule in COX-2 leaves a gap in the wall of the channel, giving access to a side pocket, which is thought to be the binding site of many selective drugs. The bulkier isoleucine at 523 in COX-1 is large enough to block access to the side pocket.

Both rofecoxib and celecoxib have been examined in clinical trials large enough to have sufficient statistical power for detection of clinical specificity. The results fulfilled expectations that COX-2 specific inhibitors could achieve efficacy equal to nonselective NSAIDs with less side effects.

As previously said, in addition to the well-established pathophysiological role that COX-2 plays in inflammation, it has been established that this isoform may also be involved in tumorigenic process. Pharmacological studies consistently demonstrate that COX-2 inhibitors dose-dependently inhibit tumor growth and metastasis in various relevant animal model of cancer. Several investigators have also shown that COX-2 inhibitors may act additively or synergistically with currently used anticancer drugs.

The anti-tumoral effects of coxibs have been studied on *in vitro* and *in vivo* experimental MPM models. Marrogi and collaborators [Marrogi A. et al., 2000] studied the effects of NS398, a COX-2 specific inhibitor, on MPM cell lines established and derived from previously untreated patients. NS398 treatment produced a significant reduction of proliferation levels and FACS analysis showed a clear reduction in the S-phase fraction and a large increase of cells in the G_2-M phase of the cell cycle, suggesting that NS398 antiproliferative effects is not mediated by increases of apoptosis. These data suggest that inhibition of COX-2 does not account for all the antiproliferative activity of NS398 into mesothelioma cell lines.

In 2004 Catalano and collaborators [Catalano A. et al., 2004] characterized the effects of nonsteroidal anti-inflammatory agents on *in vitro* and *in vivo* experimental mesothelioma models. Celecoxib and NS398, selective COX-2 inhibitors, and indometacin inhibited cell proliferation of three mesothelioma cell lines obtained from previously untreated patients, but no effect was observed with normal primary mesothelial cells that resulted resistant to the growth inhibitory effect of each treatment. Celecoxib was more efficient in inhibiting mesothelioma cell growth than acetylsalicylic acid, indometacin and NS398; indometacin was the least efficient, and NS398 had an intermediate effect. This variability may be not associated with COX-2 protein levels, suggesting that the higher antineoplastic effect of celecoxib in respect to the other NSAIDs is not only due to prostaglandin synthesis inhibition but also to other non-COX targets. Catalano et al. also demonstrated that celecoxib induced MPM cell apoptosis, in a dose- and time-dependent manner, through a decreased Akt phosphorilation, loss of Bcl-2 and survivin protein expression and caspase-3 activation.

Moreover Catalano and collaborators investigated the growth-inhibitory effects of NSAIDs also in soft agar. All NSAIDs were be able to inhibit colony formation in a dose-dependent manner but with differential inhibitory effects. In fact, the cells used in this work were less sensitive to the inhibitory effect of indometacin, showed an intermediate sensitivity to NS398, and were more inhibited by celecoxib treatment. These results indicate that celecoxib is the most effective NSAID to some MPM cells, followed by NS398 and indometacin.

The authors studied the inhibitory effect of celecoxib also *in vivo*, in an orthotopic mouse model of MPM. Also in this experiment the inhibitory effect of celecoxib was evidenced: in fact, the drug led to a significant increase in median survival of treated mice and did not cause any evident toxic side effects.

Another important result with regard to MPM inhibitory effects of celecoxib has been obtained with combination of celecoxib with a vascular endothelial growth factor (VEGF) receptor inhibitor (SU-1498). VEGF is an important autocrine growth factor for MM cells and its autocrine/paracrine loop protects MM cells from celecoxib-induced apoptotic effects. Consequently, the use of SU-1498 in combination with celecoxib can enhance the sensitivity to celecoxib of MM cells *in vitro*. Catalano et al. demonstrated a supra-additive effect using celecoxib in combination with SU-1498, indicating that the chemosensitivity to celecoxib could be synergistically enhanced in MM cells by the co-treatment of anti-VEGF agents, such as SU-1498.

Another interesting study was carried out by DeLong and collaborators [DeLong P. et al., 2003]. They started from some considerations:

[1] Different studies suggest that mesothelioma may be susceptible to immunotherapy [Odaka M. et al., 2001; Bielefeldt-Ohmann H. et al., 1994; Bielefeldt-Ohmann H. et al., 1995].

[2] Success was reported in treating small mesothelioma tumors in mice with liposomes containing immunogenic cDNA [Lanuti M. et al., 2000] and even more impressive response with Ad IFN-β, an adenovirus expressing murine IFN-β [Odaka M. et al., 2001; Odaka M. et al., 2002].

[3] One of the effects of COX-2 inhibition is the reduction of immunosuppressive environment within the tumour.

On the basis of these consideration, the authors investigated the effect of COX-2 inhibition combined with Ad IFN-β in mice bearing small and large tumours. As COX-2 inhibitor they used rofecoxib. Rofecoxib alone was shown to reduce tumoral growth in mice inoculated with mesothelioma cells into the flanks. This anti-tumour effect seems to be attributable to immunological effects because inhibition is completely lost in immunodeficient mice. Unfortunately, the inhibitory effect of rofecoxib was observed only in small tumors and not when mice carried on moderate or large tumours. This suggests that COX-2 inhibition in patients with MPM would only be effective in those patients with minimal disease or as adjuvant therapy after surgical debulking. Therapeutic combination of rofecoxib with Ad IFN-β resulted in recovery of small tumours, significant inhibition of the growth of large established tumours, and inhibition of the growth of metastatic tumour foci after surgical debulking. The additive effect of a COX-2 inhibitor and Ad IFN-β demonstrated in this work could represent the rational to combine COX-2 inhibition with immuno- and immunogene therapy approaches in human clinical trials of treatment of malignant mesothelioma.

Finally, our research group recently evaluated both the *in vitro* and *in vivo* effects of piroxicam, a widely used non-steroidal anti-inflammatory drug (NSAID), alone and in combination with cisplatin (CDDP), on cell growth of mesothelioma cells [Spugnini E.P. et al., 2006]. Interestingly, we found a marked tumour growth inhibition and an extended survival of mice treated with a combination of piroxicam and CDDP in peritoneal mesotheliomas induced by MSTO-211H cells. Moreover, geneChip® array analysis of MSTO-211H mesothelioma cell line revealed that piroxicam treatment caused up-regulation of metabolic pathway associated genes and down-regulation of genes related to RNA processing apparatus. Of note, among the down-regulated genes there was that for Epidermal Growth Factor Receptor (EGFR), one of the new biological targets of chemotherapy for mesothelioma. Among the up-regulated genes there was HtrA1, a serine-protease recently shown to be an endogenous mediator of cisplatin cytotoxicity. These data suggest that piroxicam sensitizes mesothelioma cells to cisplatin-induced cytotoxicity by modulating the expression of several target genes. Therefore, piroxicam in combination with CDDP might potentially be useful in the treatment of patients with mesothelioma.

References

Appleby S.B., Ristimaki A., Neilson K., Narko K. and Hla T. (1994). Structure of the human yclo-oxygenase-2 gene. *Biochem. J.* 302: 723-727.

Baldi A., Santini D., Vasaturo F., Santini M., Vicidomini G., Di Marino M.P., Esposito V., Groeger A.M., Liuzzi G., Vincenti B., Tonini G., Piccoli M., Baldi F. and Scarpa S. (2004). Prognostic significance of cyclooxygenase-2 (COX-2) and expression of cell cycle inhibitors p21 and p27 in human pleural malignant mesothelioma. *Thorax* 59: 428-433.

Bansal P. and Sonnenberg A. (1995). Pancreatitis is a risk factor for pancreatic cancer, *Gastroenterology* 109: 247-251.

Bielefeldt-Ohmann H., Fitzpatrick D.R., Marzo A.L., Jarnicki A.G., Himbeck R., Davis M., Manning L.S. and Robinson B.W. (1994). Patho- and immunobiology of malignant mesothelioma: characterisation of tumour infiltrating leucocytes and cytokine production in a murine model. *Cancer Immunol. Immunother.* 39: 347-359.

Bielefeldt-Ohmann H., Fitzpatrick D.R., Marzo A.L., Jarnicki A.G., Musk A.W. and Robinson B.W. (1995). Potential for interferon-α-based therapy in mesothelioma: assessment in a murine model. *J. Interferon Cytokine Res.* 15: 213-223.

Bissonnette E., Carre B., Dubois C. and Rola-Pleszczynski M. (1990). Inhibition of alveolar macrophage cytotoxicity by asbestos: possible role of prostaglandins. *Leukoc. Biol.* 47: 129-134.

Boerboom D. and Sirois J. (1998). Molecular characterization of equine prostaglandin G/H synthase-2 and regulation of its messenger ribonucleic acid in preovulatory follicles. *Endocrinology* 139: 1662–1670.

Bozza P.T., Yu W., Penrose J.F., Morgan E.S., Dvorak A.M. and Weller P.F. (1997). Eosinophil lipid bodies: specific, inducible intracellular sites for enhanced eicosanoid formation. *J. Exp. Med.* 186: 909-920.

Campbell I.D. and Bork P. (1993). Epidermal growth factor-like modules. *Curr. Opin. Struct. Biol.* 3: 385-92.

Cardillo I., Spugnini E.P., Verdina A., Galati R., Citro G. and Baldi A. (2005). Cox and mesothelioma: an overview. *Histol. Histopathol.* 20: 1267-1274.

Catalano A., Graciotti L., Rinaldi L., Raffaelli G., Rodilossi S., Betta P., Gianni W., Amoroso S. and Procopio A. (2004). Preclinical evaluation of the nonsteroidal anti-inflammatory agent celecoxib on malignant mesothelioma chemoprevention. *Int. J. Cancer.* 109: 322-328.

Chan C.C., Boyce S., Brideau C., Charleson S., Cromlish W., Ethier D., Evans J., Ford-Hutchinson A.W., Forrest M.J., Gauthier J.Y., Gordon R., Gresser M., Guay J., Kargman S., et al. (1999). Rofecoxib [Vioxx, MK-0966; 4-(4'-methylsulfonylphenyl)-3-phenyl-2-(5H)-furanone]: a potent and orally active cyclooxygenase-2 inhibitor. Pharmacological and biochemical profiles. *J. Pharmacol. Exp. Ther.* 290: 551-560.

Chan G., Boyle J.O., Yang E.K., Zhang F., Sacks P.G., Shah J.P., Edelstein D., Soslow R.A., Koki A.T., Woerner B.M., Masferrer J.L. and Dannenberg A.J. (1999). Cyclooxygenase-2 expression is up-regulated in squamous cell carcinoma of the head and neck. *Cancer Res.* 59: 991-994.

Chan T.A., Morin P.J., Vogelstein B. and Kinzler K.W. (1998). Mechanisms underlying nonsteroidal antiin£ammatory drug-mediated apoptosis. *Proc. Natl. Acad. Sci. USA* 95: 681-686.

Coffey R.J., Hawkey C.J., Damstrup L., Graves-Deal R., Daniel V.C., Dempsey P.J., Chinery R., Kirkland S.C., DuBois R.N., Jetton T.L. and Morrow J.D. (1997). Epidermal growth factor receptor activation induces nuclear targeting of cyclooxygenase-2, basolateral release of prostaglandins, and mitogenesis in polarizing colon cancer cells. *Proc. Natl. Acad. Sci. USA* 94: 657-662.

Cylwik B., Nowak H.F., Puchalski Z. and Barczyk J. (1998). Epithelial anomalies in chronic pancreatitis as a risk factor of pancreatic cancer. *Hepatogastroenterology* 45: 528-532.

Degen G.H. (1990). Role of prostaglandin-H synthase in mediating genotoxic and carcinogenic e¡ects of estrogens. *Environ. Health Perspect.* 88: 217-223.

DeLong P., Tanaka T., Kruklitis R., Henry A.C., Kapoor V., Kaiser L.R., Sterman D.H. and Albelda S.M. (2003). Use of cyclooxygenase-2 inhibition to enhance the efficacy of immunotherapy. *Cancer Res.* 63: 7845-7852.

DeWitt D. and Smith W.L. (1995). Yes, but do they still get headaches? *Cell* 83: 345-348.

DeWitt D.L., El-Harith E.A., Kraemer S.A., Andrews M.J., Yao E.F, Armstrong R.L. and Smith W.L. (1990). The aspirin and heme-binding sites of ovine and murine prostaglandin endoperoxide synthases. *J. Biol. Chem.* 265: 5192-5198.

Edwards J.G., Faux S.P., Plummer S.M., Abrams K.R., Walker R.A., Waller D.A. and O'Byrne K.J. (2002). Cyclooxygenase-2 Expression is a novel Prognostic Factor in Malignant Mesothelioma. *Clin. Cancer Res.* 8: 1857-1862.

Egan K.M., Stampfer M.J., Giovannucci E., Rosner B.A. and Colditz G.A. (1996). Prospective study of regular aspirin use and the risk of breast cancer. *J. Natl. Cancer Inst.* 88: 988-993.

Ekbom A., Helmnick C., Zack M. and Adami H.O. (1990). Ulcerative colitis and colorectal cancer. A population based study, *New Engl. J. Med.* 323: 1228-1233.

Farrow D.C., Vaughan T.L., Hansten P.D., Stanford J.L., Risch H.A., Gammon M.D., Chow W.H., Dubrow R., Ahsan H., Mayne S.T., Schoenberg J.B., West A.B., Rotterdam H., Fraumeni J.F. Jr and Blot W.J. (1998). Use of aspirin and other nonsteroidal anti-inflammatory drugs and risk of esophageal and gastric cancer. *Cancer Epidemiol. Biomarkers Prev.* 7: 97-102.

Fujita T., Matsui M., Takaku K., Uetake H., Ichikawa W., Taketo M.M. and Sugihara K. (1998). Size- and invasion-dependent increase in cyclooxygenase 2 levels in human colorectal carcinomas. *Cancer Res.* 58: 4823-4826.

Funk C.D., Funk L.B., Kennedy M.E., Pong A.S. and Fitzgerald G.A. (1991). Human platelet/erythroleukemia cell prostaglandin G/Hsynthase: cDNA cloning, expression, and gene chromosomal assignment. *FASEB J.* 5: 2304-2312.

Garavito R.M., Malkowski M.G. and DeWitt D.L. (2002). The structures of prostaglandin endoperoxide H synthases-1 and -2. *Prostaglandins Other Lipid Mediat.* 68: 129–152.

Garavito R.M., Picot D. and Loll P.J. (1994). Prostaglandin H synthase. *Curr. Opin. Struct. Biol.* 4: 529-535.

Gierse J., McDonald J., Hauser S., Rangwala S. and Seibert K. (1996). A single amino acid difference between cyclooxygenase-1 (COX-1) and -2 (COX-2) reverses the selectivity of COX-2 specific inhibitors. *J. Biol. Chem.* 271: 15810-15814.

Guo Q. and Kulmacz R.J. (2000). Distinct influences of carboxyl terminal segment structure on function in the two isoforms of prostaglandin H synthase. *Arch. Biochem. Biophys.* 384: 269-279.

Harris R.E., Kasbari S. and Farrar W.B. (1999). Prospective study of nonsteroidal anti-inflammatory drugs and breast cancer. *Oncol. Rep.* 6: 71-73.

Harris R.E., Namboodiri K.K. and Farrar W.B. (1996). Nonsteroidal antiinflammatory drugs and breast cancer. *Epidemiology* 7: 203-205.

Harvey P., Clark I.M., Jaurand M.C., Warn R.M. and Edwards D.R. (2000). Hepatocyte growth factor/scatter factor enhances the invasion of mesothelioma cell lines and the expression of matrix metalloproteinases. *Br. J. Cancer.* 83: 1147-1153.

Hida T., Yatabe Y., Achiwa H., Muramatsu H., Kozaki K., Nakamura S., Ogawa M, Mitsudomi T., Sugiura T., Takahashi T. (1998). Increased expression of cyclooxygenase 2 occurs frequently in human lung cancers, specifically in adenocarcinomas. *Cancer Res.* 58: 3761-3764.

Hla T. and Neilson K. (1992). Human cyclooxygenase-2 cDNA. *Proc. Natl. Acad. Sci. USA.* 89: 7384-7388.

Hla T., Bishop-Bailey D., Liu C.H., Schaefers H.J. and Trifan O.C. (1999). Cyclooxygenase-1 and -2 isoenzymes. *Int. J. Biochem. Cell Biol.* 31: 551-557.

Hla T., Ristimaki A., Appleby S. and Barriocanal J.G. (1993). Cyclooxygenase gene expression in inflammation and angiogenesis. *Ann. NY Acad. Sci.* 696: 197-204.

Huang M., Sharma S., Mao J.T. and Dubinett S.M. (1996). Non-small cell lung cancer-derived soluble mediators and prostaglandin E2 enhance peripheral blood lymphocyte IL-10 transcription and protein production. *J. Immunol.* 157: 5512-5520.

Inoue H., Yokoyama C., Hara S., Tone Y., Tanabe T. (1995). Transcriptional regulation of human prostaglandin-endoperoxide synthase-2 gene by lipopolysaccharide and phorbol ester in vascular endothelial cells. Involvement of both nuclear factor for interleukin-6 expression site and cAMP response element. *J. Biol. Chem.* 270: 24965-24971.

Jones D.A., Carlton D.P., McIntyre T.M., Zimmerman G.A. and Prescott S.M. (1993). Molecular cloning of human prostaglandin endoperoxide synthase type II and demonstration of expression in response to cytokines. *J. Biol. Chem.* 268: 9049-9054.

Kamp D.W. and Weitzman S.A. (1999). The molecular basis of asbestos induced lung injury. *Thorax* 54: 638-652.

Kinzler K.W. and Vogelstein B.W. (1996). Lessons from hereditary colorectal cancer. *Cell* 87: 159-170.

Klein G., Powers A. and Croce C. (2002). Association of SV40 with human tumors. *Oncogene* 21: 1141-1149.

Kosaka T., Miyata A., Ihara H., Hara S., Sugimoto T., Takeda O., Takahashi E. and Tanabe T. (1994). Characterization of the human gene (PTGS2) encoding prostaglandin-endoperoxide synthase 2. *Eur. J. Biochem.* 221: 889-897.

Kraemer S.A., Meade E.A. and DeWitt D.L. (1992). Prostaglandin endoperoxide synthase gene structure: identification of the transcriptional start site and 5'-flanking regulatory sequences. *Arch. Biochem. Biophys.* 293: 391-400.

Kujubu D.A., Fletcher B.S., Varnum B.C., Lim R.W. and Herschman H.R. (1991). TIS10, a phorbol ester tumor promoter-inducible mRNA from Swiss 3T3 cells, encodes a novel prostaglandin synthase/cyclooxygenase homologue. *J. Biol. Chem.* 266: 12866-12872.

Kulmacz R.J., van der Donk W.A. and Tsai A.L. (2003). Comparison of the properties of prostaglandin H synthase-1 and -2. *Prog. Lipid Res.* 42: 377-404.

Kurumbail R.G., Stevens A.M., Gierse J K., McDonald J.J., Stegeman R.A., Pak J.Y., Gildehaus D., Miyashiro J.M., Penning T.D., Seibert K., Isakson P.C. and Stallings W.C. (1996). Structural basis for selective inhibition of cyclooxygenase-2 by anti-inflammatory agents. *Nature* 384: 644-648.

Kutchera W., Jones D.A., Matsunami N., Groden J., McIntyre T.M., Zimmerman G.A., White R.L. and Prescott S.M. (1996). Prostaglandin H synthase 2 is expressed abnormally in human colon cancer: evidence for a transcriptional effect. *Proc.Natl. Acad. Sci. USA* 93: 4816-4820.

Kyriazis A. and Kyriazis A.P. (1980). Preferential sites of growth of human tumors in nude mice following subcutaneous transplantation. *Cancer Res.* 40: 4509-4511.

Langerak A.W., De Laat P.A., Van Der Linden-Van Beurden C.A., Delahaye M., Van Der Kwast T.H., Hoogsteden H.C., Benner R. and Versnel M.A. (1996). Expression of platelet-derived growth factor (PDGF) and PDGF receptors in human malignant mesothelioma in vitro and in vivo. *J. Pathol.* 178: 151-60.

Lanuti M., Rudginsky S., Force S., Lambright E., Siders W., Chang M., Amin K., Kaiser L., Scheule R. and Albelda S. (2000). Cationic lipid: bacterial DNA complexes elicit adaptive cellular immunity in murine intraperitoneal tumor models. *Cancer Res.* 60: 2955-2963.

Lashner B.A. (1994). Colorectal cancer in ulcerative colitis patients: survival curves and surveillance, Clevel. *Clin. J. Med.* 61: 272-275.

Leikauf G.D., Fink S.P., Miller M.L., Lockey J.E. and Driscoll K.E. (1995). Refractory ceramic fibers activate alveolar macrophage eicosanoid and cytokine release. *J. Appl. Physiol.* 78: 164-171.

Liou J.Y., Deng W.G., Gilroy D.W., Shyue S.K. and Wu K.K. (2001). Colocalization and interaction of cyclooxygenase-2 with caveolin-1 in human fibroblasts. *J. Biol. Chem.* 276: 34975-34982.

Liou J.Y., Shyue S.K., Tsai M.J., Chung C.L., Chu K.Y. and Wu K.K. (2000). Colocalization of prostacyclin synthase with prostaglandin H synthase-1 (PGHS-1). but not phorbol ester-induced PGHS-2 in cultured endothelial cells. *J. Biol. Chem.* 275: 15314-15320.

Longo W.E., Grossmann E.M., Erickson B., Panesar N., Mazuski J.E., Kaminski D.L. (1999). The effect of phospholipase A2 inhibitors on proliferation and apoptosis of murine intestinal cells. *Surg. Res.* 84: 51-56.

Luong C., Miller A., Barnett J., Chow J., Ramesha C. and Browner M.F. (1996). The structure of human cyclooxygenase-2; conservation and flexibility of the NSAID binding site. *Nat. Struct. Biol.* 3: 927-933.

Marnett L.J. (1990). Prostaglandin synthase-mediated metabolism of carcinogens and a potential role for peroxyl radicals as reactive intermediates. *Environ. Health Perspect.* 88: 5-12.

Marnett L.J. (1992). Aspirin and the potential role of prostaglandins in colon cancer. *Cancer Res.* 52: 5575-5589.

Marnett L.J., Goodwin D.C., Rowlinson S.W., Kalgutkar A.S. and Landino L.M. (1999). In *Comprehensive Natural Products Chemistry* (Poulter C., ed.) Vol. 5, pp. 225-261, Elsevier Science Publishers Ltd., Oxford.

Marnett L.J., Rowlinson S.W., Goodwin D.C., Kalgutkar A.S., Lanzo C.A. (1999). Arachidonic acid oxygenation by COX-1 and COX-2. *J. Biol. Chem.* 274:22903-22906.

Marrogi A., Pass H.I., Khan M., Metheny-Barlow L.J., Harris C.C. and Gerwin B.I. (2000). Human mesothelioma samples overexpress both cyclooxygenase-2 (COX-2). and inducible nitric oxide synthase (NOS2): in vitro antiproliferative effects of a COX-2 inhibitor. *Cancer Res.* 60: 3696-3700.

Marzo A.L., Fitzpatrick D.R., Robinson B.W. and Scott B. (1997). Antisense oligonucleotides specific for transforming growth factor beta2 inhibit the growth of malignant mesothelioma both in vitro and in vivo. *Cancer Res.* 57: 3200-3207.

Mestre J.R., Mackrell P.J., Rivadeneira D.E., Stapleton P.P., Tanabe T. and Daly J.M. (2001). Redundancy in the signalling pathways and promoter elements regulating cyclooxygenase-2 gene expression in endotoxin-treated macrophage/monocytic cells. *J. Biol. Chem.* 276: 3977-3982.

Mestre J.R., Rivadeneira D.E., Mackrell P.J., Duff M., Stapleton P.P., Mack-Strong V., Maddali S., Smyth G.P., Tanabe T. and Daly J.M. (2001). Overlapping CRE and E-box promoter elements can independently regulate COX-2 gene transcription in macrophages. *FEBS Lett.* 496: 147-151.

Miyamoto T., Ogino N., Yamamoto S. and Hayaishi O. (1976). Purification of prostaglandin endoperoxide synthetase from bovine vesicular gland microsomes. *J. Biol. Chem.* 251: 2629-2636.

Morris J.K. and Richards J.S. (1996). An E-box region within the prostaglandin endoperoxide synthase-2 (PGS-2) promoter is required for transcription in rat ovarian granulosa cells. *J. Biol. Chem.* 271: 16633-16643.

Mossman B.T. and Churg A. (1998). Mechanisms in the pathogenesis of asbestosis and silicosis. *Am. J. Respir. Crit. Care Med.* 157: 1666-1680.

Muscat J.E., Stellman S.D. and Wynder E.L. (1994). Nonsteroidal antiinflammatory drugs and colorectal cancer. *Cancer* 74: 1847-1854.

Odaka M., Sterman D.H., Wiewrodt R., Zhang Y., Kiefer M., Amin K., Gao G.P., Wilson J. M., Barsoum J., Kaiser L.R. and Albelda S.M. (2001). Eradication of intraperitoneal and distant tumor by adenovirus-mediated interferon-ß gene therapy is attributable to induction of systemic immunity. *Cancer Res.* 61: 6201-6212.

Odaka M., Wiewrodt R., DeLong P., Tanaka T., Zhang Y., Kaiser L. and Albelda S. (2002). Analysis of the immunologic response generated by Ad.IFN-ß during successful intraperitoneal tumor gene therapy. *Mol. Ther.* 6: 210-218.

O'Kane S.L., Cawkwell L., Campbell A. and Lind M.J. (2005). Cyclooxygenase-2 expression predicts survival in malignant pleural mesothelioma. *Eur. J. Cancer.* 41: 1645-1648.

Orlov S.N., Thorin-Trescases N., Dulin N.O., Dam T.V., Fortuno M.A., Tremblay J. and Hamet P. (1999). Activation of cAMP signaling transiently inhibits apoptosis in vascular smooth muscle cells in a site upstream of caspase-3. *Cell Death Differ.* 6: 661-672.

Otto J. and Smith W. (1996). Photolabeling of prostaglandin endoperoxide H synthase-1 with 3-trifluoro-3-(m-[125I]iodophenyl) diazirine as a probe of membrane association and the cyclooxygenase active site. *J. Biol. Chem.* 271: 9906-9910.

Otto J., DeWitt D. and Smith W. (1993). Nglycosylation of prostaglandin endoperoxide synthases-1 and -2 and their orientations in the endoplasmic reticulum. *J. Biol. Chem.* 268: 18234-18242.

Patrono C., Patrignani P. and Garcia Rodriguez L.A. (2001). Cyclooxygenase-selective inhibition of prostanoid formation: transducing biochemical selectivity into clinical read-outs. *J. Clin. Invest.* 108: 7-13.

Picot D., Loll P.J. and Garavito R.M. (1994). The X-ray crystal structure of the membrane protein prostaglandin H_2 synthase-1. *Nature* 367: 243-249.

Prescott S.M. and Fitzpatrick F.A. (2000). Cyclooxygenase and carcinogenesis. *Biochim. Biophys. Acta* 1470: M69-78.

Prescott S.M. and White R.L. (1996). Self-promotion? Intimate connections between APC and prostaglandin H synthase-2. *Cell* 87: 783-786.

Reddy S.T., Wadleigh D.J. and Herschman H.R. (2000). Transcriptional regulation of the cyclooxygenase-2 gene in activated mast cells. *J. Biol. Chem.* 275: 3107-3113.

Ristimaki A., Garfinkel S., Wessendorf J., Maciag T. and Hla T. (1994). Induction of cyclooxygenase-2 by interleukin-1 alpha, evidence for post-transcriptional regulation. *J. Biol. Chem.* 269: 11769-11775.

Ristimaki A., Honkanen N., Jankala H., Sipponen P. and Harkonen M. (1997). Expression of cyclooxygenase-2 in human gastric carcinoma. *Cancer Res.* 57: 1276-1280.

Robert A. (1983). Cytoprotection of the gastrointestinal mucosa. *Adv. Intern. Med.* 28: 325-337.

Rourke I.J., Hansen T.V., Nerlov C., Rehfeld J.F. and Nielsen F.C. (1999). Negative cooperativity between juxtaposed E-box and cAMP/TPA responsive elements in the cholecystokinin gene promoter. *FEBS Lett.* 448: 15-18.

Schreinemachers D.M. and Everson R.B. (1994). Aspirin use and lung, colon, and breast cancer incidence in a prospective study. *Epidemiology* 5: 138-146.

Sheng H., Shao J., Dixon D.A., Williams C.S., Prescott S.M., DuBois R.N., Beauchamp R.D. (2000). Transforming growth factor-beta1 enhances Ha-ras-induced expression of cyclooxygenase-2 in intestinal epithelial cells via stabilization of mRNA. *J. Biol. Chem.* 275: 6628-6635.

Sheng H., Shao J., Kirkland S.C., Isakson P., Coffey R.J., Morrow J., Beauchamp R.D. and DuBois R.N. (1997). Inhibition of human colon cancer cell growth by selective inhibition of cyclooxygenase-2. *J. Clin. Invest.* 99: 2254-2259.

Sheng H., Shao J., Morrow J.D., Beauchamp R.D. and DuBois R.N. (1998). Modulation of apoptosis and Bcl-2 expression by prostaglandin E2 in human colon cancer cells. *Cancer Res.* 58: 362-366.

Shimada T., Hiraishi H. and Terano A. (2000). Hepatocyte growth factor protects gastric epithelial cells against ceramide-induced apoptosis through induction of cyclooxygenase-2. *Life Sci.* 68: 539-546.

Simmons D.L., Xie W., Chipman J.G. and Evett G.E. (1991). In *Prostaglandins, Leukotriems, Lipoxins, and PAF* (Bailey J.M., ed.) pp. 67-78, Plenum Press, New York.

Sirois J. and Richards J.S. (1992). Purification and characterization of a novel, distinct isoform of prostaglandin endoperoxide synthase induced by human chorionic gonadotropin in granulosa cells of rat preovulatory follicles. *J. Biol. Chem.* 267: 6382-6388.

Smith B.J., Curtis J.F. and Eling T.E. (1991). Bioactivation of xenobiotics by prostaglandin H synthase. *Chem. Biol. Interact.* 79: 245-264.

Smith W.L. and DeWitt D.L. (1996). Prostaglandin endoperoxide synthases-1 and -2. In *Advances in Immunology* (Dixon F.J., ed.) pp. 167-215, San Diego: Academic.

Smith W.L. and Langenbach R. (2001). Why there are two cyclooxygenase isozymes. *J. Clin. Invest.* 107: 1491-1495.

Smith W.L., DeWitt D.L. and Garavito R.M. (2000). Cyclooxygenases: structural, cellular, and molecular biology. *Annu. Rev.Biochem.* 69: 145-182.

Smith W.L., Garavito R.M. and DeWitt. D.L. (1996). Prostaglandin endoperoxide H synthases (cyclooxygenses)-1 and -2. *J. Biol. Chem.* 271: 33157-33160.

Song I. and Smith W.L. (1996). C-terminal Ser/Pro-Thr-Glu-Leu tetrapeptides of prostaglandin endoperoxide H synthases-1 and -2 target the enzymes to the endoplasmic reticulum. *Arch. Biochem. Biophys.* 334: 67-72.

Spencer A.G., Thuresson E., Otto J.C., Song I., Smith T., DeWitt D.L., Garavito R.M. and Smith W.L. (1999). The membrane binding domains of prostaglandin endoperoxide H synthases 1 and 2. Peptide mapping and mutational analysis. *J. Biol.Chem.* 274: 32936-32942.

Spugnini E.P., Cardillo I., Verdina A. , Crispi S., Saviozzi S., Calogero R., Nebbioso A., Altucci L., Cortese G., Galati R., Chien J., Shridhar V., Vincenzi B., Citro G., Cognetti F., Sacchi A. and Baldi A. (2006). Piroxicam and cisplatin in a mouse model of peritoneal mesothelioma. *Clin. Cancer Res.* 12: 6133-6143.

Stolina M., Sharma S., Zhu L., et al. (2000). Lung cancer cyclooxygenase-2 dependent inhibition of dendritic cell maturation and and function. *Proc. Am. Assoc. Cancer Res.* 41: 619.

Subbaramaiah K., Telang N., Ramonetti J.T., Araki R., DeVito B., Weksler B.B. and Dannenberg A.J. (1996). Transcription of cyclooxygenase-2 is enhanced in transformed mammary epithelial cells. *Cancer Res.* 56: 4424-4429.

Suh O., Mettlin C. and Petrelli N.J. (1993). Aspirin use, cancer, and polyps of the large bowel. *Cancer* 72: 1171-1177.

Surette M.E., Fonteh A.N., Bernatchez C. and Chilton F.H. (1999). Perturbations in the control of cellular arachidonic acid levels block cell growth and induce apoptosis in HL-60 cells. *Carcinogenesis* 20: 757-763.

Surette M.E., Winkler J.D., Fonteh A.N. and Chilton F.H. (1996). Relationship between arachidonate-phospholipid remodelling and apoptosis. *Biochemistry* 35: 9187-9196.

Tanabe T. and Tohnai N. (2002). Cyclooxygenase isozymes and their gene structures and expression. *Prostaglandins Other Lipid Mediat.* 68: 95–114.

Tay A., Squire J.A., Goldberg H. and Skorecki K. (1994). Assignment of the human prostaglandin-endoperoxide synthase 2 (PTGS2) gene to 1q25 by fluorescence in situ hybridization. *Genomics* 23: 718-719.

Tazawa R., Xu X.M., Wu K.K. and Wang L.H. (1994). Characterization of the genomic structure, chromosomal location and promoter of human prostaglandin H synthase-2 gene. *Biochem. Biophys. Res. Commun.* 203: 190-199.

Thun M.J. (1996). NSAID use and decreased risk of gastrointestinal cancers. *Gastroenterol. Clin. North. Am.* 25: 333-348.

Thun M.J., Namboodiri M.M., Calle E.E., Flanders W.D. and Heath C.W. Jr (1993). Aspirin use and risk of fatal cancer. *Cancer Res.* 53: 1322-1327.

Tsujii M. and DuBois R.N. (1995). Alterations in cellular adhesion and apoptosis in epithelial cells overexpressing prostaglandin endoperoxide synthase 2. *Cell* 83: 493-501.

Tsujii M., Kawano S., Tsuji S., Sawaoka H., Hori M. and DuBois R.N. (1998). Cyclooxygenase regulates angiogenesis induced by colon cancer cells. *Cell* 93: 705-716.

Tucker O.N., Dannenberg A.J., Yang E.K., Zhang F., Teng L., Daly J.M., Soslow R.A., Masferrer J.L., Woerner B.M., Koki A.T. and Fahey T.J. (1999). Cyclooxygenase-2 expression is up-regulated in human pancreatic cancer. *Cancer Res.* 59: 987-990.

Van der Ouderaa F.J., Buytenhek M., Nugteren D.H. and van Dorp D.A. (1977). Purification and characterization of prostaglandin endoperoxide synthetase from sheep vesicular glands. *Biochim. Biophys. Acta* 487: 315-331.

Vane J.R., Bakhle Y.S. and Botting R.M. (1998). Cyclooxygenases 1 and 2. *Annu. Rev. Pharmacol. Toxicol.* 38: 97-120.

Vesterinen E., Pukkala E., Timonen T. and Aromaa A. (1993). Cancer incidence among 78 000 asthma patients. *Int. J. Epidemiol.* 22: 976-982.

Wadleigh D.J., Reddy S.T., Kopp E., Ghosh S. and Herschman H.R. (2000). Transcriptional activation of the cyclooxygenase-2 gene in endotoxin-treated RAW 264.7 macrophages. *J. Biol. Chem.* 275: 6259-6266.

Whelton A. (1999). Nephrotoxicity of nonsteroidal anti-in£ammatory drugs: physiologic foundations and clinical implications. *Am. J. Med.* 106: S13-S24.

Wolff H., Saukkonen K., Anttila S., Karjalainen A., Vainio H. and Ristimaki A. (1998). Expression of cyclooxygenase-2 in human lung carcinoma. *Cancer Res.* 58: 4997-5001.

Xie W., Chipman J.G., Robertson D.L., Erikson R.L. and Simmons D.L. (1991). Expression of a mitogen-responsive gene encoding prostaglandin synthase is regulated by mRNA splicing. *Proc. Natl. Acad. Sci. USA*. 88: 2692-2696.

Xie W. and Herschman H.R. (1996). Transcriptional regulation of prostaglandin synthase 2 gene expression by platelet-derived growth factor and serum. *J. Biol. Chem.* 271: 31742-31748.

Xie W., Merrill J.R., Bradshaw W.S. and Simmons D.L. (1993). Structural determination and promoter analysis of the chicken mitogen-inducible prostaglandin G/H synthase gene and genetic mapping of the murine homolog. *Arch. Biochem. Biophys.* 300: 247-252.

Xu X.M., Tang J.L., Chen X., Wang L.H. and Wu K.K. (1997). Involvement of two Sp1 elements in basal endothelial prostaglandin H synthase-1 promoter activity. *J. Biol. Chem.* 272: 6943-6950.

Yokoyama C. and Tanabe T. (1989). Cloning of human gene encoding prostaglandin endoperoxide synthase and primary structure of the enzyme. *Biochem. Biophys. Res. Commun.* 165: 888-894.

Zeng J. and Fenna R.E. (1992). X-ray crystal structure of canine myeloperoxidase at 3 A resolution. *J. Mol. Biol.* 226: 185-207.

In: Mesothelioma from Bench Side to Clinic
Editor: Alfonso Baldi, pp. 243-264

ISBN: 978-1-60021-789-0

Chapter XII

The SV40 Hypothesis: Evidence against a Role for SV40 in the Pathogenesis of Mesothelioma

James J. Manfredi
Department of Oncological Sciences, Mount Sinai School of Medicine,
New York (NY), USA

Abstract

Simian virus 40 (SV40) has been implicated in the etiology of 40-60% of human mesotheliomas. These studies could have important medical implications concerning possible sources of human infection and potential therapies if this agent does, indeed, induce human tumors. Epidemiological studies have examined the possible increased incidence of disease among different populations known to be exposed to contaminated poliovirus vaccines. No clear association has yet been demonstrated. Indeed, examination of specific populations known to have been exposed to contaminated vaccines failed to show any increased risk of malignancy. Careful analysis of studies using serological data suggests that reported presence of seropositivity for SV40 in many cases is likely due to cross-reactivity with the closely related JC and BK viruses. Taken together, population-based studies do not support a role for SV40 in human disease. Studies that report positivity for SV40 typically only find it in a subset of tumor cells. As there is little published evidence consistent with a "hit and run" model of T antigen-dependent transformation, it is unclear the relevance of such findings. Recent studies have suggested that cases of SV40 positivity may be due to laboratory contamination. Utilization of highly sensitive assays under appropriately controlled conditions does not confirm the presence of SV40. Taken together, these findings strongly argue against a role of SV40 by any known transformation mechanism in the etiology of the majority of human malignant mesotheliomas.

Introduction

Batches of poliovaccine were shown to be contaminated with simian virus 40 (SV40). As millions of people had been possibly exposed to the virus in the vaccine, SV40 was the focus of research to determine whether it played a role as a human pathogen. Early epidemiological studies failed to show any correlation between exposure to the vaccine and human disease. Laboratory studies however clearly demonstrated that SV40 was capable of transforming rodent cells and inducing tumor formation in animals. SV40 rapidly became a model organism of choice in the study of DNA replication, transcription, and cellular transformation. Indeed, many of the seminal findings in each of these areas were made through the use of SV40 as an experimental tool. In particular, it was studies of SV40 that established a clear tumor suppressor role for both the p53 protein as well as the product of the retinoblastoma susceptibility gene, pRb. Thus, mechanistic insight into the functions of these two important proteins was also gained through experimental manipulations of SV40. Exposure to asbestos has been clearly implicated in the etiology of human mesothelioma, but a role for other environmental factors has been suggested. Recently, numerous reports have appeared identifying either SV40 DNA or protein in human tumors, most notably mesotheliomas. This raises important public health issues and medical implications and therefore is a critical issue that needs to be rigorously addressed.

The detailed and insightful studies of SV40 have revealed a great deal about the underlying mechanisms for SV40-induced tumorigenesis. Much of this knowledge provides a sound molecular basis for viral-mediated transformation. However, the data that has been generated implicating SV40 in human mesothelioma is not consistent with known mechanisms of action of the virus. More recent studies using highly sensitive methods of detection have failed to confirm the findings of SV40. Further, additional epidemiological evidence has yet to support a significant role for SV40. In order to address the possible relevance of SV40 in the generation of human mesothelioma, the molecular biology of SV40-dependent transformation will first be reviewed. With this insight, possible explanations for the published reports detecting SV40 in human mesothelioma samples will be explored. It will be argued that the findings to date are incompatible with a role for SV40 in the etiology of human mesothelioma.

The Mechanism of SV40-Mediated Transformation Involves Inactivation of the P53 and PRB Tumor Suppressors

The SV40 genome is a small circular DNA that encodes two sets of transcripts, expressed either early or late in infection (Figure 1). Two tumor antigens are expressed from the early region, large T and small t (Figure 2). Since SV40 DNA synthesis utilizes many of the enzymes and activities of the host cell, the virus needs to drive the cell into S phase for successful generation of new viral genomes. Cell cycle progression is largely mediated through a series of phosphorylation events mediated by cyclin-dependent kinases. These kinases rely upon an interaction with a regulatory subunit, the cyclin, for their activity.

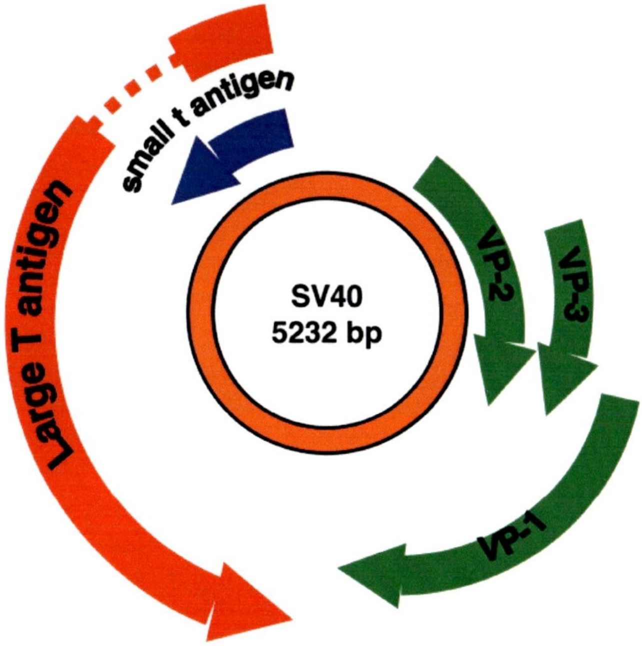

Figure 1. The SV40 genome is a compact circular DNA. The SV40 genome is 5232 bp and can be divided into two main regions. The early region encodes the two tumor antigens, small t and large T, which are responsible for regulation of viral DNA replication. The late region encodes three proteins, VP-1, VP-2, and VP-3 that are involved in viral assembly.

SV40 expresses its large T antigen that, in part, contributes to facilitated entry into S phase through the regulation of cyclin-dependent kinase activity. The ability of SV40 to transform rodent cells in vitro was shown to be dependent upon expression of this large T antigen. Large T antigen directly interacts in cells with both the p53 and pRb tumor suppressors as well as the related pRb family members, p130 and p107. T antigen interacts with p53 through two non-contiguous stretches of amino acids near its carboxyl end (Figure 3). This interaction has been shown to stabilize p53 protein thereby increasing its half-life. The p53 protein is a transcription factor that mediates the cellular response to genomic DNA damage. p53 protein levels are increased in response to such stress leading to its binding to specific sites in genomic DNA and effects on gene expression. p53 will trigger mainly either a cell cycle arrest or an apoptotic response depending upon the cell type and conditions. Cell cycle arrest is predominantly mediated by upregulation of the cyclin-dependent kinase p21 whereas the cell death appears to be mediated by transcriptional activation of the bcl-2 related proteins PUMA and Noxa. The binding of T antigen to p53 inhibits its ability to bind to DNA and to activate gene expression, thereby inactivating its function . It has been hypothesized that viral infection triggers a stress that activates p53 leading to an increase in its expression level. For the virus to successfully replicate its DNA, the host cell needs to enter S phase. Large T antigen inactivates p53 thereby abrogating the viral-induced effects on p53 and allowing cell cycle progression to proceed. This ability of T antigen to interact with p53 is required for its ability to transform cells both in vitro and in vivo.

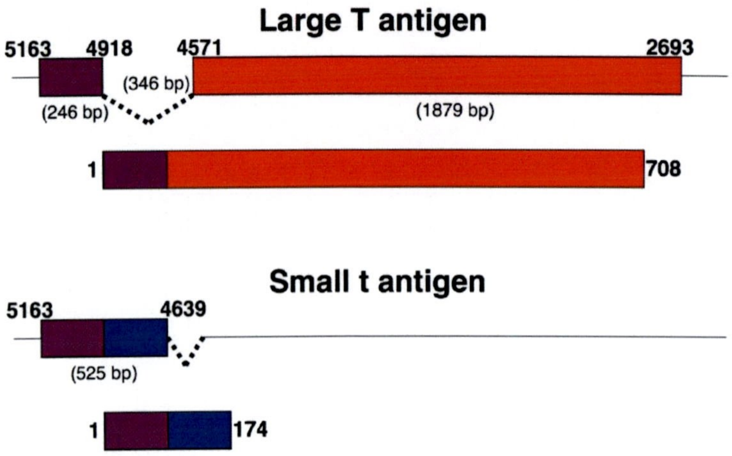

Figure 2. The SV40 early region encodes two distinct tumor antigens due to alternate splicing. The structure of the large T and small t messenger RNA and corresponding proteins is shown. The SV40 large T antigen is a 708 amino acid protein that is expressed from a messenger RNA derived from two exons (bases 5163-4918 and 4571-2693). The small t antigen is a 174 amino acid protein that is expressed from a messenger RNA encoded by a single exon (bases 5163-4639). Small t antigen shares the sequence of exon 1 of large T and thus also the N-terminal region the large T antigen protein. There are two additional key features of this genomic structure. First, genomic DNA that spans the intron of large T encodes the C-terminus of small t. Second, the intron of small t includes part of the coding region of large T antigen derived from its second exon (bases 4639-4571).

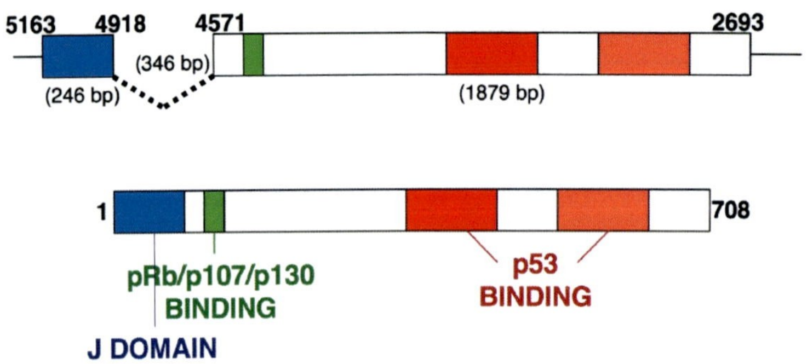

Figure 3. Four regions of the SV40 large T antigen contribute to its ability to transform cells. The structure of the SV40 large T antigen messenger RNA and its encoded protein are shown. Mutagenesis has demonstrated that four regions of the large T protein are needed for its ability to induce cellular transformation. The region responsible for binding to the product of the retinoblastoma susceptibility gene, pRb, and is family members p107 and p130 is shown in green (amino acids 102-115). Two regions gave been identified that are involved in the binding to the tumor suppressor p53 and are shown in two shades of red (amino acids 351-450 and 533-626). A region at the amino terminus shown in blue is referred to as the J domain (amino acids 1-82). This region is shared with small t antigen and also has been implicated in the ability of large T to affect cellular transformation.

The interaction of large T antigen with pRb appears to have a similar goal, that is, facilitating entry of the host cell into S phase. Prior to DNA synthesis, the pRb protein is found in complex with members of the E2F family of transcription factors. Binding of pRb inhibits the ability of E2Fs to activate gene expression. Binding of large T antigen to pRb leads to the release of E2Fs. The pRb binding site on large T antigen is near the amino end, just beyond the sequences that are shared with the small t antigen (Figure 3). The relevant transcriptional targets in this context are genes that encode enzymes that are required for successful entry into S phase. Such genes include thymidylate synthetase, ribonucleotide reductase, as well as thymidine kinase. In addition, cyclins E and A are upregulated which allow for further activation of cyclin-dependent kinases (notably cdk2) that are involved in cell cycle progression as well. During the normal cell cycle, pRb function is inactivated through its phosphorylation by cyclin-dependent kinases. Large T antigen is capable of inactivating the function of pRb in the absence of such phosphorylation via its direct binding. Thus, expression of large T antigen also facilitates S phase entry, enhancing viral DNA synthesis and subsequent virus production. The amino terminal end of SV40 large T antigen has also been implicated in its transforming activity. This so-called " J domain" was shown to play an essential role in the ability of T antigen to inactivate the function of pRb and its family members. The large T antigen has an apparent molecular weight of 90 kd and is localized to the nucleus (Figure 4).

In permissive cells in which viral DNA can be replicated, the role of p53 and pRb binding to large T antigen is to enable S phase entry. Upon successful replication of the viral genome, virus particle production can ensue.

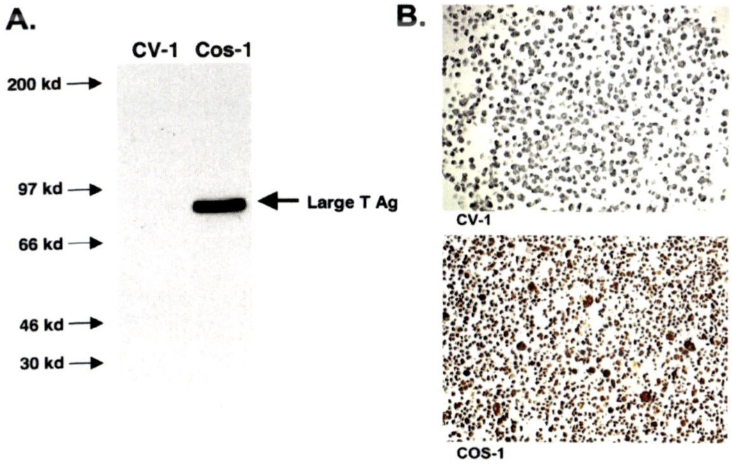

Figure 4. A monoclonal antibody (mAb 101) is highly specific and detects SV40 large T antigen in the nucleus. Cos-1 cells are green monkey kidney cells containing a single integrated copy of the SV40 genome. CV-1 is a corresponding cell line that does not contain any SV40 sequences. mAb 101 is a highly specific monoclonal antibody which interacts with an epitope in the C-terminal end of SV40 large T antigen . (A) Extracts of Cos-1 and CV-1 cells were electrophoresed on an SDS polyacrylamide gel and transferred to nitrocellulose. Immunoblotting was performed with the monoclonal antibody mAb 101 demonstrating a single detectable band of the appropriate molecular weight. (B) CV-1 and Cos-1 cells were formaldehyde-fixed and paraffin embedded. Immunohistochemical staining using mAb 101 demonstrates that SV40 large T antigen is readily detectable in Cos-1 cells and is nuclear.

In cells which are non-permissive for viral DNA synthesis, rodent cells and in many cases those of human origin, there is no viral DNA replication. However, large T antigen still is capable of inactivating the functions of p53 and pRb thus leading to uncontrolled proliferation and cellular transformation.

Expression of SV40 Large T Antigen Is Required for Both the Initiation and Maintenance of Cellular Transformation

The expression of large T antigen alone was sufficient to fully transform primary rodent cells. A mutant SV40 which showed temperature-sensitive behavior was originally used to demonstrate that the large T antigen was the key transforming activity. Use of such a temperature-sensitive T antigen demonstrated that continuous expression of functional protein was needed in order to maintain the transformed phenotype in vitro as well as for the cells to form tumors in animals. Large T antigen has also been expressed under control of an inducible promoter. Downregulation of T antigen by removal of the inducing agent led to a reversal of cellular transformation. Use of Cre recombinase to remove a large T antigen gene flanked by loxP sites also inhibited tumor cell proliferation. Maintenance of the immortalized state in human fibroblasts was shown to be strictly dependent upon continued expression of functional large T antigen. Most notably, levels of T antigen expression directly correlate with transformation.

Both Large and Small Tumor Antigens of SV40 Are Required for Full Transformation of Human Cells

Alternative splicing of the early region pre-messenger RNA leads to expression of either the large T or small t antigen. Studies demonstrated that large T expression was sufficient to immortalize and transform primary rodent cells in culture. However, the small t antigen has also been implicated in playing a role in cellular transformation by SV40. Its role has been most clearly revealed in recent studies that have determined the requirements for transformation of a variety of different primary human cell types. Expression of an activated Ras protein, the reverse transcriptase subunit of telomerase, as well as both large T and small t antigen has been shown to be necessary for full transformation of primary human fibroblasts. An obligatory role for small t antigen has also been demonstrated for human mammary epithelial cells as well. The mechanism of action of the small t antigen is related to its ability to interact with two subunits of protein phosphatase 2A, thereby presumably altering the phosphorylation state of key regulatory proteins. Although the importance of binding to protein phosphatase 2 A is clear, the detailed downstream effectors that mediate this effect of small t have yet to be fully elucidated. It also remain unclear what are the corresponding mechanisms, if any, that target protein phosphates 2A and its pathway in human tumors. Nevertheless, the persistent expression of both SV40 tumor antigens is clearly a necessary step in SV40-mediated transformation of human cells in vitro.

SV40 Has Been Implicated in a Subset of Human Mesotheliomas

Immediately following the detection of SV40 in batches of poliovaccine, a burst of studies ensued attempting to determine the potential role of the virus in human disease. It was only approximately thirty years later that the first publications appear in which SV40 genomic DNA was detected in human tumor samples, initially in bone cancer and lymphoma. These were subsequently followed by studies showing the presence of viral DNA in human mesotheliomas. There are several possible explanations for this lag time. First, it is well accepted that human cancer is a multi-step process. Thus, a period of time was necessary for tumors that were initiated by exposure to SV40 to sustain the multiple genetic changes that were required for full, pathological neoplasia. Second, and perhaps most important, was advances in technology. The main methodology for detection of SV40 is the use of polymerase chain reaction (PCR), a technique that has only become readily available and easily performed in the last 10-15 years.

The initial findings of the presence of SV40 genomic DNA using PCR analysis were followed by a series of confirmatory studies. Notably, use of laser-capture microdissection was able to show the presence of the viral DNA in tumor tissue but not in adjacent normal cells . Southern blotting has been used to detect SV40 genomic DNA, albeit in osteosarcomas . Sequencing of the PCR products detected from human mesothelioma samples showed that these were distinct from those found in laboratory strains of SV40. The large T antigen protein was detected in a subset of mesothelioma samples. Although in one cases, the T antigen was localized to the cytoplasm, while it is known to exert its effects in the nucleus. The protein detected in mesothelioma samples was shown to interact with both p53 and the pRb family members, suggesting that it was indeed functional. Strikingly, antisense to SV40 large T antigen was used to inhibit the proliferation of mesothelioma cell lines which had been shown to express detectable T antigen. These studies were also consistent with the observation that human mesothelioma rarely presents with mutation of either p53 or pRb. It is to be expected that an SV40-mediated transformation mechanism would obviate the need for genetic alterations in either of these two pathways. In support of this, no evidence of overexpression of the negative regulator of p53, Mdm2 was detected in human mesothelioma. Taken together, these published studies were intriguing in their implication of a role for SV40, albeit, tentative and in need of confirmation and validation.

Laboratory studies supported the relevance of SV40 in the genesis of mesothelioma. Intraperitoneal injection of SV40 caused formation of mesotheliomas in a hamster model. Use of mutant mice which lack p53 expression demonstrated that loss of p53 enhanced asbestos-induced mesothlioma, arguing that loss of p53 function is important in this neoplasm. Human fibroblasts are not readily transformed by SV40 in vitro. In contrast, primary human mesothelial cells were reported to undergo SV40-dependent transformation at a high rate. It should be noted, however, that this latter report is in contrast to an earlier study in which human mesothelial cells escaped senescence but remained non-tumorigenic upon introduction of the SV40 early region.

To address the significance of detection of SV40 genomic DNA in human mesothelioma samples in a more definitive way, two studies were performed at multiple institutions to examine the same samples in different laboratories. The published reports showed positivity for SV40 in multiple samples, but there was a lack of reproducibility between laboratories, raising important concerns about the validity of their conclusions.

Detection of SV40 in Only a Subset of Cells in Human Mesotheliomas Has Led to the Idea of Novel Transformation Mechanisms

Studies which showed detectable SV40 large T antigen DNA or protein, only found that a small subset of tumor cells were positive. This could account for the wide variability in the incidence of SV40 detection. Less than a single copy per cell was not to be expected based upon previous studies of SV40-induced transformation, leading to a variety of possible explanations. First, it was proposed that SV40 infection could lead to chronic cellular stress, similar to the mechanism of action that has been proposed for viral hepatitis-associated liver cancer. Second, the notion has been presented that expression of SV40 large T antigen induces gene expression changes resulting in upregulation of expression of growth factors. Cells that now constitutively express these growth factors become engaged in an autocrine loop, leading to their own transformation, as well as the induction of tumorigenicity in surrounding cells which lack SV40 expression, but that are influenced by the increased local concentration of growth factors. Third, it has been suggested that a stem cell population is the key target for SV40-mediated transformation. Fourth, it was noted that some studies of large T antigen-dependent transformation have revealed maintenance of the tumorigenic phenotype in the absence of persistent large T antigen protein expression. However, it should be noted that in two of these mouse models, loss of T antigen expression was accompanied by the appearance of missense mutations in p53. This is in contrast to the striking lack of p53 mutation that is seen in human mesothelioma. It should be added that this so-called "hit and run" model for SV40-mediated transformation is consistent with studies showing that the viral proteins can enhance chromosomal instability.

There is also a technical issue that needs to be addressed. If SV40 sequences are present in a sufficiently low enough number of cells in a given sample, it is likely that there will be an inherent lack of reproducibility from assay to assay. A given PCR reaction may contain the equivalent of tumor cells which is below the reported frequency of positivity. Hence, it should not be expected that there will be equivalent results from samples derived from adjacent sections of tumor. For example, the more sensitive assays have been shown to detect as little as 1 positive cell in a sample of 5000 cells. If a typical PCR reaction contains DNA derived from less than 5000 cells, there should not be reproducibility of results from samples derived from adjacent tissue. Although studies have noted the low level of positive cells in a given sample, this has not been clearly quantitated. It will be critical in the future for published studies to carefully note the number of genome equivalents per cell that are detected and relate this to the sample size for detection.

The Known Mechanism of SV40-Mediated Transformation Is Inconsistent with Its Expression in a Subset of Tumor Cells

Infection with SV40 or expression of the SV40 large T antigen was shown to be sufficient to immortalize primary human fibroblasts, although the resulting cells remain non-transformed. Use of a temperature-sensitive mutant of large T led to the observation that expression of this oncoprotein was required for maintenance of the immortalized state. Thus, at the non-permissive temperatures, these established fibroblasts cell lines would cease proliferation. Use of a negative selection strategy in which T antigen expression is selectively lost also resulted in inhibition of cell proliferation. These results from in vitro cell culture argue that persistent expression of large T antigen is required for long-term proliferation.

A comparison of the results involving SV40 in human cancer with what is known about other DNA tumor viruses with clear relevance to human tumors is informative. For example, the role of the oncogenic variants of human papillomaviruses (HPV) in human cervical cancer is well-established. The HPV E6 and E7 proteins have been shown to be necessary and sufficient for transformation. The E6 protein binds and targets p53 for degradation whereas the E7 protein binds and inactivates pRb function. Thus, the combination of E6 and E7 is functionally equivalent to the large T antigen of SV40. In human cervical cancer, persistence of expression of both E6 and E7 is found and this occurs in virtually all of the cells in the tumor. Similarly, the presence of Epstein-Barr viral proteins is found in human lymphomas and typically occurs in a majority of the cancer cells. In light of these well-documented findings, especially involving the clear etiologic role of HPV in cervical cancer, it is to be expected that should SV40 have relevance in human disease, large T antigen should be detected in most cells in the tumor.

As was noted, it is also to be expected that transformation mediated by SV40 large T antigen would obviate the need for mutation or loss of either p53 or pRb. This has indeed been shown to be the case for most mesotheliomas. However, numerous studies in a variety of tumor types have argued that it is alterations in the pathways involving these tumor suppressors that are key rather than direct genetic alteration per se. Loss of the cyclin-dependent kinase inhibitor p16, overexpression or mutation of the cyclin-dependent kinase cdk4 or cdk6 as well as upregulation of the regulatory subunit of this kinase, cyclin D1 have been considered to be redundant with direct alterations of pRb. The genetic locus that encodes p16 also expresses the $p14^{ARF}$ protein which has been shown to antagonize the negative regulation of p53 by its ubiquitin ligase Mdm2. Thus, deletions of this CDKN2A locus can serve to inactivate both p53 and pRb pathways. Alterations in the CDKN2A locus are found in a majority of human mesotheliomas . It is unclear why this should be the case, if large T antigen is a critical player in these tumors. These findings involving p16 and $p14^{ARF}$ argue against a role for SV40 in the genesis of this tumor type. Indeed, one study has even failed to show a correlation between detection of SV40 DNA and the pRb or p53 status of the mesotheliomas.

The SV40 DNA Sequences Commonly Detected in Human Mesothelioma Derive from the Small T Intron, an Element Often Present in Laboratory Vectors

Early attempts to develop vectors that ectopically express proteins at a high level relied on the inclusion of SV40 genomic sequences. The SV40 origin of replication was included in some vectors to enhance the copy number. By cotransfecting a plasmid that expressed SV40 large T antigen or using cell lines which constitutively express T antigen, the replication of the expression vector was enhanced thereby increasing its ability to express exogenously introduced proteins. It was also found that splicing of messenger RNA enhanced its expression which led to the incorporation of the sequence from the small t intron into many such vectors. This latter genomic sequence overlaps with the region of the large T antigen sequence which encodes the part of T antigen which binds to pRb and its family members. This is also the genomic region which is amplified by the commonly used primers to detect SV40 in human mesotheliomas. Many laboratories that may never have worked with SV40 itself are therefore likely to have used plasmids that contain SV40 sequences. This notion had been proposed in the past and was directly tested recently. Indeed, the frequency of positive detection of SV40 in primary tumor samples was higher when primers were used that hybridize to the region containing the small t intron. In contrast, use of primers that amplify other genomic SV40 sequences failed to show products. BLAST searches confirmed that a large number of widely used vectors included the commonly utilized pGL2 series are capable of being amplified when such primers are used. These findings raise important concerns about a number of the studies that have detected SV40 genomic DNA using a PCR amplification approach.

Sensitive Detection Methods Fail to Confirm the Presence of SV40 in Human Tumor Samples

There are now a growing number of studies that fail to detect SV40 genomic DNA or expression of SV40 large T antigen in human mesothelioma. Similar negative findings have recently been reported in other tumor types. Several of these studies have presented data to argue that the PCR-based assays that are used therein are quite sensitive. Similar findings have now been reported for other tumor types as well. It should be noted that there is a debate in the literature over the methodologies employed in some of these studies. It has become clear however that variations in protocols between laboratories have contributed to the confusion and there is a need for standardization of assay conditions.

Two recent studies established highly sensitive assays to detect the presence of genomic SV40 DNA using a PCR-based approach. In one case, it was estimated that one copy of SV40 could be detected in a sample containing 10,000 cells. The second group was able to demonstrate that as little as a single copy in 5,000 cells using formalin-fixed preparations could be detected. Use of these highly sensitive approached detected little or no SV40 DNA in the cases of mesothelioma that were analyzed. Further, there was no evidence of either early region messenger RNA by RT-PCR or large T antigen protein by immunohistochemistry. A sensitive protein detection assay was established using a highly specific monoclonal antibody to large T antigen (Figure 4) under conditions in which 1 positive cell in 50 could be detected. Under these conditions, there was no detectable large T antigen in a subset of mesothelioma cell lines which had previously been reported to contain it.

Epidemiological Evidence Argues against a Role for SV40 in Human Mesothelioma

After thirty years of follow-up, there is no evidence of increased mesothelioma or other cancers in birth cohorts likely to have received the SV-40 contaminated poliovaccine as compared to controls. Similar results have been obtained by analysis of other populations. One study reported an association between maternal exposure to poliovaccine and tumor formation in children, but a follow-up analysis failed to detect significant seropositivity for SV40 in these mothers. More recently, use of sensitive assays for SV40 antibodies revealed no connection between maternal SV40 seropositivity, exposure of the mothers to poliovaccine, or the status of their children. Adenovirus vaccines given to US Army recruits were also shown to be contaminated with SV40. No correlation was observed between exposure to these vaccines and the incidence of several cancers including mesothelioma. Taken together, attempts to correlate serological positivity for SV40 and incidence of cancer have failed to show any association. Indeed, studies in rodent models have shown that SV40 triggers a strong immune response that readily clears the virus. Should this be the case in humans as well, these results argue against the notion of a persistent SV40 infection in individuals who are not immune-compromised.

A review of the published literature reveals that there is generally quite a low frequency of seropositivity in populations that have been exposed to the vaccine. Where seropositivity was detected, the titer of antibodies were low. In addition, there are two related human viruses, JC and BK which share considerable similarity to SV40. Exposure of humans to these viruses has been well-documented with disease association occurring largely in immunocompromised individuals. Circulating antibodies to JC and BK have been shown to cross-react frequently with SV40, suggesting that where SV40 seropositivity is detected, it may be due to exposure to the related human polyomaviruses.

A variety of epidemiological studies have addressed the association of cancer with exposure to the SV40-contaminated vaccines. None of these showed a clear increase in incidence of tumors related to being a vaccine recipient. It has been argued that these studies do not directly address vaccine exposure as this is inferred rather than rigorously documented. However, this has been countered by noting the widespread use of vaccines that were known to be contaminated and that studies which utilized serum markers of SV40 exposure failed to show a cancer increase. One recent study suggested that SV40 enhances the risk of asbestos-associated mesothelioma, although this finding utilized a PCR approach to detect SV40 DNA. It should be noted that a published study by the Immunization Safety Review Committee of the Institute of Medicine concluded that existing evidence is inadequate to address this issue sufficiently.

Conclusion

There is a lack of experimental evidence to support a mechanism of transformation by SV40 in which only a minor fraction of cells express the viral oncoproteins. Comparisons to the mode of action of human papilloma virus in human cancer also question this as well. There are important concerns about laboratory contamination and the over-reliance on PCR-based approaches, especially as highly sensitive assays fail to detect SV40 at the frequency reported by others. Taken together, the published literature that argues in favor of an etiologic role for SV40 in human cancer, is, in fact, quite inconclusive. This has led some to propose that further studies are necessary. Nevertheless, the available data to date does not clearly implicate a role for SV40 in the etiology of human mesothelioma and in many cases suggests quite the opposite.

Acknowledgements

This work was supported by the International Environmental Research Foundation and NCI grants CA86001 and CA080058 from the National Institutes of Health. The advice and assistance of Stuart Aaronson, Charles Axten, David Burstein, Philippe Chahinian, Jianli Dong, Luciana Giono, Wen-jun Liu, Dana Lukin, Robert Nolan, Sejal Patel, Rui Qiao, Amy Ream, Lois Resnick-Silverman, and Shohreh Varmeh-Ziaie is grateful acknowledged.

References

Ahuja, D., Saenz-Robles, M.T. and Pipas, J.M. SV40 large T antigen targets multiple cellular pathways to elicit cellular transformation. (2005). *Oncogene*, 24, 7729-7745.

Ali, S.H. and DeCaprio, J.A. Cellular transformation by SV40 large T antigen: interaction with host proteins. (2001). *Semin. Cancer Biol.,* 11, 15-23.

Anderson, J.L. and Martin, R.G. SV40 transformation of mouse brain cells: critical role of gene A in maintenance of the transformed phenotype. (1976). *J. Cell Physiol.*, 88, 65-76.

Bargonetti, J. and Manfredi, J.J. Multiple roles of the tumor suppressor p53. (2002). *Curr. Opin. Oncol.*, 14, 86-91.

Bergsagel, D.J., Finegold, M.J., Butel, J.S., Kupsky, W.J. and Garcea, R.L. DNA sequences similar to those of simian virus 40 in ependymomas and choroid plexus tumors of childhood. (1992). *N. Engl. J. Med.*, 326, 988-993.

Bikel, I., Mamon, H., Brown, E.L., Boltax, J., Agha, M. and Livingston, D.M. The t-unique coding domain is important to the transformation maintenance function of the simian virus 40 small t antigen. (1986). *Mol. Cell Biol.*, 6, 1172-1178.

Bocchetta, M., Di Resta, I., Powers, A., Fresco, R., Tosolini, A., Testa, J.R., Pass, H.I., Rizzo, P. and Carbone, M. Human mesothelial cells are unusually susceptible to simian virus 40-mediated transformation and asbestos cocarcinogenicity. (2000). *Proc. Natl. Acad. Sci. USA*, 97, 10214-10219.

Bocchetta, M., Miele, L., Pass, H.I. and Carbone, M. Notch-1 induction, a novel activity of SV40 required for growth of SV40-transformed human mesothelial cells. (2003). *Oncogene,* 22, 81-89.

Brouchet, L., Valmary, S., Dahan, M., Didier, A., Galateau-Salle, F., Brousset, P. and Degano, B. Detection of oncogenic virus genomes and gene products in lung carcinoma. (2005). *British Journal of Cancer,* 92, 743-746.

Brugge, J.S. and Butel, J.S. Role of simian virus 40 gene A function in maintenance of transformation. (1975). *J. Virol.*, 15, 619-635.

Butel, J.S. and Lednicky, J.A. Cell and molecular biology of simian virus 40: implications for human infections and disease. (1999). *J. Natl. Cancer Inst.*, 91, 119-134.

Cacciotti, P., Barbone, D., Porta, C., Altomare, D.A., Testa, J.R., Mutti, L. and Gaudino, G. SV40-dependent AKT activity drives mesothelial cell transformation after asbestos exposure. (2005). *Cancer Res.*, 65, 5256-5262.

Cacciotti, P., Libener, R., Betta, P., Martini, F., Porta, C., Procopio, A., Strizzi, L., Penengo, L., Tognon, M., Mutti, L. *et al.* SV40 replication in human mesothelial cells induces HGF/Met receptor activation: a model for viral-related carcinogenesis of human malignant mesothelioma. (2001). *Proc. Natl. Acad. Sci. USA*, 98, 12032-12037.

Capello, D., Rossi, D., Gaudino, G., Carbone, A. and Gaidano, G. Simian virus 40 infection in lymphoproliferative disorders [21]. (2003). *Lancet,* 361, 88-89.

Carbone, M., Bocchetta, M., Cristaudo, A., Emri, S., Gazdar, A., Jasani, B., Lednicky, J., Miele, L., Mutti, L., Pass, H.I. *et al.* SV40 and human brain tumors. (2003). *Int. J. Cancer,* 106, 140-142; author reply 143-145.

Carbone, M., Kratzke, R.A. and Testa, J.R. The pathogenesis of mesothelioma. (2002). *Semin. Oncol.*, 29, 2-17.

Carbone, M., Pass, H.I., Rizzo, P., Marinetti, M., Di Muzio, M., Mew, D.J., Levine, A.S. and Procopio, A. Simian virus 40-like DNA sequences in human pleural mesothelioma. (1994). *Oncogene,* 9, 1781-1790.

Carbone, M., Rdzanek, M.A., Rudzinski, J.J., De Marco, M.A., Bocchetta, M., Ramos Nino, M., Mossman, B. and Pass, H.I. SV40 detection in human tumor specimens. (2005). *Cancer Res.*, 65, 10120-10121.

Carbone, M., Rizzo, P., Grimley, P.M., Procopio, A., Mew, D.J., Shridhar, V., de Bartolomeis, A., Esposito, V., Giuliano, M.T., Steinberg, S.M. *et al.* Simian virus-40 large-T antigen binds p53 in human mesotheliomas. (1997). *Nat. Med.,* 3, 908-912.

Carbone, M., Rizzo, P., Procopio, A., Giuliano, M., Pass, H.I., Gebhardt, M.C., Mangham, C., Hansen, M., Malkin, D.F., Bushart, G. *et al.* SV40-like sequences in human bone tumors. (1996). *Oncogene*, 13, 527-535.

Carroll, R.B. and Gurney, E.G. Time-dependent maturation of the simian virus 40 large T antigen-p53 complex studied by using monoclonal antibodies. (1982). *J. Virol.*, 44, 565-573.

Chellappan, S., Kraus, V.B., Kroger, B., Munger, K., Howley, P.M., Phelps, W.C. and Nevins, J.R. Adenovirus E1A, simian virus 40 tumor antigen, and human papillomavirus E7 share the capacity to disrupt the interaction between transcription factor E2F and the retinoblastoma gene product. (1992). *Proc. Natl. Acad. Sci. USA*, 89, 4549-4553.

Cheng, J.Q., Jhanwar, S.C., Klein, W.M., Bell, D.W., Lee, W.C., Altomare, D.A., Nobori, T., Olopade, O.I., Buckler, A.J. and Testa, J.R. p16 alterations and deletion mapping of 9p21-p22 in malignant mesothelioma. (1994). *Cancer Res*, 54, 5547-5551.

Cicala, C., Pompetti, F. and Carbone, M. SV40 induces mesotheliomas in hamsters. (1993). *Am. J. Pathol.*, 142, 1524-1533.

Cristaudo, A., Foddis, R., Vivaldi, A., Buselli, R., Gattini, V., Guglielmi, G., Cosentino, F., Ottenga, F., Ciancia, E., Libener, R. *et al.* SV40 enhances the risk of malignant mesothelioma among people exposed to asbestos: a molecular epidemiologic case-control study. (2005). *Cancer Res.*, 65, 3049-3052.

Cristaudo, A., Vivaldi, A., Sensales, G., Guglielmi, G., Ciancia, E., Elisei, R. and Ottenga, F. Molecular biology studies on mesothelioma tumor samples: preliminary data on H-ras, p21, and SV40. (1995). *J. Environ. Pathol Toxicol Oncol.*, 14, 29-34.

Cutrone, R., Lednicky, J., Dunn, G., Rizzo, P., Bocchetta, M., Chumakov, K., Minor, P. and Carbone, M. Some oral poliovirus vaccines were contaminated with infectious SV40 after 1961. (2005). *Cancer Research,* 65, 10273-10279.

David, H., Mendoza, S., Konishi, T. and Miller, C.W. Simian virus 40 is present in human lymphomas and normal blood. (2001). *Cancer Lett,* 162, 57-64.

De Luca, A., Baldi, A., Esposito, V., Howard, C.M., Bagella, L., Rizzo, P., Caputi, M., Pass, H.I., Giordano, G.G., Baldi, F. *et al.* The retinoblastoma gene family pRb/p105, p107, pRb2/p130 and simian virus-40 large T-antigen in human mesotheliomas. (1997). *Nat. Med.*, 3, 913-916.

De Sanjose, S., Shah, K.V., Domingo-Domenech, E., Engels, E.A., De Sevilla, A.F., Alvaro, T., Garcia-Villanueva, M., Romagosa, V., Gonzalez-Barca, E. and Viscidi, R.P. Lack of serological evidence for an association between simian virus 40 and lymphoma. (2003). *International Journal of Cancer,* 104, 522-524.

Deppert, W., Steinmayer, T. and Richter, W. Cooperation of SV40 large T antigen and the cellular protein p53 in maintenance of cell transformation. (1989). *Oncogene,* 4, 1103-1110.

Dhaene, K., Verhulst, A. and Van Marck, E. SV40 large T-antigen and human pleural mesothelioma. Screening by polymerase chain reaction and tyramine-amplified immunohistochemistry. (1999). *Virchows Arch.*, 435, 1-7.

Doerries, K. Human polyomavirus JC and BK persistent infection. (2006). *Adv. Exp. Med. Biol.,* 577, 102-116.

Dyson, N. The regulation of E2F by pRB-family proteins. (1998). Genes Dev, 12, 2245-2262.

Dyson, N., Howley, P.M., Munger, K. and Harlow, E. The human papilloma virus-16 E7 oncoprotein is able to bind to the retinoblastoma gene product. (1989). *Science,* 243, 934-937.

Elenbaas, B., Spirio, L., Koerner, F., Fleming, M.D., Zimonjic, D.B., Donaher, J.L., Popescu, N.C., Hahn, W.C. and Weinberg, R.A. Human breast cancer cells generated by oncogenic transformation of primary mammary epithelial cells. (2001). *Genes Dev,* 15, 50-65.

Emri, S., Kocagoz, T., Olut, A., Güngen, Y., Mutti, L. and Baris, Y.I. Simian Virus 40 is not a cofactor in the pathogenesis of environmentally induced malignant pleural mesothelioma in Turkey. (2000). *Anticancer Research,* 20, 891-894.

Engels, E.A. Cancer risk associated with receipt of vaccines contaminated with simian virus 40: epidemiologic research. (2005). Expert Rev Vaccines, 4, 197-206.

Engels, E.A. Does simian virus 40 cause non-Hodgkin lymphoma? A review of the laboratory and epidemiological evidence. (2005). *Cancer Invest,* 23, 529-536.

Engels, E.A., Chen, J., Viscidi, R.P., Shah, K.V., Daniel, R.W., Chatterjee, N. and Klebanoff, M.A. Poliovirus vaccination during pregnancy, maternal seroconversion to simian virus 40, and risk of childhood cancer. (2004). *Am. J. Epidemiol.,* 160, 306-316.

Engels, E.A., Gravitt, P.E., Daniel, R.W., Quezado, M. and Shah, K.V. Re: Absence of simian virus 40 in human brain tumors from northern India; Response to Letter From Carbone et al. (2003). *Int. J. Cancer,* 106, 143-145.

Engels, E.A., Katki, H.A., Nielsen, N.M., Winther, J.F., Hjalgrim, H., Gjerris, F., Rosenberg, P.S. and Frisch, M. Cancer incidence in Denmark following exposure to poliovirus vaccine contaminated with simian virus 40. (2003). *Journal of the National Cancer Institute,* 95, 532-539.

Engels, E.A., Sarkar, C., Daniel, R.W., Gravitt, P.E., Verma, K., Quezado, M. and Shah, K.V. Absence of simian virus 40 in human brain tumors from northern India. (2002). *Int. J. Cancer,* 101, 348-352.

Epstein-Baak, R., Lin, Y., Bradshaw, V. and Cohn, M. Inducible transformation of cells from transgenic mice expressing SV40 under lac operon control. (1992). *Cell Growth Differ,* 3, 127-134.

Ewald, D., Li, M., Efrat, S., Auer, G., Wall, R.J., Furth, P.A. and Hennighausen, L. Time-sensitive reversal of hyperplasia in transgenic mice expressing SV40 T antigen. (1996). *Science,* 273, 1384-1386.

Fraumeni, J.F., Jr., Ederer, F. and Miller, R.W. An evaluation of the carcinogenicity of simian virus 40 in man. (1963). *Jama,* 185, 713-718.

Frizelle, S.P., Grim, J., Zhou, J., Gupta, P., Curiel, D.T., Geradts, J. and Kratzke, R.A. Re-expression of p16INK4a in mesothelioma cells results in cell cycle arrest, cell death, tumor suppression and tumor regression. (1998). *Oncogene,* 16, 3087-3095.

Galateau-Salle, F., Bidet, P., Iwatsubo, Y., Gennetay, E., Renier, A., Letourneux, M., Pairon, J.C., Moritz, S., Brochard, P., Jaurand, M.C. *et al.* SV40-like DNA sequences in pleural mesothelioma, bronchopulmonary carcinoma, and non-malignant pulmonary diseases. (1998). *J. Pathol.,* 184, 252-257.

Garcea, R.L. and Imperiale, M.J. Simian virus 40 infection of humans. (2003). *J. Virol.,* 77, 5039-5045.

Gaudray, P., Rassoulzadegan, M. and Cuzin, F. Expression of simian virus 40 early genes in transformed rat cells is correlated with maintenance of the transformed phenotype. (1978). *Proc. Natl. Acad. Sci. USA*, 75, 4987-4991.

Gazdar, A.F., Butel, J.S. and Carbone, M. SV40 and human tumours: myth, association or causality? (2002). *Nat. Rev. Cancer*, 2, 957-964.

Gordon, G.J., Chen, C.J., Jaklitsch, M.T., Richards, W.G., Sugarbaker, D.J. and Bueno, R. Detection and quantification of SV40 large T-antigen DNA in mesothelioma tissues and cell lines. (2002). *Oncology reports*, 9, 631-634.

Griffiths, D.J., Nicholson, A.G. and Weiss, R.A. Detection of SV40 sequences in human mesothelioma. (1998). *Dev. Biol. Stand.*, 94, 127-136.

Gurney, E.G., Harrison, R.O. and Fenno, J. Monoclonal antibodies against simian virus 40 T antigens: evidence for distinct subclasses of large T antigen and for similarities among nonviral T antigens. (1980). *J. Virol.*, 34, 752-763.

Hahn, W.C., Counter, C.M., Lundberg, A.S., Beijersbergen, R.L., Brooks, M.W. and Weinberg, R.A. Creation of human tumour cells with defined genetic elements. (1999). *Nature*, 400, 464-468.

Hahn, W.C., Dessain, S.K., Brooks, M.W., King, J.E., Elenbaas, B., Sabatini, D.M., DeCaprio, J.A. and Weinberg, R.A. Enumeration of the simian virus 40 early region elements necessary for human cell transformation. (2002). *Mol. Cell Biol.*, 22, 2111-2123.

Heinonen, O.P., Shapiro, S., Monson, R.R., Hartz, S.C., Rosenberg, L. and Slone, D. Immunization during pregnancy against poliomyelitis and influenza in relation to childhood malignancy. (1973). *Int. J. Epidemiol.*, 2, 229-235.

Hirvonen, A., Mattson, K., Karjalainen, A., Ollikainen, T., Tammilehto, L., Hovi, T., Vainio, H., Pass, H.I., Resta, I.D., Carbone, M. *et al.* Simian virus 40 (SV40)-like DNA sequences not detectable in Finnish mesothelioma patients not exposed to SV40-contaminated polio vaccines. (1999). *Molecular Carcinogenesis,* 26, 93-99.

Hubner, R. and Van Marck, E. Reappraisal of the strong association between simian virus 40 and human malignant mesothelioma of the pleura (Belgium). (2002). *Cancer Causes Control,* 13, 121-129.

Jasani, B., Cristaudo, A., Emri, S.A., Gazdar, A.F., Gibbs, A., Krynska, B., Miller, C., Mutti, L., Radu, C., Tognon, M. *et al.* Association of SV40 with human tumours. (2001). *Seminars in Cancer Biology*, 11, 49-61.

Jasani, B., Jones, C.J., Radu, C., Wynford-Thomas, D., Navabi, H., Mason, M., Adams, M. and Gibbs, A. Simian virus 40 detection in human mesothelioma: reliability and significance of the available molecular evidence. (2001). *Front Biosci,* 6, E12-22.

Ke, Y., Reddel, R.R., Gerwin, B.I., Reddel, H.K., Somers, A.N., McMenamin, M.G., LaVeck, M.A., Stahel, R.A., Lechner, J.F. and Harris, C.C. Establishment of a human in vitro mesothelial cell model system for investigating mechanisms of asbestos-induced mesothelioma. (1989). *Am. J. Pathol.,* 134, 979-991.

Kim, J.Y.H., Koralnik, I.J., LeFave, M., Segal, R.A., Pfister, L.A. and Pomeroy, S.L. Medulloblastomas and primitive neuroectodermal tumors rarely contain polyomavirus DNA sequences. (2002). *Neuro-Oncology,* 4, 165-170.

Kimura, G. and Itagaki, A. Initiation and maintenance of cell transformation by simian virus 40: a viral genetic property. (1975). *Proc. Natl. Acad. Sci. USA*, 72, 673-677.

Kitamura, F., Araki, S., Suzuki, Y., Yokoyama, K., Tanigawa, T. and Iwasaki, R. Assessment of the mutations of p53 suppressor gene and Ha- and Ki-ras oncogenes in malignant mesothelioma in relation to asbestos exposure: a study of 12 American patients. (2002). *Ind. Health*, 40, 175-181.

Kitamura, F., Araki, S., Tanigawa, T., Miura, H., Akabane, H. and Iwasaki, R. Assessment of mutations of Ha- and Ki-ras oncogenes and the p53 suppressor gene in seven malignant mesothelioma patients exposed to asbestos--PCR-SSCP and sequencing analyses of paraffin-embedded primary tumors. (1998). *Ind. Health*, 36, 52-56.

Klein, G., Powers, A. and Croce, C. Association of SV40 with human tumors. (2002). *Oncogene,* 21, 1141-1149.

Knowles, W.A. Discovery and epidemiology of the human polyomaviruses BK virus (BKV) and JC virus (JCV). (2006). *Adv. Exp. Med. Biol.*, 577, 19-45.

Knowles, W.A., Pipkin, P., Andrews, N., Vyse, A., Minor, P., Brown, D.W.G. and Miller, E. Population-based study of antibody to the human polyomaviruses BKV and JCV and the simian polyomavirus SV40. (2003). *Journal of Medical Virology*, 71, 115-123.

Kratzke, R.A., Otterson, G.A., Lincoln, C.E., Ewing, S., Oie, H., Geradts, J. and Kaye, F.J. Immunohistochemical analysis of the p16INK4 cyclin-dependent kinase inhibitor in malignant mesothelioma. (1995). *J. Natl. Cancer Inst.*, 87, 1870-1875.

Law, M.F., Martin, J.D., Takemoto, K.K. and Howley, P.M. The colinear alignment of the genomes of papovaviruses JC, BK, and SV40. (1979). *Virology,* 96, 576-587.

Lednicky, J.A. and Butel, J.S. Simian virus 40 regulatory region structural diversity and the association of viral archetypal regulatory regions with human brain tumors. (2001). *Semin.Cancer Biol.*, 11, 39-47.

Lednicky, J.A. and Butel, J.S. Tissue culture adaptation of natural isolates of simian virus 40: changes occur in viral regulatory region but not in carboxy-terminal domain of large T-antigen. (1997). *J. Gen. Virol.*, 78 (Pt 7), 1697-1705.

Lednicky, J.A., Garcea, R.L., Bergsagel, D.J. and Butel, J.S. Natural simian virus 40 strains are present in human choroid plexus and ependymoma tumors. (1995). *Virology,* 212, 710-717.

Leithner, A., Weinhaeusel, A., Windhager, R., Schlegl, R., Waldner, P., Lang, S., Dominkus, M., Zoubek, A., Popper, H.H. and Haas, O.A. Absence of SV40 in Austrian tumors correlates with low incidence of mesotheliomas. (2002). *Cancer biology and therapy*, 1, 375-379.

Levine, A.J. and Burger, M.M. A working hypothesis explaining the maintenance of the transformed state by SV40 and polyoma. (1972). *J. Theor. Biol.*, 37, 436-446.

Levrero, M. Viral hepatitis and liver cancer: the case of hepatitis C. (2006). *Oncogene,* 25, 3834-3847.

Li, R.M., Branton, M.H., Tanawattanacharoen, S., Falk, R.A., Jennette, J.C. and Kopp, J.B. Molecular identification of SV40 infection in human subjects and possible association with kidney disease. (2002). *J. Am. Soc. Nephrol.*, 13, 2320-2330.

Ilei, P.B., Rusch, V.W., Zakowski, M.F. and Ladanyi, M. Homozygous deletion of CDKN2A and codeletion of the methylthioadenosine phosphorylase gene in the majority of pleural mesotheliomas. (2003). *Clinical Cancer Research*, 9, 2108-2113.

Lopez-Rios, F., Illei, P.B., Rusch, V. and Ladanyi, M. Evidence against a role for SV40 infection in human mesotheliomas and high risk of false-positive PCR results owing to presence of SV40 sequences in common laboratory plasmids. (2004). *Lancet,* 364, 1157-1166.

MacKenzie, J., Wilson, K.S., Perry, J., Gallagher, A. and Jarrett, R.F. Association between simian virus 40 DNA and lymphoma in the United Kingdom. (2003). *JNCI,* 95, 1001-1003.

MacLachlan, D.S. SV40 in human tumors: new documents shed light on the apparent controversy. (2002). *Anticancer Res.*, 22, 3495-3499.

Manfredi, J.J. and Prives, C. The transforming activity of simian virus 40 large tumor antigen. (1994). *Biochim. Biophys. Acta*, 1198, 65-83.

Manfredi, J.J., Dong, J., Liu, W.J., Resnick-Silverman, L., Qiao, R., Chahinian, P., Saric, M., Gibbs, A.R., Phillips, J.I., Murray, J. *et al.* Evidence against a role for SV40 in human mesothelioma. (2005). *Cancer Res.*, 65, 2602-2609.

Martin, R.G. and Chou, J.Y. Simian virus 40 functions required for the establishment and maintenance of malignant transformation. (1975). *J. Virol.*, 15, 599-612.

Mayall, F., Barratt, K. and Shanks, J. The detection of Simian virus 40 in mesotheliomas from New Zealand and England using real time FRET probe PCR protocols. (2003). *Journal of Clinical Pathology*, 56, 728-730.

McConnell, E.E. and Carbone, M. A comparison of pleural mesotheliomas induced by asbestos or SV40 virus in Syrian golden hamsters. (2000). *Inhalation Toxicology*, 12 (Supplement 3), 173-181.

Mendoza, S.M., Konishi, T. and Miller, C.W. Integration of SV40 in human osteosarcoma DNA. (1998). *Oncogene,* 17, 2457-2462.

Metcalf, R.A., Welsh, J.A., Bennett, W.P., Seddon, M.B., Lehman, T.A., Pelin, K., Linnainmaa, K., Tammilehto, L., Mattson, K., Gerwin, B.I. *et al.* p53 and Kirsten-ras mutations in human mesothelioma cell lines. (1992). *Cancer Res.*, 52, 2610-2615.

Modi, S., Kubo, A., Oie, H., Coxon, A.B., Rehmatulla, A. and Kaye, F.J. Protein expression of the RB-related gene family and SV40 large T antigen in mesothelioma and lung cancer. (2000). *Oncogene*, 19, 4632-4639.

Mor, O., Yaron, P., Huszar, M., Yellin, A., Jakobovitz, O., Brok-Simoni, F., Rechavi, G. and Reichert, N. Absence of p53 mutations in malignant mesotheliomas. (1997). *Am. J. Respir. Cell Mol. Biol.*, 16, 9-13.

Morgan, D.O. Principles of cdk regulation. (1995). *Nature*, 374, 131-134.

Mortimer, E.A., Jr., Lepow, M.L., Gold, E., Robbins, F.C., Burton, G.J. and Fraumeni, J.F., Jr. Long-term follow-up of persons inadvertently inoculated with SV40 as neonates. (1981). *N. Engl. J. Med.*, 305, 1517-1518.

Mulatero, C., Surentheran, T., Breuer, J. and Rudd, R.M. Simian virus 40 and human pleural mesothelioma. (1999). *Thorax,* 54, 60-61.

Olin, P. and Giesecke, J. Potential exposure to SV40 in polio vaccines used in Sweden during 1957: no impact on cancer incidence rates 1960 to 1993. (1998). *Dev. Biol. Stand.,* 94, 227-233.

Osborn, M. and Weber, K. Simian virus 40 gene A function and maintenance of transformation. (1975). *J. Virol.*, 15, 636-644.

Pagano, J.S. Viruses and lymphomas. (2002). N Engl J Med, 347, 78-79.

Paracchini, V., Garte, S., Pedotti, P. and Taioli, E. Review of prevalence of Simian Virus 40 (SV40) genomic infection in healthy subjects. (2006). *Mutat. Res.*, 612, 77-83.

Pass, H.I. and Mew, D.J. In vitro and in vivo studies of mesothelioma. (1996). *J. Cell Biochem. Suppl.*, 24, 142-151.

Pepper, C., Jasani, B., Navabi, H., Wynford-Thomas, D. and Gibbs, A.R. Simian virus 40 large T antigen (SV40LTAg) primer specific DNA amplification in human pleural mesothelioma tissue. (1996). *Thorax*, 51, 1074-1076.

Pilatte, Y., Vivo, C., Renier, A., Kheuang, L., Greffard, A. and Jaurand, M.C. Absence of SV40 large T-antigen expression in human mesothelioma cell lines. (2000). *Am. J. Respir. Cell Mol. Biol.,* 23, 788-793.

Pipas, J.M. and Levine, A.J. Role of T antigen interactions with p53 in tumorigenesis. (2001). *Semin. Cancer Biol.*, 11, 23-30.

Porcu, P., Ferber, A., Pietrzkowski, Z., Roberts, C.T., Adamo, M., LeRoith, D. and Baserga, R. The growth-stimulatory effect of simian virus 40 T antigen requires the interaction of insulinlike growth factor 1 with its receptor. (1992). *Mol. Cell Biol.,* 12, 5069-5077.

Price, T.N., Moorwood, K., James, M.R., Burke, J.F. and Mayne, L.V. Cell cycle progression, morphology and contact inhibition are regulated by the amount of SV40 T antigen in immortal human cells. (1994). *Oncogene,* 9, 2897-2904.

Prins, J.B., Williamson, K.A., Kamp, M.M.K., Van Hezik, E.J., Van Der Kwast, T.H., Hagemeijer, A. and Versnel, M.A. The gene for the cyclin-dependent-kinase-4 inhibitor, CDKN2A, is preferentially deleted in malignant mesothelioma. (1998). *International Journal of Cancer,* 75, 649-653.

Radna, R.L., Caton, Y., Jha, K.K., Kaplan, P., Li, G., Traganos, F. and Ozer, H.L. Growth of immortal simian virus 40 tsA-transformed human fibroblasts is temperature dependent. (1989). *Mol. Cell Biol.,* 9, 3093-3096.

Ramael, M., Nagels, J., Heylen, H., De Schepper, S., Paulussen, J., De Maeyer, M. and Van Haesendonck, C. Detection of SV40 like viral DNA and viral antigens in malignant pleural mesothelioma. (1999). *Eur. Respir. J.*, 14, 1381-1386.

Rizzo, P., Bocchetta, M., Powers, A., Foddis, R., Stekala, E., Pass, H.I. and Carbone, M. SV40 and the pathogenesis of mesothelioma. (2001). *Semin. Cancer Biol.*, 11, 63-71.

Rizzo, P., Carbone, M., Fisher, S.G., Matker, C., Swinnen, L.J., Powers, A., Di Resta, I., Alkan, S., Pass, H.I. and Fisher, R.I. Simian virus 40 is present in most United States human mesotheliomas, but it is rarely present in non-Hodgkin's lymphoma. (1999). *Chest,* 116, 470S-473S.

Rollison, D.E., Page, W.F., Crawford, H., Gridley, G., Wacholder, S., Martin, J., Miller, R. and Engels, E.A. Case-control study of cancer among US Army veterans exposed to simian virus 40-contaminated adenovirus vaccine. (2004). *Am. J. Epidemiol.,* 160, 317-324.

Rollison, D.E.M., Helzlsouer, K.J., Alberg, A.J., Hoffman, S., Hou, J., Daniel, R., Shah, K.V. and Major, E.O. Serum antibodies to JC virus, BK virus, simian virus 40, and the risk of incident adult astrocytic brain tumors. (2003). *Cancer Epidemiology Biomarkers and Prevention,* 12, 460-463.

Rosa, F.W., Sever, J.L. and Madden, D.L. Absence of antibody response to simian virus 40 after inoculation with killed-poliovirus vaccine of mothers of offspring with neurologic tumors. (1988). *N. Engl. J. Med.*, 318, 1469.

Rovigatti, U. and Basilico, C. Expression of the SV40-transformed phenotype in hybrids between conditional and wild-type transformants. (1977). *Exp. Cell Res.*, 106, 277-284.

Rundell, K. and Parakati, R. The role of the SV40 ST antigen in cell growth promotion and transformation. (2001). *Semin. Cancer Biol.*, 11, 5-13.

Rybkin, II, Markham, D.W., Yan, Z., Bassel-Duby, R., Williams, R.S. and Olson, E.N. Conditional expression of SV40 T-antigen in mouse cardiomyocytes facilitates an inducible switch from proliferation to differentiation. (2003). *J. Biol. Chem.,* 278, 15927-15934.

Salewski, H., Bayer, T.A., Eidhoff, U., Preuss, U., Weggen, S. and Scheidtmann, K.H. Increased oncogenicity of subclones of SV40 large T-induced neuroectodermal tumor cell lines after loss of large T expression and concomitant mutation in p53. (1999). *Cancer Res*., 59, 1980-1986.

Scheffner, M., Werness, B.A., Huibregtse, J.M., Levine, A.J. and Howley, P.M. The E6 oncoprotein encoded by human papillomavirus types 16 and 18 promotes the degradation of p53. (1990). *Cell*, 63, 1129-1136.

Schell, T.D. and Tevethia, S.S. Control of advanced choroid plexus tumors in SV40 T antigen transgenic mice following priming of donor CD8(+) T lymphocytes by the endogenous tumor antigen. (2001). *J. Immunol.*, 167, 6947-6956.

Schell, T.D. and Tevethia, S.S. Cytotoxic T lymphocytes in SV40 infections. (2001). Methods Mol Biol, 165, 243-256.

Schuler, F., Dolken, S.C., Hirt, C., Dolken, M.T., Mentel, R., Gurtler, L.G. and Dolken, G. No evidence for simian virus 40 DNA sequences in malignant non-Hodgkin lymphomas. (2006). *International Journal of Cancer*, 118, 498-504.

Shah, K. and Nathanson, N. Human exposure to SV40: review and comment. (1976). *Am. J. Epidemiol.*, 103, 1-12.

Shah, K.V. Does SV40 infection contribute to the development of human cancers? (2000). *Rev. Med. Virol.*, 10, 31-43.

Shah, K.V., Galloway, D.A., Knowles, W.A. and Viscidi, R.P. Simian virus 40 (SV40) and human cancer: a review of the serological data. (2004). *Rev. Med. Virol.*, 14, 231-239.

Sherr, C.J. The INK4a/ARF network in tumour suppression. (2001). *Nature Reviews Molecular Cell Biology*, 2, 731-737.

Sherwood, R.W., Buescher, E.L., Nitz, R.E. and Cooch, J.W. Effects of adenovirus vaccine on acute respiratory disease in U. S. Army recruits. (1961). *JAMA*, 178, 1125-1127.

Shimizu, E., Coxon, A., Otterson, G.A., Steinberg, S.M., Kratzke, R.A., Kim, Y.W., Fedorko, J., Oie, H., Johnson, B.E., Mulshine, J.L. *et al.* RB protein status and clinical correlation from 171 cell lines representing lung cancer, extrapulmonary small cell carcinoma, and mesothelioma. (1994). *Oncogene*, 9, 2441-2448.

Shivapurkar, N., Wiethege, T., Wistuba, II, Milchgrub, S., Muller, K.M. and Gazdar, A.F. Presence of simian virus 40 sequences in malignant pleural, peritoneal and noninvasive mesotheliomas. (2000). *Int. J. Cancer,* 85, 743-745.

Shivapurkar, N., Wiethege, T., Wistuba, II, Salomon, E., Milchgrub, S., Muller, K.M., Churg, A., Pass, H. and Gazdar, A.F. Presence of simian virus 40 sequences in malignant mesotheliomas and mesothelial cell proliferations. (1999). *J. Cell Biochem.*, 76, 181-188.

Simsir, A., Fetsch, P., Bedrossian, C.W., Ioffe, O.B. and Abati, A. Absence of SV-40 large T antigen (Tag) in malignant mesothelioma effusions: an immunocytochemical study. (2001). *Diagn. Cytopathol*, 25, 203-207.

Steinberg, B., Pollack, R., Topp, W. and Botchan, M. Isolation and characterization of T antigen-negative revertants from a line of transformed rat cells containing one copy of the SV40 genome. (1978). *Cell,* 13, 19-32.

Stewart, A.R., Lednicky, J.A., Benzick, U.S., Tevethia, M.J. and Butel, J.S. Identification of a variable region at the carboxy terminus of SV40 large T-antigen. (1996). *Virology,* 221, 355-361.

Stratton, K., Alamario, D.A. and McCormick, M.C. (eds.) (2003) *Immunization Safety Review: SV40 Contamination of Polio Vaccine and Cancer, Institute of Medicine of the National Academies*. The National Academies Press, Washington, D.C.

Strickler, H.D. A multicenter evaluation of assays for detection of SV40 DNA and results in masked mesothelioma specimens. (2001). *Cancer Epidemiol Biomarkers Prev*, 10, 523-532.

Strickler, H.D. and Goedert, J.J. Exposure to SV40-contaminated poliovirus vaccine and the risk of cancer--a review of the epidemiological evidence. (1998). *Dev. Biol. Stand,* 94, 235-244.

Strickler, H.D., Goedert, J.J., Devesa, S.S., Lahey, J., Fraumeni Jr, J.F. and Rosenberg, P.S. Trends in U.S. pleural mesothelioma incidence rates following simian virus 40 contamination of early poliovirus vaccines. (2003). *Journal of the National Cancer Institute*, 95, 38-45.

Strickler, H.D., Goedert, J.J., Fleming, M., Travis, W.D., Williams, A.E., Rabkin, C.S., Daniel, R.W. and Shah, K.V. Simian virus 40 and pleural mesothelioma in humans. (1996). *Cancer Epidemiol. Biomarkers Prev.*, 5, 473-475.

Strickler, H.D., Rosenberg, P.S., Devesa, S.S., Hertel, J., Fraumeni, J.F., Jr. and Goedert, J.J. Contamination of poliovirus vaccines with simian virus 40 (1955-1963) and subsequent cancer rates. (1998). *JAMA*, 279, 292-295.

Symonds, H., Krall, L., Remington, L., Saenz-Robles, M., Lowe, S., Jacks, T. and Van Dyke, T. p53-dependent apoptosis suppresses tumor growth and progression in vivo. (1994). *Cell,* 78, 703-711.

Testa, J.R. and Giordano, A. SV40 and cell cycle perturbations in malignant mesothelioma. (2001). *Semin Cancer Biol*, 11, 31-38.

Testa, J.R., Carbone, M., Hirvonen, A., Khalili, K., Krynska, B., Linnainmaa, K., Pooley, F.D., Rizzo, P., Rusch, V. and Xiao, G.H. A multi-institutional study confirms the presence and expression of simian virus 40 in human malignant mesotheliomas. (1998). *Cancer Res*., 58, 4505-4509.

Thomas, M., Pim, D. and Banks, L. The role of the E6-p53 interaction in the molecular pathogenesis of HPV. (1999). *Oncogene*, 18, 7690-7700.

Thu, G.O., Hem, L.Y., Hansen, S., M¯ller, B., Norstein, J., N¯kleby, H. and Grotmol, T. Is there an association between SV40 contaminated polio vaccine and lymphoproliferative disorders? An age-period-cohort analysis on Norwegian data from 1953 to 1997. (2006). *International Journal of Cancer*, 118, 2035-2039.

Tognon, M., Martini, F., Corallini, A. and Barbanti-Brodano, G. SV40 and human cancers. (2004). *Int. J. Cancer,* 110, 778-779; author reply 780.

Tsuyama, N., Miura, M., Kitahira, M., Ishibashi, S. and Ide, T. SV40 T-antigen is required for maintenance of immortal growth in SV40-transformed human fibroblasts. (1991). *Cell Struct. Funct.*, 16, 55-62.

Tzeng, Y.J., Zimmermann, C., Guhl, E., Berg, B., Avantaggiati, M.L. and Graessmann, A. SV40 T/t-antigen induces premature mammary gland involution by apoptosis and selects for p53 missense mutation in mammary tumors. (1998). *Oncogene,* 16, 2103-2114.

Ungar, S., Van de Meeren, A., Tammilehto, L., Linnainmaa, K., Mattson, K. and Gerwin, B.I. High levels of MDM2 are not correlated with the presence of wild-type p53 in human malignant mesothelioma cell lines. (1996). *Br. J. Cancer,* 74, 1534-1540.

Vaslet, C.A., Messier, N.J. and Kane, A.B. Accelerated progression of asbestos-induced mesotheliomas in heterozygous p53+/- mice. (2002). *Toxicol. Sci.*, 68, 331-338.

Villunger, A., Michalak, E.M., Coultas, L., Mullauer, F., Bock, G., Ausserlechner, M.J., Adams, J.M. and Strasser, A. p53- and Drug-Induced Apoptotic Responses Mediated by BH3-Only Proteins Puma and Noxa. (2003). *Science,* 302, 1036-1038.

Volter, C., zur Hausen, H., Alber, D. and de Villiers, E.M. A broad spectrum PCR method for the detection of polyomaviruses and avoidance of contamination by cloning vectors. (1998). *Dev. Biol. Stand.*, 94, 137-142.

Vousden, K.H. and Lu, X. Live or let die: the cell's response to p53. (2002). *Nat. Rev. Cancer,* 2, 594-604.

Waheed, I., Guo, Z.S., Chen, G.A., Weiser, T.S., Nguyen, D.M. and Schrump, D.S. Antisense to SV40 early gene region induces growth arrest and apoptosis in T-antigen-positive human pleural mesothelioma cells. (1999). *Cancer Res.*, 59, 6068-6073.

Werness, B.A., Levine, A.J. and Howley, P.M. Association of human papillomavirus types 16 and 18 E6 proteins with p53. (1990). *Science*, 248, 76-79.

Xiao, S., Li, D., Vijg, J., Sugarbaker, D.J., Corson, J.M. and Fletcher, J.A. Codeletion of p15 and p16 in primary malignant mesothelioma. (1995). *Oncogene,* 11, 511-515.

Yamamoto, H., Nakayama, T., Murakami, H., Hosaka, T., Nakamata, T., Tsuboyama, T., Oka, M., Nakamura, T. and Toguchida, J. High incidence of SV40-like sequences detection in tumour and peripheral blood cells of Japanese osteosarcoma patients. (2000). *Br. J. Cancer,* 82, 1677-1681.

Zalvide, J., Stubdal, H. and DeCaprio, J.A. The J domain of simian virus 40 large T antigen is required to functionally inactivate RB family proteins. (1998). *Mol. Cell Biol.*, 18, 1408-1415.

zur Hausen, H. Papillomaviruses in human cancer. (1987). *Cancer,* 59, 1692-1696.

zur Hausen, H. SV40 in human cancers: response. (2004). *Int. J. Cancer,* 110, 780.

zur Hausen, H. SV40 in human cancers--an endless tale? (2003). *Int. J. Cancer,* 107, 687.

In: Mesothelioma from Bench Side to Clinic
Editor: Alfonso Baldi, pp. 265-278
ISBN: 978-1-60021-789-0

Chapter XIII

Pathology of Malignant Mesothelioma

Luigi M. Terracciano, Florinda Feroce and Luigi Tornillo
Department of Pathology
University of Basel, Basel, Switzerland

Abstract

Mesothelioma is an uncommon diffuse neoplasm that originates from the mesothelial cells lining body cavities, in particular pleura and peritoneum. Rarely, pleural mesothelioma may be localized and readily resectable for cure. However the great majority of mesothelioma are highly aggressive and treatment-resistant malignant tumours.

Approximately 90-95% of mesotheliomas arise in the pleural cavity and 5-10% in the peritoneal cavity. Rare mesotheliomas arise in the pericardium and in the tunica vaginalis. Unlike many neoplasms, mesotheliomas grow in a diffuse distribution and tend to encase the organs in the various body cavities. A combination of histochemical, immunohistochemical, and ultrastructural features are often necessary to obtain an accurate diagnosis.

Gross Features

Malignant pleural mesotheliomas are typically “diffuse” tumors characterized in the early stages by multiple small tumor nodules studding the visceral and parietal pleural surface. These nodules range from 1 mm to occasionally 1cm. Progression of the tumor results in coalescence of the nodules to form plaques and, ultimately, a continuous sheet of tumor with encasement of the underlying organ. Encasement by a rind of tumor is usually a sign of advanced disease and with time this process may obliterate the pleural, pericardial or peritoneal cavity. Pleural mesotheliomas frequently invade chest wall skeletal muscle and sometimes skin and subcutaneous tissue. They quite often invade the hemidiaphragms and extend into the abdominal cavity. In the pleural cavity they typically infiltrate along the fissures between the lobes of the lung, along biopsy tracks or surgical incisions.

Metastases are late but they may be widespread at death. Occasionally, pleural mesotheliomas metastasize to hilar lymph nodes and produce an hilar mass. In peritoneal cavity, tumor encasement of the bowel is seen in advanced disease. Sometimes encasement may be so extensive that the abdominal organs appear noticeably atrophic. Most peritoneal mesotheliomas, like pleural mesotheliomas, are initially associated with an effusion.

Primary mesotheliomas that arise in the tunica vaginalis often present as a mass in that location. They can remain localized, but more frequently they invade the peritoneal cavity.

Primary pericardial mesotheliomas are rare. They frequently invade the myocardium. However, before performing the diagnosis of primary pericardial mesothelioma a pericardial extension of a pleural mesothelioma should be excluded.

Rarely, mesotheliomas occur as a localized mass rather than a diffuse involvement of a body cavity. These types occur most frequently in the pleural cavity and are called *localized malignant mesotheliomas*. However, the general rule of thumb is that the gross finding of a rather localized than diffuse disease should prompt one to doubt about the diagnosis of mesothelioma.

Microscopic Subtypes

Malignant mesotheliomas are subtyped into three major categories: epithelial, sarcomatoid and biphasic (mixed) type. Moreover, among the sarcomatoid mesotheliomas, one should distinguish the desmoplastic type, which is particularly aggressive. On the other hand, no general agreement exists on the nomenclature of other morphologic subtypes. Recognition of histologic subtypes is indeed important for the morphologic diagnosis, but they do not show an important clinical significance.

Among epithelial mesothelioma several histologic subtypes have been reported (Table 1). Furthermore, it is frequent, mainly in epithelial mesothelioma, to observe two or more histologic patterns. One can often see 5 or 6 histologic subtypes of differentiation by the tumor and the more sections one takes, the more likely the tumor is found to be biphasic.

Table 1. Epithelial Mesothelial Subtypes

1	Tubulopapillary	10	Glomeruloid
2	Glandula	11	In association with excessive amounts of hyaluronic acid/proteoglycan
3	Histiocytoid	12	Small cell
4	Adenoid cystic	13	Poorly differentiated (large cell) / pleomorphic
5	Microcystic	14	Deciduoid
6	Macrocystic	15	Mucin positive
7	Signet ring	16	Gaucher cell-like
8	Single file	17	*In situ*
9	Diffuse-NOS		

Mesotheliomas are aggressive tumors; notwithstanding, their histologic aspect is quite bland and monotonous so that differentiating them from benign reactive mesothelial proliferations can be difficult. The number of mitoses is not a criterion, as well as the presence of necrosis. Furthermore no standard grading schemes have been adopted.

Epithelial Mesothelioma

As mentioned above, epithelial mesotheliomas are deceptively bland. They are formed by cuboidal or polygonal (sometimes flattened) cells, with moderate amounts of eosinophilic cytoplasm and round nuclei containing a single, often evident nucleolus. In most epithelial mesotheliomas the cells are sharply demarcated and often they form tubular structures. Mitoses are infrequent. These morphologic features are quite different from those of metastatic carcinomas, which generally display more pleomorphic cytological features and often show columnar differentiation. Moreover, in carcinomas, necrosis is more frequent and the mitotic index is higher. On the other hand, it could be difficult to differentiate this form from benign mesothelial proliferations. Benign mesothelial cells are usually smaller and do not infiltrate fat and muscle. Furthermore, it must be remembered that longstanding pleural effusions are associated with reactive proliferation of mesothelial cells, which may appear in needle biopsy as loose aggregates in a fibrinous background. The presence of papillae in such biopsies is suggestive of mesothelioma but by no means pathognomonic.

Morphologic Subtypes of Epithelial Mesothelioma

Deciduoid mesothelioma. This pattern, first described in the peritoneum of young women, was initially thought to represent a bizarre benign decidual reaction as a form of endometriosis. Subsequently, it has been shown, by immunohistochemical and ultrastructural evidence, that these cells are indeed mesothelial and behave as a malignancy. Moreover they can also occur in the pleura. Typically deciduoid mesotheliomas are composed by large polygonal cells with eosinophilic cytoplasm that somewhat resemble decidua.

Tubulopapillary mesothelioma. This is one of the most frequent patterns of epithelial mesothelioma . It consists of small tubules and papillary structures with fibrovascular cores, lined by uniform, polygonal, cuboidal or flattened cells that are cytologically bland. Sometimes the cells are peg-shaped, with only a narrow base. A in other papillary neoplasms, psammoma bodies can be also seen, but they are not frequent.

The cells of epithelial mesothelioma can show cytoplasmic vacuoles that are typically diastase-PAS negative. This finding can help in the diffferential diagnosis with carcinoma.

Microcystic (adenomatoid, microglandular) mesothelioma. This form is histologically characterized by lace-like spaces lined by flattened cells. In these spaces a pale haematoxyphilic material is sometimes observed. It stains with Alcian blue pH 2.5 and is removed by hyaluronidase. Occasionally this material can form lakes so that on gross examination the tumors may appear cystic. Rarely, the differential diagnosis can be made with adenomatoid tumor, that are however very rare in the pleura and do not show a propensity to infiltrate.

Small cell mesothelioma. This pattern is very rarely observed . The tumor is composed by very small cells in sheets and can be similar to small cell carcinoma of the lung . On the other hand, the cells do not form neither rosettes nor nests and do not stain for chromogranin. Mitoses are rare and chromatin is clear. Crushing artifacts are usually not observed and the tumor shows in other areas typical patterns of epithelial mesotheliomas.

Solid (well-differentiated) pattern. This is a very common histologic pattern. It is characterized by round or polygonal cells with abundant granular cytoplasm and round nuclei with evident nucleoli and a very low mitotic index. Particularly, this histologic subtype can be difficult to differentiate from reactive mesothelial proliferation. In general, the lacking of clear evidence of infiltration should make one hesitate before diagnosing a malignat mesothelioma.

Solid (poorly-differentiated) pattern. It consists of discohesive polygonal cells with large cytoplasm and quite monotonous nuclei, arranged in sheets and nests. The differential diagnosis is with large cell lymhoma or large cell carcinoma.

Clear cell mesothelioma. It is characterized by cells with clear cytoplasm. The differential diagnosis is with other clear cell tumors metastatic to the serosa (clear cell carcinoma of the kidney, clear cell carcinoma of the lung, clear cell melanoma, etc.).

Mucin-positive epithelial mesotheliomas. In general, mesotheliomas do not produce neutral mucins and therefore they are negative for PAS diastase, mucicarmine and Alcian blue/colloidal iron. Epithelial mesotheliomas frequently contain glycogen and are PAS-positive with this reaction eradicated with pretreatment with diastase. The production of hyaluronic acid is highlighted by Alcian blue pH 2.5 that is normally removed by pretreatment with hyaluronidase . In 2-5% of cases however, epithelial mesotheliomas may stain positive also after pretreatment with hyluronidase. These tumors are referred to as *mucin-positive epithelial mesotheliomas*. This intracellular material probably represents cristallized proteoglygcans. These tumors may also show immunohistochemical positivity for markers as CEA,m LeuM1 and B72.3 , making the differential diagnosis with lung adenocarcinoma particularly difficult.

Gaucher Cell-Like

Rare mesotheliomas may display a Gaucher-like appearance that ultrastructurally is associated with a unique crystalloid material within the cisternae of rough endoplasmic reticulum of the neoplastic cells

Sarcomatoid (Fibrous) Mesothelioma

Sarcomatoid mesotheliomas may show a very broad range of appearances. Generally, they tend to be more pleomorphic and cytologically atypical than the epithelial types.

Sarcomatoid mesotheliomas are composed by spindle cells that may vary from bland to anaplastic appearance. A storiform "fibrous histiocytoma-like" pattern may be observed, together with giant cells or interlacing, fibrosarcoma-like bundles. Elements of osseous, chondroid, and, rarely leiomyomatous or rhabdomyosarcomatous metaplasia are observed.

They are set in a varying amount of collagenised stroma and the cellularity varies greatly. When scanty, bland spindle cells are widely scattered in a densely collagenised stroma the distinction from scar tissue may be very difficult, whilst more cellular tumours may resemble granulation tissue. At the other end of the spectrum, markedly pleomorphic, cellular foci are indistinguishable from other forms of undifferentiated sarcoma.

Morphologic Patterns of sarcomatoid Mesothelioma

Transitional mesothelioma. These are tumors in which the cells appear both spindle and very plump, depending on the plane of the section. It is therefore very difficult to assign them to the sarcomatoid or to the epithelial category. They behave like other sarcomatoid mesotheliomas.

Lymphohistiocytoid mesothelioma. This pattern is characterized by an intense inflammatory infiltrate (lymphocytes, plasma cells, eosinophils). Tumor cells are large, spindle or polygonal, with a somehow granular cytoplasm, vesicular nuclei and evident nucleoli. It is important not to overlook the tumor cells, that can be covered by the inflammatory cells and leading to the diagnosis of inflammatory process. Moreover, rare cases showing a marked lymphohistiocytoid reactive infiltrate, have been misdiagnosed as lymphomas.

Desmoplastic mesothelioma. Desmoplastic mesotheliomas are probably the most difficult of all mesotheliomas to diagnose. They should not be diagnosed from a needle core biopsy. After the first description in 1980, further small series have been reported. By definition, this tumor consists mostly of paucicellular, dense fibrous tissue. It occurs typically in the pleura. It shows a storiform or a so-called "patternless" pattern in at least 50% of the tumour, with few elongated, bland cells in the spaces between the collagen bundles. Because of these histological features, the primary differential diagnosis is fibrosing pleuritis. Therefore for diagnosing desmoplastic mesothelioma, the typical paucicellular pattern should be associated with at least one of the following one: invasion of the subparietal pleural fat/chest wall or invasion of the lung (most important), focal areas of stellate bland necrosis, areas of increased cellularity (sarcomatous foci) or distant metastases. Infiltrating cells are immunohistochemically keratin-positive. Invasion of the lung may result in an image somehow similar to organizing pneumonia. Bland necrosis is necrosis without cellular reaction. In sarcomatous foci the lesion is not distinguishable from typical sarcomatous mesothelioma. Therefore an area of high cellularity in a obviously fibrotic pleura should be regarded as suspicious and the lesion should be appropriately sampled. Rarely, the first manifestation of the tumour can be a metastasis.

An additional important histological feature are the so-called expansile stromal nodules: they have pushing borders and stain differently from the surrounding stroma. Interestingly, they are not present in organizing pleuritis. Rarely, osseous or cartilagineous metaplasia can be observed.

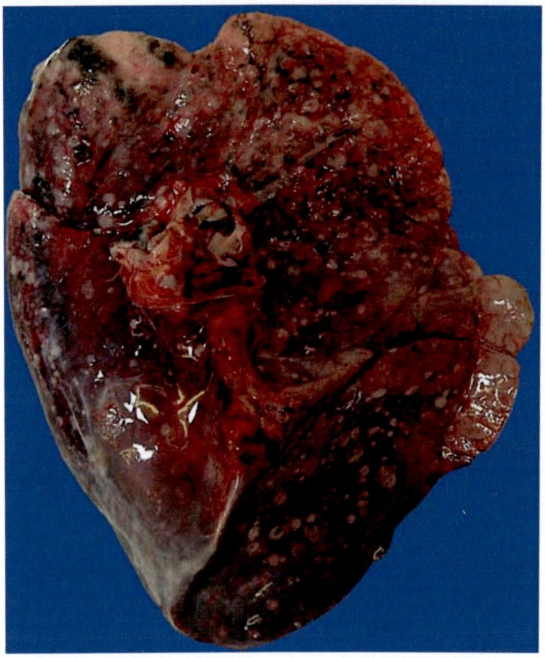

Figure 1. Malignant pleural mesothelioma appears as small tumor nodules.

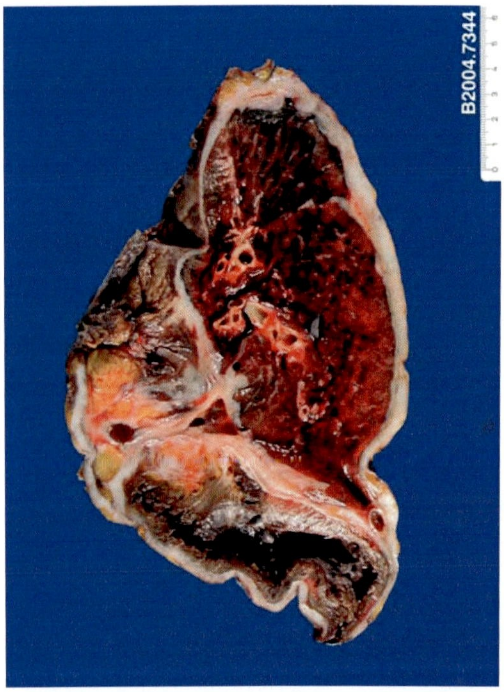

Figure 2. The tumor almost completely encases the lung extends along the major fissures.

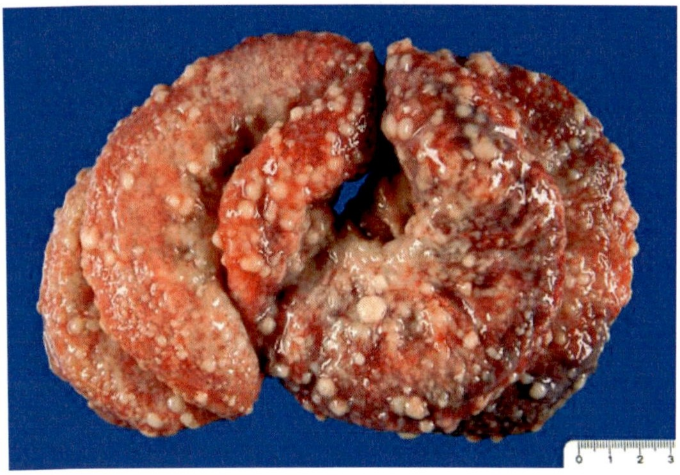

Figure 3. Malignant peritoneal mesothelioma showing small intestinal loop studded by multiple withish tumor nodules.

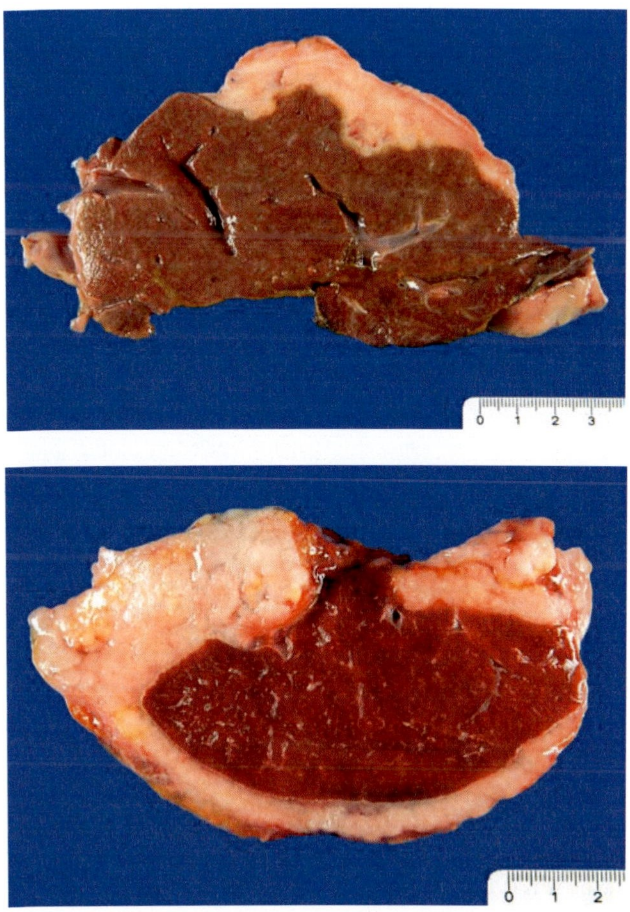

Figure 4. Malignant peritoneal mesothelioma encases visceral organs as liver (4a) and spleen (4b).

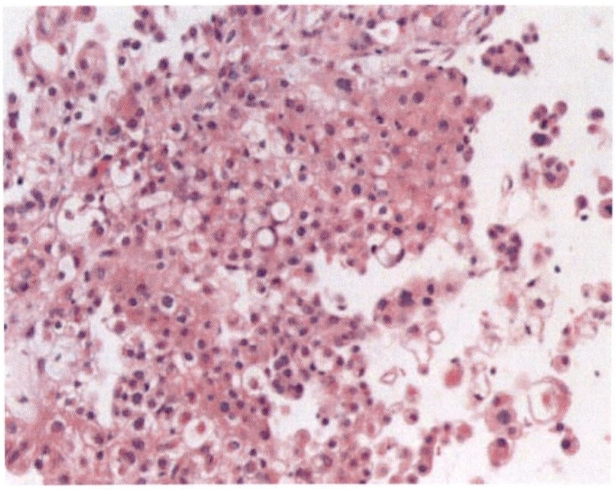

Figure 5. Malignant mesothelioma epithelial type showing monotonous and rather bland cytology.

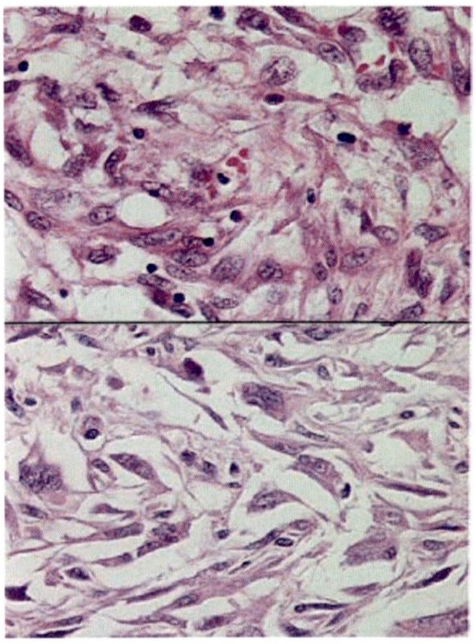

Figure 6. Malignant mesothelioma sarcomatous type characterized by plump spindle cells with little atypia.

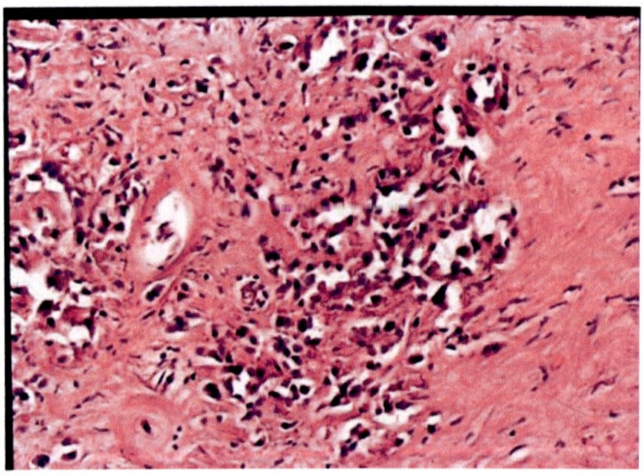

Figure 7. Desmoplastic mesothelioma consisting of paucicellular, densely collagenized tissue.

Mixed (Biphasic) Epithelial/Sarcomatous Mesothelioma

Any combination of the above described patterns can be observed. Mixed mesotheliomas account for nearly 30% of all malignant mesotheliomas. The transition between the epithelioid and the spindle component can be abrupt or gradual. Merging of the components of the tumour can often be seen, the transition from epithelial to spindle cells morphology being accompanied by dissociation of the tumour cells and an increase in the stroma.

Mesotheliomas of the Tunica Vaginalis

They are tin he two thirds of cases epithelial and in the remaining cases of mixed subtype. There are no morphologic differences with pleural or peritoneal tumours.

Mesothelioma of Pericardium

They are similar to mesotheliomas in other localizations.

Histochemistry of Mesothelioma

Mucin Stains

Diastase-PAS stains neutral mucins, which should be negative in mesotheliomas, with the exception of mucin-positive epithelioid mesotheliomas (see above), and is positive in carcinomas.

Alcian-blue pH 2.5 stains hyaluronic acid that disappears after pretreatment with hyaluronidase. Positivity after pretreatment is a hallmark of carcinomas. Most importantly, the positive staining should be intracellular (mucin droplets) or as lakes of mucin in cystic mesotheliomas. A positive stromal staining has obviously no meaning, because all stromas may contain hyaluronic acid.

Special Types of Mesothelioma

Well-Differentiated Papillary Mesothelioma

These are indolent tumours without tendency to invasion. They are typical of female peritoneal cavity, but may also be observed in pleura, pericardium and tunica vaginalis.

Histologically, well-differentiated papillary mesothelioma is composed by broad papillae covered by a single layer of flattened mesothelial cells. The fibrovascular core can sometimes be myxoid in appearance. Rarely, psammoma bodies are observed. The tumor cells are cytologically deceptively bland. Neither mitoses nor necrosis are present. In most of cases there is no invasion. It should be kept in mind that some epithelial malignant mesotheliomas may have areas looking like well-differentiated papillary mesotheliomas. Therefore, caution is needed in making such a diagnosis on scarse material (e.g. small pleural biopsies).

Localized Malignant Mesothelioma

Rare pleural tumours appear as a sharply circumscribed mass arising from the visceral or parietal pleura. Histologically, immunohistochemically and ultrastructurally the tumours are similar to diffuse malignant mesothelioma, but they do not spread over the pleura. It can locally recur and rarely metastasize. The diagnosis of localized malignant mesothelioma needs therefore evidence that the process is localized. Localized malignant mesotheliomas should be separated from the diffuse one because of their local presentation, quite different biologic behavior and far better prognosis.

Differential Diagnosis of Malignant Mesothelioma

Diffuse malignant mesothelioma should be differentiated from other tumors metastasizing to serosal membranes and from benign mesothelial processes.

Tumours Metastasizing to the Serosal Membranes

Epithelial mesotheliomas have to be differentiated from adenocarcinomas and other epithelial neoplasms. All malignant tumours can spread to the serosal membranes. Lung adenocarcinomas, lung squamous cell carcinomas and small cell carcinomas, thymomas, renal cell carcinomas, thyroid carcinoma, sarcomas, melanomas and lymphomas can grow in the pleura entrapping the lung, in a pattern that has been called *pseudomesotheliomatous*. Metastatic carcinomas of the gastrointestinal tract, the ovary, of the lung, the breast, the uterus and many sarcomas may grow in nodules or entrap the organs. In most cases the distinction is obvious. In difficult cases the histochemical and immunohistochemical features may be of help. Peculiar cases are the *primary serous papillary tumours of the peritoneum/metastatic serous papillary tumours of the ovary*. These are common tumours that grow in small nodules on the peritoneum. Histologically, they have atypical cells growing on delicate papillae with stratification. Frequently psammoma bodies are observed. Unlike mesotheliomas, they do not form gland-like structures and often show necrosis. In mesothelioma, stratification is usually not observed. Some of them may produce mucin droplets. With respect to sarcomatoid mesotheliomas, one has to be aware that sarcomatoid carcinomas of the kidney and pancreas can metastasize to the lung and form a macroscopic pattern characteristic of a mesothelioma (pseudomesotheliomatous metastatic sacrmatoid carcinoma).

Vascular tumors. The histologic distinction is sometimes very difficult, but they stain for CD31, CD34 or factor VIII, that are negative in mesotheliomas.

Synovial sarcoma. Some synovial sarcoma fairly extensively involve the pleura and can be extremely difficult to differentiate from a sarcomatoid mesothelioma or a biphasic mesothelioma. The spindle cells of this tumour are smaller than those of sarcomatoid mesotheliomas. In biphasic tumours there are often cleft-like spaces that are only occasionally observed in mesothelioma. The immunophenotype is not very helpful: synovial sarcomas may also stain for calretinin. They are often positive for BerEp4, that is not commonly positive in mesotheliomas. The detection of the fusion transcripts SYT-SSX1 or SYT-SSX2 by RT-PCR is quite specific for synovial sarcoma.

Differential Diagnosis with Benign Mesothelial Processes

This is a particularly difficult topic, as is shown by the results of the United States-Canadian Mesothelioma Reference Panel. For this differential diagnosis appropriate clinical and radiologic information are essential. If the clinician tells of a localized process, the diagnosis of diffuse malignant mesothelioma should be made with caution.

Epithelial-Type Proliferations

Proliferations Limited to the Surface

In hyperplasia of the mesothelium, the cells are not flattened, but rather cuboidal, with a monotonous appearance, sometimes with small nucleoli. It is the result of irritation of the serosa (ascites, endometriosis, inflammatory processes, other tumours). In some cases, the mesothelial proliferation may be florid, with some degree of cytological atypia, enlarged nuclei, prominent nucleoli and mild pleomorphism. These cases should be termed "atypical mesothelial hyperplasia", but no certain issue can be made on the biological and clinical meaning of these lesions. It is possible that some of these lesions may represent premalignant stages of malignant mesothelioma. So far, however, there are no reliable morphologic criteria to diagnose premalignant mesothelial lesions. It is well known for instance that benign mesothelial processes can also show severe cytologic atypia. In such cases, the diagnosis of "atyipical mesothelial proliferation" should be rendered.

Proliferations Invading Underlying Tissue

Probably the most reliable morphologic clue for the diagnosis of malignant mesothelioma is invasion of underlying tissue. Invasion is often straightforward to recognize. Many inflammatory processes, however, tend to "entrap" mesothelial cells in granulation tissue or in fibrosis. Such an "entrapment" can be difficult to differentiate from true invasion. Benign mesothelial proliferations usually do not invade the whole thickness of the pleura; malignant processes on the contrary extend to the chest wall or fat. Therefore it can be stated, that "the deeper the invasion, the more likely the process is to be malignant". A clear zonal distribution of the cellularity can be seen in benign proliferation: the cellularity is progressively lost (and fibrosis increased) moving away from the free serosal surfaces. This pattern is called "zonation". The presence of fibrin, inflammatory infiltrate and granulation tissue strongly favors a benign process, even if the mesothelial cells show atypical features (nucleoli, pleomoprhism, etc,). In inflammatory processes linear arrays of mesothelial cells or gland-like structures are common. In these cases a clue too the diagnosis is that they have always the same depth of penetration. In mesothelioma the cells invade disorderly the tissue, without any preferential orientation. Invasion of fat or muscle may be considered always as a sign of malignancy. All these considerations need of course a large biopsy specimen. When dealing with small biopsies, the orientation is doubtful and it is possible that apparent invasion may be merely the result of tangential orientation of the specimen. The presence of mesothelial lining on two surfaces is a good sign of such an orientation. Additional useful criteria are the presence of nodular stromal expansion and of bland necrosis (see above).

Spindle Cell Proliferations

Fibrosing (Organizing) pleuritis. This process is defined as the organization of a fibrinous or hemorrhagic effusion of an empyema. The pleura is always thickened and showed the phenomenon of "zonation" (see above), i.e. a loss of cellularity toward the depth of the tissue, with a contemporary loss of cytological atypia and increase of fibrosis. The spindle cells are often arranged in layers parallel to the surface, a pattern that is different from desmoplastic mesothelioma. The presence of capillaries parallel to the surface is a featture typical of a benign process. Sometimes the process may also extend into fat and also striated muscle. The process is however usually paucicellular. This feature is quite different from desmoplastic mesothelioma (see above). Features typical of desmoplastic mesothelioma that are not seen in organizing pleuritis are again bland necrosis, expansile stromal nodules and true invasion.

References

Allen, T. C. (2005). "Recognition of Histopathologic Pattens of Diffuse Malignant Mesothelioma in Differential Diagnosis of Pleural Biopsies." 2005 129(11): 1415-1420.

Allen, T. C., P. T. Cagle, et al. (2005). "Localized malignant mesothelioma." *Am. J. Surg. Pathol.* 29(7): 866-73.

Attanoos, R. L. and A. R. Gibbs (2003). "'Pseudomesotheliomatous' carcinomas of the pleura: a 10-year analysis of cases from the Environmental Lung Disease Research Group, Cardiff." *Histopathology* 43(5): 444-52.

Attanoos, R. L., R. Webb, et al. (2002). "Value of mesothelial and epithelial antibodies in distinguishing diffuse peritoneal mesothelioma in females from serous papillary carcinoma of the ovary and peritoneum." *Histopathology* 40(3): 237-44.

Attems, J. H. and F. Lintner (2001). "Pseudomesotheliomatous adenocarcinoma of the lung with rhabdoid features." *Pathol. Res. Pract.* 197(12): 841-6.

Aubry, M. C., J. A. Bridge, et al. (2001). "Primary monophasic synovial sarcoma of the pleura: five cases confirmed by the presence of SYT-SSX fusion transcript." *Am. J. Surg. Pathol.*25(6): 776-81.

Butnor, K. J., T. A. Sporn, et al. (2001). "Well-differentiated papillary mesothelioma." *Am. J. Surg. Pathol.* 25(10): 1304-9.

Cagle, P. T. and A. Churg (2005). "Differential diagnosis of benign and malignant mesothelial proliferations on pleural biopsies." *Arch. Pathol. Lab. Med.* 129(11): 1421-7.

Cantin, R., M. Al-Jabi, et al. (1982). "Desmoplastic diffuse mesothelioma." *Am. J. Surg. Pathol.* 6(3): 215-22.

Chetty, R. (1992). "Well differentiated (benign) papillary mesothelioma of the tunica vaginalis." J Clin Pathol 45(11): 1029-30.

Churg, A., P. T. Cagle, et al. (2006). Diffuse Malignant Tumors of the Serosal Membranes. *Tumors of the Serosal Membranes*. Siilver Spring, MD, ARP Press. 3: 33-82.

Churg, A., T. V. Colby, et al. (2000). "The separation of benign and malignant mesothelial proliferations." *Am. J. Surg. Pathol.* 24(9): 1183-200.

Churg, A., V. Roggli, et al. (2004). *Mesothelioma. Tumours of the Lung, Pleura, Thymus and Heart.* W. D. Travis, E. Brambilla, H. K. Müller-Hermelink and C. C. Harris. Lyon, IARC Press. 7: 128-136.

Crotty, T. B., J. L. Myers, et al. (1994). "Localized malignant mesothelioma. A clinicopathologic and flow cytometric study." *Am. J. Surg. Pathol.* 18(4): 357-63.

Del Frate, C., K. Mortele, et al. (2003). "Pseudomesotheliomatous angiosarcoma of the chest wall and pleura." *J. Thorac. Imaging.* 18(3): 200-3.

Dessy, E., M. Falleni, et al. (2001). "Unusual clear cell variant of epithelioid mesothelioma." *Arch. Pathol. Lab. Med.* 125(1588-1590).

Gomez-Roman, J. J., R. Mons-Lera, et al. (2002). "Flow cytometric analysis of a localized malignant mesothelioma." *Ann. Thorac. Surg.* 73(4): 1292-4.

Granville, L., A. C. Laga, et al. (2005). "Review and Update of Uncommon Primary Pleural Tumors. A practical approach to diagnosis." *Arch. Pathol. Lab. Med.* 129: 1428-1442.

Guru, P. K., S. Phillips, et al. (2005). "Pseudomesotheliomatous presentation of primary signet ring cell carcinoma of lung." *Indian J. Chest Dis. Allied Sci.* 47(3): 209-11.

Hammar, S. P. (2006). "Macroscopic, Histologic, Immunohistochemical and Ultrastructural Features of Mesothelioma." *Ultr. Pathol.* 30: 3-17.

Henderson, D. W., H. D. Attwood, et al. (1988). "Lymphohistiocytoid mesothelioma: a rare lymphomatoid variant of predominantly sarcomatoid mesothelioma." *Ultrastruct Pathol.* 12(367-384).

Henderson, D. W., K. B. Shilkin, et al. (1998). "Reactive mesothelial hyperplasia vs mesothelioma, including mesothelioma in situ: a brief review." *Am. J. Clin. Pathol.* 110(3): 397-404.

Hirano, H., S. Takeda, et al. (2003). "Localized pleural malignant mesothelioma." *Pathol. Int.* 53(9): 616-21.

Imura, J., K. Ichikawa, et al. (2002). "Localized malignant mesothelioma of the epithelial type occurring as a primary hepatic neoplasm: a case report with review of the literature." *Apmis* 110(11): 789-94.

Jones, M. A., R. H. Young, et al. (1995). "Malignant mesothelioma of the tunica vaginalis. A clinicopathologic analysis of 11 cases with review of the literature." *Am. J. Surg. Pathol.* 19(7): 815-25.

Kannerstein, M. and J. Churg (1980). "Desmoplastic diffuse malignant mesothelioma." *Prog. Surg. Pathol.* 1: 19-27.

Kaplan, M. A., H. D. Tazelaar, et al. (1996). "Adenomatoid tumors of the pleura." *Am. J. Surg. Pathol.* 20(1219-1223).

Khalidi, H. S., L. J. Medeiros, et al. (2000). "Lymphohistiocytoid mesothelioma. An often misdiiagnosed variant of sarcomatoid malignant mesothelioma." *Am. J. Clin. Pathol.* 113: 649-654.

Kiyozuka, Y., H. Miyazaki, et al. (1999). "An autopsy case of malignant mesothelioma with osseous and cartilgineous differentiation: bone morphogenetic protein-2 in mesothelial cells and its tumors." *Dig. Dis. Sci.* 44: 1612-1631.

Koss, M., W. Travis, et al. (1992). "Pseudomesotheliomatous adenocarcinoma: a reappraisal." *Semin. Diagn. Pathol.* 9(2): 117-23.

Mangano, W. E., P. T. Cagle, et al. (1998). "The diagnosis of desmoplastic malignant mesothelioma and its distinction from fibrous pleurisy: a histologic and immunohistochemical analysis of 31 cases including p53 immunostaining." *Am. J. Clin. Pathol.* 110(2): 191-9.

Mayall, F. G. and A. R. Gibbs (1992). "The histology and immunohistochemistry of small cell mesothelioma." *Histopathology* 20: 47-51.

Ordonez, N. G., M. Myhre, et al. (1996). "Clear cell mesothelioma." *Ultrastruct Pathol.* 20: 331-336.

Perez-Ordonez, B. and J. R. Srigley (2000). "Mesothelial lesions of the paratesticular region." *Semin. Diagn. Pathol.* 17(4): 294-306.

Plas, E., C. R. Riedl, et al. (1998). "Malignant mesothelioma of the tunica vaginalis testis: review of the literature and assessment of prognostic parameters." *Cancer* 83(12): 2437-46.

Schreiner, S. R., B. D. Kirkpatrick, et al. (1998). "Pseudomesotheliomatous adenocarcinoma of the lung in a patient with HIV infection." *Chest* 113(3): 839-41.

Serio, G., A. Scattone, et al. (2002). "Malignant deciduoid mesoothelioma of the pluera." *Histopathology* 40: 348-352.

Shah, I. A., J. R. Salvatore, et al. (1999). "Pseudomesotheliomatous carcinoma involving pleura and peritoneum: A clinicopathologic and immunohistochemical study of three cases." *Ann. Diagn. Pathol.* 3(3): 148-59.

Shukunami, K., S. Hirabuki, et al. (2000). "Well-differentiated papillary mesothelioma involving the peritoneal and pleural cavities: successful treatment by local and systemic administration of carboplatin." *Tumori* 86(5): 419-21.

Stout, A. P. (1971). "Tumors of the pleura." *Harlem Hosp. Bull.* 5: 54-57.

Truong, L. D., M. L. Maccato, et al. (1990). "Serous surface carcinoma of the peritoneum: a clinicopathologic study of 22 cases." *Hum. Pathol.* 21(1): 99-110.

Wilson, G. E., P. S. Hasleton, et al. (1992). "Desmoplastic malignant mesothelioma: a review of 17 cases." *J. Clin. Pathol.* 45(4): 295-8.

Yousem, S. A. and L. Hochhoolzer (1987). "Malignant mesotheliomas with osseous and cartilagineous differentiation." *Arch. Pathol. Lab. Med.* 111: 62-66.

In: Mesothelioma from Bench Side to Clinic
Editor: Alfonso Baldi, pp. 279-294
ISBN: 978-1-60021-789-0

Chapter XIV

The Immunohistochemical Picture of Mesothelioma

Feliciano Baldi, Florinda Feroce, Pasquale Mellone, Maria Pia Di Marino and Alfonso Baldi[1]
Department of Biochemistry, Section of Pathology,
Second University of Naples, Naples, Italy

Abstract

The number of immunohistochemical markers that can help the distinction between epithelioid pleural mesotheliomas and pulmonary peripheral adenocarcinomas are continuously increasing. The aim of this chapter is to describe the diagnostic value of the most commonly used markers.

Introduction

The differentiation of primary from metastatic pleural neoplasms is an area that has been deeply investigated in the discipline of immunohistochemistry. In fact, immunohistochemistry is the predominant technique used for diagnosing mesotheliomas accurately and differentiating them from primary lung cancer that invade the pleura and from primary lung cancers and neoplasms outside the chest cavity that metastatize to pleura. A number of antibodies have been used to this end. They can be simply divided into two main categories: a) antibodies that are relatively specific for mesothelioma cells and mesotheliomas, which serve a positive markers for mesothelioma; b) antibodies that show no reaction for mesothelioma cells or mesotheliomas and serve as negative markers for mesothelioma.

[1] Corresponding Author: "Alfonso Baldi" alfonsobaldi@tiscali.it

Positive Markers

Calretinin

It is considered one of the best and most frequently used in the diagnosis of mesothelioma. Calretinin is a calcium-binding protein similar to S-100 protein with a molecular weight of 29 kd. It is detected in the nervous system and in several non-neural cells, such as steroid-producing cells of ovaries and testes, fat cells, renal tubular epithelial cells, eccrine glands, thymic epithelial cells, and logically mesothelial cells [1]. Calretinin strong and diffuse positivity is generally found in the great majority of mesothelioma samples, while only a small fraction of lung adenocarcinomas can exhibit focal reactivity, limited to small areas or to a few scattered cells [2-24]. Therefore, a negative staining for this marker should be interpreted as a strong indicator that the tumor most likely does not have mesothelial differentiation. As with S-100 protein, the immunostaining pattern of calretinin is both cytoplasmic and nuclear [see figure 1). It should be noted that reactive, multipotential sub-serosal spindle cells express calretinin.

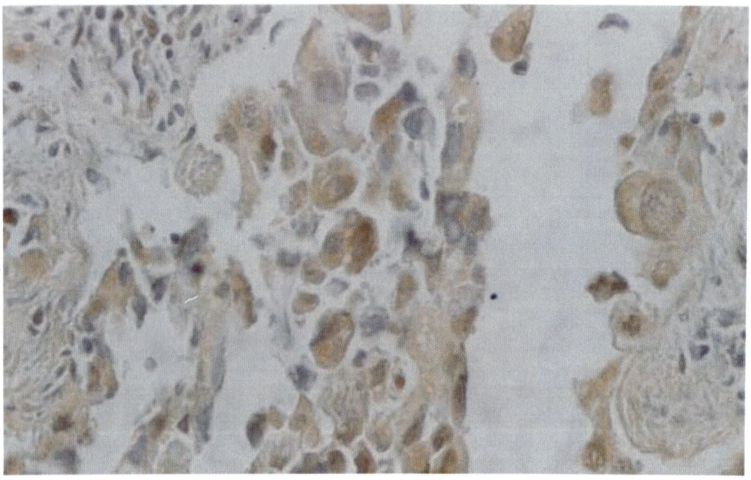

Figure 1. Immunohistochemical expression of Calretinin in an epithelioid mestothelioma.

Keratins

Keratins are found in nearly 100% of mesotheliomas. In particular, some cytokeratins, including cytokeratins 5 and 6 are present in epithelioid mesotheliomas but not in lung adenocarcinomas. Generally, the positivity is diffuse with a peculiar perinuclear distribution, but cases with reactivity limited to small areas or to a few cells have been reported [12,19,24-31]. To note, squamous carcinomas of the lung commonly espress cytokeratin 5/6.

WT1

Wilms' tumor suppressor gene is mapped on the chromosome 11p13 and its inactivation causes susceptibility to Wilms' tumor. This gene is found predominantly in tissues of mesodermal origin. Several investigations have confirmed that WT1 is mainly expressed in mesothelioma cells, while very few cases of lung adenocarcinomas show WT1 expression. It should also noted that WT1 is commonly expressed in serous carcinomas of the ovary and peritoneum; therefore it could not be used for distinguish these malignancies from mesotheliomas [18, 19, 24, 32-34].

Thrombomodulin (CD141)

Thrombomodulin is a plasma membrane-related glycoprotein that has anticoagulant activity. It is found in several cell types, including mesangial cells, synovial cells, mesothelial cells, endothelial cells, megakaryocytes, and some squamous epithelial cells. It has been demonstrated by different observations that this antigen is expressed in the great majority of epithelioid mesotheliomas, while lung adenocarcinomas are generally negative. The typical positivity for CD141 is a thick cell membrane staining, while reactive mesothelial cells display a thin cell membrane staining and some carcinomas a cytoplasmic staining [2,5,6,10,12,15,16,18,20,24,30,35-41].

Mesothelin

Mesothelin is a 40-kDa surface glycoprotein of unknown function that is strongly expressed in mesothelial cells and mesotheliomas (see figure 2). To note, mesothelin is expressed also in a great percentage of lung adenocarcinomas and also in other carcinomas, especially serous carcinomas of the ovary, pancreatica adenocarcinomas, and some squamous carcinomas.

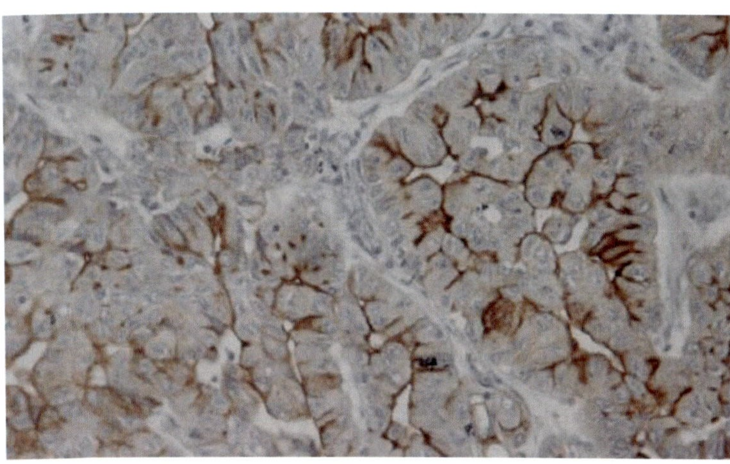

Figure 2. Immunohistochemical expression of Mesotelin-1 in an epithelioid mesothelioma.

Therefore, mesothelin is considered a very sensitive positive marker for mesothelioma, and a negative staining for this marker can be considered a strong indication against a diagnosis of mesothelioma [42-44].

N-Cadherin

Cadherins are a family of adhesion proteins important in sorting cells into specialized tissues during morphogenesis. In particular, N-cadherin is a protein found in nerve cells, developing muscle cells and mesothelioma cells. Despite the first promising results, the last observations support the conclusion that N-cadherin immunostaining has not value for separating epithelioid mesothelioma from lung adenocarcinomas [9, 17, 24, 45, 46]

HBME-1

It is a monoclonal antibody generated from the mesothelioma cell line SPC11, that reacts with an antigen of unknown nature present on the villous surface of the mesothelioma cells producing a membranous staining pattern (see figure 3). Nevertheless, it is strongly expressed also in lung adenocarcinomas, even if the expression pattern is usually cytoplasmic. Its value as specific marker for mesothelioma is limited [5,6,10,13,16,20,24,30,38,39,41,47-55].

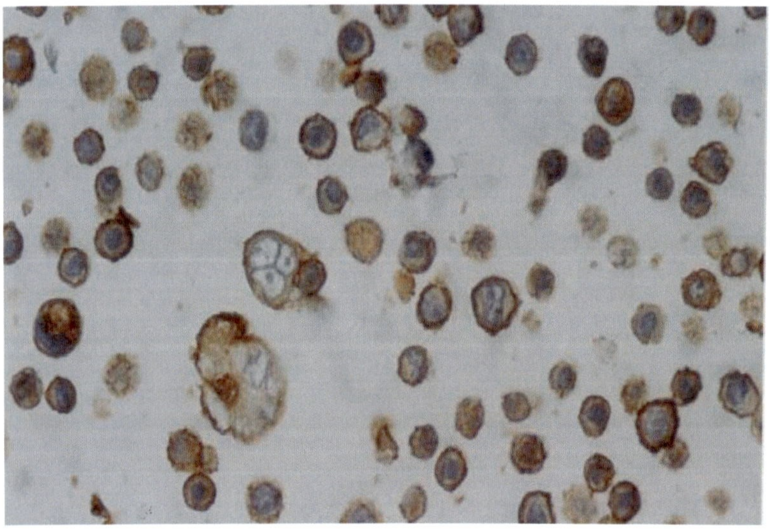

Figure 3. Immunocytochemical expression of HBME-1 in a cytological sample of mesothelioma.

Negative Markers

MOC-31

It is a monoclonal antibody that reacts with an epithelial-associated transmembrane glycoprotein on small cell lung carcinoma known as epithelial glycoprotein-2. It is strongly expressed by lung adenocarcinomas and a only by a little portion of epithelioid mesotheliomas. Additionally, the reactivity in adenocarcinomas is usually strong and diffuse, while the mesothelioma staining is limited to small areas or even to a few scattered cells. For these reasons MOC-31 is considered one of the most useful negative markers for the diagnosis of mesothelioma [6, 7, 13, 15, 24, 56-63].

E-Cadherin

It is a 120-kd cell adhesion molecule expressed in epithelial cells. Loss of expression of E-cadherin is associated with a higher degree of invasiveness and an increase in malignant potential in several carcinomas. Recent works have proposed this antigen as a negative marker for mesothelioma, but this observation has been denied by other investigator, therefore E-cadherin is not actually considered a very helpful marker in discriminating epithelioid mesotheliomas from lung adenocarcinomas [7, 9, 17, 24, 30, 34, 45, 46, 64-68].

BG-8

It is a moclonal antibody that recognizes the blood group Lewis^{y} . This antigen is strongly expressed in lung adenocarcinomas, while epithelioid mesotheliomas are generally negative or show only focal positivity. It is considered a good negative marker for mesothelioma [5, 24, 34, 69-71].

TTF-1

It is a tissue-specific transcription factor that is expressed in the normal lung and thyroid as well as in the tumors derived from these organs. Because of this high specificity of TTF-1 for lung adenocarcinomas, it has been successfully proposed as a negative marker for mesotheliomas [34,72-75].

CEA

Carcinoembryonic antigen (CEA) is a glycoprotein of 200 kd. It is often referred to as an oncofetal antigen, but it is expressed in normal adult tissues and in a variety of epithelial neoplasms. CEA is negative in most epithelial mesotheliomas, while it is found in a high percentage of lung adenocarcinomas (85 to 100%). Because of its high sensitivity and specificity, CEA is considered one of the best negative mesothelioma markers [2,15,16,20,24,30,36,50,52,56, 60,76-95]. To note, while CEA immunostaining is very useful in distinguishing between lung adenocarcinomas and mesotheliomas, the diagnostic value of CEA expression is more limited for discriminating mesothelioma from serous carcinomas of the ovary and peritoneum, because less than half of these tumors express this marker.

B72.3

It is an antibody that recognizes a high molecular weight glycoprotein complex derived from a membrane-enriched fraction of human metastatic breast carcinoma. This antibody stains the great majority of lung adenocarcinomas, while it gives negative results in most of the mesotheliomas. However, some controversy exists regarding the percentage of adenocarcinomas and mesotheliomas that are positive for this antigen and, therefore, on its value as negative marker for mesothelioma [5, 7, 16, 24, 36, 52-54, 60, 85, 89, 91-93, 96-103].

LEU-M1 (CD15)

It is a monoclonal antibody against the membrane-related trisaccharide fucosyl-N-acetyl-lactosamine on myelomonocityc cells. Several investigations have shown that this antigen is commonly expressed in lung adenocarcinomas, while is generally not expressed in mesotheliomas. Actually, its value as negative marker for mesothelioma is not universally accepted, since controversial results are reported in the scientific literature [2, 5-7, 10, 16, 20, 24, 30, 35, 36, 47, 50, 52-55, 60, 84, 89, 90-92, 97-106]

Ber-EP4

It is a monoclonal antibody that recognizes the protein moiety of two glycopolypeptides on human epithelial cells. Latza and collegues [107] were the first to report that most lung adenocarcinomas stains positively for this antibody (99%), while mesotheliomas are generally negative. Although this observation was confirmed in subsequent investigations, some disagreement exists regarding the percentage of Ber-EP4 expression in mesotheliomas, which could reach, accordingly to the most recent publications, one-third of the cases [2, 5-7, 15-17, 19, 20, 24, 30, 37, 50, 52, 53, 55, 59, 60, 93, 95, 101, 103, 105-113].

CA19-9

Ordoñez was the first showing the value of CA19-9 as a marker for distinguishing between epithelioid mesothelioma and lung adenocarcinoma [89]. Since that time, several other studies confirmed this data [6,50,54,116]. However, it should be mentioned that this marker has an high specificity for lung adenocarcinomas, but a low sensitivity. Neverrtheless, CA19-9 is often expressed in serous carcinomas of the ovary and peritoneum and can be an useful marker in distinguishing these tumors from epithelioid peritoneal mesotheliomas.

VIMENTIN

Starting from the first observation of Churg [114], some other investigators have shown that vimentin could be a good negative marker for mesothelioma. However, a large number of studies have been published reaching conflicting results. To date, the scientific community does not consider this marker useful in discriminating between lung adenocarcinomas and mesotheliomas [5,6,10,17,20,24,36,55,83,88-93,102,106,114-118].

Conclusion

There are actually many immunohistochemical markers available for the differential diagnosis between lung adenocarcinoma and epithelioid mesothelioma. Table 1 summarizes the most recent data from the literature on this topic. From a practical point of view, a panel of four markers (two positive and two negative for mesothelioma) should be used for the distinction between lung adenocarcinoma and mesothelioma. Based on specificity and sensitivity, the best choice, according to our experience and to the recent literature, should include calretinin and cytokeratin 5/6 (or WT1) for the positive markers and CEA and MOC-31 (or either B72.3 or Ber-EP4) for the negative markers. When considering non pulmonary adenocarcinomas, it should be mentioned that WT1 is strongly expressed in serous carcinomas of the ovary, while CEA is often negative.

***Table 1. Studies using the largest number of markers for distinguishing epithelioid mesothelioma from lung adenocarcinoma**

Reference	Markers investigated	Conclusion
Brown et al. [36]	CEA, B72.3, leu-M1, thrombodulin vimentin, CA-125	CEA and B72.3 are the best markers
Moch et al. [93]	CEA, B72.3, leu-M1, Ber-EP4, CK7 CK18, vimentin, amylase, HEA125 PLAP, BMA-120, Blood group-related antigens A,B,H	Ber-EP4, HEA125, Blood group- related antigens A,B,H and CEA are the best marker in descending order
Skov et al. [117]	CEA, B72.3, leu-M1, Ber-EP4, EMA vimentin	The best panel is CEA, Ber-EP4, B72.3
Kortsik et al. [118]	CEA, EMA, vimentin, HEA125, IOB3 CK4, CK7, CK8, CK10, CK14, CK18 CK19, CK5/6, CK 13/16, CK8/18/19	The best panel is CEA and IOB3
Ordoñez [52]	CEA, B72.3, leu-M1, HBME-1, SM3 Ber-EP4, thrombomodulin, 443A6	The best markers are CEA, B72.3 leu-M1 and thrombomodulin

Table 1. (Continued)

Reference	Markers investigated	Conclusion
Riera [57]	CEA, B72.3, leu-M1, BG-8, HMFG-2 HBME-1, Ber-EP4, thrombomodulin, vimentin, calretinin	The best markers are CEA, BG-8 Ber-EP4
Chenard-Neu [6]	CEA, leu-M1, HBME-1, Ber-EP4, AUA1, thrombomodulin, calretinin, MOC-31, CA19.9, CA-125	The best panel is CEA, CA19.9 MOC-31 and vimentin
Garcia-Prats [95]	CEA, B72.3, leu-M1, Ber-EP4, EMA, vimentin, CAM 5.2, ,34βE12, Ber-H2desmin, CK20	The best markers are vimentin and Ber-EP4
Leers [7]	CEA, B72.3, leu-M1, Ber-EP4, MOC31 Calretinin, E-cadherin	The best markers are calretinin, and E-cadherin
Brockstedt [10]	CEA, leu-M1, HBME-1, calretinin, EMA, Ber-EP4, thrombomodulin, vimentin, CK MNF116, Sialosyl-TN	The best panel is CEA, EMA, calretinin and leu-M1
Comin [16]	CEA, B72.3, leu-M1, HBME-1, Ber-EP4, thrombomodulin, CD44H, calretinin EMA	The best markers are calretinin thrombomodulin, leu-M1 and CEA
Oates [13]	Leu-M1, MOC31, HBME-1, calretinin, WT1	The best markers are MOC31 and WT1
Carella [15]	CEA, Ber-EP4, thrombomodulin, CK5/6 calretinin, MOC31, 34βE12	The best panel is Ber-EP4, CK5/6 and calretinin
Gonzales-Lois [55]	CEA, B72.3, leu-M1, HBME-1, MOC31, vimentin, desmin	The best markers are HBME-1 and MOC31
Roberts [20]	CEA, leu-M1, HBME-1, EMA, p53, CAM 5.2, Ber-EP4, thrombomodulin, calretinin, CD44H, vimentin, p-170gp, PDGFR-beta	Using two positive markers for adenocarcinoma and two for me- sothelioma
Abutaily [30]	CEA, leu-M1, HBME-1, Ber-EP4, thrombomodulin, calretinin, SP-A, CK5/6, E-cadherin, N-cadherin, TTF-1	The primary panel is TTF-1 and E-cadherin
Ordoñez [24]	calretinin, CK5/6, thrombomodulin, WT1, meosthelin, CD44S, HBME-1, N-cadherin, E-cadherin, TTF-1, BG-8 MOC31, CEA, Ber-EP4, B72.3, EMA, Leu-M1, CA19.9	The best panel is calretinin,CEA, CK5/6 and MOC31

* modified form reference 24.

Acknowledgements

Research in our laboratory is supported by grants from FUTURA-onlus, ISSCO, AIRC,Ministry of Health and Second University of Naples.

References

[1] Andersen C, Blumcke I, Celio MR. Calcium-binding proteins: selective markers of nerve cells. *Cell Tissue Res.* 1993; 271: 181-208.

[2] Doglioni C, Dei Tos AP, Laurino L, et al. Calretinin: a novel immunocytochemical marker for mesothelioma. *Am. J. Surg. Pathol.* 1996;20:1037-46.

[3] Gotzos V, Vogt P, Celio MR. The calcium binding protein calretinin is a selective marker for malignant pleural mesotheliomas of the epithelial type. *Pathol. Res. Pract.* 1996;192:137-47.

[4] Barberis MCP, Faleri M, Veronese S, et al. Calretinin: a selective marker of normal and neoplastic mesothelial cells in serous effusions. *Acta Cytol.* 1997;41:1757-61.

[5] Riera JR, Astengo-Osuna C, Longmate JA, et al. The immunohistochemical diagnostic panel for epithelial mesothelioma: a reevaluation after heat-induced epitope retrieval. *Am. J. Surg. Pathol.* 1997;21:1409-19.

[6] Chenard-Neu MP, Kabou A, Mechine A, et al. L'immunohistochimie dans le diagnostic différentiel entre mésothéliome et adénocarcinome: évaluation de 5 nouveaux anticorps et réévaluation de 6 anticorps traditionnels. *Ann. Pathol.* 1998;18:460-5.

[7] Leers MPG, Aarts MMJ, Theunissen PHMH. E-cadherin and calretinin: a useful combination of immunochemical markers for differentiation between mesothelioma and metastatic adenocarcinoma. *Histopathology* 1998;32:209-16.

[8] Ordóñez NG. Value of calretinin immunostaining in differentiating epithelial mesothelioma from lung adenocarcinoma. *Mod. Pathol.* 1998;11:929-33.

[9] Simsir A, Fetsch P, Mehta D, et al. E-cadherin, N-cadherin, and calretinin in pleural effusions: the good, the bad, the worthless. *Diagn. Cytopathol.* 1999; 20:125-30.

[10] Brockstedt U, Gulyas M, Dobra K, et al. An optimized battery of eight antibodies that can distinguish most cases of epithelial mesothelioma from adenocarcinoma. Am. *J. Clin. Pathol.* 2000;114:203-9.

[11] Chhieng DC, Yee H, Schaefer D, et al. Calretinin staining pattern aids in the differentiation of mesothelioma from adenocarcinoma in serous effusions. *Cancer* (Cancer Cytopathol) 2000;90:194-200.

[12] Cury PM, Butcher DN, Fisher C, et al. Value of the mesothelium-associated antibodies thrombomodulin, cytokeratin 5/6, calretinin, and CD44H in distinguishing epithelioid pleural mesothelioma from adenocarcinoma metastatic to the pleura. *Mod. Pathol.* 2000;13:107-12.

[13] Oates J, Edwards C. HBME-1, MOC-31, WT1 and calretinin: as assessment of recently described markers for mesothelioma and adenocarcinoma. *Histopathology* 2000;36:341-7.

[14] Wieczorek TJ, Krane JF. Diagnostic utility of calretinin immunohistochemistry in cytologic cell block preparations. *Cancer* (Cancer Cytopathol) 2000;90:312-9.

[15] Carella R, Deleonardi G, D'Errico A, et al. Immunohistochemical panels for differentiating epithelial malignant mesothelioma from lung adenocarcinoma: a study with logistic regression analysis. *Am. J. Surg. Pathol.* 2001;25:43-50.

[16] Comin CE, Novelli L, Boddi V, et al. Calretinin, thrombomodulin, CEA, and CD15: a useful combination of immunohistochemical markers for differentiating pleural epithelial mesothelioma from peripheral pulmonary adenocarcinoma. *Hum. Pathol.* 2001;32:529-36.

[17] Davidson B, Nielsen S, Christensen J, et al. The role of desmin and N-cadherin in effusion cytology: a comparative study using established markers of mesothelial and epithelial cells. *Am. J. Surg. Pathol.* 2001;25:1405-12.

[18] Foster MR, Johnson JE, Olson SJ, et al. Immunohistochemical analysis of nuclear versus cytoplasmic staining of WT1 in malignant mesotheliomas and primary pulmonary adenocarcinomas. *Arch. Pathol. Lab. Med.* 2001;125:1316-20.

[19] Miettinen M, Limon J, Niezabitowski A, et al. Calretinin and other mesothelioma markers in synovial sarcoma: analysis of antigenic similarities and differences with malignant mesothelioma. *Am. J. Surg. Pathol.* 2001;25:610-7.

[20] Roberts F, Harper CM, Downie I, et al. Immunohistochemical analysis still has a limited role in the diagnosis of malignant mesothelioma: a study of thirteen antibodies. *Am. J. Clin. Pathol.* 2001;116:253-62.

[21] Simsir A, Fetsch P, Abati A. Calretinin immunostaining in benign and malignant pleural effusions. *Diagn. Cytopathol.* 2001;24:149-52.

[22] Tot T. The value of cytokeratins 20 and 7 in discriminating metastatic adenocarcinomas from pleural mesotheliomas. *Cancer* 2001;92:2727-32.

[23] De Leij L, Broers J, Ramaekers F, et al.Monoclonal antibodies in clinical and experimental pathology of lung cancer. In: Ruiter DJ, Fleuren GJ, Warnaar SO, eds. Application of Monoclonal Antibodies in Tumor Pathology. *Dordrecht: Martinus Nijhoff*, 1987:191-210.

[24] Ordóñez NG. The immunohistochemical diagnosis of mesothelioma: a comparative study of epithelioid mesothelioma and lung adenocarcinoma. *Am. J. Surg. Pathol.* 2003;27(8): 1031-51.

[25] Clover J, Oates J, Edwards C. Anti-cytokeratin 5/6: a positive marker for epithelioid mesothelioma. *Histopathology* 1997;31:140-3.

[26] Ordóñez NG. Value of cytokeratin 5/6 immunostaining in distinguishing epithelial mesothelioma of the pleura from lung adenocarcinoma. *Am. J. Surg. Pathol.* 1998;22:1215-21.

[27] Attanoos RL, Webb R, Dojcinov SD, et al. Malignant epithelioid mesothelioma: anti-mesothelial marker expression correlates with histological pattern. *Histopathology* 2001;39:584-8.

[28] Kaufmann O, Fietze E, Mengs J, et al. Value of p63 and cytokeratin 5/6 as immunohistochemical markers for the differential diagnosis of poorly differentiated and undifferentiated carcinomas. *Am. J. Clin. Pathol.* 2001;116:823-30.

[29] Tot T. The value of cytokeratins 20 and 7 in discriminating metastatic adenocarcinomas from pleural mesotheliomas. *Cancer* 2001;92:2727-32.

[30] Abutaily AS, Addis BJ, Roche WR. Immunohistochemistry in the distinction between malignant mesothelioma and pulmonary adenocarcinoma: a critical evaluation of new antibodies. *J. Clin. Pathol.* 2002;55:662-8.

[31] Chu PG, Weiss LM. Expression of cytokeratin 5/6 in epithelial neoplasms: an immunohistochemical study of 509 cases. *Mod. Pathol.* 2002;15:6-10.

[32] Amin KM, Litzky LA, Smythe WR, et al. Wilms'tumor 1 susceptibility (WT1) gene products are selectively expressed in malignant mesothelioma. *Am. J. Pathol.* 1995;146:344-56.

[33] Kumar-Singh S, Segers K, Rodeck U, et al. WT1 mutation in malignant mesothelioma and WT1 immunoreactivity in relation to p53 and growth factor receptor expression, cell-type transition, and prognosis. *J. Pathol.* 1997;181:67-74.

[34] Ordóñez NG. Value of thyroid transcription factor-1, E-cadherin, BG8, WT1, and CD44S immunostaining in distinguishing epithelial pleural mesothelioma from pulmonary and nonpulmonary adenocarcinoma. *Am. J. Surg. Pathol.* 2000;24:598-606.

[35] Collins CL, Ordóñez NG, Schaefer R, et al. Thrombomodulin expression in malignant pleural mesothelioma and pulmonary adenocarcinoma. *Am. J. Pathol.* 1992;141:827-33.

[36] Brown RW, Clark GM, Tandon AK, et al. Multiple-marker immunohistochemical phenotypes distinguishing malignant pleural mesothelioma from pulmonary adenocarcinoma. *Hum. Pathol.* 1993;24:347-54.

[37] Ascoli V, Scalzo CC, Taccogna S, et al. The diagnostic value of thrombomodulin immunolocalization in serous effusions. *Arch. Pathol. Lab. Med.* 1995;119:1136-40.

[38] Attanoos RL, Goddard H, Gibbs AR. Mesothelioma-binding antibodies: thrombomodulin, OV 632 and HBME-1 and their use in the diagnosis of malignant mesothelioma. *Histopathology* 1996;29:209-15.

[39] Kennedy AD, King G, Kerr KM. HBME-1 and antithrombomodulin in the differential diagnosis of malignant mesothelioma of pleura. *J. Clin. Pathol.* 1997;50:859-62.

[40] Ordóñez NG. Value of thrombomodulin immunostaining in the diagnosis of mesothelioma. H*istopathology* 1997;31:25-30.

[41] Fetsch PA, Abati A, Hijazi YM. Utility of the antibodies CA19-9, HBME-1, and thrombomodulin in the diagnosis of malignant mesothelioma and adenocarcinoma in cytology. *Cancer* (Cancer Cytopathol) 1998;84:101-8.

[42] Chang K, Pai LH, Pass H, et al. Monoclonal antibody K1 reacts with epithelial mesothelioma but not with lung adenocarcinoma. *Am. J. Surg. Pathol.* 1992;16:259-68.

[43] Chang K, Pastan I. Molecular cloning of mesothelin, a differentiation antigen present on mesothelium, mesotheliomas, and ovarian cancers. *Proc. Natl. Acad. Sci. USA* 1996;93:136-40.

[44] Chang K, Pastan I, Willingham MC. Isolation and characterization of a monoclonal antibody, K1, reactive with ovarian cancers and normal mesothelium. *Int. J. Cancer* 1992;50:373-81.

[45] Han AC, Filstein MR, Hunt JV, et al. N-cadherin distinguishes pleural mesotheliomas from lung adenocarcinomas: a ThinPrep immunocytochemical study. *Cancer* (Cancer Cytopathol) 1999;87:83-6.

[46] Han AC, Peralta-Soler A, Knudsen KA, et al. Differential expression of N-cadherin in pleural mesotheliomas and E-cadherin in lung adenocarcinomas in formalin-fixed, paraffin-embedded tissues. *Hum. Pathol.* 1997;28:641-5.

[47] Miettinen M, Kovatich AJ. HBME-1: a monoclonal antibody useful in the differential diagnosis of mesothelioma, adenocarcinoma, and soft tissue and bone tumors. *Appl. Immunohistochem.* 1995;3:115-22.

[48] Renshaw AA, Pinkus GS, Corson JM. HBME-1 aids in distinguishing mesotheliomas and adenocarcinomas of the lung and breast [Abstract]. *Mod. Pathol.* 1995;8:152.

[49] Savera AT, Raju U, Linden MD. Mesothelioma vs adenocarcinoma: diagnostic utility of HBME-1 [Abstract]. *Lab. Invest* 1996;74:162.

[50] Bateman AC, Al-Talib RK, Newman T, et al. Immunohistochemical phenotype of malignant mesothelioma: predictive value of CA125 and HBME-1 expression. *Histopathology* 1997;30:49-56.

[51] Donna A, Betta P-G, Chiodera P, et al. Newly marketed tissue markers for malignant mesothelioma: immunoreactivity of rabbit AMAD-2 antiserum compared with monoclonal antibody HBME-1 and a review of the literature on so-called antimesothelioma antibodies. *Hum. Pathol.* 1997;28:929-37.

[52] Ordóñez NG. Value of antibodies 44-3A6, SM3, HBME-1 and thrombomodulin in differentiating epithelial pleural mesothelioma from lung adenocarcinoma: a comparative study with other commonly used antibodies. *Am. J. Surg. Pathol.* 1997;21:1399-408.

[53] Wilson JD, Merino MJ, Harris C, et al. Mesothelioma vs adenocarcinoma: does immunohistochemistry help? *Lab. Invest.* 1997;76:174A.

[54] Ordóñez NG. Role of immunohistochemistry in distinguishing epithelial peritoneal mesotheliomas from peritoneal and ovarian carcinomas. *Am. J. Surg. Pathol.* 1998;22:1203-14.

[55] González-Lois C, Ballentín C, Sotelo MT, et al. Combined use of novel epithelial (MOC-31) and mesothelial (HBME-1) immunohistochemical markers for optimal first line diagnostic distinction between mesothelioma and metastatic carcinoma in pleura. *Histopathology* 2001;38:528-34.

[56] Delahaye M, Hoogsteden HC, van der Kwast TH. Immunocytochemistry of malignant mesothelioma: OV632 as a marker of malignant mesothelioma. *J. Pathol.* 1991;165:137-43.

[57] Ruitenbeek T, Gouw ASH, Poppema S. Immunocytology of body cavity fluids: MOC-31, a monoclonal antibody discriminating between mesothelial and epithelial cells. *Arch. Pathol. Lab. Med.* 1994;118:265-9.

[58] Edwards C, Oates J. OV632 and MOC31 in the diagnosis of mesothelioma and adenocarcinoma: an assessment of their use in formalin-fixed and paraffin wax embedded material. *J. Clin. Pathol.* 1995;48:626-30.

[59] Kuenen-Boumeester V, van Loenen P, de Bruijn EMCA, et al. Quality control of immunocytochemical staining of effusions using a standardized method of cell processing. *Acta Cytol.* 1996;40:475-9.

[60] Delahaye M, van der Ham F, van der Kwast TH. Complementary value of five carcinoma markers for the diagnosis of malignant mesothelioma, adenocarcinoma metastasis, and reactive mesothelium in serous effusions. *Diagn. Cytopathol.* 1997;17:115-20.

[61] Sosolik RC, McGaughy VR, De Young BR. Anti-MOC-31: a potential addition to the pulmonary adenocarcinoma versus mesothelioma immunohistochemistry panel. *Mod. Pathol.* 1997;10:716-9.

[62] Ordóñez NG. Value of the MOC-31 monoclonal antibody in differentiating epithelial pleural mesothelioma from lung adenocarcinoma. *Hum. Pathol.* 1998;29:166-9.

[63] Morgan RL, De Young BR, McGaughy VR, et al. MOC-31 aids in the differentiation between adenocarcinoma and reactive mesothelial cells. *Cancer* (Cancer Cytopathol) 1999;87:390-4.

[64] Peralta-Soler A, Knudsen KA, Jaurand MC, et al. The differential expression of N-cadherin and E-cadherin distinguishes pleural mesotheliomas from lung adenocarcinomas. *Hum. Pathol.* 1995;26:1363-9.

[65] Kitazume H, Kitamura K, Mukai K, et al. Cytologic differential diagnosis among reactive mesothelial cells, malignant mesothelioma, and adenocarcinoma: utility of combined E-cadherin and calretinin immunostaining. *Cancer* (Cancer Cytopathol) 2000;90:55-60.

[66] Thirkettle I, Harvey P, Hasleton PS, et al. Immunoreactivity for cadherins, HGF/SF, met, and erb-2 in pleural malignant mesotheliomas. *Histopathology* 2000;36:522-8.

[67] Tot T. The value of cytokeratins 20 and 7 in discriminating metastatic adenocarcinomas from pleural mesotheliomas. *Cancer* 2001;92:2727-32.

[68] Laskin WB, Miettinen M. Epithelial-type and neural-type cadherin expression in malignant noncarcinomatous neoplasms with epithelioid features that involve the soft tissues. *Arch. Pathol. Lab. Med.* 2002;126:425-31.

[69] Jordon D, Jagirdar J, Kaneko M. Blood group antigens, Lewisx and Lewisy, in the diagnostic discrimination of malignant mesothelioma versus adenocarcinoma. *Am. J. Pathol.* 1989;135:931-7.

[70] Battifora H. Diffuse malignant mesothelioma. In: Battifora H, McCaughey WTE, eds. *Atlas of Tumor Pathology: Tumors of the Serosal Membranes,* 3rd series, fascicle 15. Washington, DC: Armed Forces Istitute of Pathology, 1995:71.

[71] Wieczorek TJ, Kranc JF. Diagnostic utility of calretinin immunohistochemistry in cytologic cell block preparations. *Cancer* (Cancer Cytopathol) 2000;90:312-9.

[72] Khoor A, Whitsett JA, Stahlman MT, et al. Utility of surfactant protein B precursor and thyroid transcription factor 1 in differentiating adenocarcinoma of the lung from malignant mesothelioma. *Hum. Pathol.* 1999;30:695-700.

[73] Ordóñez NG. Thyroid transcription factor-1 is a marker of lung and thyroid carcinomas. *Adv. Anat. Pathol.* 2000;7:123-7.

[74] Ordóñez NG. Immunohistochemical diagnosis of epithelioid mesothelioma: a critical review of old markers, new markers. *Hum. Pathol.* 2002;33:953-67.

[75] Yatabe Y, Mitsudomi T, Takahashi T. TTF-1 Expression in pulmonary adenocarcinomas. *Am. J. Surg. Pathol.* 2002;26:767-73.

[76] Wang NS, Huang SN, Gold P. Absence of carcinoembryonic antigen-like material in mesothelioma: an immunohistochemical differentiation from other lung cancers. *Cancer* 1979;44:937-43.

[77] Corson JM, Pinkus GS. Mesothelioma: profile of keratin proteins and carcinoembryonic antigen: an immunoperoxidase study of 20 cases and comparison with pulmonary adenocarcinomas. *Am. J. Pathol.* 1982;108:80-7.
[78] Kwee WS, Veldhuizen RW, Golding RP, et al. Histologic distinction between malignant mesothelioma, benign pleural lesion and carcinoma metastasis: evaluation of the application of morphometry combined with histochemistry and immunostaining. *Virchows Arch.* (Pathol Anat) 1982;397:287-99.
[79] Whitaker D, Sterrett GF, Shilkin KB. Detection of tissue CEA-like substance as an aid in the differential diagnosis of malignant mesothelioma. *Pathology* 1982;14:255-8.
[80] Holden J, Churg A. Immunohistochemical staining for keratin and carcinoembryonic antigen in the diagnosis of malignant mesothelioma. *Am. J. Surg. Pathol.* 1984;8:277-9.
[81] Battifora H, Kopinski MI. Distinction of mesothelioma from adenocarcinoma: an immunohistochemical approach. *Cancer* 1985;55:1679-85.
[82] Gibbs AR, Harach R, Wagner JC, et al. Comparison of tumor markers in malignant mesothelioma and pulmonary adenocarcinoma. *Thorax* 1985;40:91-5.
[83] Jasani B, Edwards RE, Thomas ND, et al. The use of vimentin antibodies in the diagnosis of malignant mesothelioma. *Virchows Arch* [Pathol Anat] 1985;406:441-8.
[84] Sheibani K, Battifora H, Burke JS. Antigenic phenotype of malignant mesotheliomas and pulmonary adenocarcinomas: an immunohistologic analysis demonstrating the value of Leu M1 antigen. *Am. J. Pathol.* 1986;123:212-9.
[85] Szpak CA, Johnston WW, Roggli V, et al. The diagnostic distinction between malignant mesothelioma of the pleura and adenocarcinoma of the lung as defined by a monoclonal antibody (B72.3). *Am. J. Pathol.* 1986;122:252-60.
[86] Dewar A, Valente M, Ring NP, et al. Pleural mesothelioma of epithelial type and pulmonary adenocarcinoma: an ultrastructural and cytochemical comparison. *J. Pathol.* 1987;152:309-16.
[87] Otis CN, Carter D, Cole S, et al. Immunohistochemical evaluation of pleural mesothelioma and pulmonary adenocarcinoma: a biinstitutional study of 47 cases. *Am. J. Surg. Pathol.* 1987;11:445-56.
[88] Pfaltz M, Odermatt B, Christen B, et al. Immunohistochemistry in the diagnosis of malignant mesothelioma. *Virchows Arch* (Pathol Anat) 1987;411:387-93.
[89] Ordóñez NG. The immunohistochemical diagnosis of mesothelioma: differentiation of mesothelioma and lung adenocarcinoma. *Am. J. Surg. Pathol.* 1989;13:276-91.
[90] O'Hara CJ, Corson JM, Pinkus GS, et al. ME1. A monoclonal antibody that distinguishes epithelial-type malignant mesothelioma from pulmonary adenocarcinoma and extrapulmonary malignancies. *Am. J. Pathol.* 1990;136:421-8.
[91] Wick MR, Loy T, Mills SE, et al. Malignant epithelioid pleural mesothelioma versus peripheral pulmonary adenocarcinoma: a histochemical, ultrastructural, and immunohistologic study of 103 cases. *Hum. Pathol.* 1990;21:759-66.
[92] Wirth PR, Legier J, Wright GL Jr. Immunohistochemical evaluation of seven monoclonal antibodies for differentiation of pleural mesothelioma from lung adenocarcinoma. *Cancer* 1991;67:655-62.
[93] Moch H, Oberholzer H, Dalquen N, et al. Diagnostic tools for differentiating between pleural mesothelioma and lung adenocarcinoma in paraffin embedded tissue: I.

Immunohistochemical findings. *Virchows Arch. Pathol. A Pathol. Anat.* 1993;423:19-27.

[94] Dejmek A, Hjerpe A. Carcinoembryonic antigen-like reactivity in malignant mesothelioma: a comparison between different commercially available antibodies. *Cancer* 1994;73:464-9.

[95] Garcia-Prats MD, Ballestin C, Sotelo T, et al. A comparative evaluation of immunohistochemical markers for the differential diagnosis of malignant pleural tumors. *Histopathology* 1998;32:462-72.

[96] Lafebvre MP, Rodriguez F, Schlom J, et al. The application of a monoclonal antibody to the differentiation of benign and malignant mesothelial proliferations from adenocarcinomas [Abstract]. *Lab. Invest* 1985;52:38.

[97] Warnock ML, Stoloff A, Thor A. Differentiation of adenocarcinoma of the lung from mesothelioma: periodic acid-Schiff, monoclonal antibodies B72.3, and Leu M1. *Am. J. Pathol.* 1998;133:30-8.

[98] Tickman RJ, Cohen C, Varma VA, et al. Distinction between carcinoma cells and mesothelial cells in serous effusions: usefulness of immunohistochemistry. *Acta. Cytol.* 1990;34:491-6.

[99] McCaughey WT, Colby TV, Battifora H, et al. Diagnosis of diffuse malignant mesothelioma: experience of a US/Canadian Mesothelioma Panel. *Mod. Pathol.* 1991;4:342-53.

[100] Nance KV, Silverman JF. Immunocytochemical panel for the identification of malignant cells in serous effusions. *Am. J. Clin. Pathol.* 1991;95:867-74.

[101] Gaffey MJ, Mills SE, Swanson PE, et al. Immunoreactivity for BER-EP4 in adenocarcinomas, adenomatoid tumors, and malignant mesotheliomas. *Am. J. Surg. Pathol.* 1992; 16:593-9.

[102] Dejmek A, Hjerpe A. Immunohistochemical reactivity in mesothelioma and adenocarcinoma: a stepwise logistic regression analysis. *APMIS* 1994;102:255-64.

[103] Bailey ME, Brown RW, Mody DR, et al. Ber-EP4 for differentiating adenocarcinoma from reactive and neoplastic mesothelial cells in serous effusions: comparison with carcinoembryonic antigen, B72.3, and Leu-M1. *Acta Cytol.*1996;40:1212-6.

[104] Sheibani K, Battifora H, Burke JS, et al. Leu-M1 antigen in human neoplasms: an immunohistologic study of 400 cases. *Am. J. Surg. Pathol.* 1986;10:227-36.

[105] Maguire B, Whitaker D, Carrello S, et al. Monoclonal antibody Ber-EP4: its use in the differential diagnosis of malignant mesothelioma and carcinoma in cell blocks of malignant effusions and FNA specimens. *Diagn. Cytopathol.* 1994;10:130-4.

[106] Dejmek A, Hjerpe A. Reactivity of six antibodies in effusions of mesothelioma, adenocarcinoma and mesotheliosis: stepwise logistic regression analysis. *Cytopathology* 2000;11:8-17.

[107] Latza U, Niedobitek G, Schwarting R, et al. Ber-EP4: new monoclonal antibody which distinguishes epithelia from mesothelia. *J. Clin. Pathol.* 1990;43:213-9.

[108] Kuhlmann L, Berghäuser K-H, Schäffer R. Distinction of mesothelioma from carcinoma in pleural effusions: an immunocytochemical study on routinely processed cytoblock preparations. *Pathol. Res. Pract.* 1991;187:467-71.

[109] Sheibani K, Shin SS, Kezirian J, et al. Ber-EP4 antibody as a discriminant in the differential diagnosis of malignant mesothelioma versus adenocarcinoma. *Am. J. Surg. Pathol.* 1991;15:779-84.

[110] Grove A, Paulsen SM, Gregersen M. The value of immunohistochemistry of pleural biopsy specimens in the differential diagnosis between malignant mesothelioma and metastatic carcinoma. *Pathol. Res. Pract.* 1994;190:1044-55.

[111] Shield PW, Callan JJ, Devine PL. Markers for metastatic adenocarcinoma in serous effusion specimens. *Diagn. Cytopathol.* 1994;11:237-45.

[112] Attanoos RL, Goddard H, Thomas ND, et al. A comparative immunohistochemical study of malignant mesothelioma and renal cell carcinoma: the diagnostic utility of Leu-M1, Ber-EP4, Tamm-Horsfall protein and thrombomodulin. *Histopathology* 1995;27:361-6.

[113] Ordóñez NG. Value of Ber-EP4 antibody in the differentiating epithelial pleural mesothelioma from adenocarcinoma: the M.D. Anderson experience and a critical review of the literature. *Am. J. Clin. Pathol.* 1998;109:85-9.

[114] Churg A. Immunohistochemical staining for vimentin and keratin in malignant mesothelioma. *Am. J. Surg. Pathol.* 1985;9:360-5.

[115] Mullink H, Henzan-Logmans SC, Alons-van Kordelaar JJM, et al. Simultaneous immunoenzyme staining of vimentin and cytokeratins with monoclonal antibodies as an aid in the differential diagnosis of malignant mesothelioma from pulmonary adenocarcinoma. *Virchows Arch.* [Cell Pathol] 1986;52:55-65.

[116] Chenard-Neu MP, Bellocq JP, Maier A, et al. Mésothéliomes malins de la plévre: analyse de leurs aspects immunohistochemiques. *Ann. Pathol.* 1990;10:20-7.

[117] Skov BG, Lauritzen AF, Hirsch FR, et al. Differentiation of adenocarcinoma of the lung and malignant mesothelioma: predictive value and reproducibility of immunoreactive antibodies. *Histopathology* 1994;25:431-7.

[118] Kortsik CS, Werner P, Freudenberg N, et al. Immunocytochemical characterization of malignant mesothelioma and carcinoma metastatic to the pleura: IOB3-a new tumor marker. *Lung* 1995;173:79-87.

In: Mesothelioma from Bench Side to Clinic
Editor: Alfonso Baldi, pp. 295-298

ISBN: 978-1-60021-789-0

Chapter XV

The Role of Cytology in the Diagnosis of Serosal Neoplasms

Antonella Rossetti
Rome American Hospital, Rome Italy

Abstract

In patients with effusions in the serous cavities, study of the fluid often provides the earliest opportunity for etiologic diagnosis. A neoplastic etiology has been found in 40 to 50 percent of pleural effusions and malignant disease is next to hepatic cirrhosis as a cause of ascites. Neoplastic involvement of the serous membranes is usually due to metastatic carcinoma: in males, carcinoma of the lung, and in females, carcinoma of the breast are the most frequent types of tumour giving rise to pleural metastases.

Carcinomas from a number of organs may involve peritoneum, with ovary and stomach being the most important sources. Over 75 percent of metastatic tumours in peritoneum are adenocarcinomas. Lymphomas also may involve the serous membranes and cause effusions. Leukemias represent the most common cause of effusions in children. Diffuse malignant mesothelioma is accompanied by effusion in a high percentage of cases. Large localized mesothelioma occasionally may give rise to an effusion.

The success rate in diagnosing neoplastic involvement of the serous cavities has varied considerably with around 60 percent being the average [1-3]. At least two or three specimens should be examined when tumour is suspected but the first cytologic diagnosis is negative. When the amount of sediment allows, cell blocks should be made. The hematoxylin and eosin stained sections prepared from these may provide valuable confirmation of the cyologic findings and show cell patterns more clearly (Table 1). Cell block sections also facilitate the application of special stains.

The general principles of malignant cell cytology are well recognized, but some further comment concerning diffuse malignant mesothelioma is appropriate. With epithelial mesotheliomas, the specimens are often cellular and there may be considerable variation in the size of the malignant cells. Cell clusters and morulae may be prominent (Figure 1).

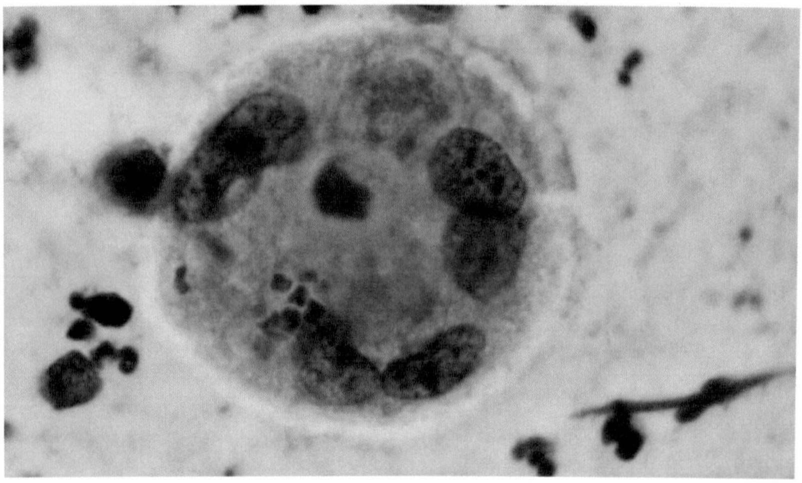

Figure 1. A single papillary cluster with nuclear abnormalities in an epithelioid mesothelioma of the pleura.

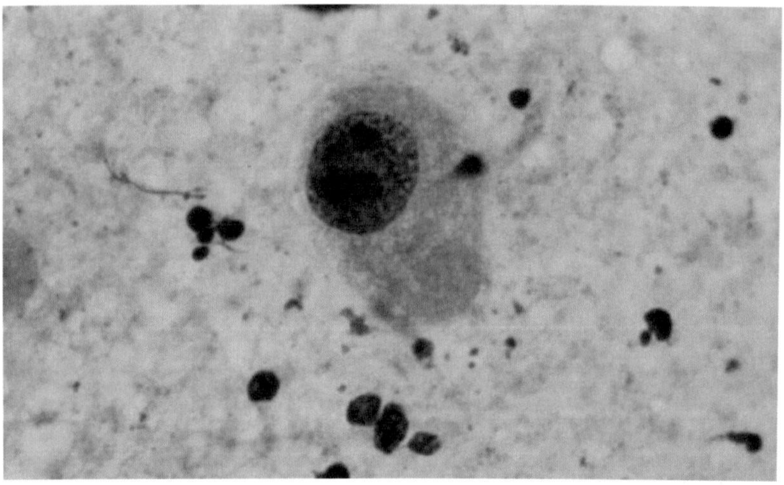

Figure 2. A tumour cell with a large, hyperchromatic nucleus and finely vacuolated cytoplasm in a peritoneal mesothelioma.

Table 1. Key cytological features in the diagnosis of malignant mesothelioma

(a) high cellularity
(b) variation in the size of malignant cells
(c) prominent cell clusters
(d) abundant dense cytoplasm, sometimes vacuolated
(e) hyperchromatic nuclei with prominent nuclei and irregular membranes.

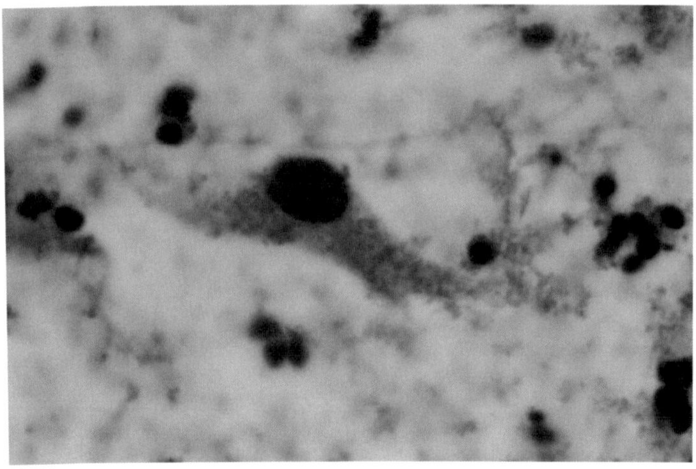

Figure 3. An elongated cancer cell with hyperchromatic nucleus in a sarcomatous mesothelioma of the pleura.

Well differentiated mesothelioma cells have abundant dense cytoplasm which is often more heavily stained than that of an adenocarcinoma and which often shows a fading away or foamy appearance at the periphery (Figure 2). Mesothelioma cells are commonly vacuolated and sometimes assume a signet ring form. Negative staining reactions for mucin distinguishes these cells from those of similar form occurring in adenocarcinoma.

Nuclear features such as increased size, hyperchromasia, prominent nucleoli and irregular staining of the nuclear membranes are indicative of malignancy in poorly differentiated mesothelial cells whereas in well differentiated lesions the nuclei may be difficult to distinguish from those of reactive mesothelial hyperplasia: however, the well differentiated tumour cells are often accompanied by more poorly differentiated transitional forms of the same populations, whose nuclear morphology indicates their malignant nature. Separation may be further assisted by the occurence in mesotheliomas of greater numbers of cells, bigger cell clusters, and larger cell size.

Histological feature in favor of malignancy include infiltration of deep tissues combined with obvious cytologic atypia, prominent groupings, as well as necrosis. The diagnosis of mesothelioma in the absence of detectable invasion (mesothelioma in situ) should be made only in the presence of clear cut cytologic aberrations. Metastatic adenocarcinoma may be associated with numerous hyperplastic mesothelial cells, but, unlike malignant mesothelioma, lacks cells which occupy and intermediate or transitional position between hyperplastic mesothelium and malignant cells. When the cell type is undifferentiated or sarcomatous (Figure 3), distinction from other malignant tumours is frequently impossible and specific diagnosis must rest on other investigations. The use of special stains and immunohistochemistry are proved of great value in the differential diagnosis between mesothelioma and adenocarcinoma.

References

[1] Lowell, J.R. *Pleural Effusions: A Comprehensive Review*, p.78. Baltimore: Univ.Park Press,1977.

[2] Bender, M.D. and Ockner, R. K. Diseases of the peritoneum, mesentery and diaphragm, p.1953. In: *Gastrointestinal Diseases*, 2nd Ed., Vol. 2 Sleisenger, M.H. and Fordtran, J. S. (Eds.) Philadelphia: W.B. Saunders Co.1978.

[3] Hirsch, A., Ruffie P., Nabut, M., Bignon, J., and Crétien, J. Pleural effusions: Laboratory tests in 300 cases. *Thorax* 34: 106-112,1979.

In: Mesothelioma from Bench Side to Clinic
Editor: Alfonso Baldi, pp. 299-322

ISBN: 978-1-60021-789-0

Chapter XVI

Non Pleural Mesotheliomas

Giuseppe Tonini, Maria E. Fratto, Bruno Vincenzi and Daniele Santini
Medical Oncology,
Campus Bio-Medico University, Rome, Italy

Abstract

In this chapter, the authors analyze in great detail the characteristics of non-pleural mesotheliomas. In particular they report the most updated aspects on the epidemiology, diagnosis, pathology, therapy and prognosis of these particular neoplasms.

Introduction

Mesotheliomas are tumors that arise from the mesothelial cells of the pleura, peritoneum, pericardium or tunica vaginalis. Although the number of new mesothelioma cases diagnosed each year in the United States seems to be decreasing, several other countries are projected to have continued increased incidence of mesothelioma over the next several years, probably as a result of a widespread exposure to asbestos, a factor with which mesothelioma is associated. Of the approximately 2500 new cases of mesothelioma in the United States each year, most are pleural mesotheliomas. The peritoneum is the second most common site of mesothelioma development and accounts for approximately 10% to 20% of all mesotheliomas. Mesotheliomas that involve the pericardium or originate from the tunica vaginalis are rare tumors. For this reason, it is difficult to obtain precise information regarding their incidence, natural history and optimal management.

Peritoneal Mesothelioma

Epidemiology

Information regarding incidence of peritoneal mesothelioma in the United States is obtained from the Surveillance, Epidemiology and End Results (SEER) Program. This database contains information from 9 cancer registries from 1973 to 1991 and 11 cancer registries from 1992 to 2000. A recent analysis of the SEER database estimated approximately 250 new cases of peritoneal mesothelioma each year in the United States. The incidence of peritoneal mesothelioma appears to be increasing in the USA and Europe, representing now 25-33% of all mesotheliomas. Although the overall incidence of mesotheliomas is higher in men than women (3:1 male/female), an higher proportion of women develop peritoneal mesothelioma compared with men. In fact peritoneal mesothelioma accounts for 17% of all mesotheliomas in women and 7% of all mesotheliomas in men.

Risk Factors

- *ASBESTOS*. Exposure to asbestos is supposed to play a role in the development of peritoneal mesothelioma. The evidence that asbestos exposure is related to the development of peritoneal mesothelioma is greater in men than women. In fact in a case control study, 88% of pleural mesotheliomas and 58% of peritoneal mesotheliomas among men were directly attributable to past asbestos exposure. For women, only 20% of cases (both pleural and peritoneal mesotheliomas) were related to past asbestos exposure. In a study using data from the Swedish Cancer Environment Registry, 35 pathologically confirmed cases of peritoneal mesothelioma were noted in Swedish men from 1961 to 1979. Almost 40% of these cases were in men who worked in the construction industry, with insulation workers at especially high risk. An increased risk of peritoneal mesothelioma among insulation workers also has been reported in other studies. In a study that examined the occupational risks for peritoneal cancer using a job-exposure matrix, researchers observed an increased incidence among male insulators and found that the risk increased significantly by probability and intensity of exposure to asbestos. Another study that prospectively followed 17, 800 asbestos insulation workers noted 175 deaths caused by mesothelioma. A higher proportion of these deaths were caused by peritoneal (64%) rather than pleural (36%) mesothelioma. Increased incidence of peritoneal mesothelioma also has been noted in workers at the Wittenoom crocidolite mines of Western Australia, although pleural mesothelioma was seven times more common in these workers than peritoneal mesothelioma. Cases of peritoneal mesothelioma caused by environmental exposure from asbestos contaminated soil in Turkey also have been reported.
- *ERIONITE*. Cases of peritoneal mesotheliomas have been reported after erionite exposure in the Cappadocia regions.

- *TREMOLITE.* Datas show that malignant mesothelioma is endemic in some rural parts of Anatolia, Turkey. Many studies have shown that the high risk of mesothelioma in this region is due to environmental exposure to asbestos-contaminated soil mixtures. Mineral analysis of these white-soil samples identified contamination predominantly with tremolite.
- *RADIATION.* A few cases of peritoneal mesothelioma after external beam radiation have been reported. They usually involved men with a history of testicular carcinoma, although cases of peritoneal mesothelioma after radiation for ovarian teratocarcinoma and cervical cancer have been described. A case of peritoneal mesothelioma after administration of thorotrast also was reported.
- *SIMIAN VIRUS 40.* Although simian virus 40 has been implicated in the causation of some mesotheliomas, its role in the causation of peritoneal mesothelioma is unclear.

Pathology

Mesothelioma is a tumor derived from cells lining the serous cavity. The tumor may be restricted to a limited area of the affected membrane or infiltrates it diffusely. Tumors confined to a small area have a papillary, cystic or adenomatoid morphology and are considered to be of low biologic aggressiveness. The *adenomatoid tumor*, a common variant in the peritoneum, is a benign tumor that forms gland-like structures. Although it could be confused with carcinomas, the cells do not exhibit nuclear atypia and mitotic figures are absent. This tumor is usually confined to the genital tract, with the epididymis being the most common site in men and the uterus, fallopian tubes and ovaries being the most common sites in women. This lesion is generally solitary and less than 2 cm in size. Clinically, patients are asymptomatic and rarely the tumor recurs after adequate excision.

The most common mesothelial tumor is *diffuse malignant mesothelioma*, an aggressive neoplasm that infiltrates serous membrane extensively and microscopically may show an epithelial, sarcomatous or mixed (biphasic) pattern. The epithelial variant can be a tubulopapillary or nonglandular (solid) variant. Histologically, this tumor shows true signs of malignancy, such as stromal invasion. Immunohistochemical markers, similar to those used in pleural mesotheliomas, help establish the diagnosis. *Deciduoid peritoneal mesothelioma* is a variant of epithelial diffuse malignant peritoneal mesothelioma, composed of cells with abundant glassy eosinophilic cytoplasm and resembles a decidual reaction. In some cases this variant has been described in patients during or after pregnancy, and researchers believe that pregnancy-induced peritoneal deciduosis and diffuse mesothelial proliferation caused by hormonal changes may be responsible. However, cases of deciduous mesothelioma also have been reported in men and elderly women. The treatment of these patients is similar to that of patients who have diffuse malignant peritoneal mesothelioma, but it is characterized by an aggressive clinical course and poor prognosis.

Occasionally, a less biologically aggressive type of diffuse mesothelioma with well-differentiated papillary or cystic characteristics is observed. On pathologic examination, *well-differentiated papillary mesothelioma* of the peritoneum is characterized by uniform appearance of tumor cells without multilayering and absence of nuclear features of malignancy. It is more common in young women and patients may present with multiple peritoneal nodules. Association with asbestos exposure is not well established. In the largest reported series, patients had a prolonged survival and, in view of the favorable prognosis, treatment is generally not recommended unless a patient is symptomatic or there is evidence of tumor progression. Anyway, there are reports that these lesions can recur or progress to malignant mesothelioma with distant metastases.

Cystic or multicystic mesothelioma is intermediate in its malignant behaviour between the localized and diffuse types. Typically these patients present with an abdominal or pelvic mass and at the time of surgery are noted to have multiple translucent, grape-like clusters of fluid-filled cysts. On microscopic examination the cysts are lined by a single layer of flattened or cuboidal mesothelial cells. It is much more common in women than men. In general, these tumors have a benign clinical course but are characterized by a high recurrence rate after surgical resection and a recent report showed malignant transformation in a patient who had multicystic mesothelioma. These tumors are believed to be hormone sensitive and some case reports have reported reduction in cyst volume and clinical improvement in patients treated with leuprolide and tamoxifen. Well-differentiated papillary and multicystic mesothelioma of the peritoneum can be of benign or of low malignant potential. But at the time of diagnosis their presentation with multiple peritoneal lesions can be confused with peritoneal carcinomatosis. Another clinically important feature of these tumors is their association with diffuse malignant mesothelioma, which underscores the necessity for adequate histologic sampling.

Another variant of a mesothelial-derived tumor is a *serous papillary tumor* that was believed to arise from the surface epithelium of the ovary and to be similar to serous papillary neoplasm of extraovarian origin. However, later studies have shown that extraovarian serous papillary tumors are a clinico-pathologically distinctive variant with a more aggressive clinical course.

Fibrous tumors are often included in the group of peritoneal tumors, but they originate from submesothelial tissues.

Table 1 shows the classification of primary tumors of serous membranes according to the Armed Forces Institute of Pathology (AFIP).

Natural History

When peritoneal mesothelioma occurs, the peritoneal surface becomes increasingly studded with numerous tumor nodules of varying sizes. Intestinal adhesions, nodularity and infiltrations of the omentum may occur at an early stage of the disease. With disease progression, massive accumulations of the tumors are observed in the omentum, in the lower abdomen, in the pelvis and beneath the right hemidiaphragm.

Tumor nodules tend to grow on the parietal peritoneum, while the visceral peritoneal surfaces remain relatively clear because peristaltic motion discourages the adherence of cancer cells to mobile surfaces. In the later stages of mesothelioma progression, tumor encases liver, spleen and even small bowel surfaces. The viscera eventually become completely encased in the tumor and the peritoneal cavity is obliterated (frozen abdomen) before intestinal obstruction occurs.

Table 1. Classification of primary tumors of serous membranes

LOCALIZED TUMORS	
MESOTHELIAL	SUBMESOTHELIAL
• Adenomatoid tumor • Cistic mesothelioma • Benign papillary mesothelioma	• Fibroma (localized fibrous mesothelioma) • Fibrosarcoma (localized fibrous malignant mesothelioma) • Angioma • Angiosarcoma • Other soft tissue tumors
DIFFUSE TUMORS	
MESOTHELIAL	SUBMESOTHELIAL
• Malignant mesothelial epithelial • Tubulopapillar • Nonglandular (solid) • Malignant mesothelial sarcomatous • Malignant mesothelial biphasic (mixed) • Malignant mesothelial undifferentiated • Papillary serous tumor • Well-differentiated papillary mesothelioma • Cystic (multicistic) mesothelioma	• Angiosarcoma

Underlying tissues can be invaded by peritoneal mesotheliomas. Invasion can involve the omentum and the dependent parts of the abdominopelvic surfaces (pelvis and right subhepatic space). Infrequently, at advanced stages of the disease, tumor infiltrates the liver capsule and extends into retroperitoneal tissues (pancreas, kidney, etc…). Although the undersurface of the diaphragm is nearly always involved by tumor masses, its full-thickness invasion is relatively uncommon. Consequently, peritoneal mesotheliomas rarely spread to the pleural cavity, while the reverse situation is common. Extension to the tunica vaginalis testis occurs frequently, while invasion of the abdominal wall is rare and is usually related to a laparotomy scar.

At autopsy, metastases are observed in 50% of peritoneal mesotheliomas, with the liver, viscera and abdominal lymph nodes being the most frequent sites. Other sites of metastases are inguinal and thoracic lymph nodes, lung, pleura, pericardium, heart and adrenal glands.

The major morbidity and mortality of this disease is caused by progression within the abdomen and pelvis. In a majority of cases peritoneal mesothelioma remains confined to the abdomen. Many reports have demonstrated that 75-80% of patients with peritoneal mesothelioma die from direct complications of the local disease, with 65-70% of deaths due to cachexia from small bowel obstruction resulting from bowel encasement by tumor.

Diagnosis

Clinical Presentation

Peritoneal mesothelioma occurs mainly in patients aged 40-65 years old, though it was described in children and young adults, as well as in a 92 years old patient. There are not specific symptoms of the disease and clinical diagnosis is difficult. In fact in a majority of patients diagnosis is postponed until laparoscopy-directed biopsy or esploratory laparotomy, which provides histologic information. According to Mohamed et al. peritoneal mesothelioma presents as a pain-predominant or ascites-predominant clinical type and 14% of patients have concomitant abdominal distension and abdominal pain. In fact patients typically present with abdominal distension, pain, bloating, alteration in bowel habits and weight loss, with ascites present in most patients at diagnosis. The abdominal pain is rarely limited to a particular region of the abdomen and it is frequently migratory and unaffected by motion and eating. Intermittent pain is invariably associated with partial or complete bowel obstruction. Other signs of advanced disease include fever, leukocytosis and thrombocytosis and they are correlated with a poor prognosis.

The onset of symptoms is usually gradual, but may be acute, with the picture of an acute abdomen, intestinal obstruction or acute testicular torsion. Peritoneal mesothelioma has also presented as a pelvic mass simulating ovarian tumor, retroperitoneal tumor or isolated lesion of the small intestine.

Laboratory Tests

Laboratory tests are not helpful in making the diagnosis of peritoneal mesothelioma. This tumor is usually associated with leukocytosis, thrombocytosis, clotting abnormalities and polyclonal hyperimmunoglobulinemia. These tumors have been reported to secrete a variety of ectopic hormones and tumor markers, but none of them can be reliably used for diagnostic purposes. A few case reports have described elevated serum CA-125, which in some instances was associated with a close correlation with tumor response.

Instrumental Procedures

- *RADIOLOGIC EXAMINATION.* Radiologic examination is an important component of patient's evaluation. The Computed Tomography (CT) is the method of choice for imaging this tumor, although it requires the use of oral and intravenous contrast agents to distinguish tumors from nearby tissues. The extent of this evaluation must be limited to chest, abdominal and pelvis CT because the incidence of distal metastasis outside this areas at presentation is low. Classic findings at CT are intraperitoneal masses, variable involvement of omentum, mesentheric thickening, peritoneal studding, signs of hemorrhage within the tumor masses and ascites. A recent study suggested that the CT scan can be a valuable aid in determining if a patient is a surgical candidate. Other findings include masses involving the bowel serosa, extensions into the liver, spleen and abdominal wall, adenopathy and distant tumor metastases. Magnetic Resonance Imaging (MRI) provides good resolution, but requires longer scan times during which respiratory motion and bowel peristalsis can blur images. Positron Emission Tomography (PET) scans may be useful and provide functional imaging, although without high resolution. However, PET-CT may be able to preserve the high resolution of CT and at the same time provides functional imaging. Contrast radiologic examination of the gastrointestinal tract in patients with peritoneal mesothelioma can reveal compression and dislocation of bowel loops by extrinsic masses, mesenteric retraction, segmental stenosis and signs of intestinal obstruction. No intraluminal abnormality is usually found. Additional radiologic techniques for detection of distant metastases should be used if there are clinical or laboratory signs of extraperitoneal spread.

- *CYTOLOGIC EXAMINATION OF ASCITIC FLUID.* Ascites is detected in up to 90% of patients. Peritoneal fluid may be a watery transudate or a viscous fluid rich in mucopolysaccarides. No diagnostic significance is attached to the character of the fluid, although a viscous ascites with high hyaluronidase levels may suggest a mesothelioma. Massive ascites may initially confuse mesothelioma with severe cirrhosis. Surprisingly, the cytologic assessment of peritoneal fluid reveals malignant cells only in 5-10% of patients. In the majority of cases diagnosis can be established only if a sufficient quantity of biopsy is submitted for histologic examination.
- *LAPAROSCOPY.* Because definitive diagnosis requires visually directed tissue sampling, a growing interest in laparoscopy has occurred. Reports on laparoscopic diagnosis of this malignancy continue to be published starting from 1966. The major role of laparoscopy is to provide bioptic material directly from peritoneal tumor nodules sufficient for histologic diagnosis. However, the following combination of features, when observed in patients without radiologic evidence of primary cancer, suggests malignant mesothelioma clinically:

  (1) Presence of homogenously spreading lesions on both parietal and visceral peritoneum.
  (2) Presence of tumor on Glisson's capsule in absence of hepatic metastases.
  (3) Absence of direct or indirect signs of other abdominal neoplasms.

Histochemical and Immunohistochemical Studies

Even if it is evident that definitive diagnosis of malignant mesothelioma can be established only by histologic examination, it is not a straightforward diagnosis in all cases and histochemistry is required for differential diagnosis. However, distinction of peritoneal mesothelioma from adenocarcinoma is sometimes impossible by routine and light microscopic studies and often classical histochemical and electron microscopic studies are not always available because of the nature of the specimen and its processing. In addition, they are not always conclusive. The spectrum of differential diagnosis is presented in Table 2.

A significant role in the histologic diagnosis of malignant mesothelioma is now played by immunohistochemical studies. A panel of monoclonal antibodies, all reactive in fixed and paraffin-embedded tissue sections, can be used in the differential diagnosis of diffuse malignant mesothelioma. This panel includes Leu-M1, B72.3, HMFG-2, carcinoembryonic antigen (CEA), keratin and some other monoclonal antibodies.

Table 2. Differential diagnosis of diffuse malignant mesothelioma of peritoneum

EPITHELIAL MESOTHELIOMA	BIPHASIC MESOTHELIOMA	SARCOMATOUS MESOTHELIOMA
• Peritoneal Carcinomatosis (from gastric, intestinal, pancreatic, breast cancer) • Well-differentiated papillary or solid mesothelial hyperplasia • Moderately differentiated tubulopapillary adenocarcinoma • Poorly differentiated carcinoma	• Other biphasic tumors • Carcinoma with cellular stroma • Mesothelial hyperplasia with serosal fibrosis	• Fibrosis • Sarcomas arising in adjacent tissues • Metastatic sarcoma • Malignant schwannoma • Malignant fibrous histiocytoma

Mesotheliomas usually stain positive for calretinin, cytokeratins 5/6, WT-1, thrombomodulin, and mesothelin but negative for the adenocarcinoma markers CEA, Leu-M1, Ber-Ep4, B72.3, Bg8 and MOC-31. Leu-M1 is a very useful marker. No cases of malignant mesothelioma express this marker, but it is present in a majority of adenocarcinomas. Therefore positive staining with this antibody excludes the diagnosis of mesothelioma. Moreover, regardless of its morphologic subtype, malignant mesothelioma is a keratin-positive tumor, so absence of keratin practically excludes the diagnosis of mesothelioma as opposed to sarcoma. However, keratin staining has not value in distinguish mesothelioma from carcinoma.

Principles of Anticancer Therapy

Surgery and Continuous Hyperthermic Peritoneal Perfusion (CHPP)

Because all surgical and autopsy series have demonstrated diffuse involvement of both parietal and visceral peritoneum, surgery is considered by most authors only as a method for tissue biopsy, for intestinal bypass or diversion in cases of intestinal obstruction and to relieve massive ascites by peritoneovenous shunting. Moreover, complete surgical removal of the tumor is rarely feasible and do not cause survival benefit without additional therapy. But patients who have peritoneal mesothelioma experience morbidity and mortality almost exclusively secondary to disease progression in the abdominal cavity and various regional therapeutic strategies have been developed to specifically control this component of disease. In general, regional therapies have the advantage of allowing intensive and directed measures to control tumor while minimizing unnecessary systemic toxicity. Until the later stages of tumor growth, peritoneal mesothelioma usually progresses as a diffuse and superficially spreading condition in the abdominal cavity that, in many circumstances, can be nearly or completely grossly resected by using systematic peritonectomy procedures or local ablative measures. In fact it has been demonstrated that patients who can be made macroscopically disease free have a greater probability of success with intraperitoneal chemotherapy.

Moreover, surgical treatment of well-differentiated papillary and cystic mesothelioma has been associated with prolonged survival despite the presence of bulky disease.

Many investigators have combined intraperitoneal (IP) administration of chemotherapeutics or biologic agents intraoperatively with hyperthermia or in the early postoperative period. There are several advantages of continuous hyperthermic peritoneal perfusion (CHPP), also commonly referred to as hyperthermic intraoperative peritoneal chemotherapy. After all or most of the peritoneal tumor has been removed and no adhesions are present is the optimal time to achieve uniform distribution of topical chemotherapy to a complex surface such as the peritoneal cavity. Conversely, topically applied intraperitoneal chemotherapy may have unpredictable or incomplete tumor penetration and may have regional toxicity, such as fibrosis. Early postoperative intraperitoneal chemotherapy shares the advantages of intraoperative chemotherapy because it is administered before the development of any intra-abdominal adhesions. Hyperthermia has established direct tumoricidal activity and can augment significantly the cytotoxicity of various chemotherapeutics.

Several centers have reported results using operative cytoreduction and CHPP for patients with peritoneal mesothelioma (Table 3). Even if there are no standard criteria for patient selection and treatment parameters, the results of these different institutional experiences have been consistent in some aspects. For example, all the series report an overall survival that seems to be better rather than the natural history of this condition. Moreover this type of therapy is clearly able to palliate the secondary malignant ascites in most individuals who present with this disease. Mongero et al. have reported preliminary results of an intensive regional therapy program that consists of initial surgical debulking, 4 months of IP chemotherapy using cisplatin and doxorubicin, and a second-look procedure to resect residual tumor and apply a CHPP using cisplatin and mitomycin C administered for 1 hour. Because the number of patients is small (n=3), meaningful interpretation of complications and outcome is difficult. A series of 19 patients who had benign and malignant peritoneal mesothelioma treated with cytoreduction and CHPP using cisplatin with either mitomycin C or doxorubicin has been reported by Dcraco et al[60]. The survival rate was 69% at a mean follow-up of 27 months. 94% of patients had complete resolution of their malignant ascites for the duration of their follow-up. A comparably sized series also was reported by Loggie et al. In their cohort of 12 patients with malignant mesothelioma, treatment consisted of cytoreduction and a 2-hour CHPP using 30 mg of mitomycin C and another 10 mg added after 1 hour of perfusion. Median survival was 34.2 months with a median follow-up of 45 months, and 86% of patients had permanent control of malignant ascites.

According to Sugarbaker et al, the overall median survival of 68 patients with peritoneal mesothelioma treated at the Washington Hospital between 1989 and 2003 was 67 months with a projected 3-year survival rate of approximately 64%. 55 of these patients were treated with cytoreduction and various regimens of CHPP using cisplatin and doxorubicin with or without early postoperative IP chemotherapy consisting of IP paclitaxel. In their series only 47% of patients had resolution of ascites. Moreover, female patients had a longer median survival and the results were also better in patients with epithelial and cystic forms of the disease. Resulting morbidities include bile leak, small bowel fistulas, and bleeding. Older patients, especially past age 70, experience an increased morbidity from the treatment.

Table 3. Studies of cytoreduction and CHPP for treatment of peritoneal mesothelioma

Study	No. of Patients	RD After Cytoreduction	CHPP Agents	Median Survival	Notes
Mongero et al.	3	NR	Cisplatin + MMC	NR	No. of patients too small to correctly understand complications and outcome
Deraco et al.	19	75%< 2,5 mm	Cisplatin + MMC/ Cisplatin + doxorubicin	NR	Survival rate after 27 months: 69%. Resolution of ascites during follow-up: 94%
Loggie et al.	12	66% < 2 cm	MMC	34,2 months	Resolution of ascites during follow-up: 86%
Sugarbaker et al.	68	60% < 2,5 cm	Cisplatin + doxorubicin	67 months	Overall survival greater for women than men. Resolution of ascites during follow-up: 47%
Feldman et al.	49	88% < 1 cm	Cisplatin	92 months	Overall survival greater for patients < 60 years. Resolution of ascites during follow-up: 57%

Abbreviations: CHPP, continuous hyperthermic peritoneal perfusion; RD, residual disease; MMC, mitomicin C; NR, mot reported.

Feldman et al. reported the results of 49 patients with malignant peritoneal mesothelioma treated with cytoreduction and CHPP using cisplatin at the National Cancer Institute. 35 patients also received early postoperative IP dwell with paclitaxel and 5-fluorouracil. At a median follow-up time of 28 months, the median overall survival was 92 months. 15 of 26 patients who presented with ascites had palliation for a median duration of 25 months.

Although morbidities after cytoreduction and CHPP are related to the operative procedure and chemotherapy, most treatment mortalities seem to be related primarily to the extent of the operative procedure rather than intraperitoneal chemotherapy and range from 0% to 7%. Many studies have demonstrated that the use of surgical resection and CHPP can palliate ascites and is associated with long-term survival and improved quality of life in many individuals. Additional studies are being conducted to refine and improve this type of approach further for patients who have peritoneal mesothelioma.

Radiotherapy

The role of radiation alone for the treatment of peritoneal mesothelioma remains unclear. Some studies have evaluated the use of external radiotherapy in combination with chemotherapy and surgery. Because this is a disease with predominantly intrabdominal spread, intraperitoneal radiotherapy with colloidal gold was considered in different studies. But the poor distribution of radioisotopes due to gravity and adhesions following previous surgery were the main reason for low complete responses and survival. Moreover, small bowel obstruction occurred in 2-10% of the patients treated. It was also mentioned that intraperitoneal radiotherapy substantially increased the risk of complications after cytoreductive surgery with intraperitoneal chemotherapy. Several groups have also used external radiation in combination with intravenous or intraperitoneal chemotherapy. But these authors stressed the advantages of intraperitoneal drug administration without clarifying the role of radiotherapy for this disease.

Intraperitoneal and Systemic Chemotherapy

Because many newly diagnosed patients who have peritoneal mesothelioma are not candidates for surgery and many of the patients treated with surgery relapse, these patients are candidates for chemotherapy. The optimal chemotherapeutic regimen or route of drug administration (intraperitoneal versus intravenous) for treatment of peritoneal mesothelioma is unclear because there have been no prospectively designed clinical trials specific for this disease. Treatment regimens that have been used incorporate drugs that have shown some activity in pleural mesothelioma. Because the disease is mostly confined to the peritoneal cavity, several studies have evaluated intraperitoneal chemotherapy in peritoneal mesotheliomas because it has the potential advantage of increased drug concentration in the peritoneal cavity with less systemic toxicity. The disadvantages of this approach include poor penetration in tumors > 1 cm and the need for an indwelling catheter with risk of complications including infection and blockage. Intraperitoneal chemotherapeutic agents that have been used include cisplatin, mitomycin, 5-fluouracil, adriamycin and paclitaxel.

Several centers have reported results using intraperitoneal (IP) or systemic chemotherapy for patients with peritoneal mesothelioma (Table 4). In one of the largest studies of IP chemotherapy in peritoneal mesothelioma performed by Markman et al., 19 patients were treated with IP administration of cisplatin (100 mg/m2 every 28 days) and mitomycin (5–10 mg/treatment given 7 days after each IP administration of cisplatin). Of the 15 patients with malignant ascites, 7 (47%) experienced control of fluid reaccumulation that ranged from 2 to more than 73 months. 4 patients survived more than 3 years from the initiation of therapy. No objective tumor responses were noted. This study showed that a subset of patients who had peritoneal mesothelioma with small volume disease after surgical resection might benefit from IP chemotherapy, especially in terms of decreasing fluid collection. Langer et al. evaluated efficacy of IP cisplatin and etoposide in patients who had peritoneal mesothelioma. Patients whose tumor was debulked to less than 2 cm before administration of chemotherapy showed a median survival of 22 months. On the contrary patients with measurable surgically inaccessible disease had a median survival of 5 months. This study showed that cisplatin-based IP chemotherapy may be of value in patients with decreased tumor bulk after cytoreductive surgery. Taub et al. demonstrated that a multimodality approach for treating peritoneal mesothelioma is effective. The treatment protocol included surgical debulking followed by intraperitoneal administration of cisplatin, doxorubicin and gamma interferon, second laparotomy with attempted resection of any residual disease and intraoperative hyperthermic perfusion with cisplatin and mitomycin followed subsequently by whole abdominal radiotherapy . The median overall survival of the 27 patients treated in this study was 68 months.

Table 4. Studies of intraperitoneal or systemic chemotherapy in peritoneal mesothelioma

Study	No. of Patients	Agents	Route	Median Survival	Notes
Markman et al.	19	Cisplatin + Mitomicin C	Intraperitoneal	9 months	Resolution of ascites during follow-up: 42%. Patients with smaller RD after resection can benefit more from IP chemotherapy.
Langer et al.	19	Cisplatin + Etoposide	Intraperitoneal	5 months (nonoperable) 22 months (if debulking)	Patients with smaller RD after resection can benefit more from IP chemotherapy.
Taub et al.	27	Cisplatin+ doxorubicin + IFNγ	Intraperitoneal	68 months	A multimodality approach for peritoneal mesothelioma is effective
Le DT et al.	17	Cisplatin + Irinotecan	Intravenous and/or intraperitoneal	Not reached	Overall Response Rate: 24% Stable Disease: 53%
Bloss et al.	98 (1056 total)	Pemetrexed +/- cisplatin	Intravenous	Not reached	Overall response rate: 26% Complete response: 5% Partial response: 21%

Abbreviations: RD, residual disease; IP, intraperitoneal.

Initial studies of systemic chemotherapy in peritoneal mesothelioma evaluated doxorubicin-containing regimens that showed some activity but also significant toxicity. A recent study by Le DT et al. tested the combination of cisplatin and irinotecan in peritoneal mesothelioma. 17 patients received the combination of intravenous (IV) or IP cisplatin, 50 or 60 mg/m2, on day 1 and irinotecan, 50 or 60 mg/m2 IV, on days 1, 8, and 15 given every 4 weeks for 6 cycles. 15 patients received two or more cycles of treatment, and 8 patients each received IV or IP cisplatin, whereas 1 patient received both IV and IP cisplatin. The treatment was well tolerated, with toxicity consisting predominately of nausea, emesis, granulocytopenia, and anemia. The overall response rate was 24%, with 4 patients achieving a partial response and 9 patients having stable disease.

Based on the results of a phase III clinical trial of cisplatin plus pemetrexed versus cisplatin alone in pleural mesothelioma that showed an increased response rate and an increase in overall survival in favour of the combination, many oncologists also would consider this regimen for the treatment of patients who have peritoneal mesothelioma who are not surgical candidates or who experience relapse after surgery. There is no published information on the effectiveness of this combination in peritoneal mesothelioma except for a nonrandomized study performed by Bloss et al. started in June 2002 designed to obtain additional efficacy and safety data on pemetrexed alone or in combination with cisplatin in mesotheliomas. Of the 1056 patients who had mesothelioma who were treated on this study, 98 (9.2%) had peritoneal mesothelioma. Newly diagnosed patients were treated with a combination of cisplatin, 75 mg/m2, and pemetrexed, 500 mg/m2, given every 21 days for a maximum of six cycles. Patients who received prior treatment were treated with pemetrexed alone. Of the 73 patients who had peritoneal mesothelioma who were evaluable for response, there were 4 complete and 15 partial responses for an overall objective response rate of 26%. The proportion of these responses in patients who received the combination treatment versus patients treated with pemetrexed alone was not described. From these limited data it is difficult to make any definitive conclusion except that pemetrexed and cisplatin seem to have activity in peritoneal mesothelioma that merits further investigation.

Biological Agents

Some patients who have peritoneal mesothelioma have been treated with biological agents usually as part of phase I studies. In a phase I study of intraperitoneal administration of recombinant human interleukin-12 in patients with peritoneal carcinomatosis a complete response was noted in a patient with epithelial papillary mesothelioma. In a phase I study of Flt3 ligand administered intraperitoneal or subcutaneous no responses were noted in the four patients with peritoneal mesothelioma treated on the study. Other biologic therapies, including immunotoxins that target the tumor antigen mesothelin, are also undergoing clinical evaluation in patients who have peritoneal mesothelioma. Mesothelin is a cell surface protein that is highly expressed in mesotheliomas and is a good target for cancer therapy given its limited expression in normal tissues. A recombinant anti-mesothelin immunotoxin, SS1P, is currently being tested in Phase I clinical trials. A total of 25 patients including 8 patients with peritoneal and 5 patients with pleural mesothelioma have been included in the study. The treatment has been well tolerated and shows promising clinical activity including resolution of ascites and stable disease in several patients. After completion of this Phase I study, Phase II studies of SS1P alone or in combination with chemotherapy are in project.

Moreover, ongoing clinical trials are evaluating the effectiveness of ZD1839, an inhibitor of Epidermal Growth Factor Receptor (EGFR), and imatinib mesylate, an inhibitor of the tyrosine kinases associated with Platelet Derived Growth Factor (PDGF) receptor, c-kit and Bcr-Abl in patients with mesothelioma. Moreover, many studies have shown that the Vascular Endothelial Growth Factor (VEGF) play an important role in mesothelioma biology.

In fact ongoing clinical trials are evaluating the role of the three VEGF inhibitors SU5416, thalidomide and bevacizumab in mesothelioma patients. Of these agents bevacizumab, an anti-VEGF monoclonal antibody is being evaluated in a randomized Phase II trial of gemcitabine plus cisplatin with bevacizumab or placebo with time to disease progression as the primary endpoint. The results of this trial will be important to determine if bevacizumab improves the outcome of patients with mesothelioma similar to that seen for other solid tumors using a combination of chemotherapy and bevacizumab.

Prognostic Factors

The favourable and unfavourable prognostic factors associated with peritoneal mesothelioma are summarized in Table 5.

Table 5. Prognostic factors in peritoneal mesothelioma

TYPE	PROGNOSTIC FACTOR	POSITIVE	NEGATIVE
CLINICAL	Age	<50	>50
	Performance Status	0-1	>2
	Previous surgery	Unexplored	Explored
	Surgical Complications	Absent	Present
	Intestinal Obstruction	Absent	Present
	Prior cytoreduction	Complete	Incomplete
RADIOLOGIC	Small bowel loops	Free, normal calibre	Entrapped, distended
	Pattern of tumor	Free ascites, redistribution	Solid tumor
	Tumor distribution	Omentum	Small Bowel
	Tumore features	Localized	Diffuse
	Tumor volume	Small	Large
HISTOLOGIC	Type	Epithelial	Sarcomatoid
	Mucin production	Present	Absent
	Grade	Low	High
	Tumor parenchyma	Cellular	Solid

The most important prognostic factor is tumor histology. It is important to separate diffuse malignant mesothelioma from the well-differentiated papillary mesotheliomas that usually have indolent behaviour and therefore a prolonged survival. Patients who have solitary tumors have a better prognosis than patients who have diffuse disease. In patients who have resectable disease who undergo extensive tumor debulking followed by intraoperative hyperthermic chemotherapy the median overall survival is longer than 5 years. Many patients are not candidates for surgical resection and prognosis of such patients is not clear. Some studies have suggested that in contrast to pleural mesothelioma, which has a uniformly poor prognosis, the prognosis of patients with diffuse epithelial peritoneal mesothelioma is varied and long-term survivors are seen.

Mesothelioma of the Tunica Vaginalis

During normal embryonic development, an outpouching of the peritoneum traverses through the inguinal canal as processus vaginalis and surrounds the testis. The processus vaginalis then atrophies, except the portion that surrounds the testis and it is called the tunica vaginalis. Histologically the cells that line the tunica vaginalis are similar to those that line the pleura, peritoneum and pericardium, so they are at risk of developing mesothelioma. Tunica vaginalis mesotheliomas are rare tumors and are mostly reported in the literature as case reports, the first described in 1957.

Epidemiology

Of the 11,629 malignant mesothelioma deaths recorded in the UK Health and Safety Executive Mesothelioma Register from 1968 to 1991, only 0.09% of the deaths were caused by mesothelioma of the tunica vaginalis. The age distribution of patients with malignant mesothelioma of the tunica vaginalis ranges from 7 to 87 years, with the highest incidence between ages 55 and 75 years (47.1%). More than two-thirds of the cases are reported in patients older than 45 years, with a median age of 60 years. The higher incidence of mesothelioma among older patients is related to longer exposure to asbestos, with a latency of 10–40 years. Although malignant mesotheliomas of the tunica vaginalis are commonly reported in older patients, 10% of the cases occurred in patients younger than 25 years. Unfortunately, especially in this young age group, there are no data on asbestos exposure, familial history of asbestos exposure or viral infection; therefore, the reasons for the development of the disease remain unclear in these cases.

Risk Factors

Although there are several mechanisms hypothesized for the development of tunical mesothelioma, the exposure to asbestos or asbestos-containing materials remains the only established risk factor. In fact occupational exposure to asbestos (shipyard and vehicle maintenance workers, engineers, building maintenance workers) is the main pathogenic factor for the illness, present in 35–45% of the cases. A previous testicular trauma, hernial repair and long lasting or recidivant hydrocele can also be related to the development of malignant tunical mesothelioma. To our knowledge, the development of tunical mesothelioma has not been reported to be secondary to radiation exposure, radiotherapy or viral infections.

Pathology

Grossly, malignant mesothelioma of the tunica vaginalis is typically a single or multinodular mass in a hydrocele or a solid tumor that surrounds the testis. In the multifocal form the nodules are fairly small, ranging from a few millimetres to 1 or 2 cm in diameter; the solitary variant tends to be larger. Microscopically, 60-75% of tunical mesotheliomas have an epithelial histology and the remainders are mixed (biphasic) epithelial and sarcomatoid lesions. The epithelial variants most commonly show a tubulopapillary growth pattern, but other patterns, including some with solid cellular sheets, are represented as well. The sarcomatoid component comprises dense aggregates of spindle cells, sometimes with fascicular or storiform growth patterns. Histologically, these neoplasms are identical to malignant mesotheliomas of the pleura and peritoneum. Purely sarcomatoid mesotheliomas are extraordinarily rare or nonexistent in the peritesticular region.

Natural History

Most of the malignant mesotheliomas typically present as papillary, exophytic excrescences of the tunica vaginalis, although they can also invade the adjacent structures. In fact the tumor may invade the testicular parenchyma, scrotal skin, epidydimis and other local structures. Tumor progression with the development of lymphatic or distant tumor metastases has been descripted several times. The incidence of primary disseminated disease has also been reported. All of these patients were older than 40 years, with a median age of 58 years. In cases of metastatic disease, retroperitoneal lymph nodes are most often involved, followed by inguinal and iliac lymph nodes. Distant tumor metastases can occur, more often in the thoracal and lumbar vertebrae, omentum, liver and lung. Primary metastatic mesothelioma occurs rarely but it should be considered and carefully looked for at the initial diagnosis.

Diagnosis

Clinical Presentation

Malignant mesothelioma of the tunica vaginalis usually presents as an unilateral testicular mass, an enlargement of the scrotum developed within several months. In most patients, the preoperative diagnosis is an hydrocele (56.3%), a testicular tumor (in 32.8%), epididymitis (3.2%), a scrotal hernia (3.2%), a spermatocele (3.2%) and a post-traumatic testicular lesion (1.6%). The right and left tunica vaginalis are involved in equal proportion, with bilateral tunica vaginalis mesothelioma being rare.

Instrumental Procedures

The major management complication lies in the difficulty of obtaining an accurate preoperative diagnosis, in fact most frequently it is achieved intraoperatively or post-operatively. However, now the diagnosis can be suggested by computed tomography or ultrasound-based imaging, that provide additional information about exophytic lesions in the tunica vaginalis when larger than 0,5 cm. In fact preoperative ultrasound can give substantial information for the determination of inhomogenous hydrocele fluid, hypoechogenecity of the fluid or exophytic tumors.

Cytological examination of aspirated hydrocele fluid has also been occasionally useful in suggesting the diagnosis, but this process is often problematic and considerable caution should be used with this type of specimen. Therefore, when the diagnosis is suspected, a biopsy should be performed.

Histochemical and Immunohistochemical Studies

By immunohistochemical staining methods, the presence of malignant mesothelioma may be determined and it is a major therapeutic advantage prior to surgical intervention.

Malignant mesothelioma of tunica vaginalis has an immunophenotype which is identical to that of mesothelioma in other anatomic locations. In fact it is reactive for broad spectrum keratin and calretinin and negative for adenocarcinoma-related markers. The differential diagnosis includes several other malignant tumors that can be encountered around the testis. Among these, the most common are "borderline" serous papillary epithelial tumors and serous papillary carcinomas. Both are typically found in hydroceles or as solid peritesticular masses, but they tend to be solitary lesions that are located between the testis and epydidimis, rather than multinodular masses in a hydrocele. Serous tumors of the testis are identical pathologically to their ovarian counterpart. They show cuboidal or columnar cells that are more pleomorphic than the cells of most epithelial mesotheliomas and serous carcinomas often show "heaped-up" epithelial cells mantling papillae. Serous borderline tumors and serous carcinomas characteristically are labeled for MOC-1, B72.3, CD15 and sometimes for other markers such as placental alkaline phosphatase. Both serous tumors and mesotheliomas may express OC125 antigen, but serous lesions are not reactive for calretinin, whereas mesotheliomas are positive for this marker. Carcinomas of the rete testis and epididymis have also been described; these tumors have the appearance of adenocarcinomas and are often histochemically positive for epithelial mucin.

Principles of Anticancer Therapy

Given the rarity of the disease, it is difficult to develop treatment guidelines based on clinical protocols developed specifically for this tumor. Surgery is the treatment of choice, especially in patients with a localized tumor. The type of surgery performed bears a relationship to local tumor recurrence. In patients who undergo only resection of the hydrocele wall, the recurrence rate is as high as 35.7% compared with recurrence rates of 10.5% and 11.5% after scrotal and inguinal orchiectomy, respectively. Because preoperative diagnosis is often difficult, most surgeons approach this as a testicular tumor and perform an inguinal orchiectomy, which avoids disruption of the scrotal lymphatics and allows complete removal of the spermatic cord. In cases in which biopsy or hydrocele surgery was performed initially, hemiscrotectomy and inguinal orchiectomy are recommended. The role of adjuvant therapy after surgery is not clear. In patients who are not surgical candidates or have tumor recurrence and metastatic disease, chemotherapy has been used with little benefit. Although mass reduction has been described in 20% of cases which received a combination of methotrexate and edatrexate, there was no effect on survival. Given the activity of cisplatin and pemetrexed combination in pleural mesothelioma, evaluation of this regimen in tunica vaginalis mesothelioma is appropriate. The treatment with radiotherapy or combined chemo-radiotherapy may be used, but the true efficacy has not yet been established. Radiotherapy seems to be more effective than chemotherapy and it should be considered for patients with locally extended mesothelioma after resection of the tumor with safe cut margins and also for patients with disseminated disease who are in good physical condition. There has also been limited experience with combined chemotherapy and radiotherapy in the treatment of malignant mesothelioma of the tunica vaginalis. However, in cases of pleural mesothelioma, no significant difference in survival was seen with radiotherapy alone compared with combined therapy. This suggests that combined chemotherapy and radiotherapy may be effective in treating disseminated disease, although the numbers are too small for any final conclusions to be drawn.

Prognostic Factors

The most important prognostic factor for survival in patients with malignant mesothelioma of the tunica vaginalis is patient's age at diagnosis. In fact patients younger than 60 years have a longer survival if compared with older patients. There is also a significant correlation between the presence of primary metastatic disease and survival. Patients with metastatic disease at diagnosis have a significantly shorter survival time than patients with organ-confined disease. Concerning the development of local recurrence, patients with a positive history of asbestos exposure have a significantly shorter interval before tumor recurrence than patients with no history. A significant survival benefit is not observed after radical orchiectomy compared with hydrocele wall resection, even if it is associated with a higher recurrence rate. In a summary of 73 cases from the literature, it was found a median of 23 months for all patients and 14 months for those whose lesions recurred.

Pericardial Mesothelioma

Epidemiology and Risk Factors

Primary tumors of the pericardium are extremely rare. Among them, pericardial mesothelioma is probably the most common type, followed by sarcoma, teratoma, fibroma, lipoma, and angioma. A study of about 500,000 autopsies revealed a pericardial mesothelioma incidence lower than 0.0022%, or about 2-3% considering only autopsies of patients died for cancer. Pericardial mesothelioma accounts for approximately 6% of all mesotheliomas; approximately 120 cases have been reported. Most of these tumors are diagnosed postmortem. Although a wide age range is affected, over half of the cases occur in the fifth to the seventh decades. There is a 2:1 male predominance. The etiology of pericardial mesothelioma is unknown, but some published series reported prior occupational exposure to asbestos in many of these patients, which suggested that like mesotheliomas at other sites, asbestos also may play a role in the development of pericardial mesotheliomas.

There have been case reports of pericardial mesothelioma occurring after mantle field radiotherapy for Hodgkin's disease.

Pathology

Grossly, most of pericardial mesotheliomas have a diffuse growth pattern, even if presentation as a mass is common. Myocardial invasion is not rare and extra-mediastinal metastases may be present. Like mesotheliomas in other sites, it can have an epithelial, mixed or sarcomatoid histology.

Natural History

Pericardial mesothelioma is commonly diagnosed at an advanced stage. It tends to infiltrate the myocardial and mediastinal structures. In fact numerous reports document that the tumor is associated with an often-bloody pericardial effusion or a diffuse mass encasing the heart and great vessels that can cause fatal hemodynamic disturbance. Invasion of cardiac chambers has been reported occasionally. Local spread usually involves pleura, lung and mediastinum. Metastases are present in about 25-45% of the cases and involve the regional lymph nodes, lungs and kidneys.

Diagnosis

Clinical Presentation

Although certain clinical manifestations can suggest a pericardial tumor, no clinical finding or set of findings is pathognomonic. Presenting signs and symptoms are non specific and arc related mostly to the compromise of cardiac function caused by tumor mass, effusion, or both. The clinical presentation can include mediastinal mass, pericardial effusion, congestive heart failure or tamponade. Symptoms due to pericardial effusion include chest pain, dyspnea, cough, fever, night sweats and sometimes paradoxical pulse. This non specificity may lead to diagnostic consideration or treatment of other disease states associated with pericardial effusion, such as rheumatic fever, metastatic disease, dissecting aortic aneurysm, viral syndrome, collagen vascular disease and tuberculosis. Patients can also develop congestive heart failure, constrictive pericarditis or cardiac tamponade because the tumor encases the heart. Due to extension of tumor into the myocardium and cardiac chambers, acute myocardial infarction or cerebral vascular accident may occur during the course of the disease.

Instrumental Procedures

Although chest radiography and echocardiography are sensitive means of detecting enlarged cardiac silhouette and effusion, they have no sensitivity in detection of pericardial mesothelioma. This likely is due to the tendency of this tumor to exhibit a diffuse growth pattern in which tumor envelopes the heart, rather than a pattern of growth as a discrete mass.

Computed tomography appears to offer a greater sensitivity for detection of the tumor. In some reports, magnetic resonance imaging successfully identified tumor, appearing a better modality for diagnosing this tumour. Finally, radionuclide imaging (with radiogallium) was reported to have been of assistance in the detection of tumor in some cases. Therefore, the diagnosis is made on the basis of cytological examination, ultrasound or CT-guided biopsy. In only 10-20% of cases can a diagnosis be made before the death of the patient. Thanks to bioptic material, it is possible differentiate between malignancy and mesothelial reactive hyperplasia associated with inflammatory disease. Features that indicate the presence of a malignancy are infiltration of deep tissues, atypical cytoplasm, necrosis and confluent forms. If deep tissue infiltration is not present, the diagnosis can be based on severely atypical cytoplasm.

Histochemical and Immunohistochemical Studies

Immunohistochemistry is useful for the differential diagnosis, but it is necessary to obtain additional information (anamnestic, clinical or radiological). Mesothelioma cells stain positive for cytokeratin, vimentin, epithelial membrane antigen (EMA) and calretinin and negative for CEA, CD15 and S-100.

Prognosis and Principles of Anticancer Therapies

Pericardial mesothelioma is an aggressive disease with poor prognosis and most patients die within a few months of diagnosis. There are no reported prospective randomized data comparing survival or symptom control in patients treated with surgery, chemotherapy, or supportive care. The optimal surgical therapy has not been established with regard to the extent of pericardial resection. However, good results have been achieved by surgical excision of a localized tumor mass. Partial excision is usually for palliation in encasing pericardial mesotheliomas. The role of radiotherapy is not clear. Pericardial mesothelioma is resistant to irradiation, but survival has been improved by partial pericardial resection and radiotherapy with radioisotopes, such as chromium phosphate, used intrapericardially for symptom relief. In cases in which chemotherapy was used, little clinical benefit was observed.

Bibliography

Acherman YI, Welch LS, Bromley CM, et al. Clinical presentation of peritoneal mesothelioma. *Tumori* 2003;89(3):269–73.

Amin A, Mason C, Rowe P. Diffuse malignant mesothelioma of the peritoneum following abdominal radiotherapy. *Eur. J. Surg. Oncol.* 2001;27(2):214–5.

Antman K, Cohen S, Dimitrov NV, et al. Malignant mesothelioma of the tunica vaginalis testis. *J. Clin. Oncol.* 1984;2(5):447–51.

Attanoos RL, Gibbs AR. Primary malignant gonadal mesotheliomas and asbestos. *Histopathology* 2000;37(2):150–9.

Bani-Hani KE, Gharaibeh KA Malignant peritoneal mesothelioma. J Surg Oncol. 2005 Jul 1;91(1):17-25.

Beck B, Konetzke G, Ludwig V, et al. Malignant pericardial mesotheliomas and asbestos exposure: a case report. *Am. J. Ind. Med.* 1982;3(2):149–59.

Berry G, de Klerk NH, Reid A, et al. Malignant pleural and peritoneal mesotheliomas in former miners and millers of crocidolite at Wittenoom, Western Australia. *Occup. Environ. Med.* 2004;61(4):e14.

Berti E, Schiaffino E, Minervini MS, Longo G, Schmid C. Primary malignant mesothelioma of the tunica vaginalis of the testis. Immunohistochemistry and electron microscopy. *Pathology.* 1997 Feb;29(1):96-9.

Bloss J, Wozniak TF, Janne PA, et al. Survival update on a subset of peritoneal mesothelioma (PM) patients in an expanded access program (EAP) of pemetrexed (P) alone combined with cisplatin in the treatment of malignant mesothelioma (MM). In: 2005 ASCO Annual Meeting Proceedings, Orlando, 2005. *J. Clin. Oncol.* 2005; 23(16S Part I):663s.

Chun PK, Leeburg WT, Coggin JT, et al. Primary pericardial malignant epithelioid mesothelioma causing acute myocardial infarction. *Chest* 1980;77(4):559–61.

Churg A. Paratesticular mesothelial proliferations. *Semin Diagn Pathol.* 2003 Nov;20(4):272-8.

Daya D, McCaughey WT. Well-differentiated papillary mesothelioma of the peritoneum. A clinicopathologic study of 22 cases. *Cancer* 1990; 65: 292–296.

Dedrick RL, Flessner MF. Pharmacokinetic problems in peritoneal drug administration: tissue penetration and surface exposure. *J. Natl. Cancer Inst.* 1997;89(7):480–7.

Deraco M, Casali P, Inglese MG, et al. Peritoneal mesothelioma treated by induction chemotherapy, cytoreductive surgery, and intraperitoneal hyperthermic perfusion. *J. Surg. Oncol.* 2003;83(3):147–53.

Eden CG, Bettochi C, Coker CB, Yates-Bell AJ, Pryor JP. Malignant mesothelioma of the tunica vaginalis. *J. Urol.* 1995 Mar;153(3 Pt 2):1053-4.

Eren NT, Akar AR. Primary pericardial mesothelioma. *Curr. Treat. Options. Oncol.* 2002 Oct;3(5):369-73.

Eryilmaz S, Sirlak M, Inan MB, et al. Primary pericardial mesothelioma. *Cardiovasc. Pathol.* 2001;10(3):147–9.

Feldman AL, Libutti SK, Pingpank JF et al. Analysis of factors associated with outcome in patients with malignant peritoneal mesothelioma undergoing surgical debulking and intraperitoneal chemotherapy. *J. Clin. Oncol.* 2003; 21: 4560–4567.

Freedman RS, Vadhan-Rai S, Butts C et al. Pilot study of Flt3 ligand comparing intraperitoneal with subcutaneous routes on hematologic and immunologic responses in patients with peritoneal carcinomatosis and mesotheliomas. *Clin. Cancer Res.* 2003; 9: 5228–5237.

Garcia de Jalon A, Gil P, Azua-Romeo J, Borque A, Sancho C, Rioja LA. Malignant mesothelioma of the tunica vaginalis. Report of a case without risk factors and review of the literature. *Int. Urol. Nephrol.* 2003;35(1):59-62.

Goldblum J, Hart WR. Localized and diffuse mesotheliomas of the genital tract and peritoneum in women: a clinicopathological study of nineteen true mesothelial neoplasms other than adenomatoid tumors, multicystic mesotheliomas and localized fibrous tumors. *Am. J. Surg. Pathol.* 1995;19(10):1124–37.

Gopez EV, Carey M, Klatt E. Cardiac tamponade as the initial manifestation of primary pericardial malignant mesothelioma. *Acta Cytol.* 2002;46(6):1171–3.

Gossinger HD, Siostrzonek P, Zangeneh M, et al. Magnetic resonance imaging findings in a patient with pericardial mesothelioma. *Am. Heart J.* 1988;115(6):1321–2.

Gupta NP, Kumar R. Malignant gonadal mesothelioma. *Curr. Treat. Options Oncol.* 2002;3(5):363–7.

Gupta NP, Agrawal AK, Sood S, et al. Malignant mesothelioma of the tunica vaginalis testis: a report of two cases and review of literature. *J. Surg. Oncol.* 1999;70(4):251–4.

Hassan R, Alexander R. Nonpleural mesotheliomas: mesothelioma of the peritoneum, tunica vaginalis, and pericardium. *Hematol. Oncol. Clin. North Am.* 2005 Dec;19(6):1067-87.

Hassan R, Alexander R., Antman K et al. Current treatment options and biology of peritoneal mesothelioma: meeting summary of the first NIH peritoneal mesothelioma conference. *Ann. Onc.* 2006 17: 1615–1619.

Hassan R, Bera T, Pastan I. Mesothelin: a new target for immunotherapy. Clin Cancer Res 2004; 10: 3937–3942.

Horn LC, Schutz A, Heinemann K, et al. Multicystic peritoneal mesothelioma of the omentum. *Eur. J. Obstet. Gynecol. Reprod. Biol.* 2004;116(2):246–7.

Iczkowski KA, Katz G, Zander DS, et al. Malignant mesothelioma of tunica vaginalis testis: a fatal case with liver metastasis. *J. Urol.* 2002;167(2 Pt 1):645–6.

Jones MA, Young RH, Scully RE. Malignant mesothelioma of the tunica vaginalis: a clinicopathologic analysis of 11 cases with review of the literature. *Am. J. Surg. Pathol.* 1995;19(7):815–25.

Kebapci M, Vardareli E, Adapinar B, et al. CT findings and serum ca 125 levels in malignant peritoneal mesothelioma: report of 11 new cases and review of the literature. *Eur. Radiol.* 2003;13(12):2620–6.

Kindler HL. Moving beyond chemotherapy: novel cytostatic agents for malignant mesothelioma. *Lung Cancer* 2004; 45S: S125–S127, 2004.

Langer CJ, Rosenblum N, Hogan M, et al. Intraperitoneal cisplatin and etoposide in peritoneal mesothelioma: favorable outcome with a multimodality approach. *Cancer Chemother Pharmacol* 1993;32(3):204–8.

Le DT, Deavers M, Hunt K, et al. Cisplatin and irinotecan (CPT-11) for peritoneal mesothelioma. *Cancer Invest* 2003;21(5):682–9.

Lenzi R, Rosenblum M, Verschraegen C, et al. Phase I study of intraperitoneal recombinant human interleukin 12 in patients with müllerian carcinoma, gastrointestinal primary malignancies and mesothelioma. *Clin. Cancer Res.* 2002;8(12):3686–95.

Lloreta-Trull J. Extrathoracic mesothelial proliferations and their mimics. *Ultrastruct Pathol.* 2006 Jan-Feb;30(1):37-51.

Loggie BW, Fleming RA, McQuellon RP, et al. Prospective trial for the treatment of malignant peritoneal mesothelioma. *Am. Surg.* 2001;67(10):999–1003.

Manavoglu O, Orhan B, Evrensel T, et al. Malignant peritoneal mesothelioma following asbestos exposure. *J. Environ. Pathol. Toxicol. Oncol.* 1996;15(2–4):191–4.

Markman M, Kelsen D. Efficacy of cisplatin-based intraperitoneal chemotherapy as treatment of malignant peritoneal mesothelioma. *J. Cancer Res. Clin. Oncol.* 1992;118(7): 547–50.

Melero M, Lloveras J, Waisman H, et al. Malignant peritoneal mesothelioma: an infrequent cause of prolonged fever syndrome and leukocytosis in a young adult. *Medicina* (B Aires) 1995;55(1):48–50.

Metintas S, Metintas M, Ucgun I, Oner U. Malignant mesothelioma due to environmental exposure to asbestos: follow-up of a Turkish cohort living in a rural area. *Chest* 2002; 122: 2224–2229.

Mohamed F, Sugarbaker PH. Peritoneal mesothelioma. *Curr. Treat. Options Oncol.* 2002 Oct;3(5):375-86.

Mongero LB, Beck JR, Kroslowitz RM, et al. Treatment of primary peritoneal mesothelioma by hyperthermic intraperitoneal chemotherapy. *Perfusion* 1999;14(2):141–5.

Nambiar CA, Tareif HE, Kishore KU, et al. Primary pericardial mesothelioma: one-year event-free survival. *Am. Heart J.* 1992;124(3):802–3.

Ordonez NG. Role of immunohistochemistry in distinguishing epithelial peritoneal mesotheliomas from peritoneal and ovarian serous carcinomas. *Am. J. Surg. Pathos.* 1998;22(10):1203–14.

Papi M, Genestreti G, Tassinari D, Lorenzini P, Serra S, Ricci M, Pasquini E, Nicolini M, Pasini G, Tamburini E, Fattori PP, Ravaioli A. Malignant pericardial mesothelioma. Report of two cases, review of the literature and differential diagnosis. *Tumori.* 2005 May-Jun;91(3):276-9.

Plas E, Riedl CR, Pfluger H. Malignant mesothelioma of the tunica vaginalis testis: review of the literature and assessment of prognostic parameters. *Cancer.* 1998 Dec 15;83(12):2437-46.

Price B, Ware A. Mesothelioma trends in the United States: an update based on surveillance, epidemiology, and end results program data from 1973 through 2003. *Am. J. Epidemiol.* 2004; 159: 107–112.

Quinn DW, Qureshi F, Mitchell IM. Pericardial mesothelioma: the diagnostic dilemma of misleading imaging. *Ann. Thorac. Surg.* 2000;69(6):1926–7.

Sane AC, Roggli VL. Curative resection of a well-differentiated papillary mesothelioma of the pericardium. *Arch. Pathol. Lab. Med.* 1995;119(3):266–7.

Sawh RN, Malpica A, Deavers MT, et al. Benign cystic mesothelioma of the peritoneum: a clinicopathologic study of 17 cases and immunohistochemical analysis of estrogen and progesterone receptor status. *Hum. Pathol.* 2003;34(4):369–74.

Sebbag G, Yan H, Shmookler BM, et al. Malignant mesothelioma of the male genital tract: report of two cases. *Urol. Oncol.* 2001;6(6):261–4.

Shah KV. Causality of mesothelioma: SV40 question. *Thorac. Surg Clin.* 2004;14(4): 497–504.

Simsek H, Kadayifci A, Okan E. High serum level of CA125 in malignant peritoneal mesothelioma. *Eur. J. Cancer* 1995;31A(1):129.

Sugarbaker PH, Welch LS, Mohamed F, Glehen O. A review of peritoneal mesothelioma at the Washington Cancer Institute. *Surg. Oncol. Clin. N. Am.* 2003; 12: 605–621.

Sugarbaker PH, Yan TD, Stuart OA, Yoo D. Comprehensive management of diffuse malignant peritoneal mesothelioma. *Eur. J. Surg. Oncol.* 2006 Aug;32(6):686-91.

Sugarbaker PH, Acherman YIZ, Brun E. Deciduoid peritoneal mesothelioma. *Contemp. Surg.* 2002;58(7):341–6.

Suman S, Schofield P, Large S. Primary pericardial mesothelioma presenting as pericardial constriction: a case report. *Heart* 2004;90(1):e4.

Taub RN, Hesdorffer ME, Keohan ML, et al. Combined resection, intraperitoneal chemotherapy, and whole abdominal radiation for malignant peritoneal mesothelioma (MPM). In: 2005 ASCO Annual Meeting Proceedings, Orlando, 2005. *J. Clin. Oncol.* 2005;23(16S Part I):664s.

Taub RN, Keohan ML, Chabot JC, Fountainks, Plitsas M. Peritoneal mesothelioma. *Curr. Treat. Options Oncol.* 2000; 1: 303–312.

Thomason R, Schlegel W, Lucca M, Cummings S, Lee S. Primary malignant mesothelioma of the pericardium. Case report and literature review. *Tex. Heart Inst. J.* 1994; 21(2):170-4.

Velissaris TJ, Tang AT, Millward-Sadler GH, et al. Pericardial mesothelioma following mantle field radiotherapy. *J. Cardiovasc. Surg.* (Torino) 2001;42(3):425–7.

Vigneswaran WT, Stefanacci PR. Pericardial mesothelioma. *Curr. Treat Options Oncol.* 2000 Oct;1(4):299-302.

Waxman AK, Gos GA, Merriam P, et al. Survival for patients with peritoneal mesothelioma: aggressive multimodality therapy for early stage disease [abstract 2223]. *Proc. Am. Soc. Clin. Oncol.* 2000;19:564a.

Whitley NO, Brenner DE, Antman KH et al. CT of peritoneal mesothelioma: analysis of eight cases. *Am. J. Roentgenol.* 1982; 138: 531–535.

Yan TD, Haveric N, Carmignani CP, et al. Abdominal computed tomography scans in the selection of patients with malignant peritoneal mesothelioma for comprehensive treatment with cytoreductive surgery and perioperative intraperitoneal chemotherapy. *Cancer* 2005;103(4):839–49.

In: Mesothelioma from Bench Side to Clinic
Editor: Alfonso Baldi, pp. 323-336

ISBN: 978-1-60021-789-0

Chapter XVII

Reactive Mesothelial Proliferations and Benign Mesotheliomas: A Practical Approach

Oscar Nappi, Amedeo Boscaino and Antonio D' Antonio
Institute of Anatomic pathology, Histopathology and Diagnostic Cytology,
"A. Cardarelli" Hospital, Naples, Italy

Abstract

Reactive mesothelial proliferations and benign mesotheliomas represent a rather broad category, encompassing well defined clinico-pathological lesions, aspecific reactive patterns and proliferating lesions of uncertain malignant potential [1, 2]. In this chapter the authors have reviewed the anatomopatological aspects of these lesions.

Mesothelial Reactive Proliferations (MRPs)

The mesothelium reacts to injuries, especially if prolonged, with epithelial and/or mesenchymal proliferative changes. Sometimes, they are so much exuberant that malignant lesions can be clinically and/or microscopically suspected. These changes are usually called mesothelial reactive proliferations (MRPs) and can exhibit patterns prevailingly involving epithelial, mesenchymal or both component of serosal membranes. Patterns are basically represented by papillary, tubular, microcystic and solid /nodular ones for epithelial proliferations [Figure 1] and spindle cell and fibrosclerotic for mesenchymal proliferations [3, 4].

Several pleural disorders can yield proliferative changes. Main of them are infectious pleuritis, pleural effusions secondary to pneumonia, post-thoracotomy syndrome, chronic hearth failure, hepatic cirrhosis, nephritic syndrome, systemic autoimmune diseases such as rheumatoid arthritis and systemic lupus erythematosus.

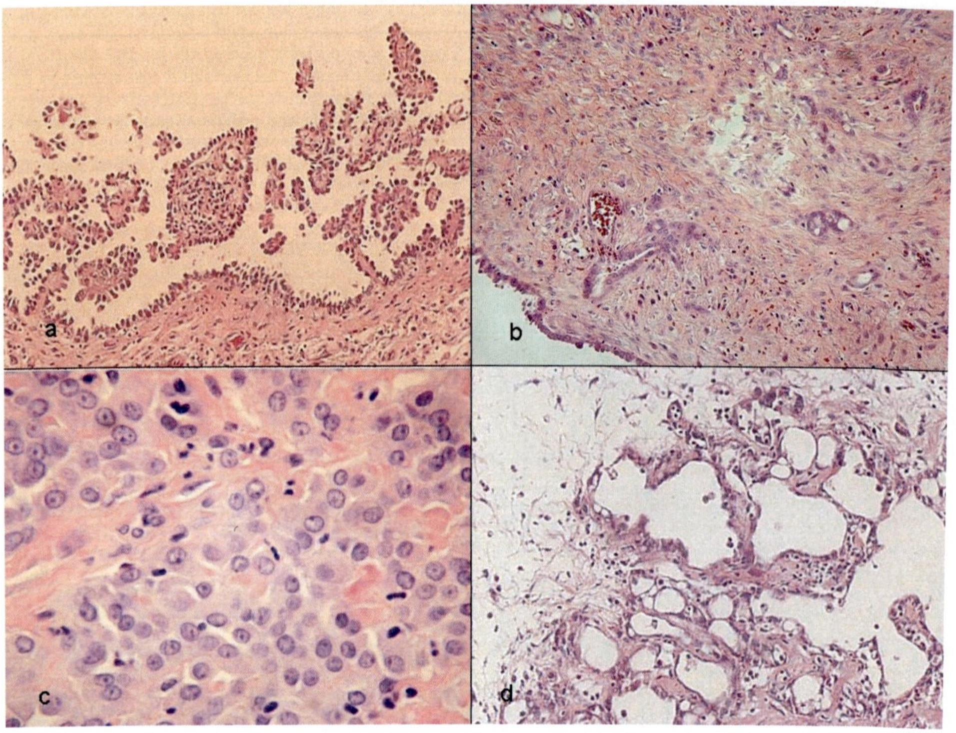

Figure 1. The four main patterns of MRPs: a.papillary; b. tubular; c. solid; d. microcystic.

Since also malignant mesotheliomas (MMs) can exhibit the same growth patterns and MRPs can present atypical changes, distinguish between benign and malignant proliferations represents often a real challenge for pathologists.

Nevertheless, two elements have to be considered in the approach to the differential diagnosis between MRPs and MMs:

(a) Clinical presentation
(b) Methodology of collecting material

Clinical Presentation

It is mandatory to be aware of the clinical and *imaging* features before making a definitive diagnosis. The awareness of a certain or suspected clinical condition favouring a mesothelial proliferation is very important as well as to know about asbestos exposure of the patient.

The imaging findings are often confusing but, obviously, the documented presence of masses suggests a neoplastic lesion. The so called "rind effect" should be typical of mesothelioma but also chronic pleurisy can feature it. Nevertheless, once again, the clinical history is useful because chronic pleurisy leads to a complete rind in much more long time (many years) than malignant mesothelioma.

Methodology of Collecting Material

A definitive diagnosis is often related to the methodology to collect tissue samples from the pleura and, of course, as much wide is the tissue sampling as much is the diagnostic reliability.

Needle core biopsy. By this is a poorly invasive but "blind" technique. Good diagnostic tissue sampling is obtained only if the material is taken from "diagnostic areas".

Pleuroscopy. Pleural lesions can be visualized and material taken more appropriately. An eventual first confirming intraoperative sample can be followed by other fragments also useful for immunohistochemical or molecular studies.

Thoracothomy. Wide sampling is allowed; a partial or total pleural decortication can be performed following the examination by frozen sections.

Moreover, also cytologic smears obtained by effusion can be diagnostic in case of a frank malignancy (in distinguish between Malignant mesotheliomas and metastatic malignant neoplasms). Cytologic criteria in distinguish between reactive mesothelial proliferations and malignant mesotheliomas have been extensively reported, in many cases this distinction can result questionable if not impossible [5].

Epithelial MRPs

Epithelial MRPs usually present as multiple small micronodules on the pleural surface , rarely as flat plaques. Microscopically, a single pattern can prevail but often mixed patterns are exhibited. MRPs with papillary pattern are relatively common and, often, associated with others; papillary growth is usually superficial while tubular, microcystic or solid ones more deeply seated.

MRPs can exhibit typical recognizable benign features but sometimes feature atypical changes. Lesions falling within this grey zone where a strong overlapping with cytohistological features of epithelial or prevailingly epithelial MMs is present, are usually called Atypical Hyperplastic proliferations (AHPs). Nuclear atypia, increased mitotic activity, pattern complexity and, in some cases, necrosis can really make hard, if not impossible, a differential diagnosis with a malignant mesothelioma. In these cases, it is absolutely mandatory to know the clinical setting in which pleural fragments have been taken and in presence of unconvincing clinical elements such as quickly developing "pleural problem" or other clinical features oriented for an inflammatory process, a final decision for a malignancy must be extremely wary and eventually implicating also repetition with a more invasive collecting technique.

In spite of the many papers published on the topic, a final diagnosis also by expert pathologists, is often suggestive or " strongly suggestive " but not definitive. Nevertheless, on the basis of our experience, an inflammatory background represented by fibrin and presence of neutrophils, although possibly present also in malignant mesotheliomas, should always suggest the possibility of a diagnosis of exclusion of malignancy.

Architectural complexity such as true papillary structures with fibrovascular core, back-to back glandular arrangement, deeply seated nodular or glandular/ pseudovascular structures are higly suspicious elements for malignancy but they can be present also in long-standing inflammatory processes. Nuclear atypia and mitotic activity can be widely observed in benign mesothelial proliferation; in particular, reactive processes are much more mitotically active than malignant mesothelioma that notoriously is a slowly growing neoplasia; of course, "atypical mitoses" are highly suspicious as also prominent nuclear atypicality, especially if found in nodules or tubular structures deeply located.

Obviously fat infiltration by epithelial structures, although very rarely reported also in reactive processes, has to be considered strongly oriented for malignancy [6, 7].

The possible contribute of immunohistochemistry to differentiating benign from malignant mesothelial epithelial proliferations, especially on small fragments, is a topic largely debated.

On the basis of our experience, no immunohistochemical maker can be today considered easily reproducible and highly specific and sensible for this differential diagnosis task.

A positivity for desmin is reported in 85% of benign and 10% of malignant lesions (Attanoos) ,a linear membranous positivity for EMA is reported in 0- 33% of benign and 80-100% of malignant mesothelial cells; a nuclear positivity for p53 is reported from 0 to 60% of benign mesothelium and 25 to 97% of malignant mesothelium; Bcl-2 is constantly absent in reactive mesothelium and expressed only in 10% of malignant mesotheliomas: consequentially, its detection although little sensible, is highly specific and useful only in selected cases.

An immunophenotype EMA- / desmin + / bcl-2 -/p53 – could be interpreted as strongly suggestive for a reactive lesion while an immunophenotype EMA+/ desmin-/p53+ could be interpreted as suggestive of malignancy and diagnostic if , in addition, Bcl-2 is positive [7, 8]. Again, to the best of our knowledge no molecular markers are, at present, available to consistently contributing to this problem.

Malignant Mesothelioma *In Situ*

For mesothelial proliferations showing frankly neoplastic cytologic features without stromal invasion, the term of malignant mesothelioma in situ has been introduced; since it is often found in proximity of invasive mesothelioma, it has been defined as a morphological precursor. Considering the poor effectiveness of any treatment of invasive mesotheliomas, the recognition of a stage 0 mesothelioma, if validated on the basis of accepted criteria, should represent a critical step in the management of this tumour. Unfortunately, so far, reliable criteria for this diagnosis have not been codified. Therefore, since mesothelial reactive proliferations often show several degrees of cellular atypia, a diagnosis of *malignant mesothelioma in situ* should be made with extreme caution because it means a radical surgical therapy. At present time we think that only in presence of a history of asbestos exposure without evidence of recognized recent inflammatory pathology and a multifocal or rather extensive mesothelial surface cell proliferations with consistent nuclear atypia, a diagnosis of *malignant mesothelioma in situ* should be suggested. Interestingly, an inmmunoreactivity for EMA and p53 similar to that of invasive mesothelioma has been found in cases of mesothelioma *in situ* associated with frankly malignant melanoma [9, 10].

Nodular Pattern

A solid pattern can be focally or extensively present as reactive change of mesothelium. Moreover it can be observed in some peculiar clinical settings:

a) Inguinal or humbelical hernia sacs [11], following chronic injury and /or incarceration of mesothelium. This feature, not infrequently found in hernia sacs of children and rarely of adults, has been defined as nodular mesothelial hyperplasia and, especially in the past has led to a misdiagnosis of malignancy.
b) Cardiac excrescences variously interpreted and called histiocytoid hemangioma-like lesions (HHLL) [12] or Mesothelial /Monocytic incidental Cardiac excrescence (MICE) [13]. These are characterized by nests of round mesothelioid cells usually detected during cardiac surgery; some authors have considered these lesions to be artefactually determined by aspirated mesothelial cells during cardiotomy suction [14].
c) Nodular aggregates found in transbronchial biopsies can represent a potential source of misdiagnosis, especially versus neuroendocrine tumours [15].

The immunohistochemical evidence that a good number, if not most, of the round mesothelioid cells present in these lesions are immunoreactive for histiocytic markers such as CD 68 and KP-1 and not for Cytokeratin, positive only in other cells, has suggested that in most cases of the above-mentioned pathological findings, a mixed proliferation of histiocytes and mesothelial cells is present. Alternatively, such evidence suggests that the mesothelial cells are entrapped and not proliferating. Consequently, a definition of Nodular histiocytic/mesothelial hyperplasia has been suggested for all of them [16].

Spindle Cell and Fibrosclerotic MRPs

Pleural plaques, round atelectasia and chronic fibrous pleurisy, with the so called Fibrothorax at the extremity of the spectrum, are the best clinically defined lesions of this type. Pleural plaques (PP) are firm, sometimes calcified lesions, present in the parietal pleura, and microscopically characterized by hypocellular collagen-rich mesenchymal proliferation with a distinctive basket-weave pattern and distrofic calcification [Figure 2]. PP can present as single or multiple lesions ranging from few millimeters to several centimetres.

A relation with asbestos exposure is widely accepted and sufficiently documented. In selected cases, association with malignant mesothelioma has been described as well. Other pneumoconiosis have been reported to be associated with PP *Round atelectasis.* It is an unusual condition often secondary to asbestosis characterized by a "radiographic peripheral opacity", often confused with a pulmonary neoplasm, due to an atelectasic area secondary to the stretching effect of a localized fibrosclerotic hypocellular proliferation of the overlying visceral pleura that presents also multiple foldings into the lung parenchyma [17].

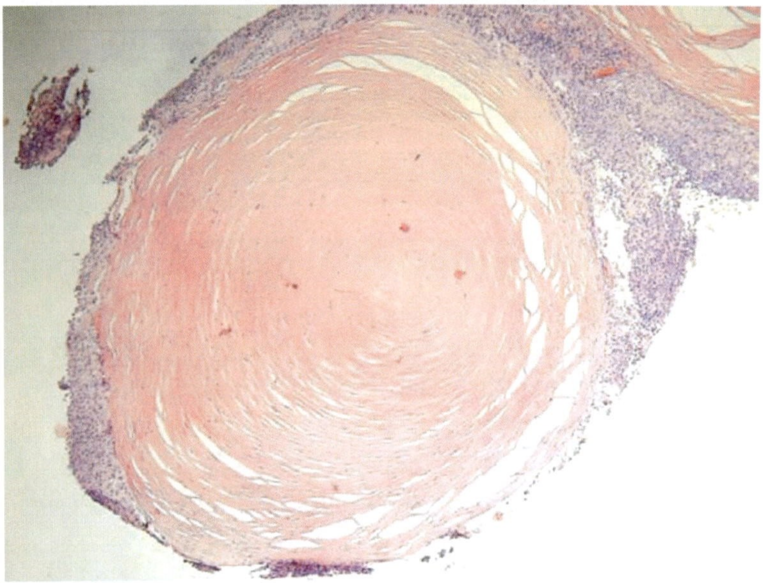

Figure 2. Pleural plaque. Hypocellular collagen-rich fibrotic proliferation with typical basket-weave feature.

Chronic fibrous pleurisy (CFP), especially in case of small biopsies, represents a hard differential diagnosis task with sarcomatous mesotheliomas, if a consistent spindle cell proliferation is present, or with desmoplastic mesotheliomas (DMM), if, as more frequently, the lesion is sclerotic and paucicellular. Proliferating cells are prevailingly spindle but also epithelioid in apparence and ganglion-like cells are sometimes present [Figure 3].

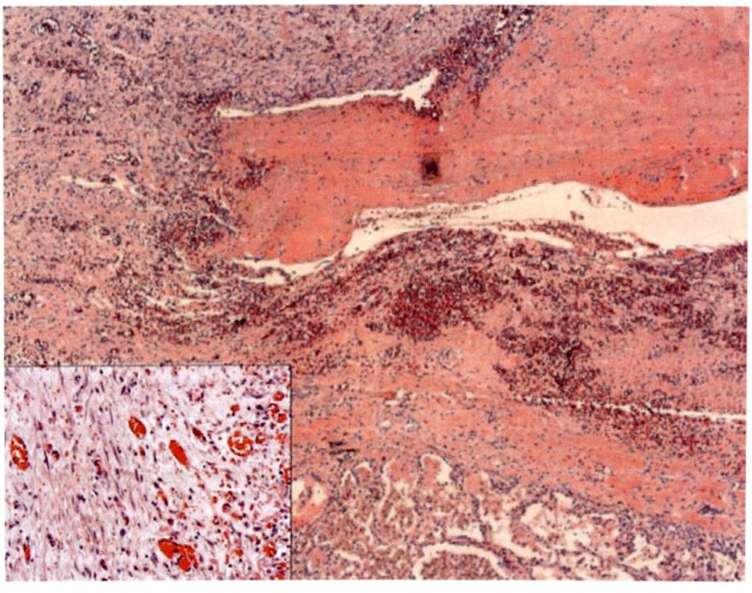

Figure 3. Fibrotic pleurisy. Fibroblastic proliferation in a collagenous background with inflammatory component and fibrin deposit. Inset: elongated slightly atypical fibrobasts with ganglion-like cells.

Reliable criteria of malignancy, in absence of frank sarcomatous overgrowths are currently considered [6, 7]: absence of a *zonal effect* (consisting in a superficial high cellularity and deep paucicellularity, usually present in chronic fibrotic reactions); invasion of surrounding tissues (adipose tissue, skeletal muscle, lung parenchyma); the so-called *bland necrosis*, typical of desmoplastic malignant mesothelioma and consisting of circumscribed areas in which necrosis is demonstrated by a poor-stained eosin; absence of elongated capillary vessel perpendicularly to serosal surface as expression of reactive granulation tissue usually present in CFP. A consistent mixed inflammatory is suggestive of chronic pleurisy. As it is well known, immunohistochemistry is of little help since after an injury causing denudation of mesothelial layers, sub-mesothelial fibroblasts normally expressed vimentin acquire immunoreactivity also for low –molecular weight cytokeratin. For this reason , in the presence of mesenchymal mesothelial proliferations the positivity for cytokeratin should not be considered as diagnostic of DMM [1, 2]. Nevertheless, a clear immunonegativity or a weakly focal positivity for cytokeratin favours the diagnosis of fibrosing pleurisy, as well as an immunopositivity of fibrosclerosing proliferation infiltrating lung parenchyma or striated muscle is suggestive for a diagnosis of DMM.

Benign Mesothelioma

This term conventionally encompasses some biologically quite defined lesions that can be divided in epithelial and mesenchymal on the basis of their morphological and immunophenotypical presentation. Epithelial mesotheliomas are represented by well differentiated papillary mesothelioma, adenomatoid tumor and multicystic mesothelioma.

A "mesenchymal" mesothelioma is historically considered the Solitary (or Localized) Fibrous Tumour (before named as fibrous mesothelioma). Today it has to be considered an ubiquitous tumour not arising from mesothelium *strictu sensu* as well as desmoid pleural tumour and calcifying fibrous pseudotumour. All of these conditions, more appropriately, can be considered benign mesenchymal lesions of the mesothelium.

Well Differentiated Papillary Mesothelioma [WDPM]

Well differentiated papillary mesothelioma (WDPM) is an intriguing tumour. It is currently considered a low grade malignant or borderline tumour because of the unfavorable outcome of several cases that in any case, have had an indolent, long clinical course.

Until the last decade WDPM have been thought to arise almost exclusively in the peritoneum of young female patients (3 0 – 40 years of age) [18, 19] with only sporadic cases described in the peritoneum and tunica vaginalis of male patients [21, 22] and pericardium and pleura of patients of both gender. Today, it has to be considered an ubiquitous mesothelial tumour. In particular, a large series of 24 cases of pleural WDPM has been recently described [20]. Clinically, the usual presentation is by serous effusion, while in abdominal and testicular cases pain is common. The exposure to the asbestos is uncommon in peritoneal cases but in the over mentioned series of pleural WDPM, 9 of 24 patients have had an occupational or para-occupational exposure.

Macroscopically, the lesion generally exhibits a superficial, sometimes multifocal vegetative proliferation. Microscopically, a papillary proliferation characterized by papillae with fibrovascular myxomatous broad stalk lined by bland, single mesothelial cells, is present [Figure 4]; mitoses are not usually detected, while in some case, psammomas bodies have been described. Occasionally adenomatoid-like microtubules in the stroma are observed.

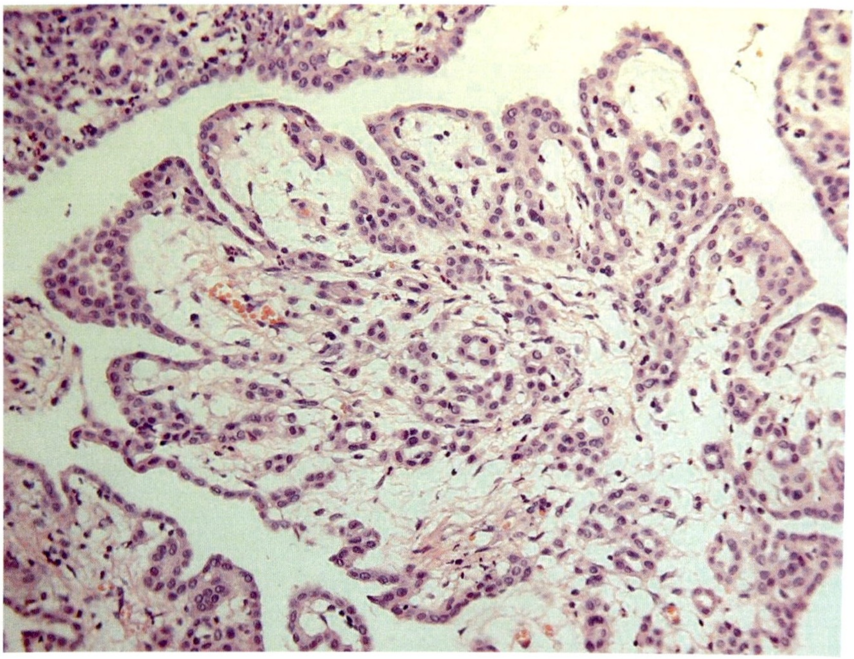

Figure 4. Well differentiated papillary mesothelioma of peritoneum. This field shows papillary projections with a fibro-myxo-vascular stalk lined by bland, flat, single mesothelial cells. In the underneath stroma a proliferation of duct-like structures is seen.

Immunohistochemically, proliferating cells are reactive for CK, CK5/6, EMA with a diffuse linear membranous pattern and mesothelial markers (Calretinin, HMBE-1); CEA is always negative; in 3 cases observed by us, desmin is resulted negative.

Especially on small biopsies, WDPM has to be differentiated from aspecific reactive mesothelial hyperplasia, epithelial malignant mesothelioma with prominent papillary pattern and serous papillary carcinoma of ovary and peritoneum. Clinical presentation is important in differentiating WDPM from reactive mesothelial hyperplasia that usually is not mass-forming and from malignant mesothelioma where the cytomorphologic features are significantly more atypical. Immunoreactivity for B72.3, Ber-Ep4, CA19.9 and Leu-M1 and negativity for calretinin and HMBE-1 are useful markers in differentiating WDPM, as well as malignant mesotheliomas, from papillary serous carcinoma of the peritoneum or of the ovary. CEA immunoreactivity is also an excellent negative marker for mesothelial neoplasia but is not always detected in papillary carcinoma [23].

Adenomatoid Tumor (AT)

Adenomatoid tumor is a benign mesothelial tumour with a basically tubular pattern but with several morphological variants [24].

This tumour usually arises from the mesothelium of the paratesticular region, from the serosal surface of the uterus wall [25] and, much less frequently, from that of the ovary, salpynx and broad ligament. Exceptionally, it can arise also from pleura [26] and pericardium [27].

Macroscopically, adenomatoid tumour is usually a small nodule not infrequently found incidentally.

Microscopically, its growth pattern is characterized by bland, flat epithelioid cells arranged in tubules, gland-like structures, microcysts, cords or pseudovascular channels. Sometimes a signet ring feature-like secondary to cytoplasmic vacuolization, is present [Figure 5].

A mesothelial origin of the AT has been definitively confirmed by ultrastructural and immunohistochemical studies [25, 26]. This tumour always expresses CK, EMA and calretinin. AT has to be histologically differentiated from adenocarcinomas and vascular tumors. Appropriate immunohistochemical reactions such as CEA and other possible markers for adenocarcinomas of specific origin and endothelial markers usually help to clarify the diagnosis. Rarely cases of AT having an infiltrating local pattern have been reported, but the behaviour of AT is usually indolent and benign.

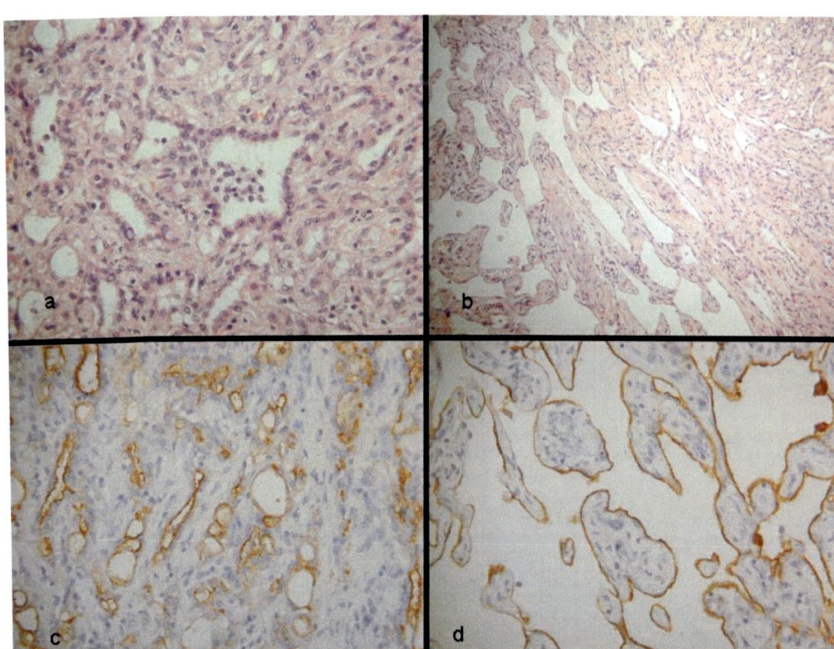

Figure 5. Adenomatoid tumor. Tubular/ pseudoglandular (a) and angiomatoid (b) patterns. Immunohistochemical positivity for calretinin (c) and cytokeratin (d).

The so-called mesothelioma of the atrioventricular node, in the past considered a mesothelioma morphologically similar to adenomatoid tumor, is not a true mesothelioma. It has been definitively accepted that it arises from a congenital heterotopia of endodermal tissue [27, 28].

Multicystic Mesothelioma

Multicystic Mesothelioma arises almost exclusively from the peritoneum. Therefore, in medical literature it is usually codified as Peritoneal Multicystic mesothelioma (PMM) [29]. Exceptional cases have been described in the pleura [30] and in testis [31]. Like the AT, the histogenesis of PMM has also been controversial, the true mesothelial origin having been confirmed only recently by ultrastructural and immunohistochemical studies.

Cystic mesotheliomas, arising from serosal peritoneal membranes, can involve also the parenchyma of single peritoneal and pelvic organs [32]. The common clinical setting is the pelvic peritoneum of young female patients; on the basis of the size of the proliferation, it presents vague symptoms or shows a palpable abdominal mass and pain; ascitis is rarely present. It can be also multifocal with synchronous or metachronous proliferating lesions in several parts of the abdomen and pelvis.

Macroscopically, more cysts with thin walls and variable size and with a fluid content are present [29].

Microscopically, the internal cystic surface is lined by bland, flat endothelioid cells [Figure 6]. They are immunoreactive for Cytokeratin, Calretinin and HMBE-1.

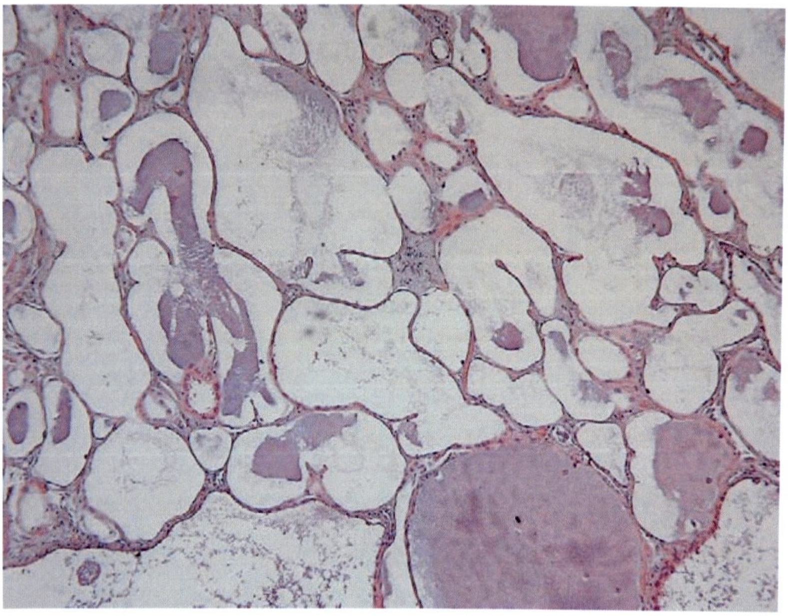

Figure 6. Peritoneal multicystic mesothelioma. Several cystic structures containing amorphous eosinophilic fluid and internally lined by flat mesothelioid cells are shown.

A common, sometimes difficult, differential diagnosis is with [multi-] cystic lymphangiomas. Immunoreactivity for endothelial markers and immunonegativity for Citokeratin addresses the correct diagnosis.

Basically, PMM is a benign tumour but surgical radicality is mandatory because of the possibility of recurrences. Follow up is needed also because of the mentioned multifocality. Cases of malignant cystic mesothelioma have been reported but cytologic and clinical features generally clarify the diagnosis.

Solitary Fibrous Tumour of the Pleura

Solitary fibrous tumour (SFT) of the pleura, although variously named, has been for many decades supposed to arise from surface mesothelial cells and, therefore, a benign mesothelioma. Actually, it is considered a pleural localization of a potentially ubiquitous lesion of mesenchymal origin [33]. SFT can arise in the pleura of patients of both sexes and of any age. Cough, pain and dyspnea are common symptoms, although in about 50% of cases, the tumour is asymptomatic and incidentally found. Typically, SFT arises in the visceral pleura and is separated from it by a peduncle, often resulting in a polypoid mass, which can also reach great size (up to 40 cm) and consistent weight. The cut surface is firmly fibrous.

Microscopically, several features have been described: sclerosing, myxoid, hemangiopericytomatous. Typically, SFT expresses CD 34 [34]. The positivity for this marker is needed to confirm the diagnosis [Figure 7]. Bcl-2 [35] and CD 99 [36], both positive in the majority of cases, are considered useful to distinguish SFT from sarcomatoid malignant mesothelioma that only sporadically express these markers.

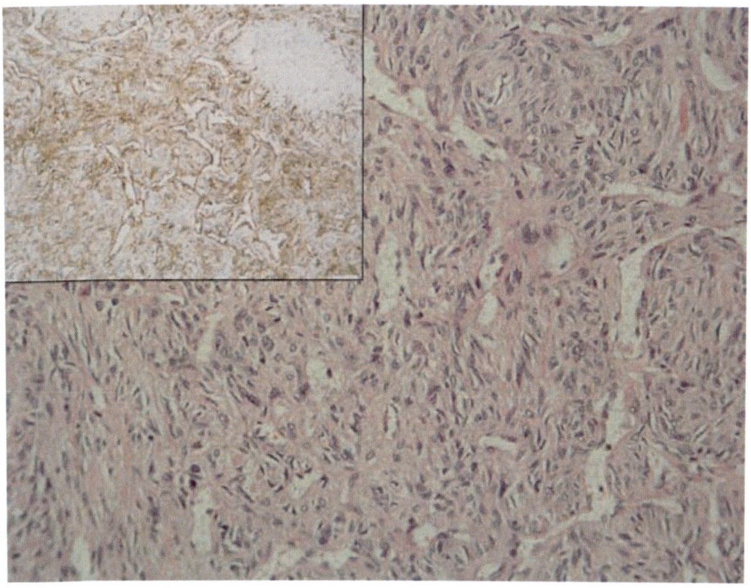

Figure 7. Solitary fibrous tumor of the pleura. The hemangiopericytoma-like pattern is shown. Inset : Spindle cells immunostained for CD 34.

Some cases of SFT have a malignant behaviour. Histological criteria for selecting them are similar to those of other mesenchymal neoplasias: an increase in cellularity, nuclear atypias, an infiltrative pattern and a greater mitotic index [more than 4 x hpf].

Solitary fibrous tumours have been described everywhere, including also pericardium [37], vaginalis testis [21], peritoneum [38].

Pleural Desmoid Tumor

Pleural desmoid tumour is a rare lesion often confusing with LFT. Like the analogous tumours arising in soft tissues, it is characterized by bland spindle tumour cells organized in parallel or interweaving bundles in a fibromyxoid matrix. Adipose tissue and skeletal fibers muscle are always infiltrated. Immunohistochemically, CD 34 is always negative, while Muscle Specific Actin and Smooth Muscle Actin are always positive. This immunophenotype allows differentiating it from LFT [39].

Calcifying Fibrous Pseudotumour

It is a rare pleural lesion similar to that arising in the somatic tissue of children and young adults, characterized microscopically by hypocellular hyalinized collagenous tissue with psammomatous calcifications and scant lymphoplasmocytic infiltrates.

Immunohistochemically, mesemchymal proliferating cells are reactive for VIM, CD 34 and Factor XIIIa, negative for EMA, CK, SMA [40].

References

[1] Battifora H, McCaughey WT E Tumors of the serosal membranes. *Atlas of tumors pathology,* third series, fasc 15 AFIP, Washington D.C., 1995.

[2] Giordano GG, Nappi O Benign mesotheliomas, mesothelial proliferations and their possible association with asbestos exposure In: Pass H, Vogelzang N, Carbone M (eds): *Malignant mesotheliomas: Advances in Pathogenesis, Diagnosis and Translational therapies.* New York, NY, Springer Science and Business Media, pp 469–480, 2005 3.

[3] Wick MR, Mills SE Mesothelial proliferations: an increasing morphologic spectrum *Am. J. Clin. Pathol.* 113: 619 – 622, 2000.

[4] Nappi O, Boscaino A, Galloro P Benign Mesotheliomas and reactive mesothelial proliferations. *A pattern approach Pathologica* 95: 301 – 302, 2003.

[5] Koss LG, *Melamed MR Koss' diagnostic cytology and its histopathologic basis 5th ed,* Philadelphia, JB Lippincott, 2005.

[6] Churg A, Roggli V, Colby TV and US-Canadian Mesothelioma Reference Panel The separation of benign and malignant mesothelial proliferations. *Am. J. Surg. Pathol* 24: 1183 – 1200, 2000.

[7] Kradin RL, Mark EJ. Distinguish benign mesothelial hyperplasia from neoplasia: a practical approach. *Sem. Diagn. Pathol.* 23: 4-14, 2006.

[8] Attanoos RL, Griffin A, Gibbs AR. The use of immunohistochemestry in distinguish reactive from neoplastic mesothelium. A novel use for desmin and comparative evaluation with epithelial membrane antigen, p53, platelet-derived growth factor-receptor, P-glycoprotein and Bcl-2. *Histopathology* 43: 231 – 238, 2003.

[9] Whitaker D, Henderson DW, Shikin KB. The concept of mesothelioma in situ: implications for diagnosis and histogenesis. *Sem. Diagn. Pathol.* 9: 151 – 161, 1992 10.

[10] Cury PM, Butcher DN, Corrin B, Nicholson AG. The use of histological and immunohistochemical markers to distinguish pleural malignant mesothelioma and in situ mesothelioma from reactive mesothelial hyperplasia and reactive pleural fibrosis. *J. Pathol.* 189: 251 – 257.

[11] Rosai J, Dehmer LP. Nodular mesothelial hyperplasia in hernia sac: a benign reactive condition simulating a neoplastic process. *Cancer:* 35:165 – 175, 1975.

[12] Luthringer DJ, Virmani R, Weiss SW, Rosai J. A distinctive cardiovascular lesion resembling histiocytoid (epithelioid) hemangioma: evidence suggesting mesothelial participation. *Am. J. Surg. Pathol.* 14: 993 – 1000, 1996.

[13] Veinot JP, Tazelaar HD, Edwards WD, Colby T V. Mesothelial/monocytic incidental cardiac excrescences (cardiac MICE). *Modern Pathol* 7: 9 –16, 1995.

[14] Courtice RW, Stinson WA, VM Walley. Tissue fragments recovered at cardiac surgery masquerading as tumoral proliferations. Evidence suggesting iatrogenic or artefactual origin and common occurrence. *Am. J. Surg. Pathol.* 18: 167 – 174,1994.

[15] Chan JKC, Loo KT, Yau BKC, Lam SY. Nodular Histocytic/Mesothelial Hyperplasia: A lesion potentially mistaken for a neoplasm in transbronchial biopsy. Am *J. Surg. Pathol.* 21: 658 – 663,1997.

[16] Ordonez NG, Ro JY, Ayala AG. Lesion described as Nodular Mesothelial Hyperplasia are primarily composed of histiocytes. *Am. J. Surg. Pathol.* 22: 285 – 292, 1998.

[17] Menzies R, Fraser R. Round atelectasis: pathologic and pathogenetic features. *Am. J. Surg. Pathol.* 11: 674 – 681, 1987.

[18] Butnor KJ, Sporn TA, Hammar SP, Roggli VL. Well differentiated papillary mesothelioma. *Am. J. Surg. Pathol.* 25: 1304 – 1309, 2001.

[19] Daya D, McCaughey WTE. Well differentiated papillary mesothelioma of the peritoneum: a clinicopathologic study of 22 cases. *Cancer* 65: 292 – 296, 1990.

[20] Xiao S-Y, Rizzo P, Carbone M. Benign papillary mesothelioma of the tunica vaginalis testis. *Arch. Pathol. Lab. Med.* 144: 143 – 147, 2000.

[21] Perez -Ordonez B, Srigley JR. Mesothelial lesions of the Paratesticular region. *Sem. Diagn. Pathol.* 17: 294 – 306, 2000.

[22] Galateau-Sallè F, Vignaud M, Burke M et al. Well differentiated papillary mesothelioma of the pleura. A series of 24 cases. *Am. J. Surg. Pathol.* 28: 534 – 540, 2004.

[23] Attanoos RL, Webb R, Dojcinov SD, Gibbs AR. Value of mesothelial and epithelial antibodies in distinguish peritoneal.Mesotheliomas in female from serous papillary carcinoma of the ovary and Peritoneum. *Histopathology* 40: 237 – 244, 2002.

[24] Lehto VP, Miettinen M, Virtanen I. Adenomatoid tumor: Immunohistological features suggesting a mesothelial origin. *Virchows Arch. B. Cell Pathol. Mol. Pathol.* 42: 153 – 159, 1983.

[25] Nogales FF, Isaac MA, Hardisson D et al. Adenomatoid tumors of the uterus: an analysis of 60 cases. *In. J. Gynecol. Pathol.* 21: 34 -40, 2002.

[26] Handra – Luca A, Couvelard A, Abd Alsamad I et al Adenomatoid tumor of the pleura. Case report. *Ann. Pathol.* 20: 369 – 372, 2000.

[27] McAllister HA Jr , Fenoglio JJ Jr. Tumors of the cardiovascular system. *Atlas of tumor pathology 2nd series*, Fasc 15. Washington D.C. AFIP, 1978.

[28] Monma N , Satodate R , Tashiro A , Segawa I. Origin of so-called mesothelioma of the atrioventricular node. An immunohistochemical study. *Arch. Pathol. Lab. Med.* 115: 1026 – 1029, 1991.

[29] Weiss SW, Tavassoli FA. Multicystic mesothelioma: an analysis of pathologic findings and biologic behaviour in 37 cases. *Am. J. Surg. Pathol.* 12 737 – 746, 1983.

[30] Ball NJ, Urbanski SJ, Green FH et al. Pleural multicystic mesothelial proliferation: the so called multicystic mesothelioma. *Am. J. Surg. Pathol.* 14: 375 – 378, 1990.

[31] Lane TM, Wilde M, Schofield J et al. Case report: Benign cystic mesothelioma of the tunica vaginalis. *Virchow Arch. B. Cell Pathol. Mol. Pathol.* 42, 153 – 159, 1999.

[32] Di Blasi A, Boscaino A. De Dominicis G et al. Multicystic mesothelioma of the liver with secondary involvment of peritoneum and inguinal region. *Int. J. Surg. Pathol.* 12: 87 – 91, 2004.

[33] Ordonez NG. Localized (Solitary) fibrous tumor of the pleura. Adv Anat Pathol 6: 327–340, 2000.

[34] van de Rijn M, Lombard CM, Rouse RV. Expression of CD 34 by solitary fibrous tumors of the pleura, mediastinum and lung. *Am. J. Surg. Pathol.* 18: 814 – 820, 1994.

[35] Chilosi M, Facchetti F, Dei Tos AP et al. Bcl-2 expression in pleural and extrapleural solitary fibrous tumors. *J. Pathol.* 181: 362 – 367, 1997.

[36] Renshaw AA. 013 (CD 99) in spindle cell tumors: reactivity with hemangiopericytoma, solitary fibrous tumor, synovial sarcoma and meningioma but rarely with sarcomatoid mesothelioma. *App. Immunohistochem* 3: 250 – 256, 1995.

[37] Altavilla G, Blandamura S, Gardiman M et al. Solitary fibrous tumor of the pericardium. *Pathologica* 87: 82 - 86, 1995.

[38] Young RH, Clement PB, McCaughey WTE. Solitary fibrous tumors ("fibrous mesotheliomas") of the peritoneum. *Arch. Pathol. Lab. Med.* 114: 493 – 495, 1990.

[39] Wilson RW, Gallateau-Sallè F, Moran CA. Desmoid tumor of the pleura: A clinico-pathologic mimic of localized fibrous tumor. *Mod. Pathol.* 12: 9 – 14, 1999.

[40] Calcifying fibrous pseudotumor of the pleura. Pinkard NB, Wilson RW, Lawless N et al. *Am. J. Clin. Pathol.* 105 : 189 – 194, 1996.

In: Mesothelioma from Bench Side to Clinic
Editor: Alfonso Baldi, pp. 337-345
ISBN: 978-1-60021-789-0

Chapter XVIII

Natural History of Human Pleural Mesothelioma

***Roberto Cassandro*[1]*, Silvia Montrasio*[1] *and Vincenzo Esposito*[2]**
[1]San Giuseppe Hospital, Service of Pneumology, Milan, Italy
[2]Third Division of Cotugno Hospital, Naples, Italy

Abstract

In this chapter, the authors report on the natural history of mesothelioma. In particular, they review the clinical symptoms at presentation, the diagnostic exams necessary to define this neoplasm, the clinical course and the complication, and finally the prognosis of this very aggressive disease.

Clinical Manifestations

Malignant pleural mesothelioma most commonly presents in the fifth to seventh decades of life and affects for 80 percent male sex. Most patients diagnosed with mesothelioma at an earlier age have a history of childhood exposure to asbestos.

The most frequent presenting symptoms of pleural malignant mesothelioma are non-pleuritic chest pain (60-70 percent), dyspnea (25 percent) and cough (20 percent). Some patients are asymptomatic at the moment of the diagnosis, with unilateral pleural effusions incidentally found on routine chest radiograph. The combination of an unexplained pleural effusion and pleural pain should raise the suspicion of malignant mesothelioma, even if the initial cytologic findings are negative [1].

Malignant mesothelioma is typically a unilateral disease: only 10 percent of patients have bilateral involvement. In more advanced stages of disease, physical findings may include unilateral dullness to percussion throughout the hemithorax, decreased breathing sounds over the base of the affected lung, palpable chest wall masses, and scoliosis towards the side of the malignancy [2, 3, 4, 5].

According to some studies, dyspnea and chest-wall pain are the first symptoms to appear and they usually persist for some months before diagnosis. Pain can be also caused by obstruction of superior abdomen as consequence of diaphragm invasion [6]. In the pathogenesis of dyspnea many factors may be involved, such as decrease in the compliance of the chest wall, controlateral shifting of the mediastinum, decrease in the ipsilateral lung volume and reflex stimulation from the lungs and chest wall [7].

Dull, weight loss, anorexia, fever, fatigue and malaise are generalized symptoms that are common later in the progression of pleural mesothelioma but are infrequent at presentation (occurring in less than 30 percent of patients). Although a cytologic diagnosis can be made quickly, malignant mesothelioma is usually not diagnosed until two or three months after the onset of symptoms; delays of diagnosis are especially frequent in centres in which the disease is uncommon. Moreover, later in the course of malignant mesothelioma a "cancer syndrome" can appear, consisting in weight loss, fatigue, cachexia, fevers and night sweats, thrombocytosis, hypoalbuminemia, an elevated erythrocyte sedimentation rate, and anemia: this syndrome should be due to circulating interleukin-6 [1].

Median survival is now 6-18 months from diagnosis as a result of combinations of severe dyspnea, chest-wall pain, abdominal distention with ascites, intestinal obstruction, pericardial tamponade, cachexia or pneumonia [8, 9].

Diagnosis

When a patient with a history of asbestos exposure begins to have cough, dyspnea, chest pain and at chest examination there is a retraction of a single emithorax, associated to a reduction of MV, some diagnostic exams can be useful.

Chest radiology: at chest x-ray, the main evidence of mesothelioma is an involvement of a single emithorax that causes a lung volume reduction. Computed tomography (CT) of chest is more sensitive to determinate mesothelioma extension, chest infiltration and lymphoadenopathy compromission. In 20% of mesothelioma cases there are pleural plaques. Mesothelioma can infiltrate pericardium and the other major vascular structures. Even if CT is often used in mesothelioma screening, there are more recent radiological techniques to better definite the tumor extension [10]. Magnetic resonance imaging (MRI) or positron emission tomography (PET) can then be used to complement CT. MRI with the use of different pulse sequences and/or with the adjunct of gadolinium can improve the detection of tumor extension. The use of PET has been described as a standard exam for mesothelioma. It defines that mesothelioma's areas are more captating than other patological areas; PET can help to show metastates areas too [11]. In conclusion, PET with 18-fluorodeoxyglucose in conjunction with computed tomography scanning has improved pre-operative imaging and staging [12]. Moreover, PET imaging is correlated to survival. In a recent study on 65 mesothelioma patients submitted to PET, the group with minor areas of captation had better survival than the others [13].

Bronchoscopy: the role of bronchoscopy is low in mesothelioma patients. It is indicated when endobronchial lesions are suspected because of hemoptysis, atelectasis or large effusions without contralateral mediastinal shift [14].

Thoracentesis: a diagnostic thoracentesis should be performed in any individual with a unilateral effusion or bilateral effusion without cardiac compromission. Only 10 percent of patients have massive pleural effusions on presentation. There are no absolute controindications to perform thoracentesis. When a thoracentesis is performed, some fluid tests are required: nucleated cell county and differential, total protein, LDH, glucose, pH, amylase, hyaluronic acid and cytology. One third of malignant effusions have a pleural fluid pH of less than 7.30 at presentation [15], this low pH is associated with glucose values of less than 60 mg/dl [16]. A pleural fluid pH less or equal 7.28 is more frequently associated to a poor survival [17]. Pleural effusions associated with mesothelioma are characteristically highly viscous, presumably because of elevated concentrations of hyaluronic acid. An increased pleural fluid hyaluronidase level is suggestive but not diagnostic of mesothelioma. But pleural fluid analyses should be used only in conjunction with others parameters as the patient's general health (performance status). However, cytology with immumoistochemical analysis is more important than the others pleural fluid test (see below).

Other invasive procedures: If abnormalities of the pleura are identified on Ct scan, CT-guided core needle biopsy has been shown to improve diagnostic accuracy. A percutaneous biopsy of the parietal pleura reports a diagnostic yield of 40 to 75 percent [18]. The relatively low yield of CT pleural biopsy is due to several factors as operator inexperience, early stage of disease with minimal pleural involvement, presence of tumor in areas not easy to biopsy [19].

Medical thoracoscopy is considered less invasive and less expensive than other surgical procedures like video thoracic surgery (VATS). It can be performed either under direct visual control through the optical shaft of the thoracoscope (a chest tube like a trocar) or by a video. With this procedure a biopsy can be performed and it is used to make diagnosis of pleural effusions and to stage the mesothelioma [20]. In a study on 208 patients with pleural effusions, the sensitivity of medical thoracoscopy was higher than that of cytology and closed pleural biopsy combined. The combined methods were diagnostic in 97% of the malignant pleural effusions [40] [21]. In conclusion, medical thoracoscopy can provide earlier diagnosis, better histological classification, finding fibrohyaline or calcified, thick, pearly white pleural plaques and/or with a biopsy, demonstrating high concentrations of asbestos fibers [22]. VATS has been shown to have a diagnostic rate of 98%. It is used in the early diagnosis and for multimodal treatment [23]. VATS is contraindicated when the patient cannot tolerate single lung-ventilation, if the pleural space contains adhesions that do not permit a thoracoscope introduction. When adhesions are not visible on chest radiograph, but only intraoperative, the surgeon must be converting VATS in an open procedure [24].

Citology and histology: Small amounts of mesothelin can be detected in the blood of some patients with a possible diagnosis of asbestos disease, follow-up of this disease and might also prove helpful for screening asbestos-exposed individuals for early evidence of mesothelioma [25]. Thoracentesis or pleural biopsy can often establish the diagnosis of pleural malignancy but may not provide enough diagnostic material to confirm the presence of mesothelioma. It' s very important the cytology of pleural fluid; immunohistochemical markers and monoclonal antibodies may be helpful to differentiate epitheloid mesothelioma from adenocarcinoma and the sarcomatoid mesothelioma from fibrosarcomas or hemangiopericytomas. Some cytopathological features of cells obtained from pleural fluid have been found to correlate well with the presence of mesothelioma, including papillary aggregates, multinucleation with atypia, cell-to-cell apposition, nuclear pleomorphism, and macronucleoli.

Malignant mesothelioma is classified into three histologic subtypes (epithelial, sarcomatoid, and biphasic). Epithelial mesothelioma have a better prognosis than sarcomatoid and biphasic forms [20] The epithelial variant is the most common (50-60%) and typical histologic appearances of this subtype include tubulopapillary, glandular and solid epitheloid patterns. The sarcomatoid pattern is composed of malignant spindle cells which may mimic malignant mesenchymal tumors, such as fibrosarcoma or leiomyosarcoma. Biphasic or mixed mesotheliomas have epithelioid and/or sarcomatoid features. At electron microscopy the predominant epithelial form is composed of polygonal cells with numerous long surface microvilli, prominent desmosomes and abundant tonofilaments. The sarcomatoid variant shows the presence of elongated nuclei and copious rough endoplasmic reticulum [20].

Immunohistochemistry: sometimes it is very difficult to establish the correct diagnosis because the three hystologic patterns and/or primary pulmonary and/or metastatic adenocarcinoma cannot be clearly differentiated. Mesothelioma cells have some molecules on their surface that react with particular antibodies There are now a lot of commercially available antibodies that can be helpful. There is no single marker that has a high sensitivity and specifity for malignant mesothelioma. In general, pathologists consider the presence of positive markers when it supports a diagnosis of malignant mesothelioma, negative when it does not do it [26]. Positive markers that can be useful for the diagnosis of malignat mesothelioma are calretin [27], the Wilms tumor-I (WT1) antigen [28] and the antibodies against cytokeratin proteins (that demonstrates diffuse cytoplasmic staining with perinuclear accentuation) like CK5/6, that is useful for differentiating mesothelioma from many sarcomas. Negative markers (not reacting with substance on cells surface) are considered the carcinoembryonic antigen (CEA), Leu-M1, Thyroid transcription factor-1 (TTF-1), Ber-EP4 and B72.3 because all of them are specific for adenocarcinoma. However the sensitivity and specificity of these negative markers is higher in the differential diagnosis from primary pulmonary adenocarcinoma, than when differential diagnosis is from metastatic lesions of kidney/ovary. Recent studies correlate mesothelioma prognosis to the vascular endothelial growth factor (VEGF), the tumor necrosis (TN) and the mitotic activity index (MAI). In particular, in 40 patients submitted to VATS or pleural decortication there was a significant correlation between VEGF staining, TN and reduce survival. In addition a positive correlation between VEGF levels and tumor stage was found. On the other hand there was no association between MAI and survival [29].

Staging: in the three following tables [28] are reported the TNM stadiation of mesothelioma, developed from the International Mesothelioma Interest Group.

Table 1. Tumor extension

Tumor	Region involved	Characteristics
T1a	Limited to the ipsilateral parietal pleura, Including the mediastinal and diaphragmatic pleurae	No involvement of the visceral pleura
T1b	Ipsilateral parietal pleura, including the mediastinal and diaphragmatic pleurae	Scattered tumor foci that also involve the visceral pleura
T2	Each ipsilateral pleural surface	At least one of the following: (1) involvement of the diaphragmatic muscle; or (2) a confluent visceral pleural tumor (including tissures) or tumor extension from the visceral pleura into the underlying pulmonary parenchyma
T3	Locally advanced but potentially resected tumor (each ipsilateral pleural surface)	At least one of the following: a) involvement of the endothoracic fascia; b) extension into mediastinal fat c) a solitary, completely respectable focus of tumor that extends into the soft issues of the chest wall:; or non-transmural involvement of the pericardium
T4	Locally advanced, technically unrescctable tumor (each ipsilateral pleural surface)	At least one of the following: a) diffuse tumor extension or multiple tumor foci in the chest wall with or without associated rib destruction b) direct transdiaphragmatic extension to the peritoneum c) direct extension to the contralateral pleura d) direct extension to the mediastinal organs e) direct extension to the spine; or f) extension to the internal surface of the pericardium with or without pericardial effusion or involvement of the myocardium

Table 2. Lymphonodes and metastasis extension

N/M	Characteristics
NX	Regional lymph nodes not accessible
N0	No regional lymph node metastases
N1	Metastases in ipsilateral bronchopulmonary or hilar lymph nodes
N2	Metastases in subcarinal or ipsilateral mediastinal lymphonodes, including ipsilateral internal mammary lymph nodes.
N3	Metastases in controlateral mediastinal, contralateral internal mammary, and ipsilateral or contralateral supraclavicular lymph nodes
MX	Distant metastases not assessable
M0	No distant metastases
M1	Distant metastases

Table 3. staging classification

Stage	Tumor	Node	Metastasis
Ia	T1a	N0	M0
Ib	T1b	N0	M0
II	T2	N0	M0
III	Any T3	Any N 1 or N2	M0
IV	Any T4	Any N3	Any M1

Clinical Course and Complications

Malignant mesothelioma exerts its morbidity and mortality via inexorable local invasion. Patients typically develop shortness of breath and chest pain as tumour and fibrosis gradually obliterate the pleural space and replace any pleural fluid. As the tumour spreads, it covers both visceral and parietal pleural surfaces, encasing the ipsilateral lung with a thick, fibrous peel that extends into interlobar fissures and occasionally into lung parenchyma. Deoxygenated blood is shunted through the trapped lung, leading to significant dyspnea and hypoxemia that is often refractory to supplemental oxygen. Dyspnea also results from abnormal chest wall mechanics secondary to tumour invasion into ribs as well as intercostals nerves and muscles. Local invasion of crucial thoracic structures can result in one or more of the following complications: dysphagia, hoarseness, cord compression, brachial plexopathy, Horner's syndrome, superior vena cava syndrome.

Patients die from local extension and respiratory failure; tumour extension below the diaphragm may result in death from small bowel obstruction. Patients may also die from arrhythmias, heart failure or stroke caused by tumour invasion of the heart or pericardium.

A number of paraneoplastic syndromes have been described in the setting of mesothelioma [24, 25] including disseminated intravascular coagulation, migratory thrombophlebitis, thrombocytosis, Coombs-positive haemolytic anemia, hypoglycemia, hypercalcemia associated with secretion of a parathyroid hormone-like peptide.

Hilar and mediastinal lymph node involvement occurs in less than 50 percent of patients but it is a marker of poor prognosis.

Distant metastatic disease by haematogenous spread is unusual in mesothelioma but may present in the opposite lung, liver, bone, brain, adrenals, thyroid, and kidney. Extension of the malignancy into the abdominal cavity may occur in patients who have prolonged survival after primary aggressive therapy of their thoracic disease, and spread throughout the abdomen in a manner similar to primary peritoneal mesothelioma may be observed. In these patients bowel obstruction can be a major problem.

Prognosis

In general a mesothelioma patient survives from first diagnosis a period of 8/12 months. Performance status and weight loss are powerful prognostic factors in mesothelioma. Others negative prognostic factors are male sex, older age, high platelet and leucocyte count .A marker of prognostic factor is the extension of the tumor and its histology. A patient with mesothelioma pattern epithelioid survives twice more than ones with mixed or sarcomatoid pattern. Sarcomatoid pattern is more invasive and aggressive. Some prognostic scoring systems have been proposed by the European Organization for research and Treatment of cancer (EORTC) [30] and by the Cancer and Leukaemia Group B (CALGB) [31]. These systems were derived from statistical analysis of large series of patients. CALGB has indicated as negative prognostic factors: LDH >500 UI/L in pleural fluid, bad performance status, chest pain, non epithelial hystologic pattern, age > 75. Instead, EORTC considers as negative prognostic factors: bad performance status, leucocitosis, sarcomatoid hystologic pattern, male sex.

Bibliography

[1] Bruces WS Robinson, Richard A Lake, Advances in malignant mesothelioma. *N. Engl. J. Med.* 2005; 353: 1591-603.

[2] Antman KH, Natural history and epidemiology of malignant mesothelioma. *Chest* 1993; 103: 373S.

[3] Pisani RJ, Colby TV, Williams DE, Malignant mesothelioma of the pleura. *Mayo Clin. Proc.* 1988; 63: 1234.

[4] Testa JR, Pass HI, Carbone M, Benign and malignant mesothelioma. In: *Principles and Practice of Oncology*, 6th Ed, 2001. p. 1937.

[5] Hillerdal G, Malignant mesothelioma 1982: Review of 4710 published cases. *Br. J. Dis. Chest* 1983; 77: 321.

[6] B. Fernandez Infante, F.J. Michel, Mesotelioma pleural maligno. *Anales cfnavarra*, Vol 28, Supl 1, 2005.

[7] Estenne M, Yernault JC, De Troyer A, Mechanism of relief of dyspnea after thoracocentesis in patients with large pleural effusion. *Am. J. Med.* 1983; 74: 813.

[8] Scagliotti GV, Novello S, State of the art in mesothelioma. *Annals of Oncolo*gy 16 (Supplement 2) 2005: ii240-ii245.

[9] Robinson BW, Musk AW, Lake RA, Malignant mesothelioma. *Lancet* 2005 Jul 30-Aug 5; 366(9483): 397-408.

[10] Wang ZJ, Reddy GP, Gotway MB et al. Malignant pleural mesothelioma : evaluation with CT, MR imaging, and PET. *Radiografics* 2004;24:105-119.

[11] Bernard F, Sterman D, Smith RJ et al. Metabolic imaging of malignant pleural with fluorodeoxiglucose positron emission tomography. *Chest* 1998,114:713-722.

[12] Sterman DH, Albelda SM. Adavances in the diagnosis, evaluation, and management of malignant pleural mesothelioma. *Respirology* 2005;10:266-83.

[13] Flores RM. The role of PET in the surgical management of malignant pleural mesothelioma. *Lung Cancer* 2005;49:S27-32.

[14] Feinsilver SH, Barrows AA, Braman SS. Fiberotic bronchoscopy and pleural effusion of unknown origin. *Chest* 1986;90:516.

[15] Rodriguez –Panadero F, Lopez-Mejias L. Low glucose and ph levels in malignant effusions; diagnostic significance and prognostic value in respect to pleurodesis. *Am. Rev. Respire Dis*. 1989;139:663.

[16] Rodriguez –Panadero F, Lopez-Mejias L. Survival time of patients with pleural metastatic carcinoma predicted by glucose and pH studies. *Chest* 1989;95:320.

[17] Heffner JE, Nietert PJ, Barbieri C. Pleural fluid pH as a predictor of survival for patients with malignant pleural effusions. *Chest* 2000;117:79.

[18] Loddenkemper R, Grosser H, Gabler A et al. Prospective evaluation of biopsy methods in the diagnosis of malignant pleural effusions: intrapatient comparison between pleural fluid cytology, blind needle biopsy and thoracoscopy. *Am. Rev. Respir. Dis.* 1983; 127 (S4):114.

[19] Canto A. Rivis J, Saumench J et al. Points to consider when choosing a biopsy method in cases of pleurisy of unknown origin. *Chest* 1983;84:176.

[20] Loddenkemper R. Thoracoscopy state of the art. *Eur. Respir. J.* 1998; 11:213.

[21] Menzies R, Charbonneau M. Thoracoscopy for the diagnosis of pleural disease. *Ann. Intern. Med.* 1991;14:271.

[22] Boutin C, Dumortier P, Rey F et al. Black spots concentrate oncogenic asbestos fibers in the parietal pleura. Thoracoscopic and mineralogic study. *Am. J. Respir. Crit. Care Med*. 1996;153:444.

[23] Pavia R., Mondello B, Barone M. et al. Malignant pleural mesothelioma: early diagnosis and multimodality management. *G. Chir*. 2005; 26:257-260.

[24] McKneally MF, Lewis RJ. Statement of the AATS/STS Joint Committee on thoracoscopic and video-assisted thoracic surgery. *Ann. Thorac. Surg.* 1992;54:1.

[25] Robinson BW, Creaney J. Lake R et al. Mesothelin-family proteins and diagnosis of mesothelioma. *Lancet* 2003;362:1612-1616.

[26] Miettinen M, Sarlomo-Rikala M. Expression of calretinin, thrombomodulin, keratin 5 and mesothelin in lung carcinomas of different types: an immunohistochemical analysis

of 596 tumors in comparison with epithelioid mesotheliomas of the pleura. *Am. J. Surg. Pathol.* 2003; 27:150.

[27] Doglioni C, Tos AP, Laurino L et al. Calretinin: a novel immunocytochemical marker for mesothelioma. *Am. J. Surg. Pathol.* 1996;20:1037.

[28] Amin KM, LItzky LA, Smythe WR et al. Wilms'tumor 1 susceptibility (WT1) gene products are selectively expressed in malignant mesothelioma. *Am. J. Pathol.* 1995;146:344.

[29] Demirag F, Unsal E, Yilmaz A et al. Prognostic significance of vascular endothelial growth factor, tumor necrosis and mitotic activity index in malignant pleural mesothelioma. *Chest* 2005; 128:3382-7.

[30] Curran D, Sahmoud T, Therasse P. Prognostic factors in patients with pleural mesothelioma: the European Organization for research and treatment of cancer experience. *J. Clin. Oncol.* 1998;16:145-152.

[31] Herndon JE, Green MR, Chainian AP et al. Factors predictive of survival among 337 patients with mesothelioma treated between 1984 and 1994 by the Cancer and Leukaemia Group B. *Chest* 1998;113:723-731.

In: Mesothelioma from Bench Side to Clinic
Editor: Alfonso Baldi, pp. 347-355

ISBN: 978-1-60021-789-0

Chapter XIX

Clinical Oncology of Mesothelioma

Francesco Cognetti, Anna Ceribelli and Fabiana Letizia Cecere
Division of Medical Oncology A,
Regina Elena National Cancer Institute, Rome, Italy

Abstract

Malignant mesothelioma (MM) is a very aggressive disease, in which the tumour develops from pleura or peritoneum resulting in an invasion/compression of the vital structure, causing symptoms which are hard to manage and which evolve rapidly. Its correlation with asbestos exposure has been proven and as a result, it is now considered a cultural and social problem. Because of the latency time in the development of this disease, incidence will increase throughout future years. Surgery is often not feasible for anatomic reasons and extent of disease at the time of diagnosis. A multimodality approach is preferable when the disease is localized. Chemotherapy recently has achieved interesting results, thanks to the clinical development of an antimetabolite drug, Pemetrexed. In combination with Cisplatin, Pemetrexed has become of standard use in cases of unresectable advanced MM. Nevertheless, MM remains an aggressive disease with a poor prognosis.

Treatment

The majority of patients with MM are not suitable for surgery, because their disease is extended/advanced or presents comorbidities. Moreover, surgery presents a high risk of morbidity and mortality.

The role of a surgeon is often limited to thoracoscopy, which not only offers tissue for diagnosis but also gives the possibility to practice pleurodesis, in order to palliate symptoms associated with effusion. Pleurodesis is a surgical procedure in which the pleural space is mechanically or pharmacologically obliterated to prevent recurrent lung collapse from pleural effusion.

Pleurectomy/decortication (P/D), which consists in the removal of parietal, visceral and pericardial pleura from the apex of the lung to the diaphragm, is possible only if the disease is diagnosed in the early stages. Only in selected Institutions with experience in this field are more aggressive procedure performed, such as extrapleural pneumonectomy, which includes resection en bloc of lung, visceral, parietal and pericardial pleura together with half of diaphragm. Initially, this kind of surgical intervention showed high rates of morbidity and mortality but recently it appears to be feasible, but should, however, be performed by skilled surgeons and in selected centres. There is, however, no impact on overall survival with aggressive procedures. The operative mortality is 5-9%, but serious complications can be seen in up to 25% . After an EPP, it is possible to deliver high doses of radiotherapy with a consequent reduction in local relapse. In the case of P/D, the presence of the lung limits high dose deliverance.

Multimodal approaches have been proposed to improve disease control. Chemotherapy or radiotherapy, either post-operative or intra-operative, seems to improve survival more than historical controls. Investigators from Brigham and Women's Hospital who favoured the use of chemotherapy or chemoradiation after EPP, in a series of 183 patients have reported 2- and 5- year survival rates of 38% and 15% respectively . CALGB is performing a multicenter clinical trial of multimodality treatment in which EPP is followed by cisplatin-pemetrexed chemotherapy and radiation therapy. Others investigators have explored a neoadjuvant approach. A Swiss group has performed a pilot neodjuvant trial with cisplatin/gemcitabine in 19 patients with T1-3 N0-2 disease.

Response rate to chemotherapy was 32%. 61% underwent surgery with a 2% operative mortality rate, and 78% received radiation after surgery. The median survival for all patients was 18 months, reaching 26 months in patients who had resection .

A multicenter neoadjuvant trial of pemetrexed cisplatin followed by EPP and hemithoracic irradiation is ongoing .

Chemotherapy

Virtually all chemotherapeutic agents have been tested in the management of MM, with response rates ranging between 0 and 30%.

Single agent doxorubicin has been the reference treatment for a long-time, reaching a 20% response rate in different studies. Other anthracyclines, such as epirubicin, have shown no advantage over doxorubicin. Overall, treatment with anthracyclines produces a 15% response rate with a median survival of 8 months .

Cisplatin at standard doses showed a response rate of 14% in the first studies in the 80s and 90s , with no evident benefit when increasing the dose. Carboplatin showed responses from 7 to 16% .

Taxanes produced low response rates and are considered to be ineffective .

Vinorelbine is the only vinca alcaloyd, which demonstrated activity in MPM. In a phase II study by Steel, vinorelbine was administered weekly to 29 patients showing 24% partial responses and an improvement in quality of life in 41% of patients.

High doses of methotrexate demonstrated a 37% response rate in a study with 60 patients with a median survival of 11 months

Combination regimens, such as platinum based or doxorubicin-based chemotherapy, have been explored in the treatment of MPM. Response rates remain around the 20% mark with a median survival rate between 6 and 12 months .

Doxorubicin-Based Chemotherapy

Doxorubicin-based chemotherapy has been tested during the past few years with differing results. Initially, there were two studies, from Germany and Italy which showed promising results (responses from 25 to 46%), but when compared to the cisplatin-mitomycin doublet, it was found to be inferior in terms of response and survival. In the study made by CALGB, in fact, patients were randomised to receive cisplatin-doxorubicin or Cisplatin-mitomycin. In the mytomicin arm, response rate was 26% vs. 14% in the doxorubicin arm, with a difference in overall survival which was not statistically significant between the two groups. A Triplet of cisplatin-cyclophosphamide and doxorubicin showed a 26% response rate with a median survival of 15 months .

Doxorubicin-ifosfamide has been tested in two studies, one of which with dose-escalation of doxorubicin, producing better responses but higher toxicity.

Platinum-Based Chemotherapy

A combination of Cisplatin at a 100 mg/mq dose at day 1 with Gemcitabine at 1000 mg/mq at days 1, 8 and 15 every 4 weeks has been tested in a single institution . In this Australian study 10 out of 21 patients (47.6%) achieved partial response, with a progression free survival of 25 weeks and overall survival of 10 months. Response was accompanied by an improvement in symptoms in 90% of patients.

Furthermore, measurement of vital capacity showed an improvement in this parameter for the entire length of the response duration.

Following these first results, a multiinstitutional Australian study, performed with the same regimen in a total of 53 patients, showed a 38% response rate and 11 month overall survival .

Median survival of 10 months with response rate of 16% was reported in another study with quite a different schedule: Cisplatin 80 mg/mq on day 1 and gemcitabine 1250 mg/mq on day 1 and 8. Carboplatin and gemcitabine produced an overall survival of 15 months and response rate of 26% .

Gemcitabine combined with oxaliplatin showed an overall response rate of 40% and a 13 month median survival .

Antimetabolites

Two phase II trials of gemcitabine from CALGB and EORTC reported response rates of 0 to 7%, respectively.

Antifolates have shown good results in different studies such as monotherapy or in combination. Of those tested pemetrexed in comination with cisplatin showed good results in phase III trials and its use in front-line therapy should be considered standard. Until the Vogelzang study, in fact, we did not have an exhaustive data supporting the use of one drug or another.

Pemetrexed is a multitarget antifolate, which inhibits different enzymes involved in purine and pyrimidines synthesis, including thimidilate synthase, dihydrofolate reductase and glycinamide ribonucleotide formyltransferase. A phase I trial with this drug indicated the recommended dose of pemetrexed in combination with cisplatin of 500 mg/mq and 75 mg/mq respectively. 5 of 11 patients in this study achieved a partial response . A phase III, randomised trial of comparison between this combination and cisplatin alone at a dose of 75 mg/mq was subsequently performed in a multi-institutional study . 456 patients were entered into this study, with 80% males and 70% of epithelial histology. Notably, improvement in overall survival was seen in the combination arm: 9.3 months for single agent versus 12.1 months observed when both drugs were administered.

One-year survival rate was 38% and 50% respectively. Also, time to progression was significantly different (3.9 to 5.7 months) and a response of 17% observed in the cisplatin arm becomes 41% in the cisplatin-pemetrexed arm.

During the trial, assessment of different characteristics of patients led to the identification of two factors related to an excessive toxicity of the drug: homocystein and methymalonic acid levels (markers of folate and vitamin B12 status respectively. After the first 70 patients treated, vitamin supplementation consisting of folic acid and vitamin B12 was administered to all patients who received treatment. Vitamin supplementation reduced incidences of toxicity, such as febrile neutropenia and gastrointestinal toxicity, without affecting the efficacy of the drug studied, as demonstrated by the efficacy parameters.

Of note, the assessment of response rates was performed accurately considering RECIST criteria. The authors, in fact, measured pleural thickness in up to three different areas on at least three different sections which were at least 2 cm apart. Partial response consisted in a 30% decrease in the sum of the unidimensional measurements.

After the presentation of this data, cisplatin and pemetrexed combination has become standard treatment of MPM. When it is not possible to administer cisplatin, some data belonging to phase I and II trials support the use of a Carboplatin-pemetrexed combination. The first one , a Phase I study, was a pilot study in which Carboplatin was given at the Auc of 5 and Pemetrexed at 500 mg/mq on day 1 every 3 weeks. In this trial, the response rate was 32% and median survival was 15 months.

Another very recent phase II trial conducted in Italy (in which our institution took part) with Carboplatin AUC 5 day 1 and Pemetrexed 500 mg/mq day 1 every three weeks showed promising results for this combination: 19 out of 102 patients (18.6%) achieved partial response, while stable disease was obtained in 48 patients (47%), resulting in an overall tumour control rate of 65.7%. Median time to progression was 6.5 months with 12.7-month median survival.

Preliminary results of gemcitabine 1250 mg/mq on day 1 and 8 in combination with pemetrexed 500 mg/mq on day 8 have been recently shown, with a response rate of 20%. Other antifolate drugs have been investigated in malignant mesothelioma, such as raltitrexed. Raltitrexed is a specific thimidilate synthase inhibitor. In a phase I study, where raltitrexed is combined with oxaliplatin, a relatively new platinum derivative, recommended doses were 3 mg/mq for raltitrexed and 130 mg/mq for oxaliplatin every three weeks. After this, a phase II trial was performed in seventy patients, fifteen pre-treated, to assess the activity of this combination .

A 20% partial response and 46% stable disease rate were observed. In chemo naive patients, median survival was 31 weeks and in pre-treated patients 44 weeks, with an overall survival of 22% and 40% respectively. A phase III has recently been published . In this study two hundred and fifty patients were randomised. Among the 213 patients with measurable disease, response rate was 13.6% (arm A) versus 23.6% (arm B; P = .056). Median overall and 1-year survival in arms A and B were 8.8 (95% CI, 7.8 to 10.8) v 11.4 months (95% CI, 10.1 to 15), respectively, and 40% v 46%, respectively (P = .048). Recently, the authors published a separate report about Quality of life in the patients treated in the previous study : the global HRQOL scale was comparable at baseline on both treatment arms (P = .848). At no point was any significant difference apparent on this end point. Both treatments led to an improvement, over time, in dyspnoea. This effect is an important clinically meaningful reduction from baseline in the cisplatin/raltitrexed arm. However, the majority of scales of the EORTC QLQ-C30 or LC13 showed stabilization of HRQOL with few clinically significant differences between the treatment arms.

REGIMEN	N	RR (%)	MTTP (months)	MEDIAN SURVIVAL (months)	REF
CISPLATINvs CISPLATIN-PEMETREXED	222	16.7	3.9	9.3	
	225	41.3	5.7	12.1	
		P<0.001	P=0.001	P=0.02	
CISPLATIN vs CISPLATIN-RALTITREXED	124	14	4	8.8	
	126	24	5.3	11.4	
		P=0.06	P=0.058	P=0.048	

New Treatment Approaches

There are some published studies of immunotherapy in MM. Despite the sensitivity of mesothelioma to immunotherapy observed in animals and clinical trials, there are yet to be any reports supporting its use apart from in clinical protocols.

Non-specific immunotherapy, such as interferons or interleukins administered systemically or intrapleurally has been studied in malignant mesothelioma. Single-agent interferon Alfa produced a response rate of 12% . Some studies with interferon and chemotherapy initially showed promising results, with a response rate of 36% and 27%, but most combination trials have shown results similar to single chemotherapy agents .

A specific immunotherapy approach is based on knowledge regarding SV40 and mesothelioma. SV40 or simian virus 40 is a DNA tumour virus, endogenous to the rhesus monkey. It is thought that the virus was present when the human population was vaccinated against polio and adenovaccines. SV40 is thought to induce tumorigenesis and many groups have found a relationship between SV40 and mesothelioma. It has been found in human mesothelioma and it has been suggested that a vaccine against SV40 could be used in the treatment of this disease and studies are ongoing in this direction. This topic is reviewed elsewhere in this book.

New targeted therapies are under evaluation in MM treatment. Of these, antiangiogenetic agents represent the most promising drugs.

In 2006, at the ASCO meeting preliminary data of 106 patients treated with cisplatin and gemcitabine with bevacizumab or placebo were presented. This study was double blinded and at the time of its first presentation remained unblinded. The median pooled PFS overall was 6.4 months; the median overall survival was 15.7 months. Correlation between VEGF baseline levels and overall survival, regardless of treatment, was statistically significant (p=. 008).

Another study of this triplet in ongoing in the United States. PTK787, an oral tyrosine kinase inhibitor of VEGF receptors flt-1 and flk-1 and PDGFRβ is under clinical evaluation in a phase II study of CALGB.

Imatinib mesylate, which inhibits both Platelet derived growth factor receptor and c-kit, showed no activity in more than three different studies . Ranpirnase is a protein of 104 amino acids with an enzymatic activity which is necessary for biological activities.

It enters the citosol through the cell surface in an active process that requires energy. In the citosol, it degrades the tRNA, resulting in a death signal for the cell and inhibition of cell growth and proliferation. The finding that tumour cells have more RNA suggests preferential activity in these cells, more than in quiescent cells, characterized by a low quantity of RNA.

In the clinical studies, toxicity was reversible and there were no toxic deaths. A phase II trial of single agent ranpirnase was published in 2002. One hundred and five patients, 37% previously treated, received ranpirnase at 480 μg/mq. Median survival was 6 months and 1- and 2- year survival rate were 34% and 22% respectively.

Among 81 patients evaluable for response, four achieved a partial response, two minor regression and thirty-five reached stabilization. Response correlated with survival.

Palliation of Mesothelioma Symptoms

Pain and dyspnoea are the most important symptoms to control. There are different kinds of pain: localised somatic pain is caused by direct invasion of the chest wall; neuropathic pain is due to vertebral or intercostal nerve invasion; lung invasion may cause visceral pain.

Opioid should be used generously in order to give pain relief without causing unnecessary side effects. Somatic pain may gain relief from non-steroidal anti-inflammatory drugs. Neuropathic pain requires anticonvulsivant drugs. In extreme cases, one should consider intratecal analgesia or nerve block. Dietary supplements or drug therapy (dexamethasone or medrossiprogesterone) may treat anorexia. We must remember that we are treating a person, so especially in the final phase of the disease, we must take care of the psychosocial aspects. Often medicolegal and bureaucratic aspects cause a lot of pain and difficulties to patients and their families. Multidisciplinary teams must be present when we want to make the life of those patients easier and more acceptable.

References

[1] Zucali PA, Giaccone G. Biology and management of malignant pleural mesothelioma. Eur J Cancer 2006.

[2] Krug LM. An overview of chemotherapy for mesothelioma. Hematol Oncol Clin North Am 2005;19(6):1117-36, vii.

[3] Weder W, Kestenholz P, Taverna C, et al. Neoadjuvant chemotherapy followed by extrapleural pneumonectomy in malignant pleural mesothelioma. J Clin Oncol 2004;22(17):3451-7.

[4] Tomek S, Emri S, Krejcy K, Manegold C. Chemotherapy for malignant pleural mesothelioma: past results and recent developments. Br J Cancer 2003;88(2):167-74.

[5] Zidar BL, Green S, Pierce HI, Roach RW, Balcerzak SP, Militello L. A phase II evaluation of cisplatin in unresectable diffuse malignant mesothelioma: a Southwest Oncology Group Study. Invest New Drugs 1988;6(3):223-6.

[6] Mintzer DM, Kelsen D, Frimmer D, Heelan R, Gralla R. Phase II trial of high-dose cisplatin in patients with malignant mesothelioma. Cancer Treat Rep 1985;69(6):711-2.

[7] Planting AS, van der Burg ME, Goey SH, et al. Phase II study of a short course of weekly high-dose cisplatin combined with long-term oral etoposide in pleural mesothelioma. Ann Oncol 1995;6(6):613-5.

[8] Raghavan D, Gianoutsos P, Bishop J, et al. Phase II trial of carboplatin in the management of malignant mesothelioma. J Clin Oncol 1990;8(1):151-4.

[9] Vogelzang NJ, Goutsou M, Corson JM, et al. Carboplatin in malignant mesothelioma: a phase II study of the Cancer and Leukemia Group B. Cancer Chemother Pharmacol 1990;27(3):239-42.

[10] Belani CP, Adak S, Aisner S, Stella PJ, Levitan N, Johnson DH. Docetaxel for malignant mesothelioma: phase II study of the Eastern Cooperative Oncology Group. Clin Lung Cancer 2004;6(1):43-7.

[11] Vorobiof DA, Rapoport BL, Chasen MR, et al. Malignant pleural mesothelioma: a phase II trial with docetaxel. Ann Oncol 2002;13(3):412-5.

[12] Steele JP, Shamash J, Evans MT, Gower NH, Tischkowitz MD, Rudd RM. Phase II study of vinorelbine in patients with malignant pleural mesothelioma. J Clin Oncol 2000;18(23):3912-7.

[13] Solheim OP, Saeter G, Finnanger AM, Stenwig AE. High-dose methotrexate in the treatment of malignant mesothelioma of the pleura. A phase II study. Br J Cancer 1992;65(6):956-60.

[14] Henss H, Fiebig HH, Schildge J, Arnold H, Hasse J. Phase-II study with the combination of cisplatin and doxorubicin in advanced malignant mesothelioma of the pleura. Onkologie 1988;11(3):118-20.

[15] Ardizzoni A, Rosso R, Salvati F, et al. Activity of doxorubicin and cisplatin combination chemotherapy in patients with diffuse malignant pleural mesothelioma. An Italian Lung Cancer Task Force (FONICAP) Phase II study. Cancer 1991;67(12):2984-7.

[16] Shin DM, Fossella FV, Umsawasdi T, et al. Prospective study of combination chemotherapy with cyclophosphamide, doxorubicin, and cisplatin for unresectable or metastatic malignant pleural mesothelioma. Cancer 1995;76(11):2230-6.

[17] Byrne MJ, Davidson JA, Musk AW, et al. Cisplatin and gemcitabine treatment for malignant mesothelioma: a phase II study. J Clin Oncol 1999;17(1):25-30.

[18] Nowak AK, Byrne MJ, Williamson R, et al. A multicentre phase II study of cisplatin and gemcitabine for malignant mesothelioma. Br J Cancer 2002;87(5):491-6.

[19] van Haarst JM, Baas P, Manegold C, et al. Multicentre phase II study of gemcitabine and cisplatin in malignant pleural mesothelioma. Br J Cancer 2002;86(3):342-5.

[20] Favaretto AG, Aversa SM, Paccagnella A, et al. Gemcitabine combined with carboplatin in patients with malignant pleural mesothelioma: a multicentric phase II study. Cancer 2003;97(11):2791-7.

[21] Schutte W, Blankenburg T, Lauerwald K, et al. A multicenter phase II study of gemcitabine and oxaliplatin for malignant pleural mesothelioma. Clin Lung Cancer 2003;4(5):294-7.

[22] Kindler HL, van Meerbeeck JP. The role of gemcitabine in the treatment of malignant mesothelioma. Semin Oncol 2002;29(1):70-6.

[23] Thodtmann R, Depenbrock H, Dumez H, et al. Clinical and pharmacokinetic phase I study of multitargeted antifolate (LY231514) in combination with cisplatin. J Clin Oncol 1999;17(10):3009-16.

[24] Vogelzang NJ, Rusthoven JJ, Symanowski J, et al. Phase III study of pemetrexed in combination with cisplatin versus cisplatin alone in patients with malignant pleural mesothelioma. J Clin Oncol 2003;21(14):2636-44.

[25] Byrne MJ, Nowak AK. Modified RECIST criteria for assessment of response in malignant pleural mesothelioma. Ann Oncol 2004;15(2):257-60.

[26] Hughes A, Calvert P, Azzabi A, et al. Phase I clinical and pharmacokinetic study of pemetrexed and carboplatin in patients with malignant pleural mesothelioma. J Clin Oncol 2002;20(16):3533-44.

[27] Ceresoli GL, Zucali PA, Favaretto AG, et al. Phase II study of pemetrexed plus carboplatin in malignant pleural mesothelioma. J Clin Oncol 2006;24(9):1443-8.

[28] Fizazi K, Doubre H, Le Chevalier T, et al. Combination of raltitrexed and oxaliplatin is an active regimen in malignant mesothelioma: results of a phase II study. J Clin Oncol 2003;21(2):349-54.

[29] van Meerbeeck JP, Gaafar R, Manegold C, et al. Randomized phase III study of cisplatin with or without raltitrexed in patients with malignant pleural mesothelioma: an intergroup study of the European Organisation for Research and Treatment of Cancer Lung Cancer Group and the National Cancer Institute of Canada. J Clin Oncol 2005;23(28):6881-9.

[30] Bottomley A, Gaafar R, Manegold C, et al. Short-term treatment-related symptoms and quality of life: results from an international randomized phase III study of cisplatin with or without raltitrexed in patients with malignant pleural mesothelioma: an EORTC Lung-Cancer Group and National Cancer Institute, Canada, Intergroup Study. J Clin Oncol 2006;24(9):1435-42.

[31] Vogelzang NJ. Emerging insights into the biology and therapy of malignant mesothelioma. Semin Oncol 2002;29(6 Suppl 18):35-42.

[32] Ong ST, Vogelzang NJ. Chemotherapy in malignant pleural mesothelioma. A review. J Clin Oncol 1996;14(3):1007-17.

[33] Purohit A, Moreau L, Dietemann A, et al. Weekly systemic combination of cisplatin and interferon alpha 2a in diffuse malignant pleural mesothelioma. Lung Cancer 1998;22(2):119-25.

[34] Soulie P, Ruffie P, Trandafir L, et al. Combined systemic chemoimmunotherapy in advanced diffuse malignant mesothelioma. Report of a phase I-II study of weekly cisplatin/interferon alfa-2a. J Clin Oncol 1996;14(3):878-85.

[35] Porta C, Mutti L, Tassi G. Negative results of an Italian Group for Mesothelioma (G.I.Me.) pilot study of single-agent imatinib mesylate in malignant pleural mesothelioma. Cancer Chemother Pharmacol 2006.

[36] Mathy A, Baas P, Dalesio O, van Zandwijk N. Limited efficacy of imatinib mesylate in malignant mesothelioma: a phase II trial. Lung Cancer 2005;50(1):83-6.

[37] Kindler HL. Moving beyond chemotherapy: novel cytostatic agents for malignant mesothelioma. Lung Cancer 2004;45 Suppl 1:S125-7.

[38] Mikulski SM, Costanzi JJ, Vogelzang NJ, et al. Phase II trial of a single weekly intravenous dose of ranpirnase in patients with unresectable malignant mesothelioma. J Clin Oncol 2002;20(1):274-81.

In: Mesothelioma from Bench Side to Clinic
Editor: Alfonso Baldi, pp. 357-366

ISBN: 978-1-60021-789-0

Chapter XX

Staging of Malignant Pleural Mesothelima

Paul Van Schil, Laurens Carp, Jeroen Hendriks and Patrick Lauwers
Department of Thoracic and Vascular Surgery and
Department of Nuclear Medicine, University Hospital of Antwerp,
Edegem, Belgium

Abstract

An ideal staging system for malignant pleural mesothelioma does not yet exist. This is mainly due to its specific growth pattern invading the pleural surfaces and neighboring structures. For this reason precise estimation of tumor volume and evaluation of local extension are particularly difficult. Different staging systems have been introduced but only the International Mesothelioma Interest Group (IMIG) system is based on TNM descriptors. Restaging of mesothelioma after induction therapy is even more complicated and still controversial. The recently described modified response evaluation criteria in solid tumors are presently the most accurate for response evaluation.

Staging of Mesothelioma: The Problem

Malignant pleural mesothelioma is a highly lethal neoplasm arising from the surface serosal cells of the pleural cavity. It has a peculiar growth pattern extending along the pleural surface invading the visceral and parietal pleura with further expansion into the lung and surrounding organs. For this reason it has a non-spherical extension witch makes estimation of precise tumor volume extremely difficult (Figure 1). However, correct staging is extremely important to make comparative studies and determine treatment and prognosis. Especially in early stages diagnosis and staging are particularly challenging [1]. Presenting symptom in these patients is often dyspnea due to a large pleural effusion (Figure 2).

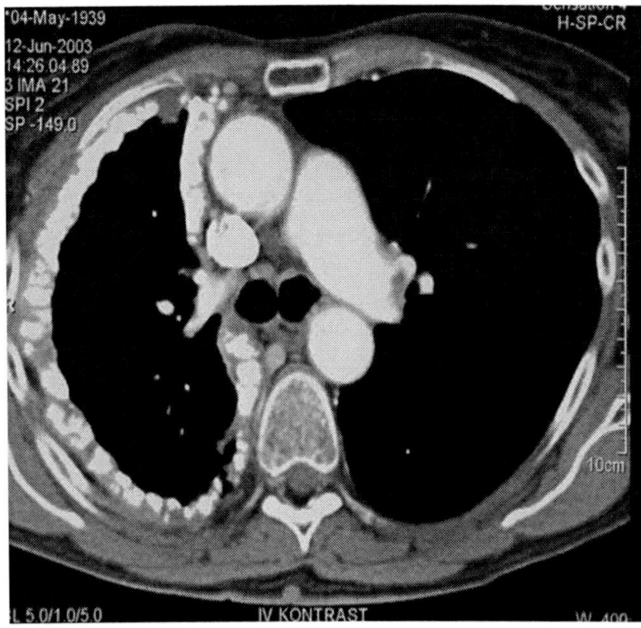

Figure 1. Calcified malignant pleural mesothelioma clearly demonstrating non-spherical growth along right pleural surface.

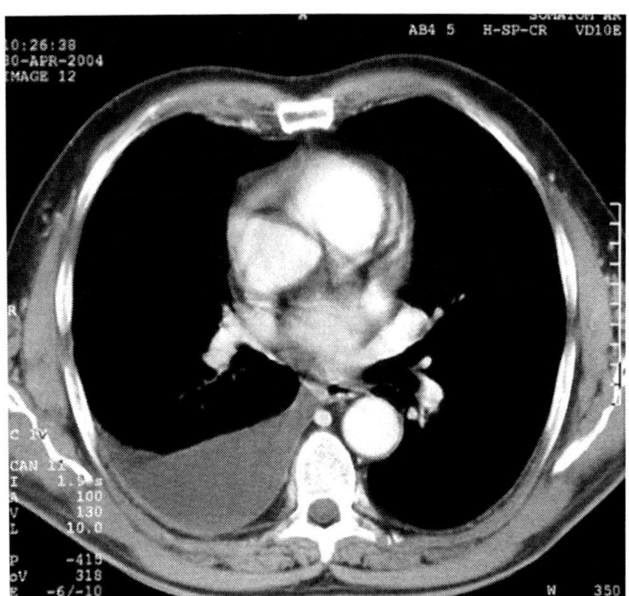

Figure 2. Patient with early stage mesothelioma presenting with large pleural effusion.

Response evaluation after chemo- or chemoradiotherapy is even more difficult and classical response criteria are insufficient. These topics are discussed separately.

Systems for Staging of Mesothelioma

At least 5 staging systems of malignant pleural mesothelioma exist. Butchart introduced a classification into 4 stages which became widely used [2]. These are described in table 1. A classification based on a multimodality approach including extrapleural pneumonectomy in 52 patients was proposed by Sugarbaker and is listed in table 2 [3]. This Brigham classification provides prognostic information and is able to stratify survival of patients treated with trimodality therapy [4]. Median survival ranged from 16 months for patients with advanced stage to 25 months for patients with early stage disease. All of these earlier staging systems including those of Butchart and Sugarbaker do not use the T, N and M descriptors as used in the classical TNM-classifications for tumors. For this reason the International Mesothelioma Interest Group (IMIG) introduced a new staging system in 1995 based on these parameters [5]. TNM-staging and stage grouping are given in tables 3 and 4. This staging system was adopted by the American Joint Committee on Cancer (AJCC) and the Union Internationale Contre le Cancer (UICC) [6]. It reconciles previous staging systems and is similar to those for other solid tumors and especially non-small cell lung cancer. It also incorporates data on the natural history and influence of TN status on overall survival. However, it relies mostly on surgical pathology and even with modern staging techniques differentiation of early stages and precise invasion in locally advanced disease remain difficult.

Table 1. Staging system by Butchart [2]

(reproduced with permission from Chest 1995; 108:1122-1128)

Stage	Description
I	Tumor confined within the "capsule" of the parietal pleura, *i.e.* involving only ipsilateral pleura, lung, pericardium, and diaphragm
II	Tumor invading chest wall or involving mediastinal structures, *e.g.* esophagus, heart, opposite pleura. Lymph node involvement within the chest
III	Tumor penetrating diaphragm to involve peritoneum; involvement of opposite pleura. Lymph node involvement outside the chest
IV	Distant blood-borne metastases

Table 2. Staging system by Sugarbaker [3]

(reproduced with permission from Chest 1995; 108:1122-1128)

Stage	Description
I	Disease confined to within capsule of the parietal pleura: ipsilateral pleura, lung, pericardium, diaphragm, or chest-wall disease limited to previous biopsy sites
II	All of stage I with positive intrathoracic (N1 or N2) lymph nodes
III	Local extension of disease into chest wall, mediastinum, heart, or through diaphragm, peritoneum with or without extrathoracic or contralateral (N3) lymph node involvement
IV	Distant metastatic disease

Table 3. IMIG staging system [4, 5]
(reproduced with permission from Chest 1995; 108:1122-1128)

Primary Tumor (T)	
TX	Primary tumor cannot be assessed
T0	No evidence of primary tumor
T1	Tumor involves ipsilateral parietal pleura, with or without focal involvement of visceral pleura
T1a	Tumor involves ipsilateral parietal (mediastinal, diaphragmatic) pleura. No involvement of the visceral pleura
T1b	Tumor involves ipsilateral parietal (mediastinal, diaphragmatic) pleura, with focal involvement of the visceral pleura
T2	Tumor involves any of the ipsilateral pleural surfaces with at least one of the following: a) confluent visceral pleural tumor (including fissure) b) invasion of diaphragmatic muscle c) invasion of lung parenchyma
T3	Tumor involves any of the ipsilateral pleural surfaces, with at least one of the following: a) invasion of the endothoracic fascia b) invasion into mediastinal fat c) solitary focus of tumor invading the soft tissues of the chest wall d) non-transmural involvement of the pericardium
T4	Tumor involves any of the ipsilateral pleural surfaces, with at least one of the following: (1) diffuse or multifocal invasion of soft tissues of the chest wall (2) any involvement of rib (3) invasion through the diaphragm to the peritoneum (4) invasion of any mediastinal organ(s) (5) direct extension to the contralateral pleura (6) invasion into the spine (7) extension to the internal surface of the pericardium (8) pericardial effusion with positive cytology (9) invasion of the myocardium (10) invasion of the brachial plexus
Regional Lymph Nodes (N)	
NX	Regional lymph nodes cannot be assessed
N0	No regional lymph node metastases
N1	Metastases in the ipsilateral bronchopulmonary and/or hilar lymph node(s)
N2	Metastases in the subcarinal lymph node(s) and/or the ipsilateral internal mammary or mediastinal lymph node(s)
N3	Metastases in the contralateral mediastinal, internal mammary, or hilar lymph node(s) and/or the ipsilateral or contralateral supraclavicular or scalene lymph node(s)
Distant Metastasis (M)	
MX	Distant metastases cannot be assessed
M0	No distant metastasis
M1	Distant metastasis

Table 4. IMIG staging system - stage grouping [4, 5]
(reproduced with permission from Chest 1995; 108:1122-1128)

Stage I	T1	N0	M0
Stage IA	T1a	N0	M0
Stage IB	T1b	N0	M0
Stage II	T2	N0	M0
Stage III	T1, T2	N1	M0
	T1, T2	N2	M0
	T3	N0, N1, N2	M0
Stage IV	T4	Any N	M0
	Any T	N3	M0
	Any T	Any N	M1

Regarding the T status, T3 implies locally advanced but potentially resectable mesothelioma, whereas T4 means an unresectable tumor as in lung cancer patients.

T1 indicates that there is usually a free pleural space and these patients often present with a large pleural effusion (Figure 2). However, the presence of pleural fluid has no effect on staging. Staging is usually done by computed tomographic (CT) scanning but also magnetic resonance imaging has an important role regarding extension along the diaphragm, the mediastinum and the apical part of the chest. Positron emission tomography has a specific value to detect distant metastases, but is less sensitive in the evaluation of locoregional extension [7].

By non-invasive staging it is rather difficult to make a distinction between T1a, T1b and T2 disease. Correct estimation of extent of disease is only possible during thoracotomy. In case of T1b disease, pleurectomy and decortication are usually feasible. In case of a T2 tumor there is more extensive involvement of the visceral pleura and lung, often necessitating an extrapleural pneumonectomy (Figure 3). The prognosis of a T4 tumor is rather similar to M1 disease and for this reason it is included in stage IV.

In the IMIG system lymph node staging is the same as for non-small cell lung cancer. The regional lymph nodes include the hilar, mediastinal, internal mammary nodes, as well as the scalene and supraclavicular lymph nodes. N2 disease includes invasion of the ipsilateral mediastinal, subcarinal or the ipsilateral internal mammary nodes, and N3 disease the contralateral hilar, mediastinal, internal mammary nodes and/or the ipsilateral or contralateral supraclavicular or scalene lymph nodes. As the pattern of spread initially involves the mediastinal lymph nodes bypassing the hilum, there is probably not a large survival difference between N1 and N2 involvement. Therefore, all patients with nodal involvement are classified as stage III (N1, N2) or stage IV (N3 disease), in contrast to non-small cell lung cancer where N1 usually belongs to stage II, and N3 disease to stage IIIB.

Precise evaluation of the superior mediastinal lymph nodes requires a cervical mediastinoscopy. In a recent study chest CT scan revealed enlarged lymph nodes in 39 % of the patients [8]. Lymph node metastases were detected by mediastinoscopy in 26 %. Overall accuracy of CT was 67 % and of mediastinoscopy 93 % [8]. Not only for mediastinal nodal involvement but also in the case of early mesothelioma tumors, there is a discrepancy between non-invasive and surgical staging.

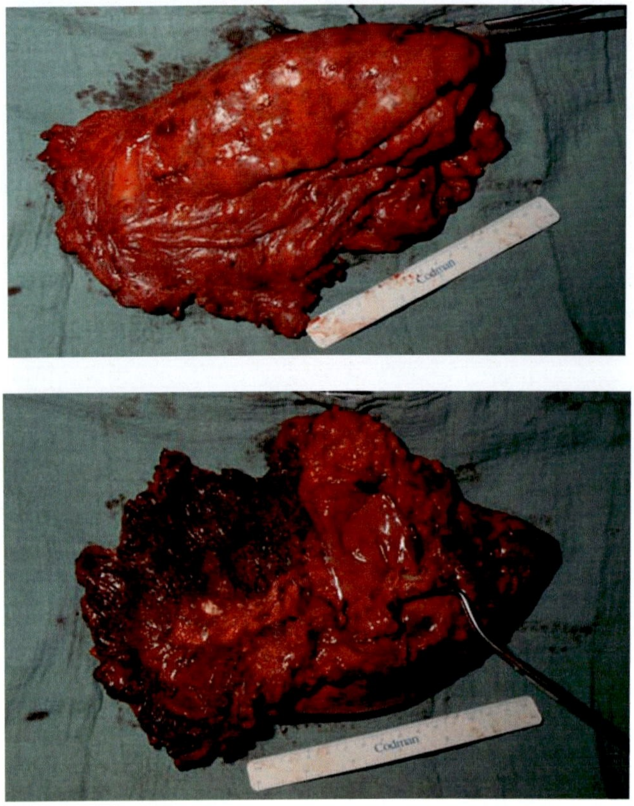

Figure 3 A and B. Extrapleural pneumonectomy for malignant pleural mesothelioma (A: view from lateral side, B: view from medial side). The resected specimen includes the ipsilateral lung, parietal pleura, diaphragm and pericardium.

The IMIG classification presumes that early tumors are evaluated surgically to determine local extension and subsequent treatment. It should also be stated that within a specific TN subset differences in tumor biology are possible, resulting in a variable prognosis within the same group. Especially with the advent of multimodality treatment, the IMIG staging system is not considered adequate anymore [1,9]. This is due to several reasons:

1. the underlying database is not known
2. it only has limited, retrospective validation
3. specific characteristics of this staging system cannot be distinguished with present-day imaging techniques as e.g. the extent of transmural involvement
4. the distinction between N1, N2 and N3 disease has been adopted form lung cancer staging which has a different nodal spread.

Restaging of Mesothelioma after Induction Therapy

Also due to its specific growth characteristics, response evaluation remains challenging in malignant pleural mesothelioma [10]. However, correct determination of this response after chemo- or chemoradiotherapy is important, especially when induction therapy is applied. With the introduction of neoadjuvant chemotherapy for mesothelioma patients, surgical treatment depends on response. Response evaluation is usually based on subsequent CT scans. The precise role of PET or combined CT-PET scanning in this setting has not been determined yet (Figure 4, 5). For response evaluation the WHO and RECIST (Response Evaluation Criteria In Solid Tumors) criteria are commonly used. Recent articles point out that as well the WHO as the RECIST criteria are inadequate for response evaluation in mesothelioma [11, 12]. The WHO criteria are difficult to apply as they require measurements of perpendicular diameters of tumor nodules. The RECIST criteria include multiple measurements of single diameter or tumor thickness which assume that tumors are spherical. However, mesotheliomas predominantly change in their perpendicular axis to the chest wall without major changes in the broader basis. For this reason modified RECIST criteria were recently introduced [13]. These include measurements perpendicular to the chest wall or mediastinum. Tumor thickness is measured in two positions at three separate levels on transverse images of CT scan. The sum of 6 measurements defines a pleural unidimensional measure. Nodal, subcutaneous and other bidimensionally measurable lesions are measured unidimensionally as in the usual RECIST criteria. Unidimensional measurements are added to obtain the total tumor measurement. *Complete response* is defined as disappearance of all target lesions with no evidence of tumor elsewhere. *Partial response* requires at least a 30 % reduction in total tumor measurement. A confirmed response requires a repeat observation on two occasions 4 weeks apart. *Progressive disease* is defined as an increase of at least 20 % in the total tumor measurement over the nadir measurement or the appearance of new lesions. *Stable disease* is present when neither the criteria for partial response nor progressive disease are met.

In a recent study of 34 mesothelioma patients the agreement between WHO and RECIST response evaluation was very poor and the RECIST criteria were found to underscore the tumor response [11]. The modified RECIST criteria perform much better than the standard WHO response and were more sensitive to detect pleural tumor response or progression. Recommendation of this study was to use the WHO criteria for bidimensional measurable lesions, RECIST for unidimensional measurable lesions and the modified RECIST criteria for response evaluation, in which the short axis perpendicular to the chest wall is used for thickened pleural rind disease [11].

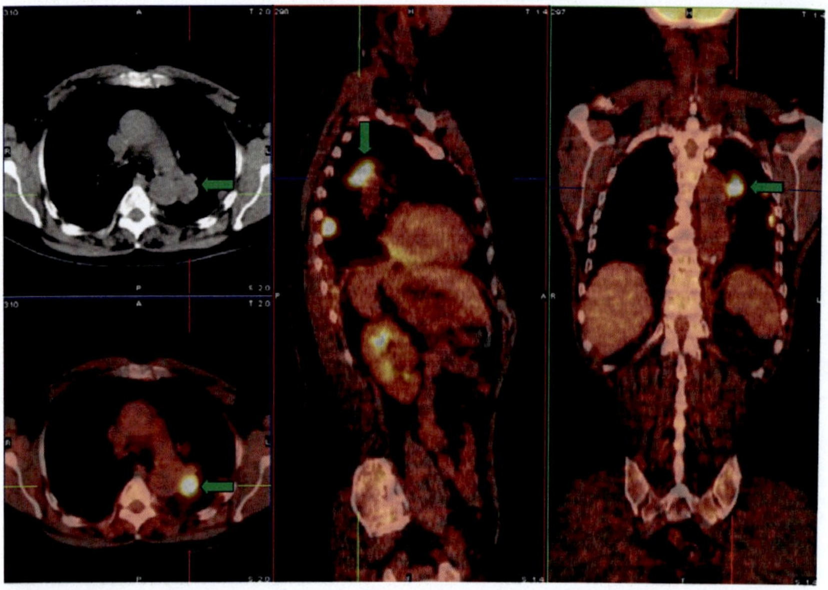

Figure 4. CT-PET images before induction chemotherapy. Arrows show involved areas along proximal descending aorta.

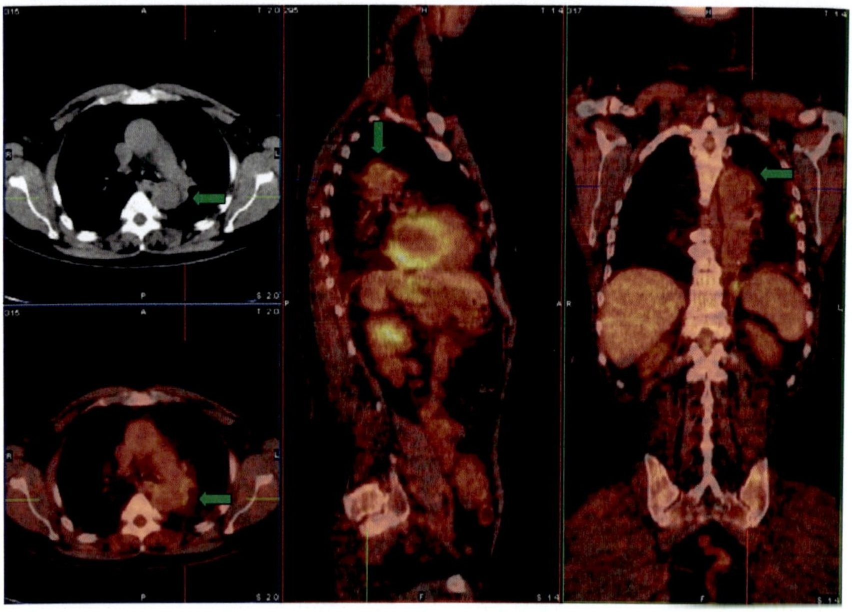

Figure 5. CT-PET images after induction chemotherapy. A clear response is noted in previously involved areas (arrows).

Conclusion

No ideal staging and restaging systems already exist for malignant pleural mesothelioma. The TNM-based classification introduced by the International Mesothelioma Interest Group in 1995 has several limitations and is mainly surgically based [5, 6]. The introduction of multimodality therapy has aggravated this staging problem which especially pertains to restaging after induction therapy when surgical resection is considered. Hopefully, the multicenter, ongoing trials will probably resolve this issue in the near future. There is a certainly a need for a new uniform clinical TNM staging system based on a large registry of patient data including those treated by multimodality therapy consisting of chemo-, radiotherapy and surgery [9]. In this way, advances can be made in the staging and treatment of this highly lethal disease.

References

[1] Neragi-Miandoab S. Multimodality approach in management of malignant pleural mesothelioma. *Eur. J. Cardiothorac. Surg*. 2006; 29:14-9.

[2] Butchart EG, Ashcroft T, Barnsley WC, Holden MP. Pleuropneumonectomy in the management of diffuse malignant mesothelioma of the pleura. Experience with 29 patients. *Thorax* 1976; 31:15-24.

[3] Sugarbaker DJ, Strauss GM, Lynch TJ, Richards W, Mentzer SJ, Lee TH, Corson JM, Antman KH. Node status has prognostic significance in the multimodality therapy of diffuse, malignant mesothelioma. *J. Clin. Oncol.* 1993;11:1172-8.

[4] Sugarbaker DJ. Macroscopic complete resection: the goal of primary surgery in multimodality therapy for pleural mesothelioma. *J. Thorac. Oncol*. 2006; 1:175-6.

[5] International Mesothelioma Interest Group. A proposed New International TNM Staging System for Malignant Pleural Mesothelioma. *Chest* 1995; 108:1122-8.

[6] American Joint Committee on Cancer. Pleural Mesothelioma. Chapter 20. *AJCC Cancer Staging Handbook.* Springer-Verlag, New York, 2002:205-9.

[7] Flores M, Akhurst T, Gonen M, Larson SM, Rusch VW. Positron emission tomography defines metastatic disease but not locoregional disease in patients with malignant pleural mesothelioma. *J. Thorac. Cardiovasc. Surg*. 2003; 126:11-6.

[8] Schouwink JH, Kool LS, Rutgers EJ, Zoetmulder FA, van Zandwijk N, v d Vijver MJ, Baas P. The value of chest computer tomography and cervical mediastinoscopy in the preoperative assessment of patients with malignant pleural mesothelioma. *Ann. Thorac. Surg*. 2003; 75:1715-8.

[9] Van Meerbeeck J, Boyer M. Consensus report: pretreatment minimal staging and treatment of potentially resectable malignant pleural mesothelioma. *Lung Cancer* 2005; 49 (suppl.1):S123-7.

[10] Van Schil P. Malignant pleural mesothelioma: staging systems. *Lung Cancer* 2005; 49 (suppl.1): S45-8.

[11] Van Klaveren RJ, Aerts JG, de Bruin H, Giaccone G, Manegold C, Van MeerbeeckJP. Inadequacy of the RECIST criteria for response evaluation in patients with malignant pleural mesothelioma. *Lung Cancer* 2004; 43:63-9.

[12] Monetti F, Casanova S, Grasso A, Cafferata MA, Ardizzoni A, Neumaier CE. Inadequacy of the new Response Evaluation Criteria in Solid Tumors (RECIST) in patients with malignant pleural mesothelioma: report of four cases. *Lung Cancer* 2004; 43:71-4.

[13] Byrne MJ, Nowak AK. Modified RECIST criteria for assessment of response in malignant pleural mesothelioma. *Ann. Oncol.* 2004; 15:257-60.

In: Mesothelioma from Bench Side to Clinic
Editor: Alfonso Baldi, pp. 367-378

ISBN: 978-1-60021-789-0

Chapter XXI

Possible Roles for Soluble Mesothelin-Related Proteins as Tumour Markers for Malignant Mesothelioma

Jenette Creaney ***and Bruce W. S. Robinson*****

*National Research Centre for Asbestos Related Diseases,
Western Australian Institute of Medical Research,
University of Western Australia, and The Australian Mesothelioma
Tissue Bank, Sir Charles Gairdner Hospital,
Verdun St, Nedlands, WA 6009, Australia

**MBBS, MD, FRACP, National Research Centre for Asbestos
Related Diseases, Western Australian Institute of Medical Research,
University of Western Australia, and The Australian Mesothelioma
Tissue Bank, Sir Charles Gairdner Hospital,
Verdun St, Nedlands, WA 6009, Australia

Abstract

The archetypical mesothelin glycoprotein is expressed predominantly on the surface of mesothelial cells lining the body's serosal cavities. Mesothelin is over-expressed in a number of malignancies including mesothelioma, non-mucinous ovarian cancer and pancreatic cancer. Little is know about the function of the protein, but it is thought to play a role in cell-adhesion and possibly in cell-cell recognition. The *MSLN* gene encodes for at least four protein products. The nomenclature used for these proteins has tended to be somewhat overlapping and complicated. However recent work by a number of laboratories has clarified the characteristics of these mesothelin-related proteins and in this review we will describe some of this evidence. The mesothelin-related proteins are promising candidates for use as tumour markers for malignant mesothelioma, a highly aggressive asbestos-induced tumour. Diagnosis of mesothelioma may be difficult, therefore a specific tumour marker would add to the currently available repertoire of

* Corresponding Author: "Jenette Creaney" creaneyj@cyllene.uwa.edu.au

tools used for its differential diagnosis. Treatment of mesothelioma is not effective, although over the past ten years there has been many new therapeutic strategies offered to patients, therefore a reliable tumour marker would provide a cost-effective way to monitor the response of patients to these various treatments whilst being minimally invasive to the patient. The significance of mesothelioma extends beyond its actual incidence; it has been estimated that compensation for this disease could reach into the hundreds of billions of dollars. If effective early intervention or preventative measures could be discovered there could be substantial reduction to this economic burden. A sensitive tumour marker would be a valuable tool in developing a screening program for asbestos-exposed individuals to detect early-stage disease. In this review will describe the data that suggest that soluble mesothelin-related proteins could be of clinical value in malignant mesothelioma.

Introduction

Malignant mesothelioma (MM) is a rare tumour that arises from mesothelial cells that line the serosal cavities of the body particularly the pleural cavity but also the peritoneum, pericardium and testicular cavities. MM is an aggressive tumour for which there are few effective treatments. As recently as ten years ago, there was considerable nihilism regarding this tumour. However, there has been upsurgeance of interest in MM from a diagnostic, a treatment and a biological standpoint although patient survival remains poor; generally less than a year after diagnosis. In this review we will examine mesothelin and mesothelin related proteins and their possible roles as tumour markers for MM.

Why Do We Need a Tumour Marker for Mesothelioma

The diagnosis of MM may present a challenge. The majority of patients present with either a pleural or peritoneal effusion, and generally with advanced stage disease. MM can present with a broad range of morphologies and patients do not necessary recall a history of asbestos exposure at initial presentation therefore MM may not be of primary consideration for diagnosis. The most common differential diagnoses include adenocarcinoma, reactive mesothelial conditions and fibrinous pleuritis. Currently clinicians and pathologists use a range of diagnostic techniques to make a definitive diagnosis of MM and in such a setting there is a role for a serum-based or effusion-based tumour marker that could provide additional information.

With an increase in therapeutic strategies being trialled for patients with MM there is a need for less expensive and less invasive methods to monitor patient's response to treatment than the currently employed radiological scans. Tumour markers represent a very attractive means of monitoring patients. Indeed it is in such a setting that serum markers have been most clinically useful.

We have proposed soluble mesothelin as a potential tumour marker for MM, both as an aid in diagnosis and in monitoring patient's response to treatment or disease progression. We are also investigating the potential of mesothelin as a marker to screen for the early detection of MM in an asbestos exposed population. The principle reason for developing a screening strategy for MM would be to commence treatment on early stage tumours which would hopefully prove more effective than treatment in more advanced disease. Although prospective studies and randomized trials would be required to test such an hypothesis.

MSLN Protein Products

The human *MSLN* gene is located on chromosome 16 and encodes a precursor protein of ~69 kDa. There is some overlap in the literature relating to the nomenclature for the *MSLN* protein products, due partially to the simultaneous identification of the protein by independent groups by independent mechanisms, the discovery of different splice forms at a molecular level and the naming of rodent homologues.

There are at least three mesothelin transcripts designated variants 1, 2, and 3. Mesothelin variant 1 is the predominant transcript (GenBank accession NM_005823) and was originally isolated from a pancreatic cell line. Variant 2 (NM_013404) was originally isolated from the cervical cancer cell line, HeLa and differs from variant 1 by the inclusion of 8 amino acids following glutamine 408. The third variant (AF180951) retains the 82 nucleotide intron between exons 16 and 17; this intron-retaining event causes a frameshift mutation and premature termination of the protein product.

Mesothelin variant 1 and 2 encode a 69kDa precursor protein which is processed and probably cleaved by furin-like proteases to produce two products. The N-terminal product designated megakaryocyte potentiating factor (MPF) and the C-terminal protein known as mesothelin. MPF is a soluble ~32kDa protein which was originally isolated from the culture supernatant of a pancreatic cancer cell line. MPF was shown to have a novel cytokine action, stimulating the colony formation of mouse bone marrow cells in the presence of interleukin-3. Mesothelin is ~40kDa glycosylated protein predominately anchored to the cell surface of normal mesothelial cells by a glycosylphosphatidyl inositol sequence. Mesothelin can be released from the cell surface, though it is not clear by what physiological mechanisms. It is in the mesothelin protein that variant 1 and 2 differ by 8 amino acids; it is not clear if there are any additional structural or functional differences between the two variants.

Mesothelin variant 3, presumably also encodes the 69kDa precursor protein which can be cleaved to form the N-terminal protein, MPF and a C-terminal protein. The C-terminal protein product of variant 3 is a soluble isoform of mesothelin, designated soluble mesothelin related protein (SMRP). SMRP has an identical N-terminal region to mesothelin but a unique C-terminal which is predicted to be hydrophilic in nature.

Rodent Mesothelin Homologues

Murine *Msln* gene is located on chromosome 17; it is slightly longer than the human homologue and has 58% identity at the amino acid level. Mesothelin knock-out mice have been generated which do not produce either MPF or mesothelin. The knock-out mice had no discernable phenotype and produced viable offspring, demonstrating that the MPF and mesothelin functions were not required for normal mouse development. Of note, the knock-out mice had equal numbers of platelets as wild-type litter mates suggesting that any possible role of MPF in platelet cell regulation was functionally redundant. Given the recent suggestion that the binding of CA125 to mesothelin may be a contributing factor to the metastatic spread of ovarian cancer it would be interesting to determine the rate of ovarian cancer metastasis in a mesothelin -/- model. Furthermore it would be interesting to determine whether these mice had impaired wound healing functions or differential susceptibility to asbestos or other carcinogenic agents.

The rat homologue of mesothelin was found to be over-expressed in Eker rats, a renal cancer model which have a germline mutation in the Tsc2 gene (a rat homologue of the human tuberous sclerosis, TSC2, gene). This rat *MSLN* homologue was designated *Erc*, expressed in renal carcinoma, and showed 90.6 and 67.6% identity with mouse and human cDNA, respectively. Importantly, the predicted *Erc* protein product shared many of the structural characteristics of the human homologue, including the putative furin-cleavage site, the signal for GPI-attachment the hydrophobic regions and three of potentially four N-linked glycosylation sites.

Mesothelin in Malignancy

Genetic studies have shown the over-expression of mesothelin in various malignancies including ovarian, pancreatic, lung, gastric and colorectal cancers. Immunohistochemical studies reveal mesothelin staining on MM, ovarian, lung, endometrial and pancreatic cancers and less frequently on oesophageal, vulval, cervix and stomach cancers.

The high expression of cell-bound mesothelin on several cancers and the limited expression on normal tissues have directed research into the use of mesothelin as a target for anti-cancer therapies. Preclinical studies using the immunotoxin SS1 (dsFv)-PE38 (SS1P), which consists of the Fv portion of a monoclonal antibody directed against mesothelin fused to a fragment of *Pseudomonas* exotoxin A, showed specific killing of mesothelin-expressing cell lines *in vitro* and regression of mesothelin-positive tumours in mice . Currently, clinical trials are underway examining the efficacy of this mesothelin directed immunotoxin in patients with mesothelin-positive tumours.

Mesothelin as a Tumour Marker

In 1992 Chang and Pastan immunized mice with ovarian cancer cells and produced a monoclonal antibody K1, they named the antigenic target CAK1. Expression of CAK1 was demonstrated on many non-mucinous ovarian cancers and on normal mesothelial cells. We now know CAK1 to be mesothelin. Chang and Pastan speculated at the time that the CAK1 antigen may be present in the serum of patients with ovarian cancer. Unfortunately their preliminary experiments using the K1 antibody as both the capture and the detecting antibody in a sandwich-type ELISA did not detect any protein in the sera of 16 patients with ovarian cancer.

Several years later the Hellstrom laboratory isolated another monoclonal antibody, OV569, following immunization of mice with ovarian cancer cells. OV569 reacted with the majority of ovarian cancers as well as a small fraction of other cancers and to normal mesothelial cells. The antigenic target of OV569 is mesothelin. Using a competitive assay they identified an additional monoclonal antibody, 4H3, which reacted to a different epitope on the OV569 antigenic target. Using these antibodies 4H3 and OV569, which notably react to different mesothelin epitopes, in a sandwich-ELISA increased levels of circulating antigen was detected in the sera of 23 of 30 ovarian cancer patients as well as a smaller percentage of patients with breast, lung, colon cancer and leukaemia compared with sera from healthy controls. Given that mesothelin is expressed on normal mesothelial cells, and is useful as a marker for malignant mesothelioma it was logical to assess whether patients with mesothelioma were also positive in this assay. Therefore, in collaboration with the Hellstrom group, we examined the sera of patients with mesothelioma and with other lung and pleural disease and found the assay to have a sensitivity of 84% and specificity of 98%.

Fujirebio Diagnostics Incorporated (Malvern, Pennsylvania) purchased the rights to the Hellstrom ELISA and the assay is currently marketed in Australia and Europe under the tradename MESOMARK ®. We repeated the measures of mesothelin levels in the samples used in the 2003 study using the MESOMARK assay and found excellent concordance in the results. Mesothelin levels were quantitated against the manufacturer's reference standard, and the median (± CI) concentration of mesothelin in patients with MM was 5.11 (± 3.8) nM; ranging from non-detectable to 78nM. For the smaller subset of twenty patients whose mesothelin was measured near the time of mesothelioma diagnosis the median level was 2.7 nM (range 0 to 35 nM). At a threshold value of 1 nM, the assay had a sensitivity of 69% and specificity 79% relative to patients with non-malignant lung or pleural disease.

Scherpereel and colleagues reported similar results using the MESOMARK assay to measure mesothelin levels in samples collected prospectively throughout France as part of a multi-centre study. In sixty MM patients the median serum level of mesothelin was 2.05 ± 2.57 nM; ranging from non-detectable to 28.84 nM. Using a threshold value of 0.93 nM, they found that the assay had a sensitivity of 80% and a specificity of 82.6% relative to patients with benign pleural lesions associated with asbestos exposure.

Recent characterisation of the 4H3 and OV569 monoclonal antibodies utilized in the MESOMARK assay demonstrated that the OV569 antibody recognises the mesothelin variants 1 and 3, and that the 4H3 antibody recognises all three variants.

Pastan and colleagues have recently developed a new panel of anti-mesothelin monoclonal antibodies. Using mesothelin-deficient mice, antibodies were raised against the pcDNA3CAK-1 plasmid (which encodes the full length pre-protein) and selected by their ability to bind mammalian expressed recombinant mesothelin protein (variant 2; NM_01340 nucleotides 937 – 1872). The resultant antibodies belong to two different topographical epitope groups and two of these antibodies were further characterised; monoclonal antibody MN belonged to the same epitope group as the previously characterised mAb K1 and the immunotoxin SSP1, and monoclonal antibody MB recognised a distinct epitope. Using the anti-mesothelin immunotoxin, SSP1 and the monoclonal antibody MB a double-determinant

ELISA was generated to detect mesothelin protein in serum. Based on levels of mesothelin in 24 healthy controls a threshold value of ≤ 9ng/ml was established. Approximately 70% of patients with advanced unresectable mesothelioma (i.e. 40/56) and with advanced ovarian cancer (i.e. 14/21) had elevated mesothelin levels in the serum.

Megakaryocyte Potentiating Factor as a Serum Marker

Although, there has been little in the literature with regards to the function of MPF given the successful detection of mesothelin and SMRP proteins in cancer patients it was compelling to see whether the MPF protein could also be detected.

In a similar approach to that taken to determine mesothelin levels, antibodies where raised against the MPF protein and a double-determinant ELISA generated. Probably at this stage the published numbers at too small to make valid conclusions but these preliminary studies suggest that the assay may be both sensitive and specific for mesothelioma patients. It is difficult to extrapolate from the published data but it appears that all seven mesothelioma patients tested had MPF levels above 10 ng/ml, whilst the 13 healthy controls were all less than 10ng/mL.

In a study published during the same time Pastan, Hassan and colleagues generated a different series of monoclonal antibodies to the MPF protein and developed a double-determinant ELISA. They defined a cut-off value for positivity in the assay as the absorbance that exceeds the mean absorbance value of sera from their cohort of 70 healthy controls by three standard deviations. Using this cut-off, 51 of 56 (i.e. 91%) of patients with advanced unresectable mesothelioma with an epithelial histology were positive.

Although not discussed in either paper it is interesting to speculate on the relationship between serum mesothelin and serum MPF levels. From a simple stoichmetric point-of-view one could assume that the assays should have equal sensitivity and specificity. However, as mesothelin must be cleaved or shed from the cell surface one could argue that MPF may be a more sensitive marker. Though using a similar argument it is possible that soluble mesothelin proteins would have greater specificity for the cancer state if those mechanisms responsible for cleaving mesothelin were part of the transformation process. We are currently investigating these relationships.

Anti-Mesothilin Antibodies as a Tumour Marker

In approximately 40% of patients with MM and epithelial ovarian cancer a spontaneous humoral immune response to mesothelin is generated. Anti-mesothelin antibodies were demonstrated to be cancer-specific as compared to 44 healthy normal blood donors and may therefore an additional tumour marker for MM. Further studies are needed to evaluate whether the formation of immune complexes between the mesothelin protein and its antibodies will distort any clinically valuable information to be derived from these markers.

The Clinical Potential of Soluble-Mesothelin Proteins as Tumour Markers in MM

Diagnosis

The sensitivity and specificity of the soluble mesothelin-related proteins are similar to those of other tumour markers currently marketed for other tumour types (Table 2). The clinical value of the soluble mesothelin-related proteins as tumour markers will be determined by studies however which examine specific clinical issues. In this respect the results of the study by Scherpereel and colleagues are most encouraging as they showed prospectively in a cohort of consecutive patients suspected of, or recently diagnosed with pleural MM that levels of soluble mesothelin-related proteins were higher in the serum and in the pleural effusions of those patients with confirmed MM than those subsequently diagnosed with benign pleural lesions associated with asbestos exposure. Recently, we have found that mesothelin protein levels were elevated in some cases in the pleural effusions collected 3 weeks to 10 months before the pathological diagnosis of MM was made (Creaney, Yeoman et al, accepted *Thorax*). Elevated effusion levels of mesothelin proteins before a definitive cytological and/or histological diagnosis may provide an early suggestion of the presence of malignancy and indicate the need for active invasive investigation such as thoracoscopy to establish a diagnosis. Of note however a negative mesothelin level does not exclude a diagnosis of mesothelioma. Early diagnosis could reduce the costs of subsequent hospitalizations and investigations and provide the opportunity for early treatment.

Monitoring

The clinical usefulness of the majority of tumour markers such as, CA125 and CA15-3 has been in monitoring the relapse of patients following successful treatment. To date little data has been published on the feasibility of using soluble mesothelin-proteins in monitoring mesothelioma patients beyond the original studies which found that the highest mesothelin levels were observed in patients with large tumours (with a width greater than 3 cm) and that levels increased with disease progression. We are currently continuing these studies to determine whether serum mesothelin levels correlate with tumour burden as assessed by PET and CT scanning.

Table 1. Published anti-mesothelin and anti-MPF antibodies

Clone(s)	Immunizing antigen	Species	Target	Reference
K1	OVCAR-3 cell line	Mouse monoclonal		
5B2	100 AA recombinant mesothelin			Nova Castra Laboratories
569	Mu immunized against hu ovarian cancer cells		Mesothelin variant 1 and 3	
4H3	Mu immunized against antigen purified from ascites via immunoadsoprtion		Mesothelin variants 1, 2 and 3	
1A6-10	Mice immunized against antigen purified from ascites via immunoadsorption		Mesothelin variant 1	
2B10	Mice immunized against mesothelin variant 2 fusion protein		Mesothelin variant 2	
8C8, 4A10 and 13HA	Mice immunized against mesothelin variant 3 fusion protein		Mesothelin variant 3	
SS1P	Anti-mesothelin Fv	Antibody phage display library	Mesothelin	
MB	full length mesothelin cDNA (NM_01340) followed by a single boost of a recombinant mesothelin-Fc fusion protein (variant 2)	Immunizing mesothelin deficient mice	Mesothelin	
MPF25	MPF (AA 1 to 291)	Immunizing mesothelin deficient mice	MPF	
MPF49	MPF (AA 1 to 291)		MPF	
7E7	Purified N-ERC/mesothelin fusion protein	Mouse monoclonal	MPF	
poAb-282	Synthetic peptide corresponding to region directly N-terminal to furin cleavage site (AA 281 to 295)	Rabbit polyclonal	MPF	

Table 2. Mesothelin and MPF levels reported in the serum of MM patients and controls

	Antibodies in Assay	Threshold value	Number of individual with elevated protein levels / total number of individuals examined				
			MM	Healthy controls	Asbestos-exposed healthy controls	Malignant disease	Non-malignant disease
	OV569 and 4H3	OD of 0.22	37/44 (84%)	0/28	*7/40	1/36	0/124
	OV569 and 4H3	0.93nM	48/60 (80%)				4/23
	OV569 and 4H3	1.85nM	35/60 (58%)			8/30	
	SS1P and MB	9ng/mL	40/56 (71%)	0/27			7/52 (13%)[a]
MPF							
	7E7 and PoAb-282	* above 10ng/ml	7/7	0/13	NA	0/3	
	MPF25 andMPF49	mean ± 3SD of controls	51/56 (91%)	0/70	NA	NA	

[a]– these 7 mesothelin positive patients had evidence of renal disease

* This value was extrapolated from the data presented by.

Screening

There is considerable interest in screening asbestos exposed individuals for the early detection of MM. Given that mesothelin levels may be elevated in some individuals up to 5 years before clinical presentation this biomarker represents a strong candidate for a screening programme. However, the sensitively of the screening programme will be limited given that at diagnosis not all individuals have detectable mesothelin proteins in their sera. Currently, methods of combining different biomarkers and a program that measures changes in biomarker values, rather than absolute values, are being evaluated.

Conclusion

One of the major issues when discussing the role of tumour markers in MM is that at present it is an incurable disease. Clearly this is most difficult from an early diagnosis point of view and indeed prospective studies and randomized trials are required to test the hypothesis that early treatment of MM may be more effective than the same therapy given later in the disease. However, there is clearly an adjunct place for tumour markers in the diagnosis and monitoring of patients with MM. Soluble mesothelin-related proteins may take on the role of tumour marker of choice for some patients with MM.

Acknowledgements

Work in our laboratory on mesothelin-related proteins has in part been supported by research grants from the National Health and Medical Council of Australia and the Insurance Commission of Western Australia, and in part by Fujirebio Diagnositic Incorporated (FDI), Malvern, PA, USA. We would like to acknowledge our many colleagues who have made this work possible.

References

Argani, P., C. Iacobuzio-Donahue, et al. (2001). "Mesothelin is overexpressed in the vast majority of ductal adenocarcinomas of the pancreas: identification of a new pancreatic cancer marker by serial analysis of gene expression (SAGE)." *Clin. Cancer Res.* 7(12): 3862-8.

Bera, T. K. and I. Pastan (2000). "Mesothelin is not required for normal mouse development or reproduction." *Mol. Cell Biol.* 20(8): 2902-6.

Chang, K., L. H. Pai, et al. (1992). "Monoclonal antibody K1 reacts with epithelial mesothelioma but not with lung adenocarcinoma." *Am. J. Surg. Pathol.* 16(3): 259-68.

Chang, K. and I. Pastan (1996). "Molecular cloning of mesothelin, a differentiation antigen present on mesothelium, mesotheliomas, and ovarian cancers." *Proc. Natl. Acad. Sci. USA* 93(1): 136-40.

Chang, K., I. Pastan, et al. (1992). "Isolation and characterization of a monoclonal antibody, K1, reactive with ovarian cancers and normal mesothelium." *Int. J. Cancer* 50(3): 373-81.

Creaney, J., H. Christansen, et al. (2006). "Soluble mesothelin related protein in mesothelioma." *Journal of Thoracic Oncology* 1(2): 172-174.

Frierson, H. F., Jr., C. A. Moskaluk, et al. (2003). "Large-scale molecular and tissue microarray analysis of mesothelin expression in common human carcinomas." *Hum. Pathol.* 34(6): 605-9.

Hassan, R., T. Bera, et al. (2004). "Mesothelin: a new target for immunotherapy." *Clin. Cancer Res.* 10(12 Pt 1): 3937-42.

Hassan, R., M. R. Lerner, et al. (2002). "Antitumor activity of SS(dsFv)PE38 and SS1(dsFv)PE38, recombinant antimesothelin immunotoxins against human gynecologic cancers grown in organotypic culture in vitro." *Clin. Cancer Res.* 8(11): 3520-6.

Hassan, R., A. T. Remaley, et al. (2006). "Detection and quantitation of serum mesothelin, a tumor marker for patients with mesothelioma and ovarian cancer." *Clin. Cancer Res.* 12(2): 447-53.

Hellstrom, I., J. Raycraft, et al. (2006). "Mesothelin variant 1 is released from tumor cells as a diagnostic marker." *Cancer Epidemiol. Biomarkers Prev.* 15(5): 1014-20.

Hippo, Y., M. Yashiro, et al. (2001). "Differential gene expression profiles of scirrhous gastric cancer cells with high metastatic potential to peritoneum or lymph nodes." *Cancer Res.* 61(3): 889-95.

Ho, M., R. Hassan, et al. (2005). "Humoral immune response to mesothelin in mesothelioma and ovarian cancer patients." *Clin. Cancer Res.* 11(10): 3814-20.

Hough, C. D., C. A. Sherman-Baust, et al. (2000). "Large-scale serial analysis of gene expression reveals genes differentially expressed in ovarian cancer." *Cancer Res.* 60(22): 6281-7.

Kojima, T., M. Oh-eda, et al. (1995). "Molecular cloning and expression of megakaryocyte potentiating factor cDNA." *J. Biol. Chem.* 270(37): 21984-90.

Miettinen, M. and M. Sarlomo-Rikala (2003). "Expression of calretinin, thrombomodulin, keratin 5, and mesothelin in lung carcinomas of different types: an immunohistochemical analysis of 596 tumors in comparison with epithelioid mesotheliomas of the pleura." *Am. J. Surg. Pathol.* 27(2): 150-8.

Muminova, Z. E., T. V. Strong, et al. (2004). "Characterization of human mesothelin transcripts in ovarian and pancreatic cancer." *BMC Cancer* 4(1): 19.

Onda, M., S. Nagata, et al. (2006). "Megakaryocyte potentiation factor cleaved from mesothelin precursor is a useful tumor marker in the serum of patients with mesothelioma." *Clin. Cancer Res.* 12(14 Pt 1): 4225-31.

Onda, M., S. Nagata, et al. (2001). "Lowering the isoelectric point of the Fv portion of recombinant immunotoxins leads to decreased nonspecific animal toxicity without affecting antitumor activity." *Cancer Res.* 61(13): 5070-7.

Onda, M., M. Willingham, et al. (2005). "New monoclonal antibodies to mesothelin useful for immunohistochemistry, fluorescence-activated cell sorting, Western blotting, and ELISA." *Clin. Cancer Res.* 11(16): 5840-6.

Ordonez, N. G. (2003). "Application of mesothelin immunostaining in tumor diagnosis." *Am. J. Surg. Pathol.* 27(11): 1418-28.

Robinson, B. W., J. Creaney, et al. (2003). "Mesothelin-family proteins and diagnosis of mesothelioma." *Lancet* 362(9396): 1612-6.

Robinson, B. W., A. W. Musk, et al. (2005). "Malignant mesothelioma." *Lancet* 366(9483): 397-408.

Robinson, B. W. S. (2003). "Soluble mesothelin-related protein-a sensitive new blood test for mesothelioma." *The American Journal of Oncology Review* 3(4): 230-233.

Rump, A., Y. Morikawa, et al. (2003). "Binding of ovarian cancer antigen CA125/MUC16 to mesothelin mediates cell adhesion." *J. Biol. Chem.*

Scherpereel, A., B. D. Grigoriu, et al. (2006). "Soluble Mesothelin-related Protein in the Diagnosis of Malignant Pleural Mesothelioma." *Am. J. Respir. Crit. Care Med.*

Scholler, N., N. Fu, et al. (1999). "Soluble member(s) of the mesothelin/megakaryocyte potentiating factor family are detectable in sera from patients with ovarian carcinoma." *Proc. Natl. Acad. Sci. USA* 96(20): 11531-6.

Shiomi, K., H. Miyamoto, et al. (2006). "Novel ELISA system for detection of N-ERC/mesothelin in the sera of mesothelioma patients." *Cancer Sci.*

Treasure, T. and A. Sedrakyan (2004). "Pleural mesothelioma: little evidence, still time to do trials." *Lancet* 364(9440): 1183-5.

Wang, K., L. Gan, et al. (1999). "Monitoring gene expression profile changes in ovarian carcinomas using cDNA microarray." *Gene* 229(1-2): 101-8.

Yamaguchi, N., K. Hattori, et al. (1994). "A novel cytokine exhibiting megakaryocyte potentiating activity from a human pancreatic tumor cell line HPC-Y5." *J. Biol. Chem.* 269(2): 805-8.

Yamashita, Y., M. Yokoyama, et al. (2000). "Mapping and determination of the cDNA sequence of the Erc gene preferentially expressed in renal cell carcinoma in the Tsc2 gene mutant (Eker) rat model." *Biochem .Biophys. Res. Commun.* 275(1): 134-40.

In: Mesothelioma from Bench Side to Clinic
Editor: Alfonso Baldi, pp. 379-388
ISBN: 978-1-60021-789-0

Chapter XXII

The Radiology of Mesothelioma

Fergus V. Gleeson
Department of Radiology, Churchill Hospital,
Oxford, United Kingdom

Abstract

Imaging and image guided intervention plays an important role throughout the care of patients with malignant pleural mesothelioma. The initial chest radiograph (CXR) may suggest the diagnosis in patients with an appropriate clinical history, and this may be confirmed and staged using computed tomography (CT). Image guided biopsy using either CT or ultrasound (US) is frequently performed to confirm the diagnosis, and magnetic resonance imaging (MRI) may be used to help stage the disease extent in some patients being considered for surgery. Recently positron emission tomography (PET) and positron emission tomography with integrated computed tomography (PET-CT) has been used to help improve staging, in targeting areas for biopsy, and providing prognostic information.

Chest Radiograph

Pleural thickening and effusion are the most frequent manifestations of mesothelioma[1]. These are most often unilateral and occur in combination [1]. The pleural thickening is frequently nodular and irregular, and extension into the oblique or horizontal fissures is present in up to 40% of cases [1]. Isolated pleural thickening without an effusion is uncommon, occurring in only 10 to 20% of cases [2, 3]. The identification of pleural thickening on CXR may be difficult due to the overlying effusion. A decrease in size of the affected hemithorax despite the presence of an effusion should raise a suspicion of pleural encasement and a possible diagnosis of mesothelioma, as should the absence of mediastinal shift in the presence of a large effusion. Rarely mesothelioma may present as a solitary mass on CXR [4].

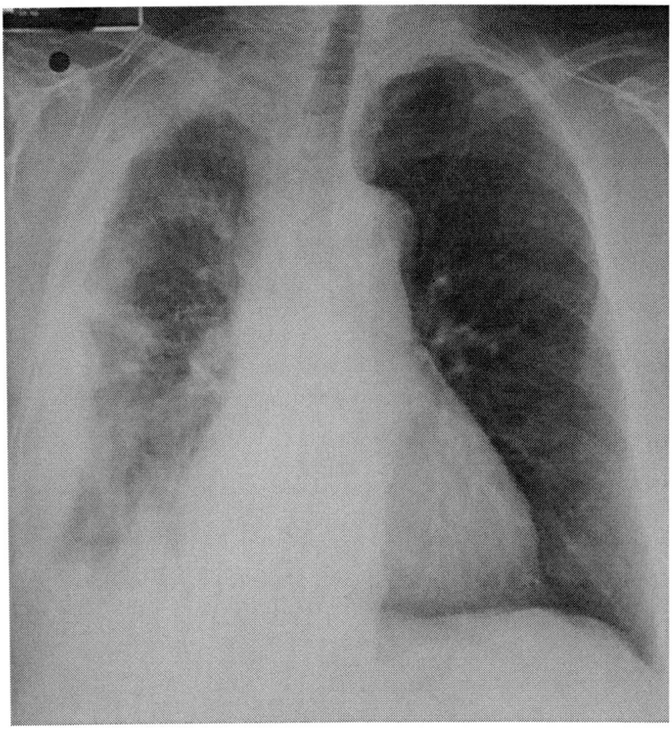

Figure 1. A CXR demonstrating irregular right sided pleural thickening and a decrease in size of the hemithorax in keeping with a mesothelioma.

Rib destruction or extension into the soft tissues of the chest wall are not commonly detected on CXR, and tend only to be identified in patients with advanced disease [3]. Pulmonary metastases are also seen on the CXR only in advanced disease, and are uncommon even then [2 3, 5]. The presence of other features of asbestos exposure such as calcified pleural plaques or pulmonary fibrosis is only identified on CXR in 20% of patients [6]. It is also important to remember that on CXR, the features may be indistinguishable from diffuse metastatic malignant pleural thickening.

Computed Tomography

CT is the imaging modality of choice for investigating patients with mesothelioma [7, 8]. CT findings include a unilateral pleural effusion in 80% of patients, nodular pleural thickening most commonly involving the lower zones in up to 50% of cases, with upper zone involvement seen in the minority of cases. Diaphragmatic thickening and fissural involvement may be present in upto 80% of patients [7, 8]. Extensive pleural thickening may result in encasement of the involved hemithorax, and a decrease in its size, readily identified by rib crowding and mediastinal shift. Mesothelioma is frequently locally aggressive with invasion of the adjacent chest wall, mediastinum and diaphragm. Features suggestive of chest wall invasion include loss of the adjacent extrapleural fat planes with extension into the intercostal muscles, and subsequent invasion of the soft tissues of the chest wall [7, 8].

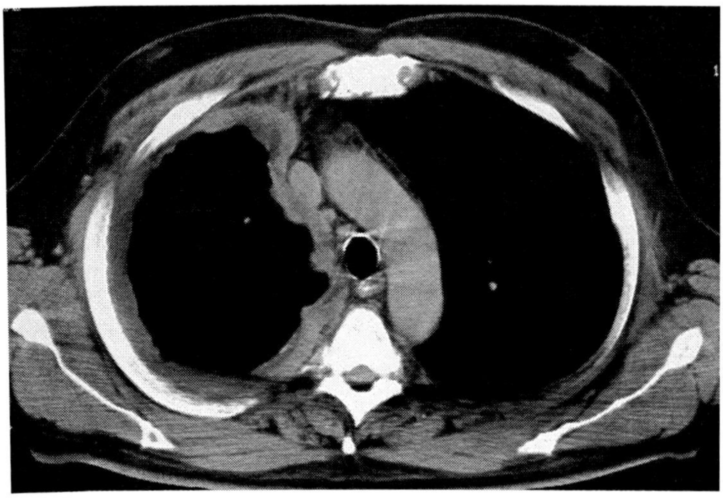

Figure 2. A contrast enhanced CT scan demonstrating circumferential nodular pleural thickening.

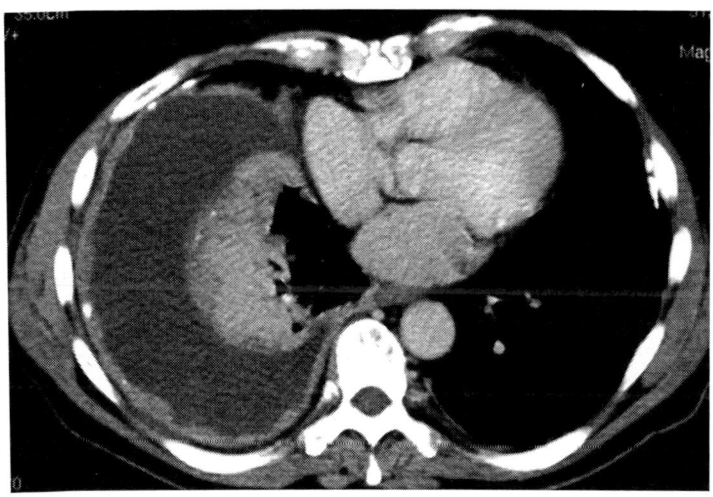

Figure 3. A contrast enhanced CT scan demonstrating a right sided pleural effusion with associated irregular pleural thickening and calcification, in keeping with prior asbestos exposure and a mesothelioma.

Advanced disease and needle tract invasion can result in extension into the subcutaneous tissues of the chest wall. Direct tumour extension into mediastinal structures occurs uncommonly, and may result in vascular or tracheal invasion [2, 7]. Pericardial involvement may be identified by the presence of nodular pericardial thickening or a pericardial effusion [2, 7, 8]. Extension through the diaphragm may occur and can be recognised by nodular diaphragmatic thickening and encasement with extracapsular hepatic indention identifiable on the right side [2, 7, 8]. Rib destruction is uncommon in mesothelioma, identified in approximately 15% of patients on CT [2, 8]. Pleural calcification and plaques may be seen in in 20% of patients, and may be encased by tumour [6, 7]. As with the CXR, metastatic pleural disease may be indistinguishable from mesothelioma. Malignant pleural thickening due to mesothelioma may be distinguished from benign pleural thickening by; thickening greater than 1 centimeter, nodular or irregular thickening, extension on to the mediastinal pleural surface, and circumferential involvement [11]. In one study of 74 consecutive patients with diffuse pleural thickening, of whom 11 had malignant mesothelioma; circumferential, mediastinal and nodular thickening was seen in 73%, 73% and 55% respectively compared to 0%, 12% and 25% in patients with benign thickening [11]. The presence of a pleural effusion, pleural plaques and ipsilateral hemithorax volume loss were not distinguishing features [11]. Pulmonary metastases occur in advanced disease and are more commonly identified on CT than on CXR. The metastases may on occasion be almost military [5], and an appearance in keeping with lymphangitis carcinomatosis has been reported [12].

Nodal involvement although present in at least 50% of patients at autopsy [13], remains difficult to evaluate on CT, as unfortunately size remains the only criteria for assessing involvement, and as with lung cancer remains suboptimal as a means of determining whether tumour involvement is present.

CT is the most commonly used modality to assess disease extent when surgery is being considered, although recent studies have also evaluated the role of MR imaging [7, 14]. CT scans should be performed using intravenous contrast, using contiguous thin sections to allow volumetric reconstruction. Multislice CT with multiplanar reformatting may be of value in assessing the degree of diaphragmatic involvement. Unfortunately, due to the mechanism of spread of mesothelioma along pleural surfaces, and its ability to invade the adjacent extrapleural fat in multiple areas, often symptomatically and asymptomatically simultaneously, and be present at initial staging, the reliable detection of invasion is difficult [7, 14]. Additionally involvement of adjacent lymphadenopathy and distinguishing this from contiguous pleural thickening may not be possible. A study comparing CT to MR in 95 patients, of whom 65 underwent CT, MR and surgery confirmed that there was no significant difference between CT and MR imaging [14]. Visualisation of hilar lymphadenopathy was unreliable, as was detection of enlarged ipsilateral mediastinal lymphadenopathy.

CT is also the modality of choice for tumour evaluation when monitoring patients being treated with chemotherapy. Both the response evaluation criteria in solid tumour (RECIST) and a modified RECIST have been used and have been shown to be more reliable than either subjective assessment, or the World Health Organisation (WHO) criteria [15, 16]. The modified RECIST criteria are: unidimensional measurements of pleural thickening, measured perpendicular to the pleural surface in three different axial locations, which sum to at least 2 centimetres should be measured. Lymphadenopathy with a diameter greater than 1 centimetre, and pulmonary metastases and other nodules with an axial diameter equal to, or greater than 1 centimetre may also be recorded. Recent studies have assessed interobserver reliability and also the use of a semiautomated software programmes for measurement, with the semiautomated programmes shown to be potentially of value [17, 18].

Magnetic Resonance Imaging

Magnetic Resonance Imaging is not routinely used in investigating patients with mesothelioma, as most patients present with advanced inoperable T4 disease, which is clearly delineated on CT [14]. Currently, MRI is performed in patients under consideration for radical surgery, as it may allow for the detection of diaphragmatic invasion, or solitary foci of chest wall invasion, enabling differentiation of T3 from T4 disease [7, 14, 19, 20].

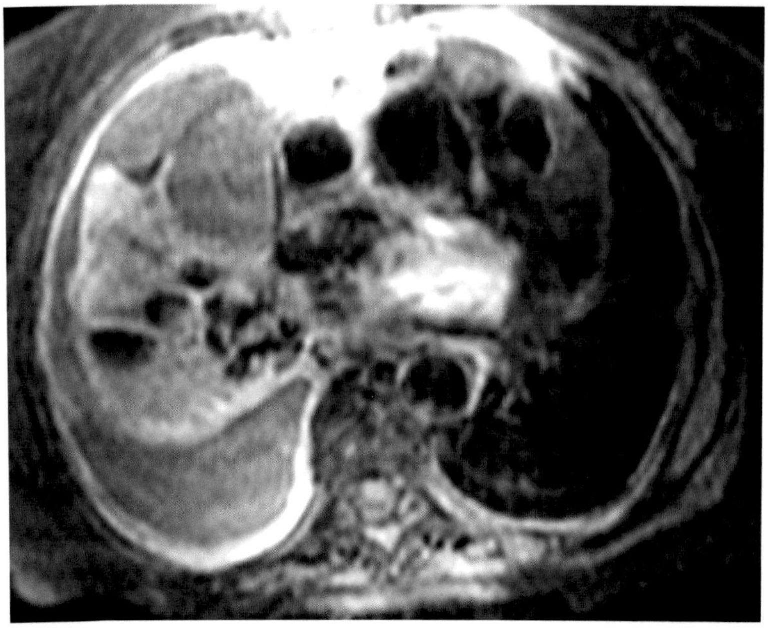

Figure 4. A contrast enhanced T1 weighted fat saturated MRI demonstrating a right sided effusion and enhancing pleural thickening.

Recently Stewart et al assessed the value of contrast enhanced MRI (CEMRI) in patients with epithelioid mesothelioma referred for surgery [21]. They found that 17 of 49 patients had unexpected unresectable disease on CEMRI that precluded surgery [21]. Mesothelioma is typically minimally hyperintense or isointense on T1-weighted images and moderately to markedly hyperintense on T2 weighted images [7, 14, 19]. It mostly demonstrates marked enhancement on contrast enhanced fat saturated T1 weighted imaging. Utilisation of the same criteria as on CT to determine the presence of invasion are used; loss of normal fat planes, extension into mediastinal fat and encasement of greater than 50% of a structure suggest tumour invasion [7].

Unfortunately neither CT nor MRI can distinguish between T1a, T1b and T2 disease since neither modality can accurately differentiate parietal from visceral involvement, or detect invasion of diaphragmatic muscle or pericardium. Similarly, assessment of metastatic nodal involvement is limited, irrespective of nodal size, with sensitivities of 50-60% [19, 20].

Positron Emission Tomography

The role of PET in the staging of mesothelioma is currently being evaluated following the advent of integrated positron emission tomography [22] and computed tomography (PET-

CT) [23]. The improved spatial and anatomical resolution available using PET-CT has increased its use and possible benefits in staging [23, 24].

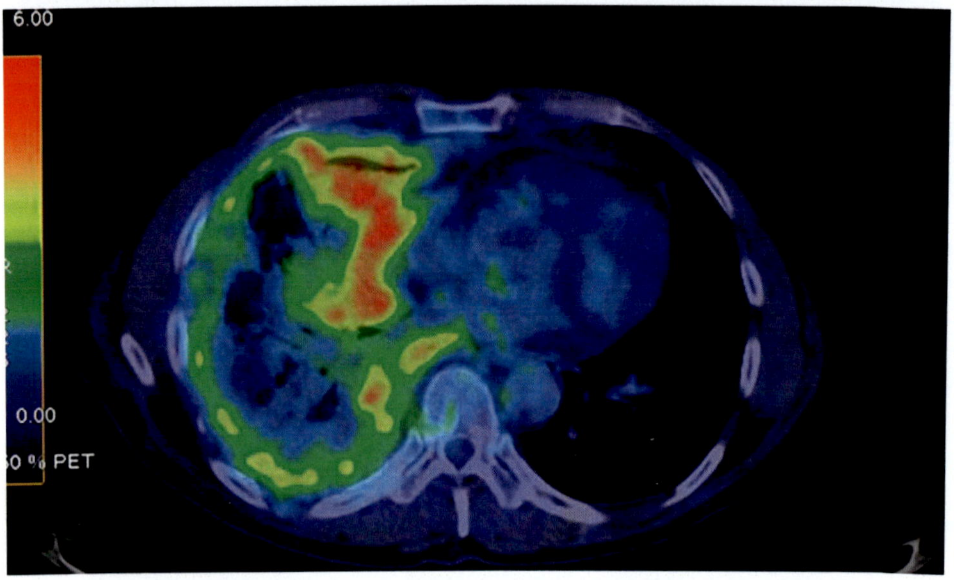

Figure 5. A PET-CT scan demonstrating increased FDG activity on the right associated with pleural thickening. A characteristic PET-CT scan appearance of a mesothelioma.

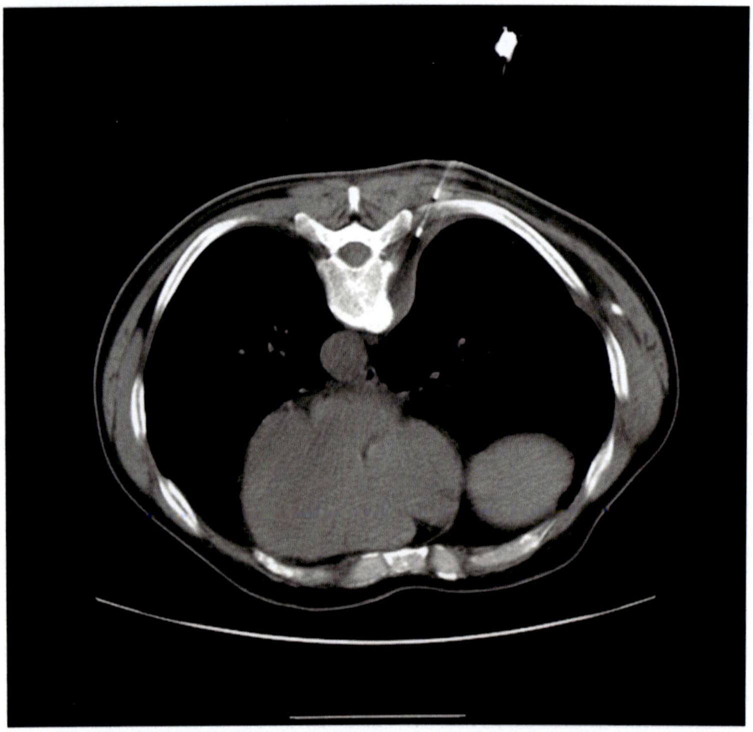

Figure 6. A CT guided biopsy of right paravertebral thickening due to mesothelioma.

Mesothelioma is characteristically ^{18}fluorodeoxyglucose (^{18}FDG) avid, and is reported to be more ^{18}FDG avid than in patients with benign pleural disease such as inflammatory pleuritis and benign asbestos related pleural thickening [22]. A recent study reported the sensitivity, specificity, negative predictive value and accuracy of PET-CT for assessing T4 disease as 67%, 93%, 86%, 82% and 83% [23]. The limitation remaining as with CT and MRI the detection of subtle T4 disease such as early transdiaphragmatic extension, and some institutions routinely perform laparoscopy to exclude this [25].

Nodal metastases are frequently found at surgical staging, and both CT and MRI continue to only be able to utilise size as the criteria for tumour involvement. Although PET-CT utilises ^{18}FDG avidity to detect nodal involvement, and is not dependent on size criteria, it is also inaccurate in the evaluation of nodal involvement [23, 26]. Erasmus et al reported that in 29 patients being considered for extrapleural pneumonectomy, the sensitivity, specificity, positive predictive value, negative predictive value and accuracy of PET-CT in lymph node staging in patients with N2 disease were 38%, 78%, 60%, 58% and 59% [23]. PET-CT remains limited as per CT and MRI in the detection of microscopic disease producing false negatives results, and may also produce false positive results due to inflammatory or infectious involvement of mediastinal lymph nodes.

Extrathoracic metastasis may be detected utilising PET and PET-CT. Erasmus et al detected metastatic disease in 25% of patients undergoing evaluation for extrapleural pneumonectomy, with >50% of these metastases undetected by routine staging and clinical evaluation [23]. Furthermore when thoracoscopic or percutaneous biopsy have been negative, PET can help demonstrate a focal area of increased uptake and a more appropriate site for biopsy.

It is possible that PET and PET-CT may be able to provide both prognostic information and be utilised to evaluate early tumour response to therapy [27, 28]. Utilising the semiquantitative method of measuring the standardise uptake value (SUV) a recent study assessed the prognostic value of PET. The authors found that a high, SUV > 4, positively correlated with decreased survival, $p=0.001$ and duration of survival, $p< 0.05$ [22]. Additionally a low SUV and epithelial histology indicate the best survival compared to a high SUV and nonepithelial histology indicating the poorest survival [27]. The use of PET to determine early tumour response has been reported by Ceresoli et al. [28]. They reported that in a study comparing CT to PET-CT in 22 patients at baseline and after 2 cycles of chemotherapy, a metabolic response detected on PET correlated significantly with median time to tumour progression, with no correlation detected utilising CT [28].

Pleural Biopsy

Confirmation of the suspected diagnosis of mesothelioma with histology is necessary in nearly all cases. Tissue may be obtained by thoracoscopy, minithoracotomy, blind pleural biopsy and image guided pleural biopsy. Blind pleural biopsies using reverse bevel Abrams and Cope needles may not achieve a tissue diagnosis, due to sampling error, when the affected pleura is missed. In experienced hands, diagnostic sensitivities of 50% are achievable for malignant disease including mesothelioma [29]. Although in patients with negative pleural fluid cytology, more typical sensitivities range from 7-27% [29, 30].

Thoracoscopic biopsy has been reported to achieve a diagnosis in up to 98% of patients [31]. A randomised double blind study comparing image guided biopsy to blind pleural biopsy reported a significantly higher diagnostic yield for malignant pleural disease with CT guidance than blind pleural biopsy, 87% versus 47% [32]. Two non-randomised case series also reported a yield of almost 90% for image guide biopsy, and confirmed that histological rather than cytological sampling is required, with core biopsy achieving a diagnosis of 93% for mesothelioma, compared to 50% on fine needle aspiration biopsy [33, 34]. Pleural biopsies are usually performed under US or CT. The choice of modality depends on the operator's personal preference and competence. No studies have directly compared the clinical utility of US to CT. If CT guidance is used, biopsy along the pleural plane allows histological cores of tissue to be achieved even in patients with pleural thickening of less than 5mm, with one study reporting a sensitivity of 75% for pleural thickness less than 5mm and 100% for thickening greater than 5mm [33].

Biopsies under ultrasound or CT can be performed in the presence or absence of a pleural effusion, although greater pleural thickening is required to perform biopsies using ultrasound guidance. The presence of an effusion reduces the risk of complications, in particular a pneumothorax.

Complications associated with percutaneous pleural biopsy occur uncommonly, < 1% of cases. Complications include pneumothorax, hemothorax, subcutaneous hematoma and laceration of the underlying upper abdominal viscera.

Tumour seeding along the needle track is relatively common with mesothelioma occurring in 20% of patients undergoing biopsy and drainage [35]. Early radiotherapy to the biopsy track has been shown to prevent tumour seeding [35].

References

[1] Muller NL. Imaging of the pleura. *Radiology* 1993;186:297-309.

[2] Miller BH, Rosado-de-Christenson ML, Mason AC et al. From the archives of the AFIP. Malignant pleural mesothelioma: radiologic-pathologic correlation. *Radiographics* 1996;16:613-644.

[3] Kawashima A, Libshitz HI. Malignant pleural Mesothelioma; CT manifestations in 50 cases. *AJR* 1990;155:965-969.

[4] Erdogan E, Demirkazik FB, Gulsam M et al. Incidental localized (solitary) mediastinal malignant mesothelioma. *Br. J. Radiol.* 20005;78:858-861.

[5] Huncharek M. Miliary mesothelioma. *Chest* 1994;106:605-606.

[6] Antman KH. Current concepts: malignant mesothelioma. *N. Engl. J. Med.* 1980;303:200-202.

[7] Wang ZJ, Reddy PJ, Gotway MB et al. Malignant Pleural Mesothelioma: Evaluation with CT, MR Imaging and PET. *Radiographics* 2004;24:105-119.

[8] Ng CS, Munden RF, Libshitz HI. Maligant pleural mesothelioma: the spectrum of manifestations on CT in 70 cases. *Clin. Radiol.* 1999;54:415-421.

[9] Patz EF Jr, Shaffer K, Piwnica-Worms DR et al. Malignant pleural mesothelioma: value of CT and MR imaging in predicting respectability. *AJR* 19992;159:961-966.

[10] Leung AN, Muller NL, Miller RR. CT in differential diagnosis of diffuse pleural disease. *AJR* 1990;154:487-492.

[11] Solomons K, Polakow R, Marchand P. Diffuse malignant mesothelioma presenting as bilateral malignant lymphangitis. *Thorax* 1985;40:682-683.

[12] Huncharek M, Smith K. Extrathoracic lymph node metastases in malignant pleural mesothelioma. *Chest* 1988;93:443-444.

[13] Heelan RT, Rusch VW, Begg CB et al. Staging of Malignant Pleural Mesothelioma: Comparison of CT and MR Imaging. *AJR* 1999;172:1039-1047.

[14] Byrne MY, Nowak AK.Modified RECIST criteria for assessment of response in malignant pleural mesothelioma. *Ann. Oncol.* 2004;15:257-260.

[15] Nowak AK. CT, RECIST, and malignant pleural mesothelioma. *Lung Cancer* 2005;49(S1):S37-40.

[16] Armato SG, Ogarek JL, Starkey A et al. Variability in Mesothelioma Tumor Response Classification. *AJR* 2006;186:1000-1006.

[17] Armato SG, Oxnard GR, Kocherginski M et al. Evaluation of semiautomated measurements of mesothelioma tumor thickness on CT scans. *Acad. Radiol.* 2005;12:1301-1309.

[18] Bonomo L, Feragalli B, Sacco R et al. Malignant pleural disease. *Eur. J. Radiol.* 2000;34:98-118.

[19] Patz EF Jr, Rusch VW, Heelan R. The proposed new international TNM staging system for malignant pleural mesothelioma: application to imaging. *AJR* 1996;166:323-327.

[20] Stewart D, Waller D, Edwards J et al. Is there a role for pre-operative contrast enhanced magnetic resonance imaging for radical surgery in malignant pleural mesothelioma? *Eur. J. Cardiothorac. Surg* .2003;24:1019-1024.

[21] Bernard F, Sterman D, Smith RJ et al. Metabolic imaging of malignant pleural mesothelioma with fluorodeoxyglucose positron emission tomography. *Chest* 1998;114:713-722.

[22] Erasmus JJ, Truong MT, Smythe WR et al. Integrated computed tomography-positron emission tomography in patients with potentially resectable malignant pleural mesothelioma: Staging implications. *J. Thorac. Cardiovasc. Surg.* 2005;129:1364-1370.

[23] Truong MT, Marom EM, Erasmus JJ. Preoperative Evaluation of Patients with Malignant Pleural Mesothelioma: role of Integrated CT-PET Imaging. *J. Thorac. Imaging* 2006;21:146-153.

[24] Rice DC, Erasmus JJ, Stevens CW et al. Extended surgical staging for potentially resectable malignant pleural mesothelioma. *Ann. Thorac. Surg.* 2005;80:1988-1992.

[25] Flores RM, Akhurst T, Gonen M et al. Positron emission tomography defines metastatic disease but not locoregional disease in patients with malignant pleural mesothelioma. *J. Thorac. Cardiovasc. Surg.* 2003;126:11-16.

[26] Benard F, Sterman D, Smith RJ et al. Prognostic value of FDG PET imaging in malignant pleural mesothelioma. *J. Nucl. Med.* 1999;40:1241-1245.

[27] Ceresoli GL, Chiti A, Zucali PA et al. Early response evaluation in malignant pleural mesothelioma by positron emission tomography with [18F] fluorodeoxyglucose. *J. Clin. Oncol.* 2006;24:4587-4593.

[28] Prakash UB, Reiman HM. Comparison of needle biopsy with cytological analysis for the evaluation of pleural effusion: analysis of 414 cases. *Mayo Clin. Proc.* 1985;60:158-164.

[29] Escudero BC, Garcia CM, Cuesta CB et al. Cytological and bacteriological analysis of fluid and pleural biopsy specimens with Cope's needle. Study of 414 patients. *Arch. Intern. Med.* 1990;150:1190-1194.

[30] Boutin C, Rey F. Thoracoscopy in pleural malignant mesothelioma: a prospective study of 188 consecutive patients – part 1: diagnosis. *Cancer* 1993;72:389-393.

[31] Maskell NA, Gleeson FV, Davies RJ. Standard pleural biopsy versus CT-guide cutting needle biopsy for diagnosis of malignant disease in pleural effusions: a randomized controlled trial. *Lancet* 2003;361-1326-1330.

[32] Adams RF, Gleeson FV. Percutaneous image-guided cutting needle biopsy of the pleura in the presence of a suspected malignant effusion. *Radiology* 2001;219:510-514.

[33] Adams RF, Gray W, Davies RJ et al. Percutaneous image-guided cutting needle biopsy of the pleura in the diagnosis of malignant mesothelioma. *Chest* 2001;120:1798-1802.

[34] Boutin C, Rey F, Viallat JR. Prevention of malignant seeding after invasive diagnostic procedures in patients with pleural mesothelioma. A randomized trial of local radiotherapy. *Chest* 1995;108:754-758.

In: Mesothelioma from Bench Side to Clinic
Editor: Alfonso Baldi, pp. 389-403
ISBN: 978-1-60021-789-0

Chapter XXIII

Instrumental Diagnosis of Mesothelioma: The Thoracoscopy

Mario Santini and Giovanni Vicidomini
Thoracic Surgery, Second University of Naples, Naples, Italy

Abstract

Diagnosis of pleural malignant mesothelioma is still a challenge for the clinicians and surgeons. Histological examination is mandatory. The thoracoscopic approach allows multiple biopsy specimens and an accurate staging of the disease. Video-assisted thoracoscopic surgery (VATS) permits a better diagnostic evaluation and offers surgical therapeutic options.

Historical Notes

Thoracoscopy is the best invasive procedure for the diagnosis of malignant mesothelioma. In fact, it yields a pathological diagnosis in at least 80% of patients [1]. However, until the early 1970s pleural biopsy was essentially percutaneous, as the use of thoracoscopy was not widely diffuse [2].

In 1910, H.C. Jacobaeus performed the first thoracoscopy using a cystoscope to lyse pleural adhesions (pneumolysis) in order to obtain lung collapse in the treatment of tuberculosis [3] (Figure 1). Widespread diffusion of the procedure was discouraged by thoracic surgeons of the time due to possible lethal complications (hemorrhage was the most frequent) [4]. Thoracoscopy was mostly performed by internists for diagnosis of pleural tumors and effusions and for treatment of tuberculosis. With the advent of antimicrobial chemotherapy and the development of pulmonary resection techniques, collapse therapy with division of pleural adhesions became obsolete and thoracoscopy was nearly forgotten. By the 1970s there was a renewed interest in the use of thoracoscopy for pleural biopsy and management of pleural tumors and effusions [5].

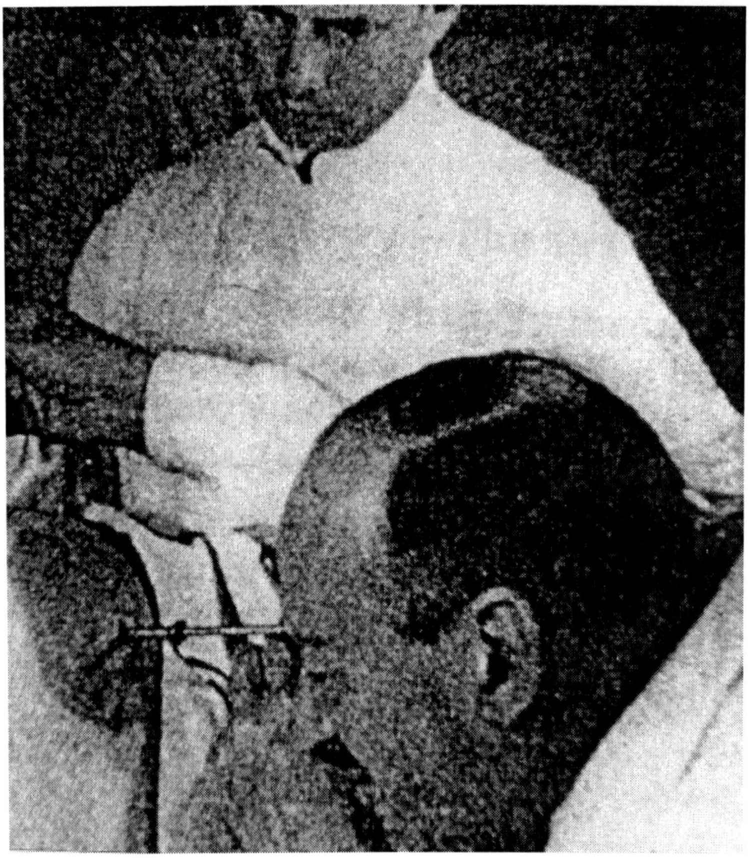

Figure 1. Hans Christian Jacobaeus (1879-1937) performs the first thoracoscopy using a cystoscope.

But it was in the 1980s that the improvements in video-technology and thoracoscopic equipment persuaded the surgeons to use thoracoscopy routinely and promoted the diffusion of the more complex video-assisted thoracoscopic surgery (VATS) that has both a diagnostic and therapeutic role [6].

Basic Operative Setting, Surgical Techniques and Equipment

The early application of thoracoscopy was performed at the patient bedside under local anesthesia and required few basic surgical instruments. Nowadays, thoracoscopy can be performed under local/regional anesthesia (medical thoracoscopy) or under general anesthesia (video-assisted thoracic surgery). The former is primarily used for differential diagnosis of pleural disease and pleurodesis [7], whereas the latter also permits a minimally invasive surgical approach [8].

Medical thoracoscopy (Figure 2). Prior to the procedure, any pleural effusion is drained and an ipsilateral pneumothorax is induced. Thoracoscopy is performed under local/regional anesthesia with spontaneous breathing and mild sedation in the operating room.

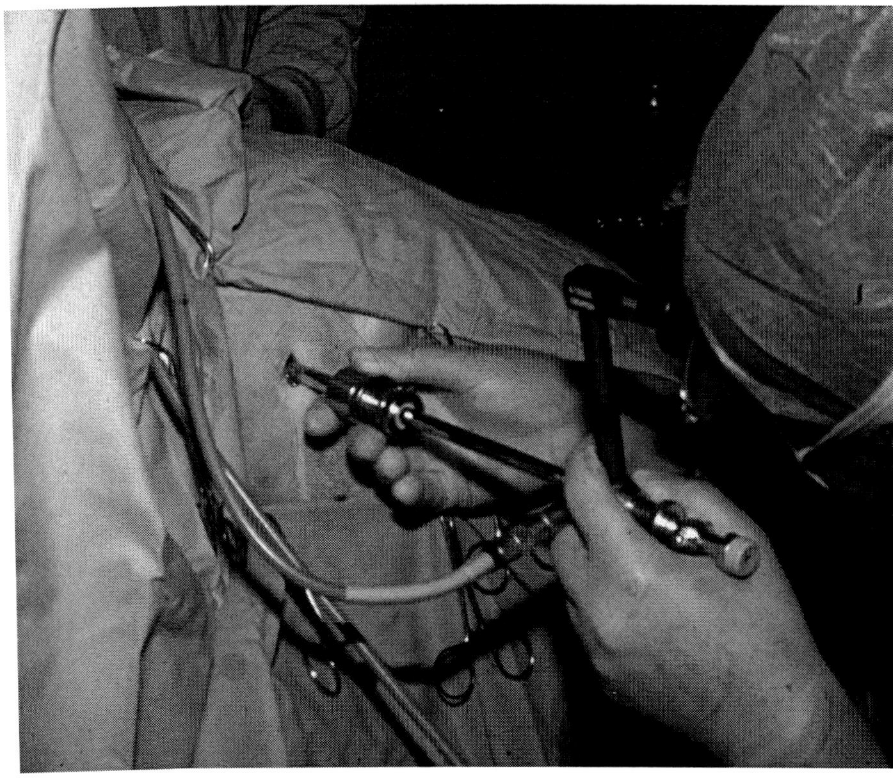

Figure 2. A medical thoracoscopy performed by an operating thoracoscope.

If indicated, surgical staff should be able to proceed with an open thoracotomy. Patient is placed in lateral decubitus position, with the involved side upward. After skin sterilization, blunt dissection is used to enter the pleural space between the third and sixth intercostal space, along the midaxillary line. A rigid thoracoscope is inserted, and the pleural cavity inspected. Adhesions between the two pleural leaves are removed when necessary. The parietal, visceral, and diaphragmatic pleura are successively inspected. Biopsies are performed under direct visual control in all suspect areas, systematically in several parts of the pleural surfaces. A chest tube is inserted before wound closure to evacuate air and fluid.

VATS (Figure 3). Most thoracoscopies are performed under general anesthesia with placement of a double-lumen endotracheal tube to allow single lung ventilation. The patient is positioned in a full lateral position and prepared for a conversion to a standard posterolateral thoracotomy. The video monitor should be positioned in front of the surgeons in order to allow the best orientation of the instruments and facilitate their handling.

The first access site must be planned to have a panoramic view of the chest and a good visualization of the lesion. This generally depends on the type of procedure being performed and on the site of lesion; however, an access through the sixth or seventh intercostal space, between the mid and the posterior axillary lines is usually adequate. Once the pleural cavity is entered, digital exploration is used to check for pleural adhesions that could impede the introduction of the thoracoscope. Although thin local adhesions can easily be separated by the finger, sometimes extensive and firm adhesions obligate the surgeon to convert the procedure to standard thoracotomy.

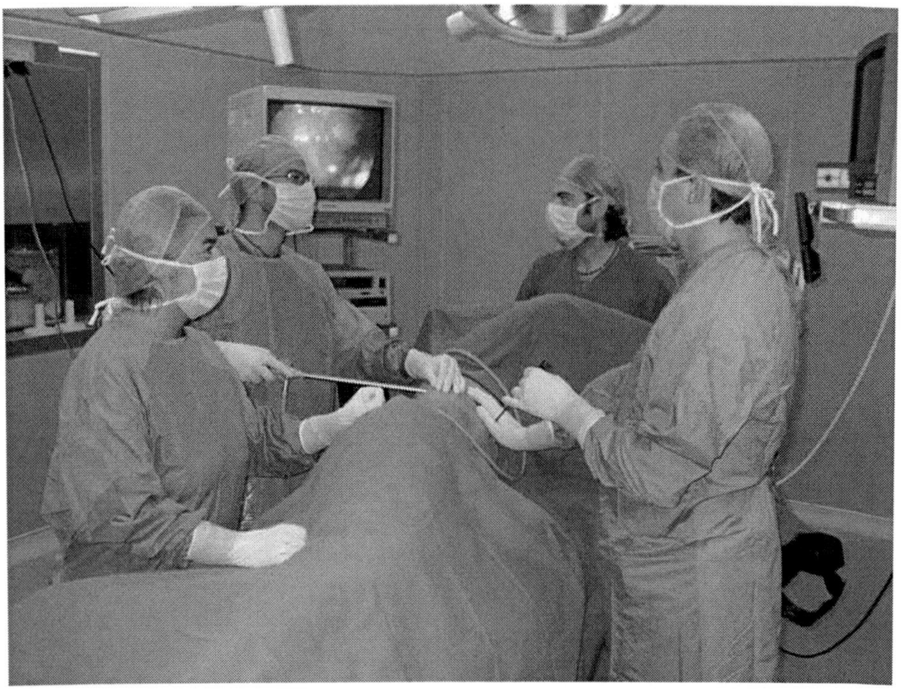

Figure 3. An operating room set-up for video-assisted thoracoscopic surgery (VATS). In addition to the standard equipment, two video monitors are needed to allow the whole surgical team to have an optimal vision of the procedure.

When an adequate pleural space has been created, a 10-mm trocar is placed through the intercostal space for the insertion of the thoracoscope. For simple procedures as pleural biopsies, a single access by the means of an operating thoracoscope may be sufficient. More complex procedures may require two or three additional trocars, inserted under direct thoracoscopic vision. The best strategy is to orient thoracoscope and additional instruments so that they face the lesion. This prevents the "mirror imaging" effect that occurs when instrument and scope are placed in opposing directions. The ports should be not too close to the lesion in order to leave adequate maneuver room. The position of the additional trocars as far as possible from the camera avoids instruments "sword-fighting" with each other during the procedure. As a general rule, the three ports are best placed in a triangular configuration, with the optic positioned centrally in the triangle. However, this configuration allows the telescope to be used through any port.

Basic Equipment

Telescopes. Standard telescopes allow excellent vision of intrathoracic structures. Currently, 10-mm videothoracoscopes are preferred with a 0-degree field of vision. A scope with a field of vision different from 0° degree (30°, 45°, 60° or greater) can allow the inspection of oblique areas of the pleural space, with a view direction that is different from the axis of the telescope. Flexible scopes are now available that allow the surgeon to guide the scope in the chest more easily; however, the image resolution is not refined as with the rigid scope and the continuous change of vision angle adds some confusion. The major advantage of angled and flexible scopes is the easier inspection of less accessible areas of the operative field, especially when extensive pleural adhesions are present.

As previously mentioned, pleural biopsies can be performed by the means of an operating thoracoscope. This incorporate a working channel that allows the passage of several instruments, like biopsy forceps; thus, the procedure can be performed with a single incision.

Cameras and monitors. In the video-assisted thoracoscopy setting, the scope is connected to a camera that transmits the image to a video screen. Some manufacturers incorporate the camera into the thoracoscope to form an integrated system that enhance the image resolution. Monitors with different diameter are available; the larger ones are preferable as they provide a magnification of the images.

Surgical Instruments

Trocar ports. The access to the thoracic cavity is obtained by insertion of trocars through stub incisions. A variety of trocars and cannulae are available, with sizes ranging from 3 to 15 mm.

Graspers. These instruments are able to hold, retract and dissect tissue. Different configurations, diameters and lengths are available. The graspers are also divided in traumatic and atraumatic.

Scissors. The thoracoscopic disposable scissors are always very sharp. Curved scissors are preferable, as they improve the visibility of the tissue within the jaws.

Electrocautery. This is used both for haemostasis and dissection. The monopolar system is the most used, with the energy transmitted through different devices, as forceps, graspers, scissors, hooks, spatulas, knives and blunt instruments. A bipolar system is also available, and it is used when wide dissection near important anatomical structures is needed. The harmonic scalpel system and the Ligasure system are other coagulation systems recently introduced, which allow good haemostasis standards with minimal damage to the surrounding tissues [9,10].

Lasers. Several laser systems are available, with different characteristics and effects on the lung tissue. The most commonly used is the Nd:YAG laser, whose effects act only on the tissue being in the same direction of the laser beam; other systems include CO_2, KTP, and Argon laser. Lasers are mainly used for tissue coagulation and air leaks sealing.

Endoscopic staplers. Endoscopic staplers are essential devices in thoracoscopic surgery. A variety of different stapling sets are available, with different characteristics based on the thickness of the tissue (parenchyma or vessel).

Other instruments. A variety of additional devices are available for different purposes. The most useful instruments include lung retractors, clip appliers, needle holders, surgical loops, suction-irrigation devices, and specimens bags. Currently, most of the surgical thoracoscopic instruments used are disposable.

Diagnostic Role of Thoracoscopy in Mesothelioma

Thoracentesis is the initial diagnostic procedure in patients with pleural effusion and suspect of mesothelioma; however, the cytologic evaluation of the fluid aspirated is positive for malignancy in only 30-50% of patients. Cytologic response from pleural fluid is unreliable since reactive mesothelial cells and neoplastic cells from other malignant tumors are often difficult to distinguish from malignant mesothelioma cells [11]. If the response is negative, pleural biopsy is mandatory in order to achieve a diagnosis. Pleural specimens can be obtained by performing a CT-guided percutaneous biopsy, but often this procedure does not provide a sufficient sample for additional studies, as immunohistochemestry and electron microscopy, which are decisive for the histological definition of the mesothelioma. Furthermore, the diagnostic yield of this procedure is often less than 85% of cases with repeat biopsies [12]. In this contest, thoracoscopy plays a fundamental role in the diagnosis and management of suspected mesothelioma. The diagnostic accuracy of thoracoscopy for mesothelioma is around 90% (from 85 to 94% in different series) [1,13]. It carries a relative low risk of complications (10%), including persistent air-leaks, hemorrhage, and infection [14].

Thoracoscopic features of malignant mesothelioma include pleural effusion, often turbid and bloodstained, that is the only visible sign in the earliest stages of the disease; pleural nodules or masses arising from parietal o visceral pleura (Figures 4,5), lardaceous pleural appearance (Figure 6), confluent sheets of tumor with pulmonary encasement, fissural spread and, finally, obliteration of most pleural space.

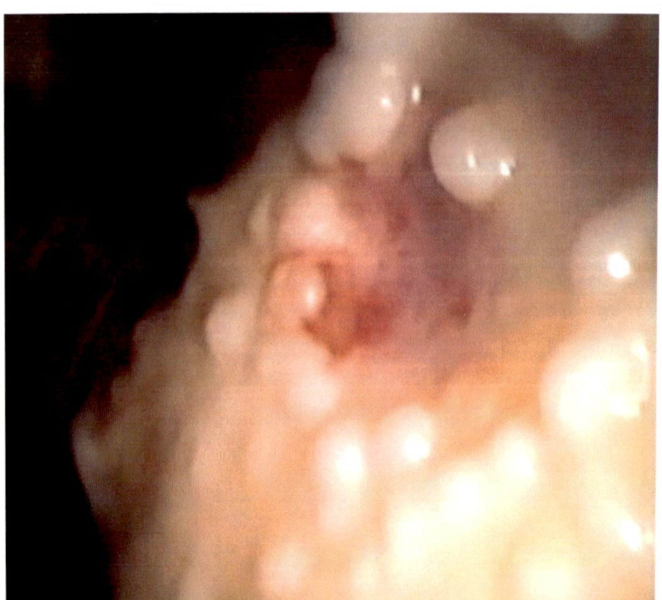

Figure 4. Malignant mesothelioma. Rounded nodules are disseminated on the parietal pleura ("en grape de raisin" appearance).

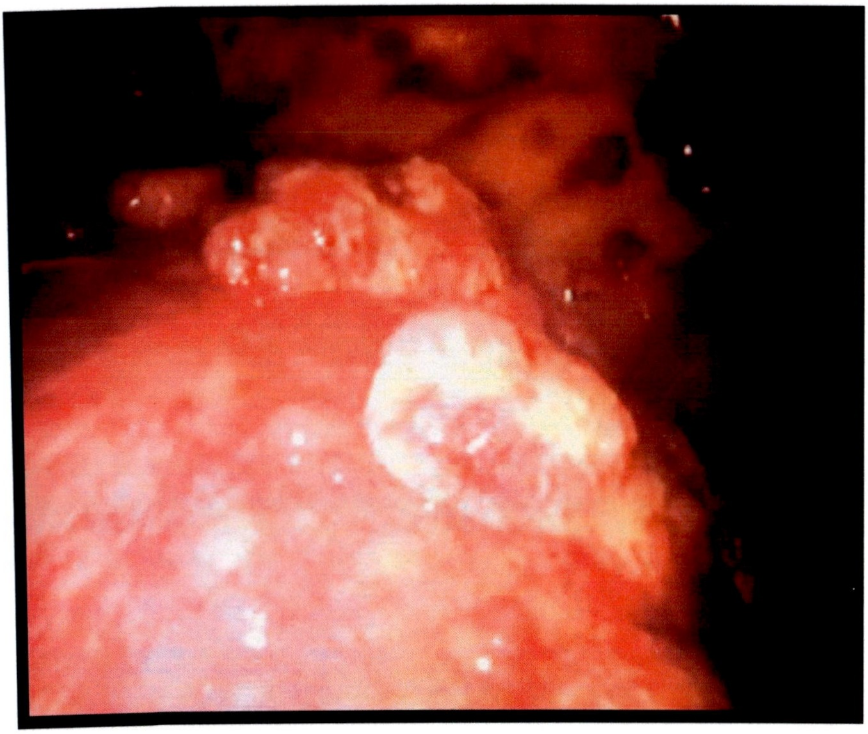

Figure 5. Malignant mesothelioma. The visceral pleura is thickened and shows several voluminous masses.

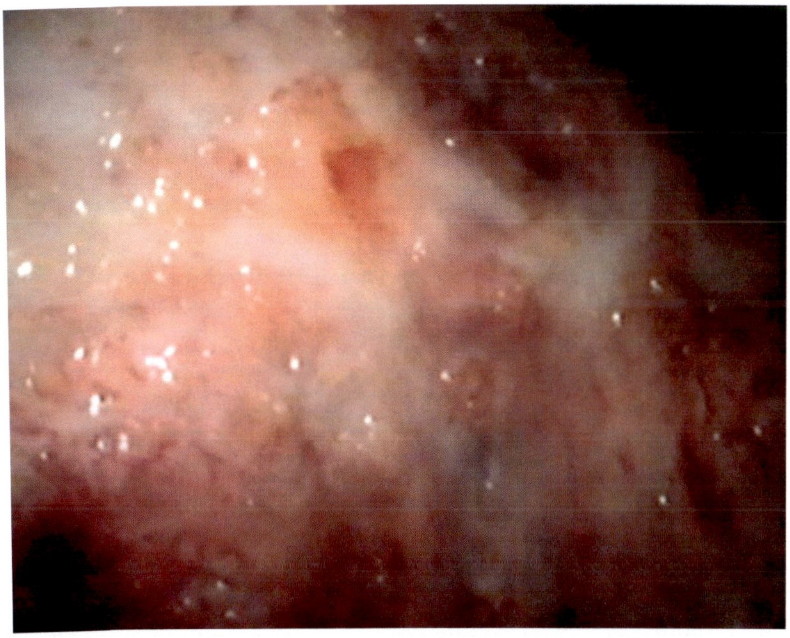

Figure 6. Malignant mesothelioma. Lardaceous appearance of the parietal pleura.

The appearance of the tumor ranges from soft, friable and hypervascular to fibrotic, depending on the cellular mixture. However, it must be underlined that macroscopic findings can be misleading; even nonspecific inflammations or apparently inoffensive plaques can mask a mesothelioma.

Pleural biopsy can be performed under direct vision by the means of single access, using an operating thoracoscope. In this case, the correct selection of the trocar site is crucial. The trocar should be inserted directly opposite to the lesion in order to achieve the most successful results. Large specimens of tissue and amounts of fluid can be obtained for diagnostic purpose. In case of loculated effusion, the operating thoracoscope lyses adhesions and allows a more extensive fluid aspiration and, if necessary, the insertion of additional trocars under direct vision. The supplementary incisions should made in the anterior axillary line (seventh and third intercostal spaces, preferably) in order to create a triangle configuration. Thoracoscopy with multiple accesses, although increases the risk of tumor cell implantation in the trocar sites [15], permits an easier pneumolysis, particularly in case of thick and vascular adhesions (Figure 7), larger pleural biopsy specimens (Figure 8) and a better hemostasis.

After the collection of the fluid and the exploration of the entire pleural space, multiple biopsies should be taken from the visible masses. As already mentioned, the appearance of the tumor varies from soft, friable and hypervascular to dense and fibrotic. However, no one of these findings is pathognomonic of malignant mesothelioma.

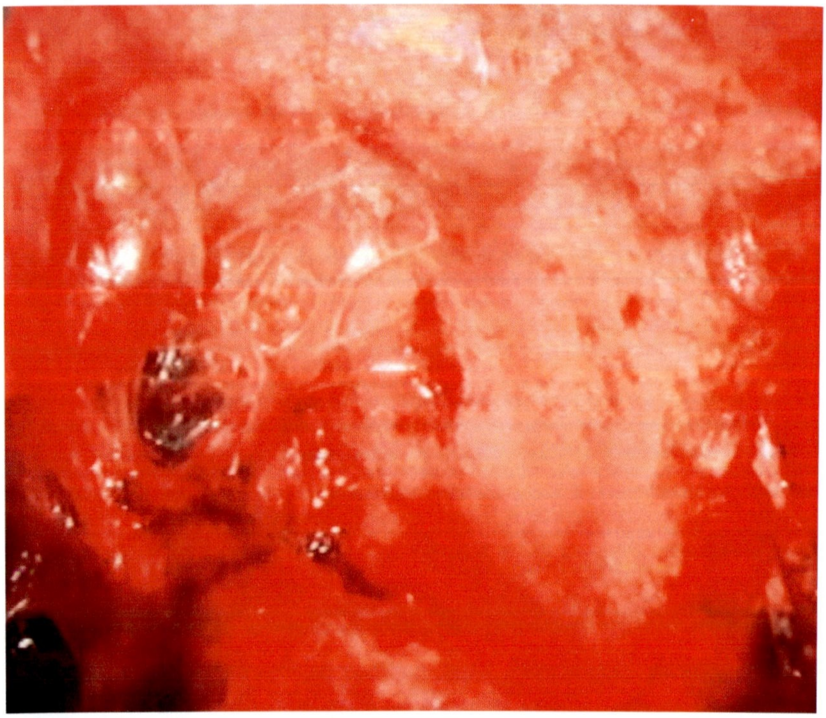

Figure 7. Malignant mesothelioma. Neoplastic nodules located on the parietal pleura are partially hidden by inflammatory adhesions.

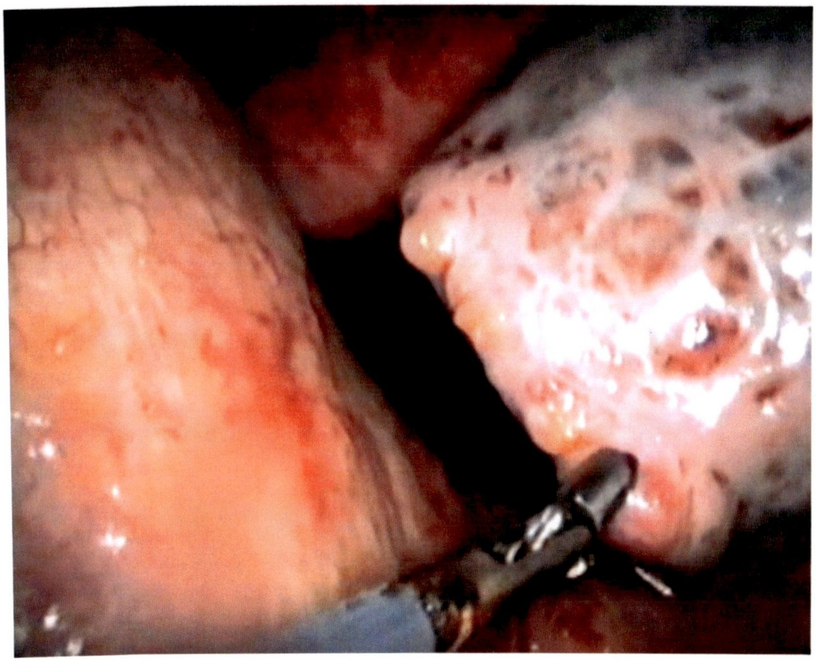

Figure 8. Visceral pleural biopsy in VATS. The approach with multiple accesses consents larger biopsy specimens.

In case of nonspecific pleural hyperemia, without any visible nodule, multiple biopsies should be randomly performed. The specimens should be as deep and large as possible; this allows the pathologist to have more tissue for additional analysis. The histologic patterns of mesothelioma include an epithelial, a sarcomatoid and a mixed one. Sometimes, the gross examination of the pleura can help the surgeon to differentiate between the histologic types. In the epithelial or mixed varieties, the most frequent findings include multiple small nodules, usually friable and vascular, often filled with a gelatinous fluid. They can be localized or spread over the entire pleural surface, or confluent in large masses. In the sarcomatous type the pleura may be only thickened, although large nodules can be found (Figures 9, 10). Immunohistochemestry is crucial in order to obtain a firm diagnosis. The presence of cytokeratin expression aids the differentiation between epithelial and sarcomatoid types, while the absence of carcinoembryonic antigen (CEA) expression exclude a metastatic adenocarcinoma, that can be often confused with a mesothelioma [16].

Diagnostic thoracotomy should not be performed to establish a definitive diagnosis in case of suspected mesothelioma, since the risk of localized wound recurrence is high in patients with this malignancy; however, thoracotomic pleural biopsy is necessary when the pleural space is obliterated by the tumor, what makes thoracoscopy technically unfeasible.

A complete and accurate inspection of pleural space is mandatory not only in the apparently negative cases, in order to detect small lesions that can be misleaded, but also for a more accurate staging of the disease. In fact, selected patients with stage I epithelial malignant mesothelioma show an improved long-term survival after an aggressive trimodality therapy, including extrapleural pneumonectomy, chemotherapy and hemithoracic irradiation [17, 18].

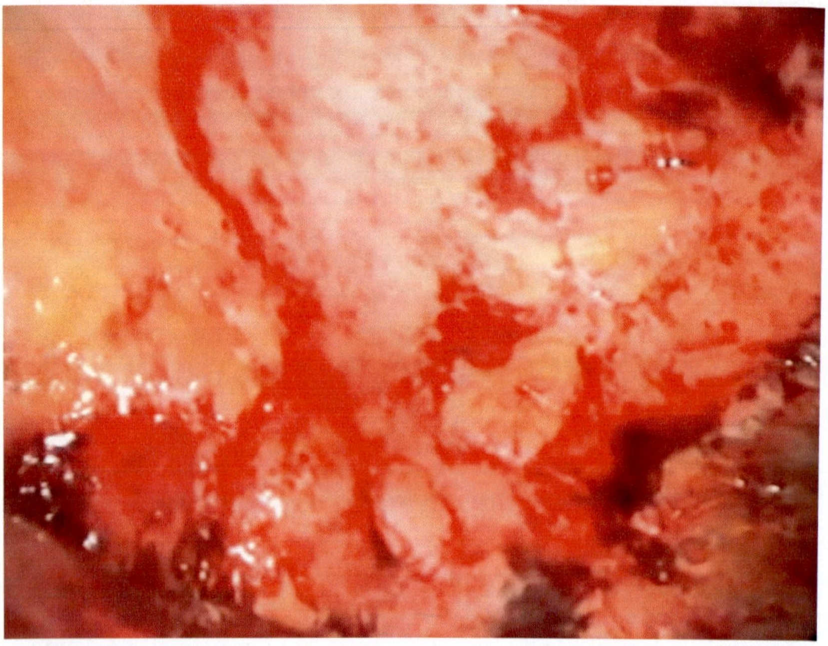

Figure 9. Malignant sarcomatous mesothelioma. Neoplastic friable nodules are disseminated on the parietal pleura.

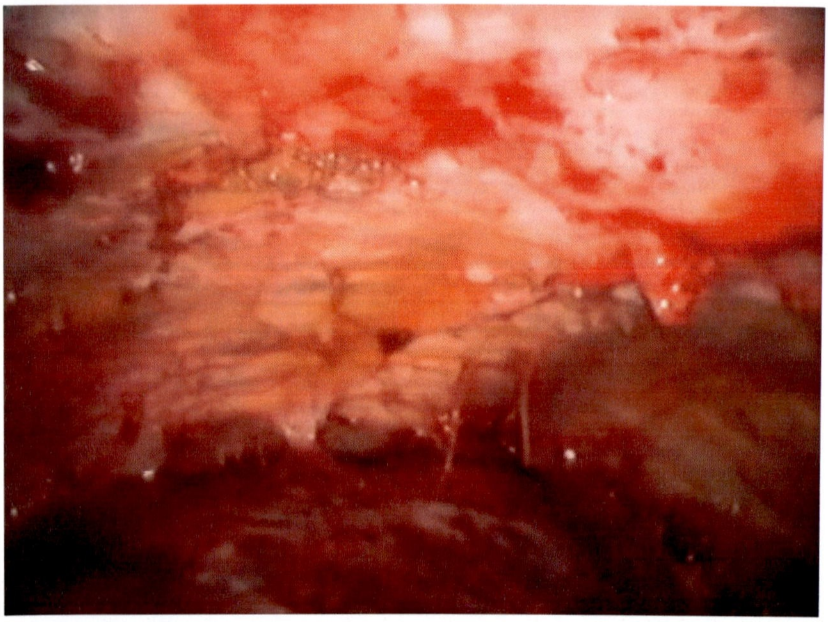

Figure 10. Malignant sarcomatous mesothelioma. Both the visceral and parietal pleural are thickened and show nodules and whitish plaques.

Because of the significant morbidity associated with this radical protocol and the limited sensitivity of the current imaging modalities, it should be emphasized the importance of an accurate surgical staging. In this contest, an extensive thoracoscopic exploration of the parietal and visceral pleura is mandatory in order to avoid a preoperative understaging that can invalidate the benefits of the trimodality therapy. Furthermore, trimodality treatment should be only performed in patients with negative examinations of mediastinum, contralateral pleura and diaphragmatic peritoneum. For this purpose, some authors routinely perform mediastinoscopy, bilateral thoracoscopy and laparoscopy [19, 20]. However, other authors advocate the use of magnetic resonance (MR) and positron emission tomography (PET) to define chest wall, diaphragm and mediastinal nodal status involvement [21]. We believe that the more aggressive surgical staging, including mediastinoscopy, bilateral thoracoscopy and laparoscopy, should be restricted and guided on the basis of imaging modalities.

Therapeutic Role of Thoracoscopy in Mesothelioma

Pleurectomy/decortication. Several therapeutic options for malignant mesothelioma are available, including surgery, radiotherapy, chemotherapy, immunotherapy, photodynamic therapy and multimodality treatments [13]. However, despite of the strategy selected, the prognosis of the disease has not significantly improved in the last years [22]. Extrapleural pneumonectomy is a potentially curative option, but is associated with significant operative mortality and morbidity rates. Furthermore, this operation is only suitable for patients with early stage disease and epithelial histologic type and it should be associated with adjuvant treatments in order to achieve better survival rates [17, 18]. In this setting, thoracoscopy (even performed bilaterally) is an essential procedure for the selection of candidates to surgery.

Pleurectomy/decortication represents a less aggressive alternative to extrapleural pneumonectomy. This treatment modality is based on the concept that reduction of tumor volume may be an important determinant of postoperative survival [23]. Usually, it is performed in patients with locally advanced disease but some authors suggest that it can be also used in early stage patients, since it provides a better life quality and its association to chemotherapy produces some survival prolongation. However, since this debulking surgical technique seems to have a primarily palliative intention [24], some authors promote the thoracoscopic approach for its minimal surgical impact [25, 26]. These authors claim that this minimally invasive approach combines well with other emerging therapeutic modalities and it is applicable to a higher proportion of patients. Moreover, avoidance of thoracotomy seems to reduce the problem of tumor seeding in the wound and to enable patients unfit for open surgery to undergo a debulking procedure. Another potential advantage of VATS is the closure of pleural space, which might reduce the incidence of postoperative complications (pleural effusion and infection). However, VATS seems to produce a higher rate of prolonged air leaks with subsequent longer hospital stay. This procedure cannot be performed in patients with lung encasement and pleural space obliteration. In conclusion, VATS pleurectomy/decortication seems to be a useful palliative strategy in mesothelioma, applicable to the majority of patients, but further studies are needed to confirm this statement and to compare VATS with open pleurectomy/decortication, a procedure that is often associated with pericardium and the diaphragm resection in order to obtain a valid debulking.

Pleurodesis. In the advanced-stage disease, thoracoscopy is routinely used for pleurodesis to palliatively treat recurrent or symptomatic pleural effusions. Several sclerosing agents can be used (*ie*, bleomycin, tetracycline, and talc) with no significant differences in efficacy [27, 28]. Talc is generally the least expensive and can be administered via a thoracoscope [29, 30] or instilled as slurry through a chest tube [31]. The thoracoscopic talc pleurodesis, both under local anesthesia (medical thoracoscopy) or through VATS requires the complete aspiration of the pleural effusion, a meticulous inspection of the entire pleural surfaces and mediastinum and the division of any pleural adhesion or loculation. At the end of this stage, a dose of 4-5 g of asbestos-free talc powder is uniformly distributed over the pleural surface using a pneumatic atomizer. The quality of pleurodesis depends on the accurate positioning of the postoperative drainage tube, as the pleural space should be persistently free from fluid. Furthermore, the patient is asked to change frequently his position in bed during the next two postoperative hours, in order to obtain an optimal distribution of the talc. Reports in the literature vary between 68% and 97% "success rate" for poudrage thoracoscopic pleurodesis [32,33]. Morbidity predominantly includes post-procedure fever, dyspnoea, and pain. About the possibility of talc migration into the lung and subsequent acute respiratory failure, the literature shows variable rates of this complication, but the risk seems to be quite low [29,31,34,35]. Pleurodesis can be obtained through talc slurry, but some authors claim that this technique does not permit a correct distribution of the talc over the pleural leaves [29]. A recent multicenter study by Dresler et al. [36] has showed no significant differences between the two techniques in the ability to prevent pleural effusion recurrences. Thoracoscopy allows the direct inspection of the pleura and the lysis of adhesions and loculations. This may be particularly indicated for patients who have had prior ipsilateral surgery or attempted pleurodesis, or for whom there is a significant possibility of a trapped lung.

Furthermore, it is to be mentioned that sometimes the rapid progression of mesothelioma and the neoplastic obliteration of the pleural cavity make unnecessary an early talc pleurodesis.

References

[1] Boutin C, Rey F. Thoracoscopy in pleural mesothelioma. A prospective study of 188 consecutive patients. Part I: diagnosis. *Cancer* 1993; 72:389-93, 1993.

[2] Mungall IP, Cowen PN, Cooke NT, Roach TC, Cooke NJ. Multiple pleural biopsy with the Abrams needle. *Thorax* 1980; 35:600-2.

[3] Jacobaeus HC. The cauterization of adhesions in pneumothorax treatment of tuberculosis. *Surg. Gynaecol. Obstet.* 1921; 32:493:500.

[4] Alexander J. *The collapse therapy of pulmonary tuberculosis.* p.313. Charles C Thomas, Springfield, IL, 1937.

[5] Boutin C, Viallat JR, Cargnino P, Farisse P. Indications actuelles de la thoracoscopie. Etude préliminaire. *Rev. Franc. Mal. Respir.* 1981; 9:309.

[6] Coltharp WH, Arnold JH, Alford WC, Burrus GR, Glassford DM, Lea JW, Petracek MR, Starkey TD, Stoney WS, Thomas CS. Videothoracoscopy: improved technique and expanded indications. *Ann. Thorac. Surg.* 1992; 53:776-9.

[7] Mathur PN, Astoul P, Boutin C. Medical thoracoscopy: technical details. *Clin. Chest Med.* 1995; 16:479-86.

[8] Mack MJ, Aronoff RJ, Acuff TE, Douthit MB, Bowman RT, Ryan WH. Present role of thoracoscopy in the diagnosis and treatment of disease of the chest. *Ann. Thorac. Surg.* 1992; 54:403-9.

[9] Yim AP, Rendina EA, Hazelrigg SR, Chow LT, Lee TW, Wan S, Arifi AA. A new technological approach to nonanatomical pulmonary resection: saline enhanced thermal sealing. *Ann. Thorac. Surg.* 2002;74:1671-6.

[10] Santini M, Vicidomini G, Baldi A, Gallo G, Laperuta P, Busiello L, Di Marino MP, Pastore V. Use of an electrothermal bipolar tissue sealing system in lung surgery. *Eur. J. Cardiothorac Surg.* 2006;29:226-30.

[11] Henderson DW, Shilkin KB, Whitaker D. Reactive mesothelial hyperplasia vs mesothelioma, including mesothelioma in situ: a brief review. *Am. J. Clin. Pathol.* 1998; 110:397-404.

[12] Metintas M, Özdemir N, Isikoy S, Kaya T, Ekici M, Erginel S, Harmanci E, Erdinc P, Ulgey N, Alatas F. CT-guided pleural needle biopsy in the diagnosis of malignant mesothelioma. *J. Comp. Assist. Tomog.* 1995; 19:370-4.

[13] Pistolesi M, Rusthoven J. Malignant pleural mesothelioma. Update, current management and newer therapeutic strategies. *Chest* 2004; 126:1318-29.

[14] Kaiser LR, Bavaria JE. Complications of thoracoscopy. *Ann. Thorac. Surg.* 1993; 56:796-8.

[15] Boutin C, Rey F, Viallat J-R. Prevention of malignant seeding after invasive diagnostic procedures in patients with pleural mesothelioma: a randomised trial of local radiotherapy. *Chest* 1995; 108:754-8.

[16] King JA, Tucker JA. Evaluation of membranous staining of mesothelioma. *Cell Vis.* 1998; 5:24-7.

[17] Sugarbaker DJ, Flores RM, Jaklitsch MT, Richards WG, Strauss GM, Corson JM, DeCamp MM Jr, Swanson SJ, Bueno R, Lukanich JM, Baldini EH, Mentzer SJ. Resection margins, extrapleural nodal status, and cell type determine postoperative long-term survival in trimodality therapy of malignant pleural mesothelioma: results in 183 patients. *J. Thorac. Cardiovasc. Surg.* 1999;117:54-65.

[18] Rusch VW, Rosenzweig K, Venkatraman E, Leon L, Raben A, Harrison L, Bains MS, Downey RJ, Ginsberg RJ. A phase II trial of surgical resection and adjuvant high-dose hemithoracic radiation for malignant pleural mesothelioma. *J. Thorac. Cardiovasc. Surg.* 2001;122:788-95.

[19] Rice DC, Erasmus JJ, Stevens CW, Vaporciyan AA, Wu JS, Tsao AS, Walsh GL, Swisher SG, Hofstetter WL, Ordonez NG, Smythe WR. Extended surgical staging for potentially resectable malignant pleural mesothelioma. *Ann. Thorac. Surg.* 2005;80:1988-93.

[20] Alvarez JM, Ha T, Musk W, Robins P, Price R, Byrne MJ. Importance of mediastinoscopy, bilateral thoracoscopy, and laparoscopy in correct staging of

malignant mesothelioma before extrapleural pneumonectomy. *J. Thorac. Cardiovasc. Surg.* 2005;130:905-6.

[21] Wang ZJ, Reddy GP, Gotway MB, Higgins CB, Jablons DM, Ramaswamy M, Hawkins RA, Webb WR. Malignant pleural mesothelioma: evaluation with CT, MR imaging, and PET. *Radiographics.* 2004;24:105-19.

[22] Butchart EG. Contemporary management of malignant pleural mesothelioma. *Oncologist* 1999;4:488-500.

[23] Pass HI, Temeck BK, Kranda K, Steinberg SM, Feuerstein IR. Preoperative tumor volume is associated with outcome in malignant pleural mesothelioma. *J. Thorac. Cardiovasc. Surg.* 1998;115:310-8.

[24] Martin-Ucar AE, Edwards JG, Rengajaran A, Muller S, Waller DA. Palliative surgical debulking in malignant mesothelioma. Predictors of survival and symptom control. *Eur. J. Cardiothorac. Surg.* 2001;20:1117-21.

[25] Grossebner MW, Arifi AA, Goddard M, Ritchie AJ. Mesothelioma - VATS biopsy and lung mobilization improves diagnosis and palliation. *Eur. J. Cardiothorac. Surg.* 1999;16:619-23.

[26] Halstead JC, Lim E, Venkateswaran RM, Charman SC, Goddard M, Ritchie AJ. Improved survival with VATS pleurectomy-decortication in advanced malignant mesothelioma. *Eur. J. Surg. Oncol.* 2005;31:314-20.

[27] Walker-Renard PB, Vaughan LM, Sahn SA. Chemical pleurodesis for malignant pleural effusions. *Ann. Intern. Med.* 1994;120:56-64.

[28] Tan C, Sedrakyan A, Browne J, Swift S, Treasure T. The evidence on the effectiveness of management for malignant pleural effusion: a systematic review. *Eur. J. Cardiothorac. Surg.* 2006;29:829-38.

[29] Viallat JR, Rey F, Astoul P, Boutin C. Thoracoscopic talc poudrage pleurodesis for malignant effusions. A review of 360 cases. *Chest.* 1996;110:1387-93.

[30] Kolschmann S, Ballin A, Gillissen A. Clinical efficacy and safety of thoracoscopic talc pleurodesis in malignant pleural effusions. Chest. 2005;128:1431-5.

[31] Kennedy L, Rusch VW, Strange C, Ginsberg RJ, Sahn SA. Pleurodesis using talc slurry. *Chest.* 1994;106:342-6.

[32] Hartman DL, Gaither JM, Kesler KA, et al. Comparison of insufflated talc under thoracoscopic guidance with standard tetracycline and bleomycin pleurodesis for control of malignant pleural effusions. *J. Thorac. Cardiovasc. Surg.* 1993;105:743–747.

[33] Yim AP, Chan AT, Lee TW, Wan IY, Ho JK. Thoracoscopic talc insufflation versus talc slurry for symptomatic malignant pleural effusion. *Ann. Thorac. Surg.* 1996;62:1655-8.

[34] Weissberg D, Ben-Zeev I. Talc pleurodesis. Experience with 360 patients. *J. Thorac. Cardiovasc Surg.* 1993;106:689-95.

[35] Marom EM, Patz EF Jr, Erasmus JJ, McAdams HP, Goodman PC, Herndon JE. Malignant pleural effusions: treatment with small-bore-catheter thoracostomy and talc pleurodesis. *Radiology* 1999;210:277-81.

[36] Dresler CM, Olak J, Herndon JE 2nd, Richards WG, Scalzetti E, Fleishman SB, Kernstine KH, Demmy T, Jablons DM, Kohman L, Daniel TM, Haasler GB,

Sugarbaker DJ; Cooperative Groups Cancer and Leukemia Group B; Eastern Cooperative Oncology Group; North Central Cooperative Oncology Group; Radiation Therapy Oncology Group. Phase III intergroup study of talc poudrage vs talc slurry sclerosis for malignant pleural effusion. *Chest* 2005;127;909-915.

In: Mesothelioma from Bench Side to Clinic
Editor: Alfonso Baldi, pp. 405-412

ISBN: 978-1-60021-789-0

Chapter XXIV

Non-Surgical Treatment of Malignant Pleural Mesothelioma: Radiotherapy and Chemotherapy

Giuseppe Sasso**, Luis E. Schiappacasse and Bahram Forouzesh
Oncology Clinical Research Unit, Townsville Teaching Hospital and
James Cook University School of Medicine;
Queensland, Australia

Abstract

This chapter aims to highlight the recent promising developments in the integrated management of mesothelioma with a special focus on non-surgical treatment schemes.

Historically, the prognosis of patients affected from malignant pleural mesothelioma (MPM), a locally invasive and rapidly fatal malignancy linked to asbestos exposure, has been uniformly poor and there has been a general sense of nihilism about its treatment.

Usually, surgical resection is possible in only a small minority of patients and diagnosis is often made late in the course of the disease resulting in fewer than 15% of these patients reported to live beyond 5 years.

Due to the lack of improved survival when comparing standard chemotherapy regimens to pain management alone, up to few years ago patients were frequently managed by supportive care only. Treatment with radiation therapy was equally disappointing, mostly because of difficulties in irradiating disease while avoiding toxicity to normal lung, cardiac, and spinal cord tissues.

But for the first time, there is now evidence that some treatments are increasing the quality and quantity of life for patients with mesothelioma with several recent randomised and non-randomized trials suggesting that multimodality therapy may improve outcome for carefully selected patients.

Chemotherapy, with the new multi-targeted antifolate drug Pemetrexed, combined with cisplatin, has shown superior survival rates in a large phase III trial when compared

* Address for correspondence: Townsville Cancer Centre, PO Box 670, Townsville QLD 4810, Australia. Tel: +61 (0) 7 4796 1626; Fax: +61 (0) 7 4796 1621; Giuseppe_Sasso@health.qld.gov.au giuseppe.sasso@jcu.edu.au

to cisplatin alone. Moreover, intensity-modulated radiotherapy (IMRT), a novel technique of irradiation which enables to spare normal tissues that are surrounded by targets with concave surfaces (as it happens for tumours of the pleura) has resulted in excellent local control when administered after extrapleural pneumonectomy.

Aim of this chapter is to provide an overview on the recent advances in multimodality treatment programs that, combining surgical cyto-reduction with novel forms of radiation therapy and more effective chemotherapy combinations, may offer significant increases in survival for certain subgroups of mesothelioma patients.

The role of symptomatic conventional radiotherapy and chemotherapy in highly palliative patients and controversy about the indication for prophylactic irradiation of the thoracotomy biopsy tract will also be discussed.

Introduction

The optimal management of patients with malignant pleural mesothelioma is still debatable. Very few patients are suitable for any potentially curative treatment and the role of radiotherapy in the management of this relatively uncommon disease is often reported as controversial. The general perception of mesothelioma being a rather radioresistant tumour is biased by past use of inadequate volumes, techniques and doses of irradiation. [1]

Comparing with other chest malignancies, human mesothelioma is actually more responsive *in vitro* to radiation therapy (RT) than non-small cell lung cancer, but not as sensitive as small cell carcinoma. In the clinical setting these observations are supported by a well known dose-response curve for mesothelioma with radiation doses of at least 40 Gray needed for palliation and above 50 Gray for local control; which is compatible with values observed in the *in vitro* studies. [2]

Theoretically its radiosensitivity makes malignant mesothelioma a good candidate for a positive response to radiation. However, due to the diffuse nature of the tumour, radical radiotherapy is technically challenging because requires delivery of tumoricidal tumour doses to large treatment volumes closely adjacent to critical organs. As a result, geographical missing or suboptimal doses were often the causes for the high rate of both infield and marginal recurrence observed in the past. [3]

Modern techniques of irradiation like intensity modulated radiation therapy (IMRT) are now able to deliver doses of above 50 Gray in standard fractionation, or biologically equivalent, to the entire hemithorax including upper mediastinum, diaphragm and pleural reflections without exceeding the radiation sensitivity of the adjacent heart, spinal cord, oesophagus, liver, and contralateral lung.

The presence of underlying ipsilateral lung, whose tolerance threshold is less than 20 Gray, remains the main obstacle to safe delivery of radical radiotherapy in patients who had pleurectomy, decortication or no surgical removal. Also, intact lung might cause under-dosage of the visceral pleura and/or dose uncertainties due to the build up effect of air at the parenchymal-pleural interface.

Further to these reasons and to the encouraging results reported in selected patients treated with extrapleural pneumonectomy (EPP), new treatment combinations of surgery followed by adjuvant radiation and chemotherapy have been tested in the attempt to overcome the failure of single modality therapy in patients with favourable prognoses. [4]

This approach, best known as trimodality treatment, benefits of the availability of new active chemotherapy regimens and avoids the risk of ipsilateral radiation pneumonitis when EPP is used as form of cytoreductive surgery. However the risk of contralateral fatal pneumonitis or severe hepatitis must not be underestimated in these patients; especially when higher radiation doses are used although with IMRT. Successful outcome always warrants careful treatment planning and meet of strict tolerance criteria for the relevant organs at risk.

Sugarbaker et al. from The Brigham and Women's Hospital, Boston (USA) reported the most impressive results amongst the groups who demonstrated improved survival using the combined modality approach. Their most recent follow up data showed a remarkable five-year survival rate of 46% in patients with epithelial histology, no mediastinal lymph node involvement and clear resection margins. Operative mortality was 4% with a major morbidity rate of 24%. [5]

Outcome for patients with unfavourable prognostic factors was much less appealing emphasising the role for thorough pre-treatment and surgical staging. Extensive preoperative evaluation includes whole body CT/PET staging, chest MRI with sagittal views to assess mediastinal and diaphragmatic involvement, full pulmonary function testing with quantitative ventilation-perfusion scanning for patients with borderline FEV1, and echocardiography to evaluate mediastinal invasion and ventricular function (which is crucial before treatment with anthracycline chemotherapy). Patients greater than 65 years of age may not be candidates for EPP, even if they meet other criteria, because of the increased perioperative mortality rate with older patients. [6]

Despite these promising results, the majority of patients have recurrent disease even after an aggressive trimodality approach to therapy. Pattern of recurrence varies between published studies and overall contributes to the uncertainties regarding the efficacy of the treatment. The value of trimodality therapy remains somewhat controversial due to concerns about selection bias and the lack of randomized trials. A randomized, controlled trial is under way in the United Kingdom comparing chemotherapy alone versus chemotherapy, EPP, and post-operative hemithoracic RT.

Regimens including intra-operative radiotherapy (IORT) or peri-operative brachytherapy have been investigated to overcome the technical challenge of delivering a radical radiation dose to patients unable to tolerate EPP. Both techniques require dedicated resources and expertise but have the theoretical advantage of being able to directly visualise the high-risk areas at the time of pleurectomy/decortication. Unfortunately, results of brachytherapy are so far disappointing because of excessive morbidity [7]. IORT is more promising and can now benefit of the availability of theatre-dedicated electron beam units that greatly simplify logistics.

Radical Radiotherapy

All patients enrolled for radical hemithoracic irradiation first undergo EPP, which includes removal of the ipsilateral lung, parietal pleura, hemidiaphragm, and pericardium with or without mediastinal lymph node dissection. Eligible patients must have no evidence of extrathoracic disease, multiple discontinuous areas of chest wall involvement, or invasion of mediastinal structures. Because of the close proximity of ipsilateral kidney to the clinical target volume (CTV), renal function should also be assessed.

Successful outcome and avoidance of severe morbidity requires careful definition of target volumes and organ at risks. Radiopaque surgical clips at intervals of 10-15mm should be used to delineate resection margins that are difficult to identify postoperatively. These include the anteromedial pleural reflection, pericardial margins, the entire outline of the resected diaphragm, and any close/positive surgical margins.

Following surgery, patients require time to recuperate and stabilize their internal anatomy. Consequently planning CT is usually performed before 4-6 week postoperatively. Pre-simulation narcotic analgesia is recommended to counterbalance the typical post surgical shoulder pain and allow the patient to hold his position in the immobilization system for the whole duration of the procedure.

All scar sites are marked with radiopaque wire and covered with 5-10mm thick tissue-equivalent bolus making sure that they don't pull away from the skin when arms are raised and lowered. All boluses should be at least 6 cm wide and extend 3 cm beyond the ends of the scar. Position and characteristics of the boluses are recorded with diagrams and photographs to ensure reproducibility.

The patient is then positioned with the arms above the head onto the immobilization system (typically a combination of a vacuum bag, overhead T-bar hand grip and headrest); aligned and 3 ball bariums (BB) are placed to define a CT reference point at the level of the sternum where the motion of the anterior BB with respiration is negligible. Respiratory gating is helpful to reduce the margins required to compensate for organ motion. Otherwise, a double helical CT acquisition with slice thickness of 3mm is performed respectively in voluntary breath hold and during quiet respiration, with the latter being the planning CT data set. The studies are then co-registered to assess organs motion in the chest cavity using the vertebral bodies and BBs as reference points. Differently from other forms of thoracic irradiation, internal motility on the ipsilateral side post EPP is greatly minimised by the reconstructed diaphragm and pericardium.

The clinical target volume (CTV) must include all surgically violated spaces but not extending to the skin other than in the scar areas. Close cooperation with the cardiothoracic surgical team is advisable. Role of elective nodal irradiation is still debatable because of its effect on the amount of contralateral lung exposed to low radiation doses which has been reported being the most significant risk factor for the development of fatal radiation pneumonitis. We do not routinely recommend extensive regional nodal irradiation, but case by case evaluation of regions at higher risk deserving inclusion.

CT-PET fusion is extremely helpful for definition of boost volumes for both patients with unresectable residual (post-operative study) and those in which a boost dose is indicated at the site of gross primary disease (pre-operative study). CTV to PTV margin varies according to the results form the dual CT scan evaluation or the availability of respiratory gating.

Standard prescribed dose ranges between 45 and 50 Gy in 25 fractions over 5 weeks with photon beams to the large post-operative volume followed by a boost with electrons up to a total dose of 54-60 Gy in 1.8-2 Gy/# to the small areas at higher risk of recurrence or residual disease.

As previously said there are many major technical challenges in the treatment planning including the cranial-caudal length of the target volumes, the sparing of the liver while maintaining an adequate dose to the surrounding CTV, minimising the dose to the contralateral lung further the excessive morbidity reported in some series. [8]

Although treatment can be successfully delivered with conventional linear accelerators using both 3D conformal and step-and-shoot intensity modulated radiotherapy [9], we believe that spiral tomotherapy is able to provide better dose distributions; therefore we do advocate its use.

Recommended dose constraints are detailed in Table 1. Special attention must be paid to the contralateral lung dose due to the risk of fatal pneumonitis especially when radiotherapy is given in combination or short sequence with chemotherapy. [10]

Table 1.

Critical organ	*Dose/Volume constraints*			
Lung (contralateral)	V20 <10%	V10 <25%	V5 <80%	MLD <9Gy
Liver	V30 <30%			
Kidney	V15 <20%			
Heart	V60 <1%	V50 <20%	V45 <30%	V40 <50%
Spinal cord	V50 <1%	V45 <10%		
Oesophagus	V50 <30%			

Prophylactic Radiotherapy

Malignant seeding along the tracts of invasive diagnostic procedures is a complication seen in around one in five mesothelioma patients undergoing cytology, needle biopsy, thoracoscopy or chest tube placement. Chest wall recurrences usually present as painful subcutaneous nodules which are often very uncomfortable and prevent patients from sleeping. Prophylactic treatment of incision sites with a short course of adjuvant radiotherapy after healing of the wound can avoid chest wall recurrences. [11]

Treatment must be delivered 10 to 15 days after thoracoscopy, thoracotomy or needle biopsy using 12 to 15 MeV electrons and 1cm bolus to encompass the skin in the 90% isodose. All procedure scars should be included. Recommended dose is 21 Gy administered in three daily fractions (3x7 Gy) which is radiobiologically equivalent to 45 Gy in conventional fractionation; a single dose of 10 Gy is ineffective. [12]

Results from study of both prophylactic irradiation and trimodality treatment contrast sharply with poor outcome of palliative radiotherapy for bulky mesothelioma. Two nonexclusive explanations have been proposed to account for this difference between treating microscopic and macroscopic disease.

The first one is known as “tumour bed effect” and is based on experimental evidence that growth of various tumour-cell lines is significantly delayed after implantation in preirradiated sites compared with normal tissue. This effect is seen after a dose of 10 Gy, with a peak between 20 and 30 Gy, and no increase in the dose response curve above 30 Gy. Although the exact mechanism is still unclear, it was suggested that alteration of blood supply in the irradiated tissue results in reduced angiogenesis, oxygen supply and growth factor release. Also radiation induced fibrosis might oppose tumour progression.

The other explanation refers to the well known correlation between radiation sensitivity and tumour size, suggesting that prophylactic radiotherapy kills vulnerable small clusters of migrating cells before they are able to form a resistant colony. [13]

Induction Chemotherapy

A Swiss group has presented encouraging preliminary experience with three cycles of induction chemotherapy with cisplatin plus gemcitabine followed by EPP within 6 weeks. Radiotherapy to incompletely resected or high-risk areas was optional. Sixty-one patients with T2N2M0 mesothelioma of all histological types were enrolled. Ninety-five percent of them completed the chemotherapy regimen as planed while 74% accomplished EPP within time schedule.

The one-year survival rate was 68% overall with a median overall survival of 18.4 months. For the group who completed treatment without delay median survival was 26 months and median time to recurrence was 14 months. Postoperative complications were seen in 62 percent of patients, with mortality rates of 2 percent, respectively. Significantly increased morbidity and mortality have been seen also in other studies of preoperative chemotherapy and EPP.

Although this study is insufficiently mature to determine the long-term "cure" rate, these results are among the best reported to date for pleural mesothelioma. [14]

Summary

Healthy patients younger than 65 years old with early-stage mesothelioma (AJCC Stage I-II), epithelioid histology, and no evidence of mediastinal lymph node involvement should be referred to specialised centres for consideration of definitive treatment with multimodality approach, including aggressive surgical cyto-reduction, radiotherapy and chemotherapy with platinum-based regimen in combination with premedtrex, paclitaxel or gemcitabine. Treatment eligibility for otherwise reasonably fit subjects with locally more advanced stages must be based on individualised case assessment.

Intensity modulated and intra-operative radiation therapy with dedicated machines has greatly increased our capability to reduce critical organ radiation-induced morbidity and supplement the dose delivered to the high-risk areas. This has given new emphasis to the role of radiotherapy in the management of MPM.

Radical radiotherapy alone should not be used as a curative option but can be used for short term symptoms palliation. Prophylactic radiotherapy to avoid the risk of seeding along the procedure tract is routinely offered to all patients.

Unfortunately, there is a lack of high-level clinical evidence supporting most of the common treatment strategies. Patients' enrolment in clinical trials is strongly recommended. Future studies should focus on confirming the value of these novel therapeutic approaches, including formal measures of quality of life and symptoms control.

Acknowledgements

To Dr Francesca Pigatto MD PhD, for her help in reviewing this manuscript.

References

[1] Chapman E, Berenstein EG, Dieguez M, Ortiz Z. Radiotherapy for malignant pleural mesothelioma. Cochrane Database Syst Rev. 2006 Jul 19;3:CD003880. Review.

[2] Carmichael J, Degraff WG, Gamson J, Russo D, Gazdar AF, Levitt ML, Minna JD, Mitchell JB. Radiation sensitivity of human lung cancer cell lines. Eur J Cancer Clin Oncol. 1989 Mar;25(3):527-34.

[3] Ahamad A, Stevens CW, Smythe WR, Vaporciyan AA, Komaki R, Kelly JF, Liao Z, Starkschall G, Forster KM. Intensity-modulated radiation therapy: a novel approach to the management of malignant pleural mesothelioma. Int J Radiat Oncol Biol Phys. 2003 Mar 1;55(3):768-75.

[4] Neragi-Miandoab S. Multimodality approach in management of malignant pleural mesothelioma. Eur J Cardiothorac Surg. 2006 Jan;29(1):14-9.

[5] Sugarbaker DJ, Flores RM, Jaklitsch MT, Richards WG, Strauss GM, Corson JM, DeCamp MM Jr, Swanson SJ, Bueno R, Lukanich JM, Baldini EH, Mentzer SJ. Resection margins, extrapleural nodal status, and cell type determine postoperative long-term survival in trimodality therapy of malignant pleural mesothelioma: results in 183 patients. J Thorac Cardiovasc Surg. 1999 Jan;117(1):54-63.

[6] Sterman DH, Albelda SM. Advances in the diagnosis, evaluation, and management of malignant pleural mesothelioma. Respirology. 2005 Jun;10(3):266-83.

[7] Gupta V, Mychalczak B, Krug L, Flores R, Bains M, Rusch VW, Rosenzweig KE. Hemithoracic radiation therapy after pleurectomy/decortication for malignant pleural mesothelioma. Int J Radiat Oncol Biol Phys. 2005 Nov 15;63(4):1045-52.

[8] Rice DC, Smythe WR, Liao Z, Guerrero T, Chang JY, McAleer MF, Jeter MD, Correa A, Vaporciyan AA, Liu HH, Komaki R, Forster KM, Stevens CW. Dose-Dependent Pulmonary Toxicity After Postoperative Intensity-Modulated Radiotherapy for Malignant Pleural Mesothelioma. Int J Radiat Oncol Biol Phys. 2007 Apr 27; [Epub ahead of print].

[9] Forster KM, Smythe WR, Starkschall G, Liao Z, Takanaka T, Kelly JF, Vaporciyan A, Ahamad A, Dong L, Salehpour M, Komaki R, Stevens CW. Intensity-modulated radiotherapy following extrapleural pneumonectomy for the treatment of malignant mesothelioma: clinical implementation. Int J Radiat Oncol Biol Phys. 2003 Mar 1;55(3):606-16.

[10] Allen AM, Czerminska M, Janne PA, Sugarbaker DJ, Bueno R, Harris JR, Court L, Baldini EH. Fatal pneumonitis associated with intensity-modulated radiation therapy for mesothelioma. Int J Radiat Oncol Biol Phys. 2006 Jul 1;65(3):640-5.

[11] Boutin C, Rey F, Viallat JR. Prevention of malignant seeding after invasive diagnostic procedures in patients with pleural mesothelioma. A randomized trial of local radiotherapy. Chest. 1995 Sep;108(3):754-8.

[12] Bydder S, Phillips M, Joseph DJ, Cameron F, Spry NA, DeMelker Y, Musk AW. A randomised trial of single-dose radiotherapy to prevent procedure tract metastasis by malignant mesothelioma. Br J Cancer. 2004 Jul 5;91(1):9-10.

[13] Summers WC, Clifton KH, Vermund H. X-irradiation of the tumor bed. A study of the indirect actions of radiation on transplantable tumors. Radiology. 1964 Apr;82:691-703.

[14] Stahel RA, Weder W, Ballabeni P, Betticher D, Schmid R, Stupp R, Ris HB, Roth A, Mingrone W, Bodis S. Neoadjuvant chemotherapy followed by extrapleural pneumonectomy for malignant pleural mesothelioma (MPM): A multicenter phase II trial of the SAKK. 2004 ASCO Annual Meeting Proceedings. J Clin Oncol. 2004 Jul 15; 22(14S):7052.

In: Mesothelioma from Bench Side to Clinic
Editor: Alfonso Baldi, pp. 413-434

ISBN: 978-1-60021-789-0

Chapter XXV

Surgical Management of Malignant Pleural Mesothelioma

Tommaso C. Mineo, Vincenzo Ambrogi and Eugenio Pompeo
Division of Thoracic Surgery
Policlinico Tor Vergata University, Rome, Italy

Abstract

Despite many years of clinical research, prognosis for malignant pleural mesothelioma remains poor. Due to the multicentric origin and the rapid local spread to vital thoracic structures the role of surgery is still controversial. At present surgery offers three options: pleurodesis, pleurectomy/decortication and extrapleural pneumonectomy. Pleurodesis is carried out as a palliative tool to arrest persistent pleural effusion in patients with advanced disease or poor general conditions. Pleurectomy/decortication is an effective symptom-relief but not-radical operation that implies preservation of the lung and is thus preferred in patients with poor residual lung function. Extrapleural pneumonectomy is the most aggressive procedure, which can be performed with acceptable morbidity and mortality in selected patients with good performance status and stage I or II. It represents an important step within a multimodality strategy, including chemo and radiotherapy, which has demonstrated to improve quality of life and survival.

Introduction

The incidence of malignant pleural mesothelioma (MPM) has increased over the past twenty years with 2,200 new cases a year in the United States [1-3]. In Western Europe the incidence ranges from 15 to 36 new cases every 100,000 inhabitants and is going to double over the next ten years [4], while for the same period annual mortality is expected to increase from 5,000 to 9,000 [5]. Incidence of MPM also has been increasing in many other parts of the world, from Australia to Egypt, leading to a truly global epidemic [6, 7].

To date, the treatment of MPM remains a particular challenge both for physicians and surgeons. The insidious presentation of the disease as well as its diffuse nature make MPM difficult to treat at early stage and no single conventional treatment has proven to be effective, with survival averaging approximately 8-10 months from diagnosis [8].

Despite recent advances in diagnostic and therapeutic fields, curative treatment continues to remain an elusive goal. Encouraging results have been achieved with multimodal approaches including extrapleural pneumonectomy (EPP) and adjuvant chemo-radiotherapy but significant mortality and morbidity have been reported with this aggressive surgical treatment and until now no randomized study supported this strategy. Nonetheless, it must be stressed that EPP is the only procedure that can provide long-term survival and cure in selected patients when associated with adjuvant chemo and radiation therapy [9]. In recent years, neoadjuvant therapy and subsequent EPP plus postoperative radiotherapy improved survival and quality of life in highly selected patients. Hence, further investigation is warranted to challenge with this lethal malignancy [10].

Surgery

The role of surgery in management of this aggressive malignancy remains controversial. Indeed, surgery is unable to eradicate a tumor arising from multiple sites on the parietal pleura and early involving both the visceral pleura and the underlying vital structures such as the lung, pericardium and diaphragm. However, surgery represents an important step within a multimodality strategy, which has recently demonstrated to improve quality of life and survival [9, 10].

Staging

Because of clinical complexity of the disease, staging of MPM is not easy to establish as demonstrated by the five different staging systems proposed in the past 25 years. As a result, it is difficult to predict survival and evaluate effectiveness of new therapeutic modalities. The various proposed staging systems were unified by the International Mesothelioma Interest Group in a unique classification [11] which can be summarized as follows.

- Stage I includes node-negative patients with tumor confined to the parietal pleura (Ia) or minimal visceral pleura involvement (Ib).
- Stage II includes node-negative patients with confluent tumor on all pleural surfaces or diaphragm or lung. Until this stage the tumor is considered resectable.
- Stage III includes hilar (N1) or ipsilateral mediastinal (N2) node-positive patients, as well as those with soft tissues, mediastinal fat or pericardium involvement (T3). It is the most common presenting form and is some instances can be resectable.
- Stage IV includes patients with distant metastasis or contralateral nodes (N3) or those with chest wall, spine, transdiaphragmatic or contralateral hemithorax involvement (T4).

Indications for Surgical Treatment

Theoretically, complete surgical resection should be considered the most effective treatment. However, because of the usual thoracic diffusion of the disease, complete resection with negative margins is rarely obtained. Hence, the term cytoredution was usually employed whatever the type of resection performed to indicate removal of the vast bulk tumor with microscopic residual left behind on the visceral pleura, mediastinum, diaphragm and chest wall [12]. The magnitude of the operation is usually tailored by taking into consideration several factors including patient's age, performance status, comorbidity and, finally, the surgeon's experience.

At present surgery offers three procedures for palliation and/or curative treatment of MPM: simple pleurodesis, pleurectomy/decortication (P/D) and EPP (Table 1).

Table 1. Surgical options

Diagnostic

- Thoracoscopy or VATS
- Mediastinoscopy
- Laparoscopy
- Open biopsy

Palliative

- Chest tube and pleurodesis
- Thoracoscopy or VATS and pleurodesis
- Pleurectomy

Potentially curative

- Pleurectomy/decortication
- Extrapleural pneumonectomy

Pleurodesis

The clinical presentation of diffuse MPM is insidious and unspecific. Dyspnea and pain are the most common symptoms occurring in 90% of the patients [13]. Greater than 95% of the patients present a pleural effusion often associated with dyspnea, cough, fever and pain [14]. The simpliest palliative treatment of this frequent condition is chest tube placement and pleurodesis. Pleural effusion is persistent and relapses rapidly following thoracentesis such that several liters may often be removed within few weeks.

If chest tube placement achieves complete evacuation of the pleural effusion and full re-expansion of the lung, 5 grams of talc in a slurry are introduced in the pleural cavity through the tube. This maneuver produces a chemical pleurodesis, which obliterates the pleural space and reduces the possibility of recurrence.

If the pleural effusion persists, redo talc pleurodesis can be performed. Amongst the different substances employed for pleurodesis including bleomycin, tetracycline, and talc, the latter agent revealed the most used and effective for this purpose [15, 16].

In recent years, pleurodesis has been performed by video-assisted thoracoscopy (VATS) [17]. This procedure offers many advantages allowing multiple biopsies for diagnosis, pleural debridment and drainage of the effusion, as well as pleurodesis by vaporized talc. Due to its safety, low invasiveness and efficacy of VATS we recommend it in patients with advanced-stage disease and comorbidity.

One potential complication is malignant growth along the catheter pathway. For this reason prophylactic irradiation of thoracostomy site has been found to be effective for seeding prevention [18].

Pleurectomy and Decortication

Originally, pleurectomy was carried out as a palliative procedure to control pleural effusion due to metastatic malignancy [19, 20].

Since macroscopic tumor is left in the pleural cavity at the end of the operation in almost 80% of instances [21], pleurectomy cannot be considered a curative procedure. However, pleurectomy constitutes a therapeutic surgical option performed within a cytoreduction strategy with surgery followed by adjuvant chemotherapy and/or radiotherapy.

It involves removal of the parietal pleura including the area over the mediastinum, pericardium and diaphragm, with or without removal of a portion of this muscle.

The indications for palliative surgery include the control or prevention of the effusion, which is symptomatic in 30% to 90% of patients [22, 23] and the amelioration of disease-related symptoms. Usually, effusion control is attempted with lesser procedures, which generally fail due to the thickened visceral pleura impairing lung re-expansion. Some surgeons perform P/D in patients with early staged disease confined to the parietal pleura [24]. Conversely, other surgeons recommend EPP even in these stage believing that the absence of the lung facilitates postoperative irradiation [9].

Pleurectomy is combined with decortication of the visceral pleura without removal of the lung. Visceral pleurectomy permits pulmonary re-expansion and facilitates pleural symphysis while parietal pleurectomy improves diaphragmatic and thoracic wall movements thus preventing fluid neoaccumulation, with amelioration of cough, dyspnea and chest pain. Soysal et al [25] performed pleurectomy in 100 patients with MPM and achieved pleural effusion control in 96 of them. Since P/D does not involve removal of the lung, it remains a valid therapeutic procedure in patients with impaired lung function and we have extensively employed this procedure as a debulking tool even in patients with locally advanced disease.

Indeed, deep neoplastic involvement of lung fissures precluding complete resection as well as involvement of the phrenic nerve causing partial or complete impairment of diaphragmatic function occur quite frequently.

Surgical Technique

Pleurectomy is technically unfeasible in about 20% of the patients with MPM, due to complete neoplastic obliteration of the pleural space [19]. In our experience, less than 10% of the patients had an unaccessible pleural space not amenable of decortication (Figure 1).

Following general anesthesia and double-lumen tube intubation, the patient is placed in the full lateral decubitus position. Arterial and central venous catheters are routinely inserted. An extended posterolateral thoracotomy incision on the sixth or seventh intercostal space is made.

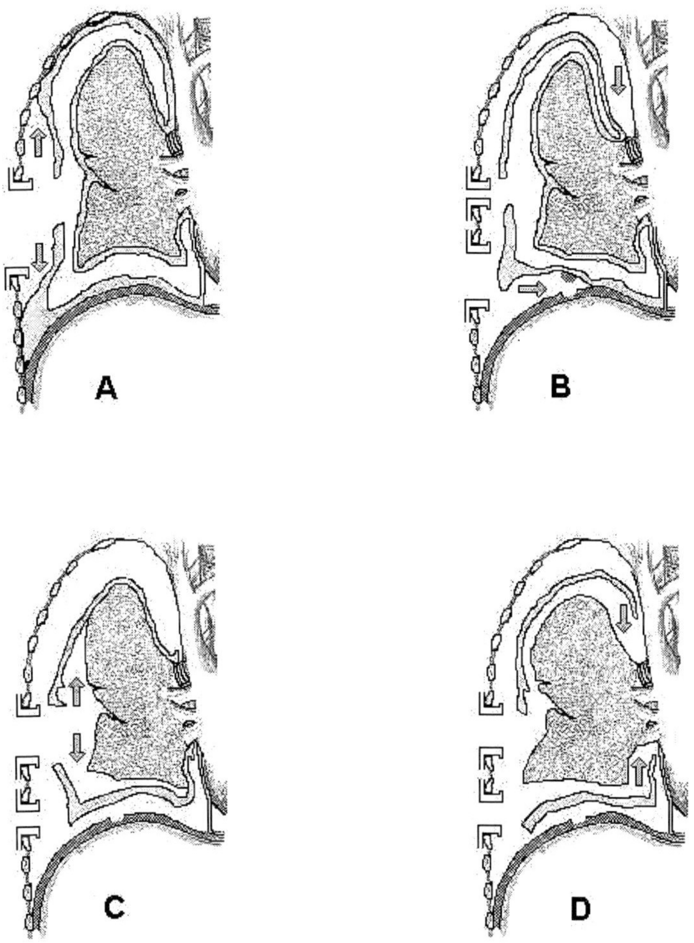

Figure 1. Schematic drawings illustrating main surgical steps of P/D. A) pleurectomy is started dissecting the neoplastic parietal pleura off the chest wall around thoracotomy incision; B) dissection is then continued towards the pericardium, which is not resected if adequate dissection plane is present, and inferiorly on the diaphragm where partial thickness muscular resection is usually carried out; C) decortication of the visceral pleura is the more demanding step of the procedure particularly when it is performed deep in the fissures and around the hilum vessels; D) the lung is finally completely freed by its neoplastic pleura envelope and the specimen is extracted.

If necessary, a counterincision through the eighth or nineth intercostal space is added to facilitate the access to the hemidiaphragm and costophrenic angle. The dissection is begun in the natural plane between endothoracic fascia and parietal pleura. The neoplastic pleura is dissected off the chest wall by blunt maneuvers to allow placement of the thoracic retractor and improve the exposure. Dissection proceeds then in a cephalad direction towards the apex. Careful dissection is necessary at the level of the subclavian vessels to avoid vascular injury that can be difficult to repair. Hemostasis is assured step by step during the ongoing procedure. For this purpose we routinely employ hot gauze packing and generous use of the argon beam coagulator in order to limit the overall blood loss. The dissection is then continued anteriorly towards the mediastinal pleura and posteriorly. On the left side, care must be devoted to dissect the pleura along the descending aorta to avoid injury to the intercostal vessels, which can be inadvertently teared off during dissection maneuvers. Subsequently, the dissection proceeds medially and the esophagus must be recognized also thanks to the previously positioned nasogastric tube. On the right side, the same careful dissection is required posteriorly along the azygos vein and anteriorly along the superior vena cava, which is gently dissected off the neoplastic pleura.

The dissection continues then onto the pericardium. A plane between the mediastinal pleura and the pericardium is usually present, whereas if pericardium is involved by tumor, it is eventually resected en bloc with the specimen and subsequently reconstructed.

Inferiorly, diaphragmatic fibres are cauterized while retracting cephalad the specimen. The dissection is then carried towards the posterior costophrenic sinus. If the diaphragm is involved superficially, a partial thickness resection is to be preferred. Conversely, deeper involvement of the diaphragm mandates a full-thickness partial resection of the muscle. In this latter case, the abdominal surface of the diaphragm must be dissected from the peritoneum taken care to avoid entering the abdomen as tumor seeding into the peritoneal cavity can occur. For this reason, any inadvertent defect in the peritoneum must be immediately repaired.

Visceral pleura is separated from the underlying lung by sharp and blunt dissection. Once the dissection is complete around the hilum, the parietal pleura is opened, the pleural envelope is entered and decortication of the visceral pleura from the underlying lung and hilar vessels is performed. Neoplastic visceral pleura is dissected off fissures by careful sharp maneuvers because they are often grossly involved by the tumor. During decortication, moderate lung inflation will allow better visualization of the right plane. The specimen including all gross tumor tissue is eventually removed. Associated atypical removal of lung areas may be necessary when local neoplastic involvement does occur (Figure 2).

Lymph node sampling is performed at the subcarinal and paratracheal site on the right and at the aortopulmonary window on the left. If enough diaphragm remains, it is usually defunctionalized and plication is carried out. On the other hand, if reconstruction of the pericardium and diaphragm are necessary, they are performed as described in the EPP paragraph.

Careful hemostasis is minutely pursued by argon beam coagulation and local packing. Aerosolized fibrin glue can also be helpful to achieve hemostasis.

Finally, two chest tubes are placed in standard manner under moderate suction to keep the lung expanded. The thoracotomy is finally closed in layers as usual.

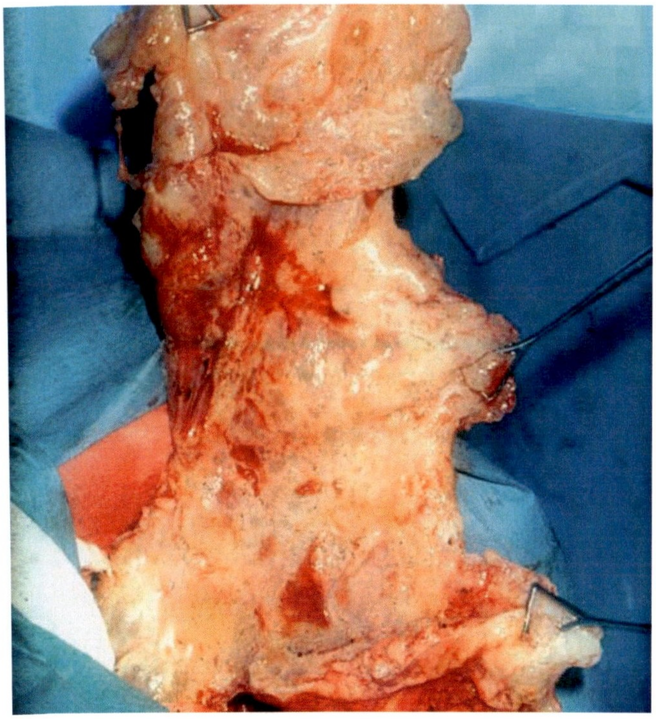

Figure 2.Pleurectomy/decortication specimen illustrating successful resection of the vast bulk of a sarcomatoid mesothelioma.

Results

Pleurectomy/decortication can be accomplished with few major complications with operative mortality rate of 1.5% to 5% and morbidity rate of 25% [12, 19, 23, 25-37]. The most common complication is the prolonged air leak occurring in 10% of the patients [13, 24]. Empyema is a rare occurrence (2% of the patients), while hemorrhage requiring re-exploration occurs in less than 1% of the patients. Pleurectomy/decortication by itself provides good palliation and prevents relapse of symptomatic effusion, but cannot avoid loco-regional recurrence, which usually occurs in 80% to 90% of the patients [38]. The median survival reached by this procedure is reported in different studies between 9 and 20 months, and 9-40% of patients survive up to 2 years (Table 2). These wide ranges are reported in different trials entailing various treatment combinations with surgery performed with or without radiation therapy and/or chemotherapy. Nevertheless, the role of pleurectomy as a curative option, even when employed in association with other therapies, remains marginal compared to EPP.

Table 2. Results of pleurectomy/decortication

	Survival rate for symptoms onset						
	No. patients	Adjuvant	Morbidity (%)	Mortality (%)	1year (%)	2 years (%)	Median (months)
Martini et al. 1975 [19]	14		NA	0	7	40	16
McCormack et al 1982 [23]	64	Radiotherapy	NA	1.5	49.0	NA	NA
Chahinian et al 1982 [26]	30		NA	0	57.0	27.0	13.0
Law et al 1984 [27]	28		NA	11.0	82	32	20
Martini et al 1987 [28]	94	Radiotherapy	NA	0	44	NA	21
Alberts et al 1988 [29]	26	Radiotherapy Chemotherapy	NA	0	NA	NA	10.9
Ruffie et al 1989 [30]	63		25	NA	NA	NA	9.8
Ball et al 1990 [31]	13		NA	NA	NA	NA	17
Brancatisano et al 1991 [32]	45		16.8	2.2	58	21	16
Allen et al 1994 [33]	56	Chemotherapy	26.8	5.4	30.4	8.9	9.0
Rusch et al 1994 [34]	27	Local chemotherapy	40	3.6	68	NA	17
Lee et al 1995 [35]	15	Local chemotherapy	13	0	NA	NA	11.5
Sauter et al 1995 [36]	13	Local chemotherapy	6	0	NA	NA	21
Takita et al 1995 [37]	22	Phototherapy	50	50	NA	NA	12
Soysal et al 1997 [25]	100		22	1	NA	NA	17
Pass et al 1997 [12]	39	Phototherapy	15	2	NA	NA	14.5

NA = not available.

Combination Treatment

Because P/D is usually unable to eradicate the whole disease, efforts at optimizing local control have been performed. Several studies included intraoperative and postoperative radiation, intrapleural and systemic chemotherapy and phototherapy.

Mc Cormack et al [23] in 1982 associated P/D with postoperative radiotherapy reporting a median survival of 12.6 months. Few year later, Hilaris et al [21] combined pleurectomy with introperative radioactive implants of iodine 125 with an increment of the median survival to 21 months.

The use of adjuvant systemic chemotherapy resulted in scant success [33]. On the contrary, intracavitary chemotherapy can provide better local control with a lower general toxicity. Rush et al in 1994 reported a series of 27 patients undergoing pleurectomy and intracavitary chemotherapy with a median survival of 17 months [34]. Lee et al [35] and Sauter et al [36] with intrapleural cisplatin and cytosine arabinoside after subtotal pleurectomy reported worse results with a median survival of 11.5 and 9 months, respectively.

Finally, photodynamic radiation delivered on the lung surface is an intraoperative treatment that has recently gained increasing attention in combination with pleurectomy. Pass and colleagues [12] have used intraoperative phototherapy in 39 patients after P/D with a slight improvement in long-term survival (14.5 months).

Extrapleural Pneumonectomy

In the late 1940, Sarot [39] first described the technique of EPP for the management of tuberculous empyema. Between 1970 and 1990, this challenging surgical procedure was extended to treat MPM, despite high perioperative mortality and morbidity initially reported [40-43].

In 1999, Sugarbaker et al [9] in a series of 183 patients with MPM who underwent EPP followed by adjuvant chemo and radiotherapy, reported significantly better results with an operative mortality of only 3.8%. This improved outcome was attributed to the advances in patients selection, preoperative assessment, surgical technique, and intra and postoperative management.

Because of the aggressive clinical course of MPM, patient's management should be performed by a multidisciplinary team. In fact, specific experience and judgement are required to appropriately select patients with potentially resectable tumors as well as to decide the most suitable operation.

Extrapleural pneumonectomy is the most aggressive surgical option aimed at radical debulking of locally advanced MPM, and is currently the only procedure, which may assure long-term survival. This operation can potentially provide complete tumor resection and allow postoperative high-doses radiotherapy due to the absence of the underlying lung. For the same reasons, EPP is considered the first and main treatment step, which must be integrated by adjuvant modalities directed at eliminating all residual disease.

Patient Selection

Before a patient is considered for EPP, careful assessment of operative risk is mandatory since this complex operation is still burdened by a mortality rate ranging around 5% and morbidity of 50% even in experienced surgical teams' series [9]. Strict selection criteria for EPP have been already outlined (Table 3) and about 10% of the patients are eligible for this operation [44].

General medical status as well as cardiac, renal and liver function tests should be evaluated as for any other thoracic operation. Although there is no definite age limit, EPP is not recommended beyond 70 years. The patient must have a Karnofsky performance status higher than 70, a room air arterial pCO_2 less than 45 mmHg, and a room air arterial pO_2 more than 65 mmHg (Table 4).

Table 3. EPP selection criteria

- Karnofsky performance status >70;
- Adequate pulmonary function to tolerate a pneumonectomy;
- Cardiac ejection fraction > 45%;
- No significant liver or renal disease or other comorbidities;
- No prior coronary bypass surgery;
- No prior pleurectomy (VATS talc pleurodesis is not a contraindication)
- Stage I or II mesothelioma (according to the International Mesothelioma Interest Group), rarely Stage III;
- Epithelial subtype mesothelioma;
- Minimal or absent chest wall pain;

Table 4. EPP preoperative assessment

- Age and performance status;
- Serum chemistries;
- Renal and liver function tests;
- Pulmonary function tests arterial blood gas, quantitative ventilation-perfusion scan;
- Echocardiography, right heart catheterization;
- CT and MRI of the chest and upper abdomen;
- FDG-PET scan;
- VATS pleural biopsy for histologic confirmation;

A forced expiratory volume in one second (FEV_1) of more than 2 liters is adequate for pneumonectomy. For patients with FEV_1 <2 liters the quantitative ventilation-perfusion scanning combined with preoperative FEV_1 proved a reliable predictor of postoperative lung function. Thus, a predicted postoperative FEV_1 of more than 0.8 liters is acceptable for EPP. Below this value we believe that P/D should be preferred.

Echocardiography is performed to assess right and left ventricular function, cardiac chamber sizes and valve motion abnormalities, and to estimate pulmonary artery pressure. Indeed, pulmonary hypertension is a contraindication to pneumonectomy and compels to accomplish right heart catheterization.

Even if ultimate assessment of local extent can be only obtained at surgery, imaging studies such as Computed Tomography (CT) and Magnetic Resonance Imaging (MRI) are useful in making an initial clinical staging. Preoperative CT and MRI of the thorax and upper abdomen are essential to assess the extent of intrathoracic and extrathoracic disease. The presence of controlateral or abdominal disease, as well as mediastinal and chest wall invasion, precludes surgical resection. According to Patz et al [45], we routinely use chest preoperative CT and MRI in all patients. Additional findings can be obtained by 18-fluorodeoxyglucose positron emission tomography (FDG-PET), which is now a fundamental staging tool and revealed particularly useful to detect N3 or M1 disease [46].

Cytologic diagnosis of mesothelioma is often possible but a definitive histologic diagnosis is mandatory before surgery. For this purpose we now privilege a single-port VATS which is a well-known safe and rapid procedure. The same technique can discriminate incidental controlateral involvements suggested by preoperative imaging studies.

The role of mediastinoscopy is controversial. There is no doubt that mediastinoscopy is more accurate than CT in determining the N-stage in most patients [47]. However, in 20% of the patients, lymph node involvement is confined in areas inaccessible by mediastinoscopy [48]. Furthermore, N2 disease should not be considered the sole criteria contraindicating EPP. Patients with distant metastases are not candidate for resection.

Adequate physiologic monitoring is important due to the complexity of the procedure. The use of a double-lumen endotracheal tube is mandatory. A nasogastric tube should also be placed to facilitate identification of the esophagus during the posterior mediastinal dissection, especially for right-sided tumors. Monitoring of arterial blood pressure should be performed by radial artery cannulation. On-line oximetry as well as insertion of central venous catheter are also useful; large-bore peripheral intravenous cannulas should be placed to facilitate replacement of the blood loss, which in some cases can reach more than 3000 mL. A thoracic epidural catheter is placed preoperatively and left in place for 3-4 days after surgery to aid deep breathing, coughing and secretion clearance.

Surgical Technique

Extrapleural pneumonectomy is an en bloc resection of the pleura, lung, pericardium, ipsilateral hemidiaphragm, and hilar and mediastinal lymph nodes (Figure 3) (Table 5).

Adequate exposure is a fundamental step for complete and safe tumor removal especially in the highest area of the apex and in the inferior portion of the diaphragm. For this purpose, the chest incision is a long posterolateral thoracotomy in the sixth interspace that extends posteriorly between the spine of the scapula and the costochondral junction, which is frequently disarticolated (Figure 4). The sixth rib can be removed to facilitate exposure of the extrapleural plane although we consider this maneuver rarely necessary. This relatively low approach is justified because the greatest neoplastic bulk is usually found in the lower half of the hemithorax.

Table 5. Surgical Sequence

- Single (6th intercostal space) or double (plus 8th intercostal space) thoracotomy incision;
- Incision and visualization of the parietal pleura;
- Blunt dissection in the extrapleural plane;
- Separation of the tumor from the chest wall, mediastinum and peritoneum;
- Division of the hilar vessels and bronchus;
- En bloc resection of the pleura with lung, pericardium and diaphragm;
- Mediastinal lymphadenectomy;
- Pericardium and diaphragm reconstruction;
- Meticolous hemostasis;
- Closure of the thoracotomy.

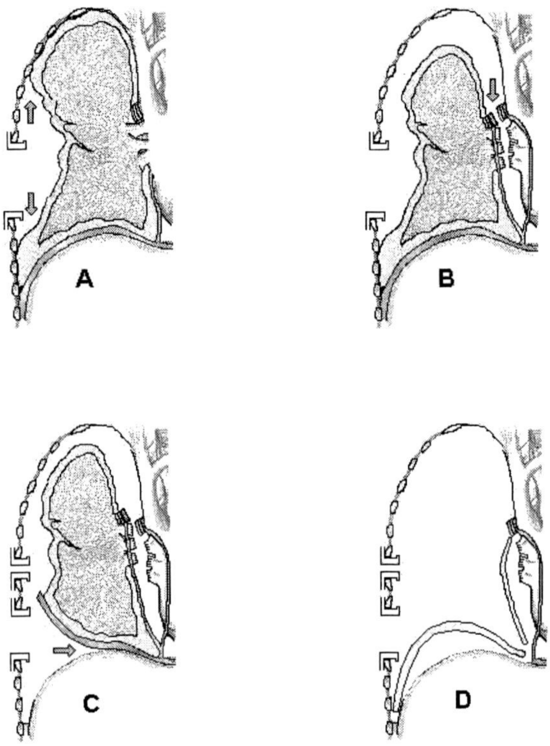

Figure 3. Schematic drawings of EPP showing: A) initial blunt dissection of the neoplastic pleura off the chest wall around thoracotomy incision; B) intrapericardial stapled section of hilar vessels and main bronchus; C) extraperitoneal en bloc resection of the diaphragm with tumor, lung and pericardium is followed by careful hemostasis; D) prosthetic reconstruction of the diaphragm is carried out by PTFE while tailored bovine pericardium patch is employed to close the pericardial defect.

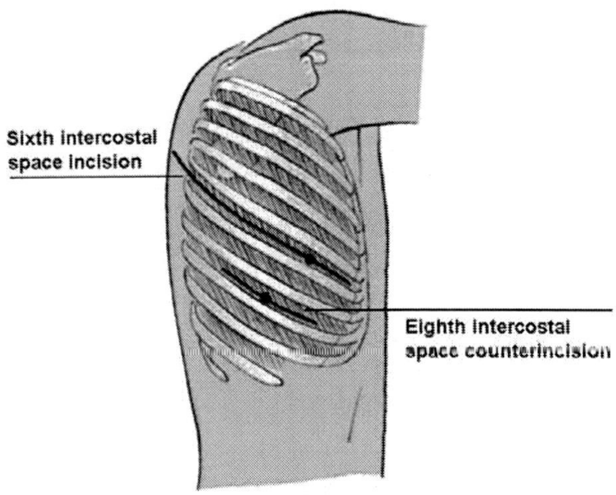

Figure 4. Posterolateral thoracotomy incision in the sixth intercostal space and lower eighth interspace counterincision incorporating the previous VATS incision or chest tube site (black circles) to ensure removal potential sites of mesothelioma implants.

The extension of the thoracotomy into a thoracoabdominal incision provides a better access to the diaphragm and an optimal visualization of the tumor extent at this level. Some surgeons perform laparoscopy to rule out neoplastic involvement of the peritoneal cavity [49] while we have found that since the advent of FDG-PET, surgical exploration of the peritoneal cavity in PET negative patients is not strictly necessary. Histologically proven peritoneal involvement mandates interruption of the surgical procedure. A complete tumor removal in the phrenocostal sulcus and diaphragmatic surface may be accomplished by a parallel lower counterincision in the eighth intercostal space. Besides, this further incision facilitates the prosthesic reconstruction of the hemidiaphragm.

Once the incision has reached the interspace, blunt dissection with the fingertips is begun in the extrapleural plane between the endothoracic fascia and the parietal pleura. This manoeuver may be initially simplified using a periosteal elevator.

The blunt dissection is then directed anteriorly to the pericardium toward the sternum and posteriorly toward the spine. Subsequently, dissection is continued inferiorly down to the diaphragm and his anterior insertion as well as superiorly toward the apex, up to approximately halfway to the apex from the incision. This step is facilitated by preoperative talc pleurodesis, which may prevent intraoperative spillage of malignant cells. In this setting we found that talc pleurodesis performed at the time of the diagnostic VATS should preceed EPP of 2-3 weeks. We usually perform single-port VATS through the eighth intercostal space because this incision can be easily incorporated into the utility counterincision during EPP.

Following this initial dissection and when the parietal pleura has been adequately mobilized away from the thoracotomy area, one or two rib retractors are placed to achieve a wider exposure and a better access into the extrapleural plane.

Despite this dissection is limited and blunt, it implies a diffuse chest wall bleeding with substantial blood loss, which may be controlled both by hot gauze packing and argon beam electrocoagulation.

The finger-dissection is now continued under direct vision progressively mobilizing the neoplastic pleura off the chest wall in all directions.

Hand dissection is a fundamental step both for progression of the operation and to feel how the plane of dissection is developing to ensure the mobilization of the neoplastic pleura from the vascular structures, keeping in mind that in the fibrosarcomatous type a degree of invasion of the adventitia will occur.

In particular, on the right side care is required when dissecting the neoplastic pleura off the azygos vein axis posteriorly and the superior vena cava anteriorly (Figure 5a).

On the left side identical care must be taken during dissection of the pleura along the descending aorta to avoid injury to the intercostal vessels, which can be inadvertently teared off if the dissection run in a deeper, wrong plane. The dissection proceeds then medially and the esophagus can be easily recognized by palpation of the nasogastric tube (Figure 5b).

At the end of the surgical dissection, the lung together with neoplastic pleura, pericardium and diaphragm are removed en bloc (Figure 6 and 7). Dissection of hilar lymph nodes and peritracheal or aorto-pulmonary window nodes in right-sided or left-sided tumors, respectively, is mandatory for post-surgical staging. Further control of the hemostasis is mandatory and can be achieved by the abovementioned tools or by aerosolized fibrin glue.

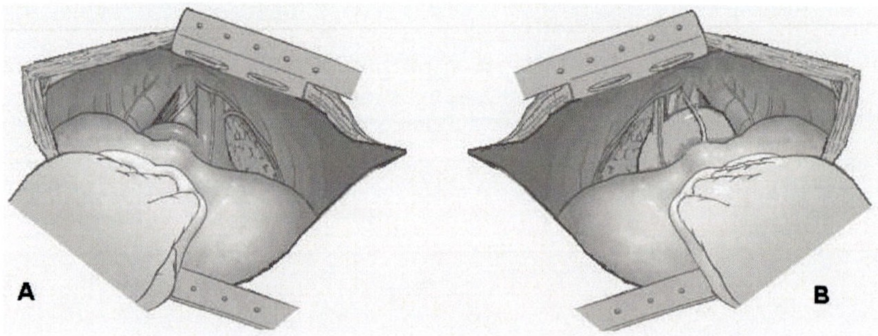

Figure 5. Schematic drawings illustrating operative view of pleural cavity during EPP on the right (A) or left (B) side with neoplastic pleura dissected off the chest wall up to the apex.

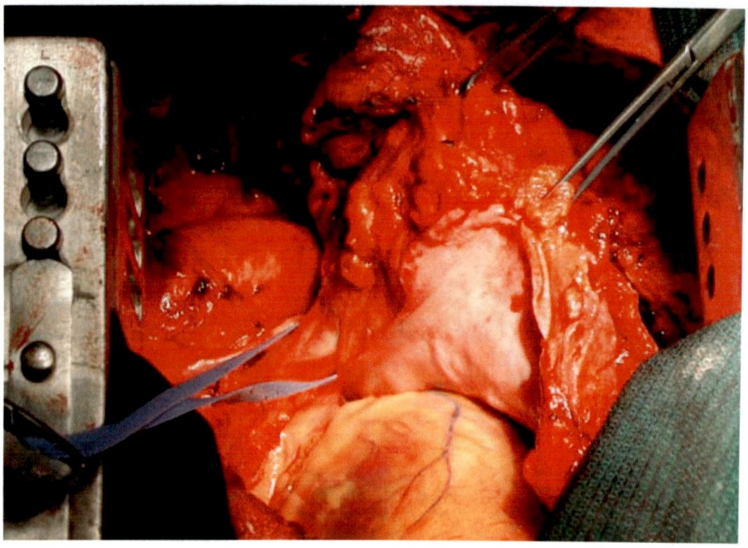

Figure 6.Operative view of ongoing EPP with radical neoplastic mass resection en bloc with the involved pericardium. Pulmonary artery is encircled.

After careful revision of the hemostasis, reconstruction of the pericardium and emidiaphragm is performed (Figure 8). Different material including polytetrafluorethylene (PTFE)(Gore-Tex, Inc., Flagstaff, AZ) and bovine pericardium can be used to repair the pericardial defect. Our preferred material is now bovine pericardium, which showed satisfactory biologic compatibility and optimal softness and malleability. Yet, this material is manufactured in different sizes allowing repair of even large defects (Bio-Vascular Inc., Saint Paul, MN). The pericardial prosthesis is tailored adequately and is sutured to the pericardium edges utilizing interrupted 2-0 nonabsorbable sutures. The key to prevent cardiac tamponade is to use a large patch, which should be fenestrated or rather sutured with stitches placed at 3-4 cm from one another to allow free passage of pericardial effusion in the early postoperative period. Furthermore, that patch should not be placed too close to the superior and inferior vena cava to avoid impairment of venous return.

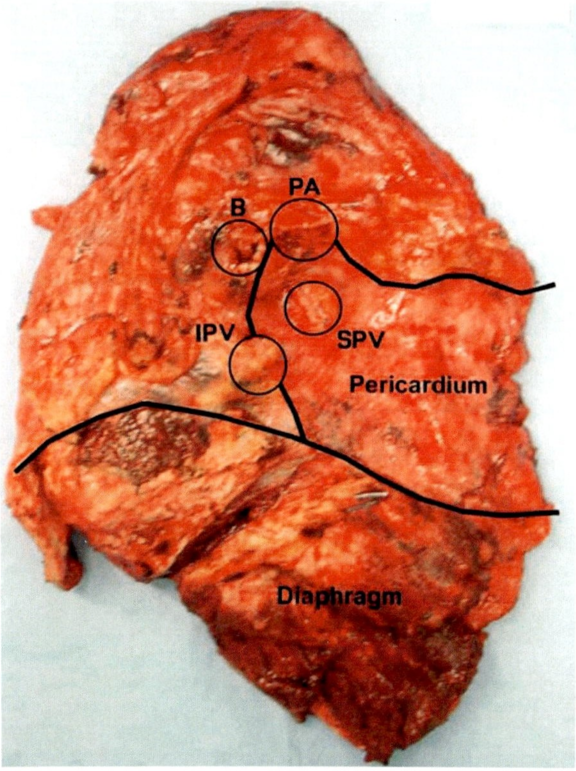

Figure 7. Extrapleural pneumonectomy specimen entailing left lung, diaphragm and pericardium resected en bloc. Interrupted hilar structures including main bronchus (B), extrapericardial section of the pulmonary artery (PA), and intrapericardial section of inferior and superior pulmonary veins (IPV and SPV, respectively) are also showed.

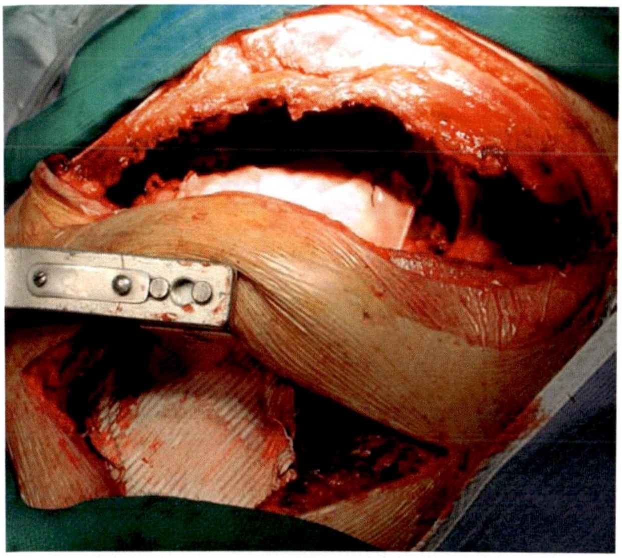

Figure 8. Operative field after successful EPP showing subtotal PTFE reconstruction of the diaphragm and large bovine pericardium patch covering the pericardial defect.

The diaphragmatic defect can be repaired with a 2-mm soft tissue PTFE patch using interrupted nonabsorbable PTFE or polypropilene sutures to help prevent patch dehiscence. By employing the lower utility thoracotomy incision excellent exposure can be obtained for placement of the diaphragmatic patch. If the emidiaphragm is excised widely and there remains not enough tissue for patch suturing, sutures are passed around the ribs inferiorly. It is important to make sure that the diaphragmatic patch is placed near the normal anatomical position of the native diaphragm to prevent intrathoracic migration of abdominal contents, which might expose them to radiation injury during subsequent adjuvant treatment.

Areas of residual neoplastic tissue that cannot be resected are outlined with metallic clips for subsequent boost doses of radiotherapy. The thoracotomy is closed in routine fashion.

Postoperative Management

Postoperative management is similar to that of patients undergoing standard pneumonectomy. Pain control and minimization of intravascular volume changes are important issues in the postoperative course.

To minimize postoperative atelectasis and frequent pulmonary dysfunction of the remaining lung, pain control is mandatory. It is obtained with the routine use of thoracic epidural analgesia for the first postoperative days. A relatively pain-free condition aids in deep breathing, coughing and secretion clearance. With this purpose in mind, chest physiotherapy is started as soon as possible, usually in postoperative day two, and frequently repeated. During the early postoperative period patients ambulate with nursing assistance at least three times per day. The nasogastric tube is removed early on postoperative day 1 or 2 to facilitate coughing. When necessary, one or more bedside fiberbronchoscopy per day can be performed to clear adequately the airways.

Patients are monitored for the first 3-4 postoperative days in the intermediate intensive care unit with continuous oximetry, arterial and central venous catheters and respiratory rate monitoring.

Deep venous thrombosis prophylaxis is achieved preferably with subcutaneous heparin. Fluid restriction in the acute postoperative period is an important to minimize capillary leak in the remaining lung, which can lead to pulmonary edema and desaturation. Atrial arrhythmias are treated aggressively to prevent cardiac dysfunction.

Daily chest radiographs are useful in the evaluation of clinical course.

Results

In reviewing the medical literature on surgery for MPM, it became quickly apparent that there is no definitive advantage for one procedure over another including EPP. However, operative morbidity and mortality of EPP have significantly decreased from the earlier series [9, 10, 30, 33, 40, 41, 50-54] because of improved patients selection, operative technique as well as intra and postoperative care (Table 6).

Table 6. Results of extrapleural pneumonectomy for diffuse malignant pleural mesothelioma

	Survival rate for symptoms onset							
	No. patients	Associated therapy	Morbidity (%)	Mortality (%)	1year (%)	2 years (%)	5 years (%)	Median (months)
Worn 1974 [40]	62	None	NA	NA	NA	37	10.0	NA
Butchart et al 1976 [41]	29	None	43	31.0	NA	10	3.5	NA
Martensson et al 1984 [51]	7	None	NA	NA	85.7	85.7	42.8	44
Ruffie et al 1989 [30]	23	None	24	14.0	NA	17.0	NA	9.3
Sugarbaker et al 1991 [50]	31	Adjuvant Radiotherapy and Chermotherapy	19	6	70	40	NA	10
Rusch et al 1991 [52]	20	None	40	15	NA	33	NA	13
Allen et al 1994 [33]	40	Adjuvant Chermotherapy	30	7.5	52.5	23	10	13.3
Sugarbaker et al 1999 [9]	183	Adjuvant Radiotherapy and Chermotherapy	50	3.8	NA	38	15	19
Weder et al 2004 [10]	16	Neoadjuvant Chemotherapy and Adjuvant Radiotherapy	31	-	79	37	NA	23
Edwards et al 2006 [53]	92	Adjuvant Radiotherapy and Chermotherapy	NA	7.6	59	34	NA	14.9
De Perrot et al 2007 [54]	50	Neoadjuvant Chemotherapy and Adjuvant Radiotherapy	NA	8	43	25	NA	11
Mineo *	26	Radiotherapy Chemotherapy	30	3.8	56	31		13

*unpublished data , NA = not available.

Sugarbaker and colleagues [9], first, in 1999, reported an operative mortality of 3.8% in 183 patients, a rate which is comparable to that of standard pneumonectomy. An improvement in survival for patients with MPM was not achieved until the trimodality therapy was introduced in 1991 [50]. This innovative approach consists in EPP followed by postoperative radio and chemotherapy. This therapeutic regimen achieved a five-year survival of 15% while patients with epithelial type of MPM, negative lymph nodes and surgical margins had a five-year survival of 46% [55]. We have also found a clearcut survival advantage for patients treated with EPP when compared with those undergoing lesser procedures. In particular, 3-year survival was 18% in patients undergoing EPP while there were no survivors amongst patients undergoing P/D.

Conclusion

There is no doubt that in this last decade the management of MPM is changing. Innovative therapeutic strategies and agents are being adopted with improvement both in quality of life and survival. New chemotherapy agents show promise against this aggressive malignancy.

Although long-term survival rates of EPP remain disappointing, it remains the most aggressive modality of treatment and at the present it can be performed with an acceptable mordibity and mortality at experienced centers.

Pleurectomy/decortication as well as EPP are cytoreductive operation aimed in selected patients to render the tumor more amenable to adjuvant therapy such as chemo and radiation therapy.

More recently, in highly selected patients with potentially operable disease EPP plus local postoperative radiotherapy can be safely performed after neoadjuvant chemotherapy. Initial promising results with this novel approach as well as further investigation into the advantagious role of neoadjuvant chemotherapy outlines better results in patients with this lethal neoplasm. Surgery combined with other therapies will continue and better survival can be achieved with high selection of patients, low operative morbidity and mortality, and with active and well tolerated chemotherapy regimens.

References

[1] Connelly RR, Spirtas R, Myers MH, Percy CL, Fraumeni JF Jr. Demographic patterns for mesothelioma in the United States. *J. Natl. Cancer Inst.* 1987;78: 1053-60.

[2] Kukreja J, Jaklitsch MT, Wiener DC, Sugarbaker DJ, Burgers S, Baas P. Malignant pleural mesothelioma: overview of the North American and European experience. *Thorac. Surg. Clin.* 2004; 14: 435-45.

[3] West D, Lee G. Management of malignant pleural mesothelioma. *Clin. Chest Med.* 2006; 27: 335-54.

[4] Pelucchi C, Malvezzi M, La Vecchia C, Levi F, Decarli A, Negri E. The mesothelioma epidemic in Western Europe: an update. *Br. J. Cancer* 2004; 90: 1022-24.

[5] Peto J, Hodgson JT, Matthews FE, Jones JR. Continuing increase in mesothelioma mortality in Britain. *Lancet* 1995; 345: 535-9.

[6] Musk AW, De Klerk NH. Epidemiology of malignant mesothelioma in Australia. *Lung Cancer* 2004; 45 (Suppl 1): S21-3.

[7] Gaafar RM, Eldin NH. Epidemic of mesothelioma in Egypt. *Lung Cancer* 2005; 49 (Suppl 2): S17-20.

[8] Rusch VW, Venkatraman E. The importance of surgical staging in the treatment of malignant pleural mesothelioma. *J. Thorac. Cardiovasc. Surg* 1996;111: 815-825.

[9] Sugarbaker D, Flores R, Jaklitsch M, Richards W, Strauss G, Corson J, DeCamp M, Swanson S, Bueno R, Lukanich J, Baldini E, Mentzer S. Resection margins, extrapleural nodal status and cell type determine postoperative long term survival in trimodality therapy of malignant pleural mesothelioma: results in 183 patients. *J. Thorac. Cardiovasc Surg*. 1999; 117: 54-65.

[10] Weder W, Kestenholz P, Taverna C, Bodis S, Lardinois D, Jerman M, Stahel RA. Neoadjuvant chemotherapy followed by extrapleural pneumonectomy in malignant pleural mesothelioma. *J. Clinl. Oncol*. 2004; 22: 3451-57.

[11] Rusch VW. A proposed new international TNM-staging system for malignant pleural mesothelioma: International Mesothelioma Interest Group. *Chest* 1995; 108:1122-1128.

[12] Pass HI, Temeck BK, Kranda K, Thomas G, Russo A, Smith P, Friauf W, Steinberg SM. Phase III randomized trial of surgery with or without intraoperative photodynamic therapy and postoperative immunochemotherapy for malignant pleural mesothelioma. *Ann. Surg. Oncol.* 1997; 4: 628-33.

[13] Pass HI, Pogrebniak HW. Malignant pleura mesothelioma. *Curr. Probl. Surg.* 1993; 30: 921-1012.

[14] Antman, KH Natural history and epidemiology of malignant mesothelioma. *Chest* 1993; 103: 373S-376S.

[15] Dresler CM, Olak J, Herndon JE, et al. Phase III intergroup study of talc poudrage vs talc slurry sclerosis for malignant pleural effusion. *Chest* 2005 ; 127: 909-15.

[16] West SD, Davies RJ, Lee YC. Pleurodesis for malignant pleural pleural effusion: current controversies and variations in pratices. *Curr. Opin. Pulm. Med.* 2004; 10: 305-10.

[17] Ismail-Kahn R, Robinson LA, Williams CC, Garret CR, Bepler G, Simon GR. Malignant pleural mesothelioma: a comprehensive review. *Cancer Control* 2006; 13: 255-263.

[18] Boutin C, Rey F, Viallat JR. Prevention of malignant seeding after invasive diagnostic procedures in patients with pleural mesothelioma: a randomized trial of local radiotherapy. *Chest* 1995; 108: 754-8.

[19] Martini N, Bains M, Beattie Jr E. Indications for pleurectomy in malignant effusion. Cancer 1975; 35: 734-738.

[20] Jensik R, Cagle Jr J, Milloy F, Perlia C, Taylor S, Kofman S, Beattie EJ Jr. Pleurectomy in the treatment of pleural effusion due to metastatic malignancy. *J. Thorac. Cardiovasc. Surg.* 1963; 46: 322-40.

[21] Hilaris BS, Nori D, Kwong E, Kutcher GJ, Martini N. Pleurectomy and intraoperative brachytherapy and postoperative radiation in the treatment of malignant pleural mesothelioma. *Int. J. Radiat. Oncol. Biol. Phys.* 1984;10:325-331.

[22] Antman K. Current concepts: malignant mesothelioma. *New Engl. J. Med.* 1980; 303: 200-2.

[23] McCormack PM, Nagasaki F, Hilaris BS, Martini N. Surgical treatment of pleural mesothelioma. *J. Thorac. Cardiovasc. Surg.* 1982; 84: 834-842.

[24] Rusch VW. Pleurectomy/decortication and adjuvant therapy for malignant mesothelioma. *Chest* 1993;103:382S-384S.

[25] Soysal O, Karaoglanoglu N, Demiracan S, Topcu S, Tastepe I, Kaya S, Unlu M, Cetin G. Pleurectomy/decortication for palliation in malignant pleural mesothelioma: results of surgery. *Eur. J. Cardiothorac. Surg.* 1997;11:210-3.

[26] Chahinian A, Pajak T, Holland J, Norton L, Ambinder R, Mandel EM. Diffuse malignant mesothelioma: prospective evaluation of 69 patients. *Ann. Intern. Med.* 1982; 6: 746-755.

[27] Law M, Gregor A, Hodson M, Bloom H, Turner-Warwick M. Malignant mesothelioma of the pleura: a study of 52 treated and 64 untreated patients. *Thorax* 1984; 39: 255-259.

[28] Martini N, McCormack PM, Bains MS, Kaiser LR, Burt ME, Hilaris BS. Pleural mesothelioma. *Ann. Thorac. Surg.* 1987;43:113-20.

[29] Alberts A, Falkson G, Goedhals L, Vorobiof D, Van der Merwe C. Malignat pleural mesothelioma: a disease unaffected by current maneuvers. *J. Clin. Oncol.* 1988; 6: 527-535.

[30] Ruffie P, Feld R, Minkin S, Cormier Y, Boutan-Laroze A, Ginsberg R, Ayoub J, Shepherd FA, Evans WK, Figueredo A, et al. Diffuse malignant mesothelioma of the pleura in Ontario and Quebec: a retrospective study of 332 patients. *J. Clin. Oncol.* 1989; 7: 1157-1168.

[31] Ball DL, Cruickshank DG. The treatment of malignant mesothelioma of the pleura: review of a 5-year experience, with special reference to radiotherapy. *Am. J. Clin. Oncol.* 1990;13:4-9.

[32] Brancatisano RP, Joseph MG, MacCaughan BC. Pleurectomy for mesothelioma. *Med. J. Aust.* 1991; 154: 455-457.

[33] Allen K, Faber L, Warren W. Malignant pleural mesothelioma: extrapleural pneumonectomy and pleurectomy. *Chest Surg. Clin. North Am.* 1994; 4: 113-126.

[34] Rusch VW, Saltz L, Venkatraman E, Ginsberg R, McCormack P, Burt M, Markman M, Kelsen D. A phase II trial of pleurectomy/decortication followed by intrapleural and systemic chemotherapy for malignant pleural mesothelioma. *J. Clin. Oncol.* 1994;12:1156-63.

[35] Lee J, Perez S, Wang H, Figlin R, Holmes C. Intrapleural chemotherapy for patients with incompletely resected malignant mesothelioma: the UCLA experience. *J. Surg. Oncol.* 1995; 60: 262-7.

[36] Sauter E, Langer C, Coia L, Goldberg M, Keller S. Optimal management of malignant mesothelioma after subtotal pleurectomy: revisiting the role of intrapleural chemotherapy and postoperative radiation. *J. Surg. Oncol.* 1995; 60: 100-5.

[37] Takita H, Dougherty T. Intracavitary photodynamic therapy for malignant pleural mesothelioma. *Semin. Surg. Oncol.* 1995; 11: 368-71.

[38] Cowan SW, Pechet TT. Pleurectomy and decortication for malignant mesothelioma. *Thorac. Surg. Clin.* 2004; 14: 517-21.

[39] Sarot I. Extrapleural pneumonectomy and pleurectomy in pulmonary tuberculosis. *Thorax* 1949; 4: 173-223.

[40] Worn H. Moeglichkeiten und Ergebnisse der chirurgischen Behandlung des malignen Pleuramesothelioms. *Thoraxchir. Vask Chir.* 1974; 22: 391-393.

[41] Butchart E, Ashcroft T, Barnsley W, Holden M. Pleuropneumonectomy in the management of diffuse malignant mesothelioma of the pleura: experience with 29 patients. *Thorax* 1976; 31: 15-24.

[42] DeLaria G, Jensik R, Faber L, Kittle C. Surgical Management of malignant mesothelioma. *Ann. Thorac. Surg.* 1978; 26: 375-82.

[43] Mineo TC. La chirurgia della pleura. I tumori maligni della pleura. Atti del XVI congresso nazionale della Società Italiana di Chirurgia Toracica. Taormina, 1978: 202-23.

[44] Kaiser LR. New therapies in the treatment of malignant pleural mesothelioma. *Semin. Thorac. Cardiovasc. Surg.* 1997; 9: 383-90.

[45] Patz EJ, Shaffer K, Piwinca-Worms D, Jochelson M, Sarin M, Sugarbaker DJ, et al. Malignant pleural mesothelioma: value of CT and MR imaging in predicted respectability. *AJR* 1992; 159: 961-6.

[46] Flores RM, Akhurst T, Gonen M, Zakowski M, Dycoco J, Larson SM, Rusch VW. Positron emission tomography predicts survival in malignant pleural mesothelioma. *J. Thorac. Cardiovasc Surg.* 2006; 132:763-8.

[47] Pilling JE, Stewart DJ, Martin-Ucar AE, Muller S, O'Byrne KJ, Waller DA. The case of routine cervical mediastinoscopy prior to radical surgery for malignant pleural mesothelioma. *Eur. J. Cardiothorac. Surg.* 2004; 25:497-501.

[48] Schouwink J, Kool L, Rutgers E, Zoetmulder F, Zandwijk N, Vijver M, Baas P. The value of chest computer tomography and cervical mediastinoscopy in the preoperative assessment of patients with malignant pleural mesothelioma. *Ann. Thorac. Surg.* 2003; 75:1715-9.

[49] Chang MY, Sugarbaker DJ. Extrapleural pneumonectomy for diffuse malignant pleural mesothelioma: techniques and complications. *Thorac. Surg. Clin.* 2004; 14: 523-30.

[50] Sugarbaker DJ, Heher E, Lee T, Couper G, Mentzer S, Corson J et al. Extrapleural pneumonectomy, chemotherapy, and radiotherapy in the treatment of diffuse malignant pleural mesothelioma. *J. Thorac. Cardiovasc. Surg.* 1991, 102: 10-14.

[51] Martensson G, Hagmar B, Zettergren L. Diagnosis and prognosis in malignant pleural mesothelioma: a prospect study. *Eur. J. Resp. Dis.* 1984; 65: 169-178.

[52] Rusch VW, Piantadosi S, Holmes EC. The role of extrapleural pneumonectomy in malignant pleural mesothelioma.Lung Cancer Study Group trial. *J. Thorac. Cardiovasc. Surg.* 1991, 102: 1-9.

[53] Edwards JG, Stewart DJ, Martin-Ucar A, Muller S, Richards C, Waller DA. The pattern of lymph node involvement influences outcome after extrapleural pneumonectomy for malignant mesothelioma. *J. Thorac. Cardiovasc. Surg.* 2006; 131: 981-7

[54] De Perrot M, Uy K, Anraku M, Tsao MS, Darling G, Waddell TK, Pierre AF, Bezjak A, Keshavjee S, Jonhston MR. Impact of lymph node metastasis on outcome after extrapleural pneumonectomy for malignant pleural mesothelioma. *J. Thorac. Cardiovasc. Surg.* 2007; 133: 111-6.

[55] Shrager JB, Sterman D, Kaiser L. Surgery and staging of malignant mesothelioma. In: Robinson B, Chahinian AP, editors. *Mesothelioma.* Martin Dunitz Ltd, London 2002: 185-99.

In: Mesothelioma from Bench Side to Clinic
Editor: Alfonso Baldi, pp. 435-441
ISBN: 978-1-60021-789-0

Chapter XXVI

Surgical Therapy of Mesothelioma: The Experience of the Regina Elena Cancer Institute

Francesco Facciolo, Enrico Melis, Felicita Corzani, Virna Cerasoli, Sandro Carlini, Gabriele Alessandrini, Michela Ricci and Micaela Maritti
National Cancer Institute "Regina Elena" (Rome)
Department of Thoracic Surgery

Abstract

In this chapter, the authors report on their own experience about the surgical treatment of pleural mesothelioma. In particular, the author describe the complete surgical protocol they use to perform extrapleural pneumonectomy.

Introduction

Malignant mesothelioma is a highly aggressive tumour arising from the serosal lining of the pleural, pericardial, and peritoneal cavity and the testicular tunica vaginalis; it exhibits a variety of histological patterns which may be confused with other types of neoplasms.

Treatment options for malignant pleural mesothelioma include surgery, radiation, chemotherapy, immunotherapy, supportive care, or some combination of these modalities. The choice of treatment is largely based on the location and/or extent of tumour and on the general conditions of patients which often present with a number of co-morbidities [1].

Complete surgical resection is the mainstay of treatment for malignant mesothelioma providing patients with the best chance for long-term survival [2]. It must be stressed, however, that radical surgery aimed at achieving macroscopic clearance of the tumour, if used as the sole form of treatment, may not entail a prognostic benefit: as a step of a multimodality treatment regime, it may however result in long-term survival. The so-called trimodality treatment (pre-operative chemotherapy (ALIMTA plus cisplatin), followed by surgery (EPP) and hemithoracic radiation) is currently the most successful therapeutic plan available for clinical stage I, II, or III (T1-3 N0-2) mesothelioma: it is intended to induce complete radiological and pathological response. of patients treated first with chemotherapy [3]. This approach stems from the traditional treatment strategy in oncology, that achieves local control with pleuropneumonectomy after a systemic chemotherapy followed by radiation therapy.

The Surgical Procedures

The role of surgery in the management of mesothelioma has largely been confined to obtaining tissue for pathological diagnosis or to achieve symptom control by pleurodesis; nevertheless, the increasing incidence of the disease together with initial reports of long-term survivors has resulted in the last few years in a more aggressive surgical approach.

Three surgical operations have been attempted and are currently available for the treatment of mesothelioma: extrapleural pneumonectomy (better known as pleuropneumonectomy), pleurectomy-decortication, and palliative limited pleurectomy [4].

Extrapleural pneumonectomy is the only procedure with a real curative rationale; it consists of an en bloc resection of the pleura, lung, ispilateral hemidiaphragm, and pericardium. Pleurectomy-decortication is an attempt to remove all grossly evident pleural disease without removing the underlying lung; the hemidiaphragm and the pericardium are also removed and reconstructed as necessary. Both pleurectomy-decortication and particularly extrapleural pneumonectomy are technically complex procedures and they are rarely performed even in referral centres.

Palliative pleurectomy involves limited resection of the parietal pleura to control pleural effusion by creating a durable pleruodesis.

Thoracoscopy and talc poudrage are only performed for strictly palliative purposes resulting in a highly effective control of effusions and providing excellent palliation for patients whose poor general conditions prevent more aggressive treatment.

Extrapleural Pneumonectomy

Extrapleural pneumonectomy has become the preferred surgical option at institutions specialized in the treatment of mesothelioma. It achieves the greatest degree of cytoreduction and allows postoperative higher radiation doses to be delivered to the ipsilateral hemithorax after the lung has been removed. It is also the only feasible procedure when a thick tumour rind obliterates the pleural space. The operative risk is largely related to the patient selection criteria and to the personal experience of the surgeon; the mortality rate ranges from 4 to 6%.

Patient Selection for Extrapleural Pneumonectomy

A careful selection and a thorough, multi-step preoperative assessment are mandatory before a patient be considered for extrapleural pneumonectomy.

1. Candidate patients need histologically proven diagnosis of stage I to III mesothelioma of the pleura (T1/T3 disease without cardiac involvement, N0/N2 disease and M0). T status can be established either clinically and radiologically or by surgical (thoracoscopic or open) chest exploration. Preoperative chest magnetic resonance imaging (MRI) and whole body computed tomography (CT) are essential in determining the extent of intrathoracic and extrathoracic disease. Testicular ultrasound must rule out any involvement of testicular tunica vaginalis.

Although PET scanning is used in some centres, it cannot yet not replace CT scan evaluation.

2. Pre-operative, pulmonary function testing, ventilation-perfusion lung scanning, and extensive, non invasive study of cardiac function are also required. More specifically, to be eligible for extrapleural pneumonectomy a patient is required to have a Karnofsky performance status higher than 70, normal liver and kidney function tests, a room air arterial PCO2 less than 45 mmHg and a room air arterial PO2 more than 65 mmHg.

Cardiac function assessment requires echocardiograpic evaluation of left and right ventricular function and must exclude t pre-existing alterations in ventricular function and/or pericardial effusion and frank invasion of pericardium. Coronary artery disease or valvular heart disease should be evaluated by radionuclide stress test (preferred) or by exercise stress test or stress echocardiogram.

In view of the restrictive nature of the pleural disease, preoperative pulmonary function tests, notably forced expiratory volume in 1 second (FEV1) and forced vital capacity (FVC), may not fully predict a patient's postoperative pulmonary function. FEV1 should be > 2L , or >35% of predicted postoperative with a DLCO > 35% of ppo FEV1 and pCO2 < 50 mmHg.

For patients in whom lung function is borderline (i.e., predicted postoperative FEV1 less than 1 L), the use of quantitative ventilation-perfusion scanning, when combined with knowledge of FEV1 and FVC, results in a reliable prediction of the postoperative lung function. (Predicted post-resection FEV1 = FEV1 x % perfusion to uninvolved lung from quantitative lung V/Q scan report).

Finally, we also perform a bronchoscopy to clean bronchial airways and allow a preoperative microbiological examination and ensure an infection risk-free surgical intervention.

VATS and Talc Pleurodesis

We perform a video assisted thoracoscopy in all patients with high degree of suspicion of malignant pleural mesothelioma. The diagnostic accuracy of thoracoscopy is comparable to open thoracotomy and the procedure is far less invasive VATS indications include need of staging, diagnosis and palliative treatment of malignant pleural mesothelioma. Thoracoscopic exploration allows examination of parietal, visceral, diaphragmatic and mediastinal pleura, inspection of pericardium and yields high quality biopsy samples. It is not uncommon to find a pleura covered by fibrinous exudate which needs to be removed to expose parietal pleural tissue adequate for biosy.

In patients undergoing extrapleural pneumonectomy, carefully selected thoracoscopic incisions should be performed along the projection line of the possible future thoracotomy as recurrences along surgical incisions often developr.

Talc poudrage results in a highly effective control of pleural effusion and provides excellent palliation for patients whose general medical condition discourage a more aggressive treatment. Nevertheless thoracoscopy and talc pleurodesis facilitates subsequent extrapleural dissection and prevent intraoperative spillage of malignant cells during extrapleural pneumonectomy.

As already mentioned, the risk of recurrences along the surgical incisions is high and these appear as painful skin nodules. They are quite radio-sensitive: early irradiation of surgical skin incisions should therefore be done on a regular basis.

Surgical Technique

After induction of anesthesia and intubation with a double lumen endotracheal tube, the patient is placed in the lateral decubitus position. Intraoperative monitoring includes use of a central venous pressure line, arterial line and a pulse oximeter.

A nasogastric tube should be placed to facilitate palpation of the esophagus during the dissection in the right pleuropneumonectomy and to maintain a decompressed stomach postoperatively, particularly in the setting of a neodiaphragm.

Thoracic epidural catheters are placed preoperatively and may be used for intraoperative management and postoperative pain control.

The patient's hemithorax is approached via an extended posterolateral thoracotomy incision along the bed of the sixth rib from 2 cm lateral to the costovertebral junction following the bed of the sixth rib to the costochondral junction; the anterior part of the sixth rib is taken down towards the costal margin to facilitate exposure to the hemidiaphragm. We always use and recommend an additional parallel incision at the 9th or 10th intercostal space posteriorly to grant a better exposition and resection of the diaphragm.

After periosteal stripping, the sixth rib is excised in its entirety to provide adequate exposure. The posterior periosteum, in the bed of the excised sixth rib, is then incised, and a widely based extrapleural dissection is advanced. The brachial triangle is exposed carefully to avoid avulsion of the subclavian artery and vein. In general, the parietal pleura thins out in this region, and special attention must be paid to the plane of dissection.

The parietal pleural tumour is mobilized away from the chest wall in the extrapleural plane, carrying the dissection to the apex of the hemithorax superiorly to the diaphragm inferiorly, to the sternum anteriorly and to the spine posteriorly. The internal mammary artery and vein must be protected from injury, because they can be easily avulsed from the the subclavian artery and superior vena cava respectively.

The dissection is carried out in the extrapleural space until the main stem bronchus and upper lobes are visualized.

Pericardium is then opened and the pericardial space is palpated to check for neoplastic invasion. Posteriorly, palapation must exclude aortic or esophageal invasion.

Once no evidence of unresectable disease is ascertain, attention is turned to the diaphragmatic resection. Dissection of the diaphragmatic tumour and diaphragm is carried from the lateral towards the medial aspect back to the pericardium, and then up on the pericardium to the level of the inferior pulmonary vein.

The diaphragm is dissected off the peritoneum by blunt dissection using a sponge stick. Sometimes the peritoneum has to be opened in a small area at the level of the central tendon of the diaphragm; if it occurs, the peritoneum should be immediately reclosed, usually with absorbable suture.

For right sided resections, particular care should be taken to identify the small branches of the front vessels which drain from the diaphragm into the inferior vena cava and to ligate and divide such branches.

After the diaphragm has been divided anteriorly to the pericardium, it is incised along the caval-esophageal hiatuses. The pericardium is incised to fully view the inferior vena cava during division of the diaphragm. Palpation of the nasogastric tube during the posterior portion of the dissection helps prevent inadvertent injury to the esophagus and facilitates mobilization of the specimen from the aorta to the esophagus. Then just lateral to the inferior vena cava and the esophagus, the posterior diaphragmatic attachments are divided. The diaphragmatic incision is now completed. Completion of the pericardial incision is performed anteromedially to the phrenic nerve and hilar vessels.

The dissection on the left side is less difficult than the right side because of the position of the caval, aortic and esophageal hiatuses. During dissection of the posteromedial aspect of the specimen, it is very important to enter the correct plane in the preaortic region to prevent avulsion of the intercostal vessels; intercostal vessels or the aorta itself may also be injured during the dissection of the aortodiaphragmatic hiatus. The assessment of the aorta is the critical step on the left side in determining tumour resecability because aortic involvement may preclude resection.

Main pulmonary arteries are dissected intrapericardially. Left main pulmonary artery, being much shorter than the right main pulmonary artery, should be dissected and divided in an extrapleural plane to prevent encroachment upon the right pulmonary artery.

The superior and inferior pulmonary veins are each stapled between two lines of vascular staples. The pericardial resection is then completed by dividing the pericardium posterior to the hilum.

At this point, a subcarinal lymph node dissection is usually carried out and the mainstem bronchus fully mobilized. Once the mainstem bronchus has been mobilized, it is dissected as far as the carina and stapled with a heavy gauge wire bronchial stapler. The left main stem bronchus must be dissected up to the carina to ensure a short bronchial stump.

The surgical specimen is then brought forward anteriorly. Radical lymph node dissection of level 8, 9 and additional levels of mediastinal lymph nodes is always performed.

A pericardial fat pad based on a superior vascular pedicle is raised and rotated over the bronchial stump. It is secured circumferentially around the stump using self-absorbing 3-0 sutures.

The pericardial defect is usually reconstructed with non-absorbable (preferably Gore-tex) patch. On the right side reconstruction is always necessary to prevent cardiac herniation. A 0.1 mm syntetic membrane (Gore-Tex) is secured to the posterior, inferior and anterior pericardial margins with running 3-0 polypropylene sutures. It is also tacked superiorly in several places to prevent superior displacement of the heart. On the left side the risk of cardiac herniation is low. The heart is tethered by the cavae and projected into the left hemithorax; therefore, although the heart can rotate or herniate into an empty right hemithorax, it will not herniate into an empty left hemithorax. Nevertheless if a small pericardial resection is carried out, risk of strangulation of the left ventricular apex exists.

The diaphragm is also always reconstructed using a prosthetic impermeable patch (2 mm Gore-Tex) that is sewn with a running monofilament 0 suture in polypropylene. The diaphragm patch is secured posteriorly to the remaining diaphragma and the endothoracic fascia, medially to the hiatal musculature and to the rim of remaining diaphragm along the pericardium, anteriorly to the chest wall with sutures placed around the ribs (8th, 9th and 10th ribs). Particular care should be taken to secure this appropriately to and around the esophagus to prevent postoperative intrathoracic herniation of abdominal contents at that level.

The prosthetic patch should be placed as low as possible to mimic the normal position of the diaphragm.

Hemostasis in the operated hemithorax is therefore completed and a chest tube is inserted and placed to balanced drainage (such as a pneumonectomy Pleur-Evac). The thoracotomic incision is closed as usual but care should be taken to achieve a completely watertight seal during the closure. It is particularly important to achieve good approximation and watertight closure of the intercostal muscles to prevent pleural fluid from leaking out of the hemithorax in the immediate postoperative period.

The chest tube is usually left in place for up to 72 hours, until the pleural fluid draining through the chest tube has become serous or serosanguinous, rather than bloody. Chest tube removal is accompanied by closure of the chest tube site with a skin suture to prevent postoperative fluid leakage from that site.

Postoperative Management

Perioperative antibiotic coverage is provided according to institutional guidelines for the entire length of time that the chest tube is in place. Perioperative antiarrhythmia prophylaxis should be considered, again according to institutional guidelines. Deep vein thrombosis prophylaxis is done with subcutaneous heparin. Pain control is vital to minimize postoperative atelectasis and its resulting pulmonary dysfunction.

Patients are placed on bedrest for 48 hours postoperatively to facilitate mediastinal stability and monitored in a thoracic stepdown unit with arterial lines, central venous lines, continuous oximetry, and respiratory rate monitors. After 48 hours, ambulation and chest physiotherapy are routine.

1-L 24 hours fluid restriction for 3 to 5 days postoperatively is routinely placed owing to the tendency of patients to retain fluid and have mild episodes of capillary leak in the remaining lung, which can lead to desaturation. Desaturation of oxygen levels is usually treated with diuresis and chest physiotherapy. If this is not effective, bronchoscopy is carried out. Daily chest radiographs are closely evaluated for mediastinal shift that might lead to tamponade or in-flow obstruction. Risk of contralateral infiltrates are treated aggressively. Because the nasogastric tube can prevent effective coughing, the tube is removed on postoperative day 1 if clinical parameters are acceptable. The patient, however should avoid any oral intake until evidence exists of return of gastric function, because aspiration has high morbidity in this group of patients.

Clinical Results

The mortality rate of extrapleural pneumonectomy is comparable, at present, to that of standard pneumonectomy, ranging about 3.8%. Accurate patient selection, advances in preoperative and intraoperative management and postoperative care are very important factors in achieving such low mortality. Cell type, adequate surgical resection margins and node status when combined with chemotherapy and radiation therapy have been shown to be of prognostic importance. Patients with epithelial cell pleural mesothelioma enjoy a survival advantage over patients with mixed or pure sarcomatous type treated with surgery, chemotherapy, and radiation therapy. The inability to obtain negative resection margins or the presence of nodal involvement at the time of surgical resection are predictors of poorer survival. At multivariate analyses, epithelial pattern, negative lymph nodes and negative resection margins are independent prognostic factor for better survival (2-year and 5-year survival 68% and 46%, respectively).

References

[1] Bruces WS Robinson, Richard A Lake, Advances in malignant mesothelioma. *N. Engl. J. Med.* 2005; 353: 1591-603.

[2] Robinson BW, Musk AW, Lake RA, Malignant mesothelioma. *Lancet* 2005 Jul 30-Aug 5; 366(9483): 397-408.

[3] Sterman DH, Albelda SM. Adavances in the diagnosis, evaluation, and management of malignant pleural mesothelioma. *Respirology* 2005;10:266-83.

[4] Scagliotti GV, Novello S, State of the art in mesothelioma. *Annals of Oncology* 16 (Supplement 2) 2005: ii240-ii245.

In: Mesothelioma from Bench Side to Clinic
Editor: Alfonso Baldi, pp. 443-467

ISBN: 978-1-60021-789-0

Chapter XXVII

Cytoreductive Surgery Combined with Perioperative Intraperitoneal Chemotherapy for Diffuse Malignant Peritoneal Mesothelioma - Prognostic Features of Long-Term Survivors

Tristan D. Yan and Paul H. Sugarbaker*
Program of Peritoneal Surface Malignancy, Washington Cancer Institute,
Washington Cancer Institute, Washington, DC, USA

Condensed Abstract

Cytoreductive surgery combined with perioperative intraperitoneal chemotherapy has shown promising survival results in patients with diffuse malignant peritoneal mesothelioma. A prospective cohort of 50 patients who underwent the combined treatment, with extended follow-up, demonstrated that female gender and adequate cytoreduction were independently associated with 3-year and 5-year survivors.

Abstract

Background: Cytoreductive surgery (CRS) combined with perioperative intraperitoneal chemotherapy (PIC) has demonstrated an improved survival in patients with diffuse malignant peritoneal mesothelioma (DMPM), as compared to historical controls. However, there have been no reported data on the characteristics of long-term survivors.

* Correspondence: Dr. Paul H. Sugarbaker, Washington Cancer Institute, 106 Irving Street, NW, Suite 3900N, Washington, DC, U.S.A. 20010; Tel #: (202) 877-3908; Fax #: (202) 877-8602 and e-mail: Paul.Sugarbaker@medstar.net

Methods: A prospective cohort of 50 DMPM patients who underwent CRS and PIC with a minimum of 5-year follow-up was analyzed for their overall survival. Univariate and multivariate analyses were performed to evaluate the correlations of clinicopathologic and treatment-related parameters with long-term survivors.

Results: The actual 3-year and 5-year survival rates were 54% and 44%, respectively. Female gender and adequate cytoreduction were independently associated with both 3-year and 5-year survivors. The actual 3-year and 5-year survival rates in female patients were 81% and 63%, respectively; in male patients were 41% and 32%, respectively; in patients who received adequate cytoreduction were 71% and 58%, respectively and in patients who received suboptimal cytoreduction were 26% and 16%, respectively.

Conclusion: CRS and PIC can achieve long-term survival in patients with DMPM. Gender and completeness of cytoreduction were most significant predictors for long-term survivors.

Keywords: *Malignant peritoneal mesothelioma, cytoreductive surgery, peritonectomy, intraperitoneal chemotherapy.*

Introduction

Diffuse malignant peritoneal chemotherapy (DMPM) is a rare disease and represents one-third of all mesotheliomas. The annual incidence of DMPM is 300 to 400 cases in the United States [1-2]. It is characterized macroscopically by thousands of whitish tumor nodules of variable size and consistency that may coalesce to form plaques or masses or layer out to uniformly cover the entire peritoneal surface (Figure 1). DMPM is a rapidly fatal disease, without aggressive surgical treatments, a long-tem survival is difficult to achieve [3-9]. Prior to the year 2000, DMPM was treated at most cancer centers with a combination of systemic chemotherapy, palliative surgery and in a few patients with total abdominal radiation. However, the DMPM patients did not seem to respond to these treatments, in that median survivals were uniformly of approximately one year [3-9]. No randomized trials were performed, but it is likely that the survival associated with this approach was little changed from the natural course of the disease. Table 1 shows the results of treatment using traditional treatment modalities for DMPM [3-9].

Because the advance of DMPM is limited to local-regional progression, an aggressive treatment plan to surgically eradicate gross disease combined with intraperitoneal chemotherapy to control residual disease has a strong rationale. As the cytoreductive surgical approach utilizing peritonectomy was expended, it was combined with intraperitoneal hyperthermic chemotherapy (IPHC) as a planned treatment strategy. Although little uniformity of the surgical approach has occurred and many different hyperthermic chemotherapy regimes exist, the results of treatment of DMPM have dramatically changed. Table 2 shows the results of treatment using CRS and IPHC. The median survival has approached 5 years and seems to improve with subsequent reports [10-18].

However, more precise long-term survival results and prognostic parameters can only be obtained by assessment of actual long-term survivors.

Table 1. Median survival of diffuse malignant peritoneal mesothelioma using traditional treatment modalities

Chief Investigators	Year	No. of patients	Median Survival (months)
Chailleux et al.[3]	1988	11/167	10*
Antman et al. [4]	1988	37/180	15*
Sridhar et al. [5]	1992	13/50	9.5*
Markman et al.[6]	1992	19	9
Yates et al.[7]	1997	14/272	14*
Neumann et al.[8]	1999	74	12 (mean)
Eltabbakl et al.[9]	1999	15**	12.5

* : Combined/pleural.

** : All females.

Table 2. Median survival of diffuse malignant peritoneal mesothelioma using combined treatment of cytoreductive surgery and hyperthermic intraoperative intraperitoneal chemotherapy

Chief Investigators	Year	No. of patients	Median Survival (months)
Park et al. [10]	1999	18	26
Loggie et al. [11]	2001	12	34
Kerrigan et al. [12]	2002	25**	30
Alexander et al. [13]	2003	49	92
Sugarbaker et al. [14]	2003	67	68
Glehen et al. [15]	2005	15	46.7
Deraco et al. [16]	2005	49	N/A
Taub et al. [17]	2005	27	68
Sugarbaker et al. [18]	2005	65***	79

N/A : median survival has not been reached.

** : All females.

***: Sixty-five out of 100 patients received cytoreductive surgery, hyperthermic intraoperative intraperitoneal chemotherapy (cisplatin+doxorubicin) and early postoperative intraperitoneal paclitaxel.

A cohort of patients with adequate length of follow-up and sufficient number of long-term survivors is prerequisite for such a study. However, cytoreductive surgery with perioperative intraperitoneal chemotherapy has only become a treatment option for DMPM over the last decade and because the disease is so rare, most centers simply do not have sufficient number of patients. To the best of our knowledge, in the current literature, there have been no reported data on the prognostic features of long-term survivors (> 5 years) after these combined treatments for DMPM. However, the elucidation of this issue is very important in the future management of these patients.

The primary aim of this study was to evaluate prognostic features of long-term survivors in a prospective cohort of 50 patients who have been observed for more than 5 years, after cytoreductive surgery with perioperative intraperitoneal chemotherapy for DMPM, at the Washington Cancer Institute, Washington DC.

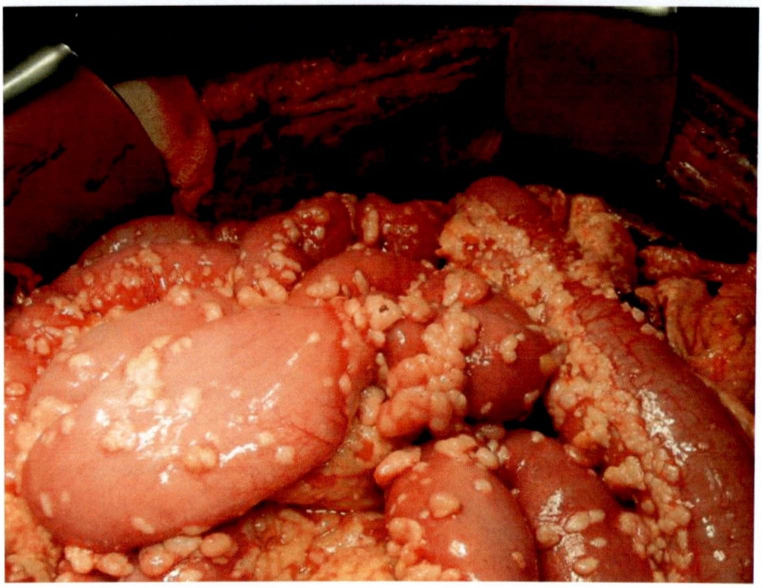

Figure 1. Intraoperative photograph of the visceral peritoneal surface of a patient with diffuse malignant peritoneal mesothelioma. Multiple whitish tumor nodules of variable sizes and shapes are distributed throughout the peritoneal surface.

Patients and Methods

Between September 1989 and November 2005, a total of 100 patients with DMPM were managed at the Washington Cancer Institute, Washington DC. Up until September 2000, 50 patients underwent cytoreductive surgery with perioperative intraperitoneal chemotherapy with an intention to achieve long-term survival. All of these 50 patients have been observed for more than 5 years from the time of cytoreductive surgery. The median follow-up was 75 months (range 61 to 144 months). These 50 patients formed the basis of this study.

Preoperative Management

All patients underwent extensive preoperative investigations, which included a physical examination, and abdominal, pelvic and chest computed tomography (CT) scans to assess the extent of the disease. Measurements of relevant tumor markers (e.g., CA 15-3, CA 19-9, CA 72-4, CA 125 and Carcino-embryonic Antigen) were also obtained. Patients with good performance status were considered for surgery. Mechanical bowel prep was performed in all patients. Oral antibiotics were not administered. Intrajugular or subclavian central venous catheters were inserted in all patients. Cefazolin 1 g every 4 hours and metronidazole 500 mg every 4 hours were began approximately 1 hour prior to the surgical procedure and were continued throughout the cytoreduction. Patients were positioned in lithotomy position with the legs extended in St. Mark's leg-holders. The weight of the legs was directed to the soles of the feet by positioning on the footrests so that minimal weight was on the calf muscles. The calves were protected with foam padding to avoid possible myonecrosis and were then wrapped with alternating-pressure boots to prevent deep venous thrombosis.

Cytoreductive Surgery

The goal of cytoreductive surgery was to maximally reduce tumor burden to a nodule size that would be penetrated by the diffusion of hyperthermic chemotherapy solution. The volume and extent of the tumor deposits were prospectively recorded in each of the 13 abdominopelvic regions (AR) using the Peritoneal Cancer Index (PCI), which is an assessment combining lesion size (LS-0 to LS-3) with tumor distribution (AR-0 to AR-12), to quantify the extent of disease as a numerical score (PCI-0 to PCI-39) (Figure 2) [19]. Lesion size-0 indicates no tumor visible; Lesion size-1 indicates nodules ≤ 5 mm; Lesion size-2 indicates nodules between 5 mm and 5 cm; and Lesion size-3 indicates nodules > 5 cm or a confluence of disease. The abdominopelvic cavity was divided with two transverse and two sagittal planes into nine regions (Abdominopelvic Region 0 to 8).

The two transverse planes were placed though the lowest aspect of the costal margin and the anterior superior iliac spine. The two sagittal planes were places through the mid-clavicular points. Abdominopelvic Regions 9 - 12 were defined as upper and lower portions of jejunum and upper and lower portions of ileum, respectively. The summation of the lesion size score in all of the 13 regions is the PCI for the individual patient.

The cytoreductive surgery was performed by using electroevaporative surgery with a ball-tipped diathermy at a maximum electrical power (Figure 3) [20]. It consisted of a series of peritonectomy procedures and visceral resections. Peritonectomy procedures included total anterior parietal peritonectomy, omentectomy ± splenectomy, right and left subphrenic peritonectomy, pelvic peritonectomy, and lesser omentectomy with stripping of the omental bursa ± cholecystectomy. The visceral resections included rectosigmoidectomy, right colectomy, total abdominal colectomy, hysterectomy and small bowel resection. The details of the techniques have been described previously [20]. All resected specimens were submitted to histopathology and all positive findings were documented. For the purpose of this study, the extent of cytoreductive surgery was determined as the number of peritonectomy procedures performed in each patient and categorized as either ≤ 4 peritonectomy procedures or > 4 peritonectomy procedures.

All sites and volumes of the residual disease following the cytoreductive surgery were also prospectively recorded using the Completeness of Cytoreduction Score (CCR) (Figure 4) [19]. A CCR-0 indicated no visible evidence of mesothelioma. CCR-1 indicated residual tumor nodule ≤ 2.5 mm in diameter. CCR-2 indicated residual tumor nodule between 2.5 mm and 2.5 cm in diameter. CCR-3 indicated residual tumor module > 2.5 cm in diameter or a confluence of tumor nodules present at any site.

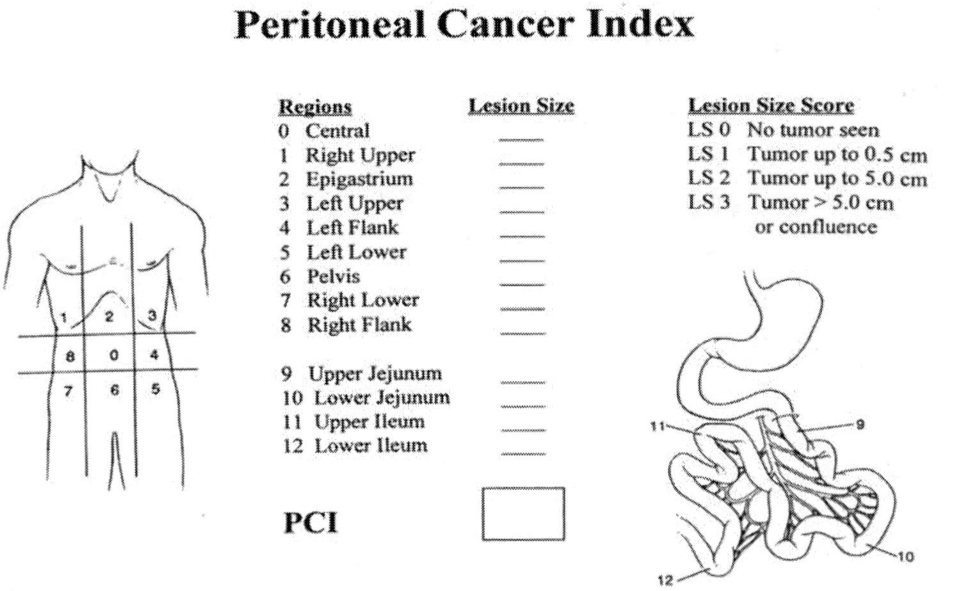

Figure 2. Peritoneal Cancer Index (PCI) – The lesion size assessment (LS-0 to LS-3) is combined with the tumor distribution assessment (13 abdominopelvic regions of AR-0 to AR-12) to quantify the extent of disease as a numerical score (PCI-0 to PCI-39).

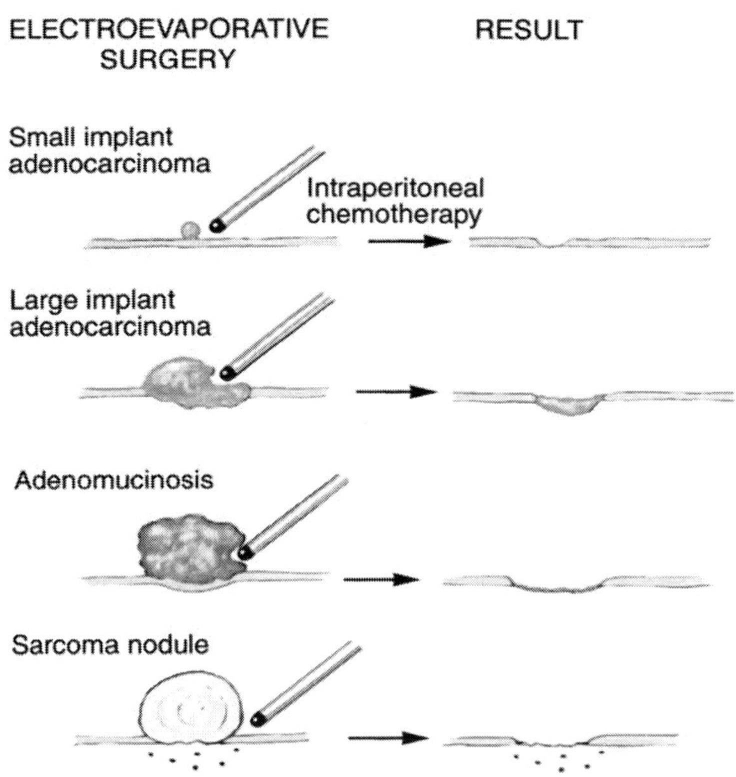

Figure 3. Diagram depicting electroevaporative surgery using a 0.3 cm diathermy tip.

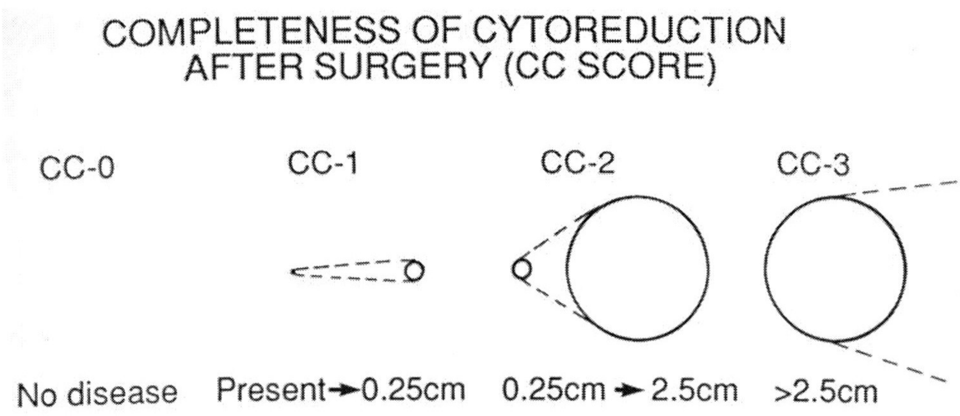

Figure 4. Completeness of Cytoreduction Score (CCR): a CCR-0 indicated no visible evidence of mesothelioma; CCR-1 indicated residual tumor nodule ≤ 2.5 mm in diameter; CCR-2 indicated residual tumor nodule between 2.5 mm and 2.5 cm in diameter; CCR-3 indicated residual tumor module > 2.5 cm in diameter or a confluence of tumor nodules present at any site.

Evolution of Perioperative Intraperitoneal Chemotherapy

Over the study period, increasingly aggressive chemotherapy regimens have evolved for DMPM at our institution [14]. The initial 9 patients were treated with induction intraperitoneal chemotherapy using cisplatin (15 mg/m^2 per day) and doxorubicin (6 mg/m^2 per day) for 5 days before CRS. They also received early postoperative intraperitoneal chemotherapy (EPIC) using mitomycin C (MMC) and 5-fluorouracil (5-FU) with or without long-term intraperitoneal chemotherapy. The next 24 patients underwent CRS combined with hyperthermic intraperitoneal chemotherapy (IPHC) using cisplatin (50 mg/m^2) and doxorubicin (15 mg/m^2) at approximately 42°C in 3 L of peritoneal dialysis solution for 90 minutes. In the remaining 17 patients, by the intention to treat principle all patients were to receive CRS, IPHC (cisplatin and doxorubicin) and additional EPIC with paclitaxel (20 mg/m^2 per day) from postoperative day 1 to day 5.

Intraperitoneal Hyperthermic Chemotherapy (IPHC)

After the cytoreduction was complete, but prior to intestinal anastomoses or repair of seromuscular tears, the abdomen and pelvis was instilled with cisplatin (50 mg/m^2) and doxorubicin (15 mg/m^2) in the operating room at approximately 42°C in 3 L of 1.5% dextrose peritoneal dialysis solution for 90 minutes [14]. The intraperitoneal chemotherapy solution was manually distributed to facilitate maximal contact and penetration of the chemotherapy into residual cancer cells. Figure 5 depicts the apparatus used for IPHC in open technique.

The pharmacokinetics of cisplatin and doxorubicin administered intraperitoneally at 42°C are illustrated in Figure 6 and Figure 7. The pharmacological data in these mesothelioma patients for cisplatin is what has been reported for this chemotherapy agent with multiple different tumor types.

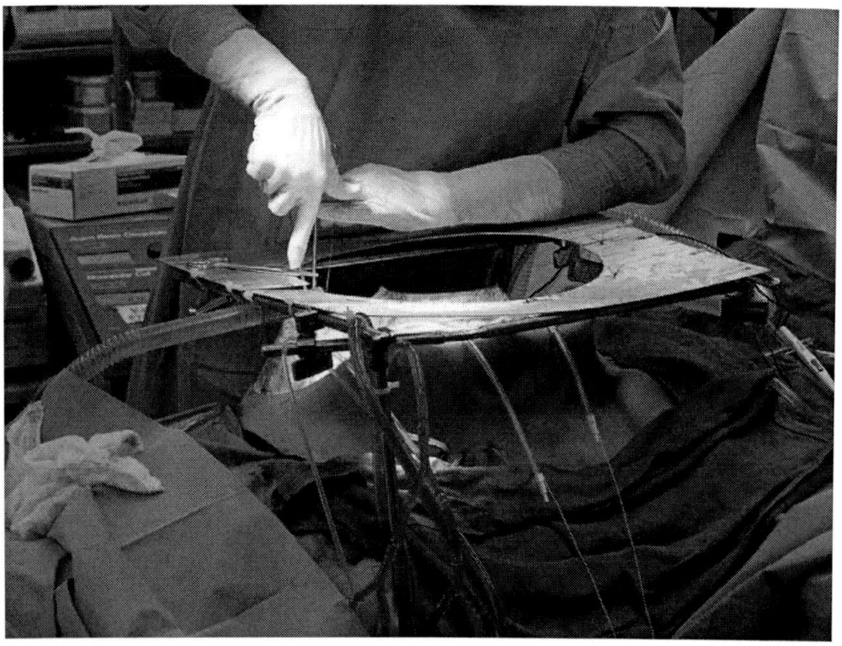

Figure 5. Photograph demonstrating the apparatus used for intraperitoneal hyperthermic chemotherapy (open technique).

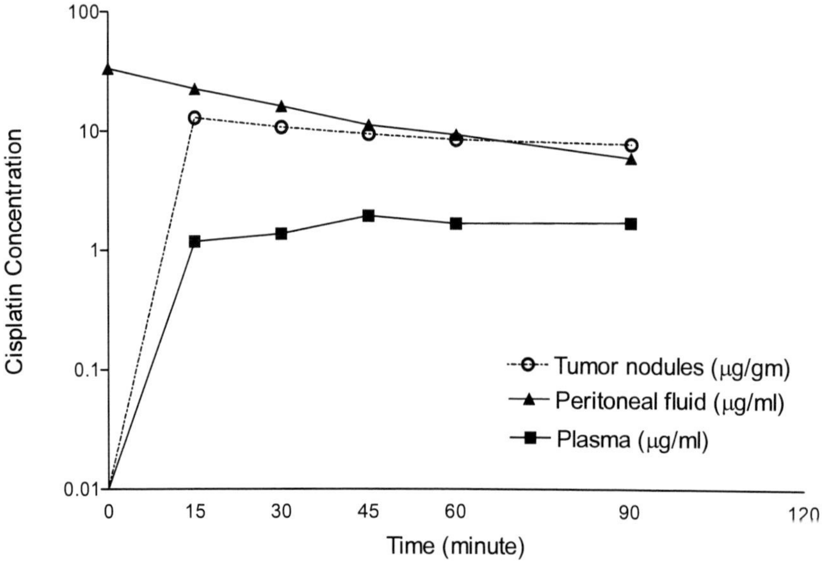

Figure 6. Pharmacokinetics of cisplatin (50 mg/m2) in 3 L of 1.5% dextrose peritoneal dialysis solution administered intraperitoneally at 42oC over 90 minutes.

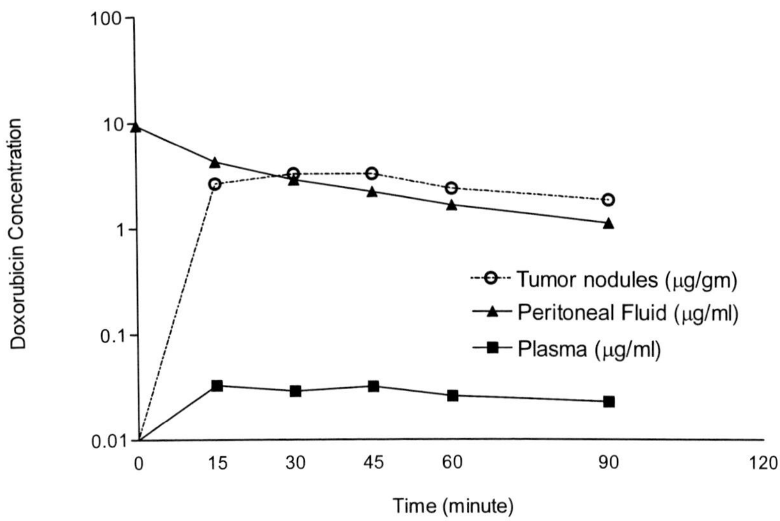

Figure 7. Pharmacokinetics of doxorubicin (15 mg/m2) in 3 L of 1.5% dextrose peritoneal dialysis solution administered intraperitoneally at 42oC over 90 minutes.

In contrast, the doxorubicin content in small mesothelioma nodules far surpasses that measured in the peritoneal fluid. An active uptake of doxorubicin by DMPM is possible and would be expected to result in a maximal response. The standardized orders for IPHC using cisplatin and doxorubicin at the Washington Cancer Institute are shown in Table 3.

Following the completion of heated intraoperative intraperitoneal chemotherapy, bowel anastomoses, plication of seromuscular tears and then abdominal closure were completed. All anastomoses and bowel closures were hand-sewn with two-layer sutures, except for colorectal anastomoses, which were performed with an intraluminal stapler of 33-mm diameter.

Table 3. Physician's orders for hyperthermic intraoperative intraperitoneal chemotherapy for mesothelioma

(1) Add cisplatin _____ mg to 2 L of 1.5% dextrose peritoneal dialysis solution. Dose of cisplatin 50 mg/m^2

(2) Add doxorubicin _____ mg to same 2 L of 1.5% dextrose peritoneal dialysis solution. Dose of doxorubicin 15 mg/m^2

(3) Send the above to operating room _____ at _____ o'clock for 90-minute irrigation at 42°C

(4) Administer with _____ ml 1.5% dextrose peritoneal dialysis solution for a total of 1.5 L/m^2 of intraperitoneal chemotherapy solution

Closed-suction drains remained in place postoperatively in all patients. One drain was placed beneath the right hemidiaphragm, another beneath the left hemidiaphragm, and two were left in the pelvis. A fifth closed-suction drain was placed within the subcutaneous space in the midline abdominal wound. Thoracostomy tubes were used whenever a patient had a subphrenic peritonectomy. The tubes were removed in the second postoperative week as drainage diminished.

Early Postoperative Intraperitoneal Chemotherapy (EPIC)

Different chemotherapy agents have variable mechanisms of actions to cause cancer cell death. Drugs used intraoperatively are chosen because they are augmented by heat and have a rapid effect to initiate cancer cell death. Other chemotherapy agents are not augmented by heat and require cell division to cause cancer cell death. Paclitaxel is an agent routinely used at the Washington Cancer Institute for DMPM.

The tubes and drains positioned for the heated intraoperative intraperitoneal chemotherapy were preserved for early postoperative intraperitoneal chemotherapy with paclitaxel at 20 mg/m^2 per day in 1 L of 1.5% dextrose peritoneal dialysis solution or 6% hetastarch solution from postoperative day 1 to day 5 [14]. After instillation, gravity distribution of the chemotherapy solution was achieved by turning the patient from the full right lateral position to the full left lateral position and back every 30 minutes for the first 6 hours. Patients were flat in bed in order to minimize pooling of chemotherapy solution in the pelvis. The intraperitoneal chemotherapy was allowed to dwell for 23 hours and was then removed by closed suction drains over the course of 1 hour. When the abdomen was cleared of fluid as completely as possible, the next instillation was commenced.

The pharmacokinetics of early postoperative intraperitoneal paclitaxel is shown in Figure 8. The large area under the curve ratio of peritoneal fluid concentration to plasma concentration is caused by the large molecule size of this drug. The drug is administered in a 6% hetastarch solution because the starch solution preserves as an artificial ascites and thereby maximizes the extent of peritoneal surface exposed. The standardized orders for early postoperative intraperitoneal paclitaxel are shown in Table 4.

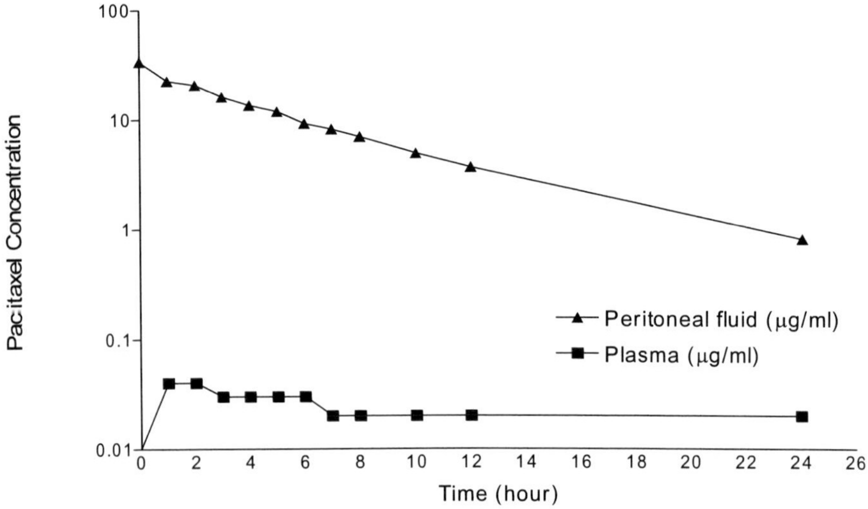

Figure 8. Pharmacokinetics of paclitaxel (20 mg/m2) in 1 L of 6% hetastarch solution administered intraperitoneally during the first 24-hour instillation.

Table 4. Physician's orders for early postoperative intraperitoneal chemotherapy with paclitaxel on postoperative day 1 to 5

(1) Paclitaxel _____ mg (20 mg/m^2 x _____ m^2) in _____ cc 6% Hetastarch via IP catheter on _____. Last dose _____
(2) Infusion as rapidly as possible via Tenckhoff catheter. Dwell for 23 hours. Drain from Tenckhoff x 15 minutes before draining all catheters for one hour prior to next instillation
(3) Continue to drain abdominal cavity after last dose until Tenckhoff catheter is removed
(4) During the initial 6 hours after chemotherapy infusion, the patient's bed should be kept flat. The patient should be on the right side during infusion. Turn at 30 minutes post infusion onto the left side and continue to change sides at 30-minute intervals for 6 hours

Monitor with pulse oximeter during the first 6 hours of intraperitoneal chemotherapy instillation.

By the "intention to treat" principle, all patients were to receive perioperative intraperitoneal chemotherapy, unless they had postoperative bleeding, hemodynamic instability or other complications early in the postoperative period were exempt from EPIC.

Study Methods

No antibiotics were used postoperatively, except to treat a specific organism causing clinically significant infection identified in follow-up. The prophylaxis for venous thrombosis and pulmonary embolus was limited to the use of sequential compression devices that were applied to the legs. These sequential compression devices were utilized throughout the hospitalization except when the patient was ambulating or up in the chair. No prophylactic anticoagulants were used; intravenous heparin was used to treat an identified venous thrombosis or pulmonary embolus. Filgastrim (Amgen, Thousand Oaks, CA) was used if the total white blood cell count fell below 2,000. The treatment was with 400 mcg a day until neutrophil counts returned to normal. Granulocyte colony stimulating factors were not used prophylactically. No pre- or post-splenectomy vaccinations were ordered on any of these patients. All patients received postoperative total parental nutrition until their caloric intake was adequate.

With an aim of constantly monitoring the postoperative and survival results in these patients, all the clinicopathologic, operative, perioperative and follow-up data were prospective collected and entered into a computerized database by a research assistant during this study period. Perioperative morbidity data were recorded at the time of a discharge summary being dictated and further stratified into different categories by their severity. For a mild adverse event, only medical treatment was required for resolution. For a moderate adverse event, an invasive intervention was required for resolution, such as a CT- or ultrasound-guided diagnostic or therapeutic intervention(s). For a severe adverse event, a definitive urgent intervention, such as returning to the operating room or returning to the surgical intensive care unit was required.

After hospital discharge, all patients were then followed at 6-monthly intervals with physical examination and measurement of serum CA-125. Abdominopelvic CT scans were performed every 6-months.

The overall survival was determined from the time of cytoreductive surgery. All patients were followed until November 2005 or until death. Institutional review board approval was obtained to review and analyze these data. Actual 3-year and 5-year survivors were analyzed by for their association with all prospective collected clinical variables. For univariate analysis, Chi-square (or Fisher's exact) test was used for categorical factors and Wilcoxon rank test was used for the comparison of difference in means of continuous factors. Logistic regression was used for the multivariate analysis to identify the independent factors predictive of 3-year and 5-year survivors. These statistical analyses were performed using SPSS for Windows (Version 11.5; SPSS GmbH, Munich, Germany). A significant difference was assumed for p values of < 0.05.

Results

Between September 1989 and September 2000, a total of 50 consecutive patients who underwent cytoreductive surgery with or without perioperative intraperitoneal chemotherapy for DMPM were prospective observed for at least 5 years. The median follow-up period was 75 months (range 61 to 144 months) and all patients were followed until November 2005 or until death. The median survival was 50 months (range 1 to 144 months). Twenty-seven patients were alive at 3 years and the actual 3-year survival was 54%. Twenty-two patients were alive at 5 years and the actual 5-year survival was 44%. The estimated 10-year survival was 35% (Figure 9).

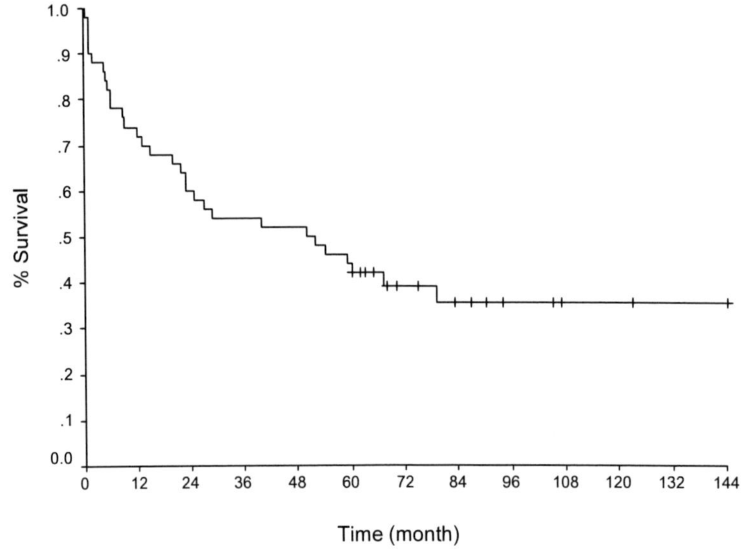

Figure 9. Overall survival curve of a prospective cohort of 50 patients who underwent cytoreductive surgery for diffuse malignant peritoneal mesothelioma, demonstrating actual survival until 60 months and actuarial survival after 60 months.

Clinicopathologic Data

There were 34 male patients (68%). The mean age at the time of the diagnosis of DMPM was 52 ±15 years. The mean age at the time of combined surgery was 52 ±15 years. Twenty patients (40%) had extensive prior surgery, with more than 5 abdominopelvic regions dissected. Nine patients (18%) had co-morbidity at the time of presentation, but this was not considered as a contraindication for undergoing cytoreductive surgery. There were 45 patients (90%) had epithelial type of DMPM and 5 patients had biphasic type of DMPM.

Treatment-Related Data

All patients underwent cytoreductive surgery with an attempt to maximally remove all visible tumors. At laparotomy, it was found that the mean number of abdominopelvic regions involved with DMPM was 11 ±4. The extent of tumor deposits was recorded as PCI (range 0 to 39), and the mean PCI was 25 ±12. The extent of cytoreductive surgery was expressed as number of peritonectomy procedures performed in each patient. The mean number of peritonectomy procedures in each patient was 4 ±2. The mean operative time was 7 ±3 hours. The mean blood loss was 712 ±984 cc. Eighteen patients (36%) had complete cytoreduction (CCR-0/CCR-1) and 13 patients (26%) had adequate cytoreduction (CCR-2). The remaining 19 patients (38%) had suboptimal cytoreduction. This happened mainly because extensive small bowel or small bowel mesenteric involvement and surgically removing all visible tumors, at the same time not sacrificing too much small bowel was almost impossible.

The overall moderate/severe perioperative morbidity rate was 38%. The incidence of moderate perioperative adverse events was 34%, with respiratory complications most common (18%). Four patients (8%) experienced severe perioperative adverse events, including 2 patients with intraabdominal bleeding and one patient with a small bowel fistula, which required returning to the operative room. The other patient had respiratory failure, which required intensive care support. Four patients (8%) died during their hospital stay, including 3 patients who died from sepsis and one patient who died from pulmonary embolism.

Univariate Analysis of Clinicopathologic Data

Table 5 demonstrates the correlation of 8 clinicopathologic parameters with actual 3-year and 5-year survivors after cytoreductive surgery for DMPM. It showed that female gender was strongly associated with both 3-year ($p = 0.014$) and 5-year survivors ($p = 0.031$).

It also showed that epithelial type of DMPM was strongly associated with 3-year survivors ($p = 0.016$) and marginally, but not statistical significantly associated with 5-year survivors ($p = 0.059$). Age at the time of diagnosis, age at the time of surgery, interval between diagnosis and surgery, time of surgery, extent of prior surgery and co-morbidity at the time of surgery were not significant in univariate analysis.

Table 5. Correlation of clinicopathologic features with actual 3-year and 5-year survivors after cytoreductive surgery for DMPM

Variable	Actual Survivors			
-	3-year n(%)	p	5-year n(%)	p
Total (n = 50)	27(54)	-	22(44)	-
Gender	-	0.014	-	0.031
Male (n = 34)	12(41)	-	11(32)	-
Female (n = 16)	13(83)	-	11(69)	-
Age at the time of diagnosis (year)	-	1.000	-	1.000
≤ 50 (n = 21)	11(52)	-	9(43)	-
> 50 (n = 29)	16(55)	-	13(45)	-
Age at the time of surgery (year)	-	0.774	-	0.733
≤ 50 (n = 20)	10(50)	-	8(40)	-
> 50 (n = 30)	17(57)	-	14(47)	-
Interval between diagnosis and surgery (month)	-	0.761	-	0.753
≤ 6 (n = 36)	20(56)	-	15(42)	-
> 6 (n = 14)	7(50)	-	7(50)	-
Time of surgery	-	0.571	-	0.393
Before January 1998 (n = 25)	12(48)	-	9(36)	-
After January 1998 (n = 25)	15(60)	-	13(52)	-
Extent of prior surgery	-	0.744	-	1.000
Laparotomy with ≤ 5 region dissected (n =30)	17(57)	-	13(43)	-
Laparotomy with > 5 region dissected (n = 20)	10(50)	-	9(45)	-
Co-morbidity at the time of surgery	-	0.394	-	1.000
No (n = 41)	23(56)	-	18(44)	-
Yes (n = 9)	4(44)	-	4(44)	-
Histopathology of peritoneal mesothelioma	-	0.016	-	0.059
Epithelial (n = 45)	27(60)	-	22(49)	-
Biphasic (n = 5)	0(0)	-	0(0)	-

Univariate Analysis of Treatment-Related Data

The correlation of 13 treatment-related parameters with actual 3-year and 5-year survivors was illustrated in Table 6. It showed that adequate cytoreduction was strongly associated with both 3-year ($p = 0.003$) and 5-year survivors ($p = 0.018$). It also showed that intraoperative blood loss of ≤ 500 cc was strongly associated with both 3-year and 5-year survivors as well. Number of abdominopelvic regions involved, peritoneal cancer index, extent of peritonectomy procedures, colonic resection, extensive enterolysis, IPHC, EPIC, duration of surgery, moderate perioperative adverse events, severe perioperative adverse events and length of hospital stay were not significant in univariate analysis.

Table 6. Correlation of operative and postoperative data with actual 3-year and 5-year survivors after cytoreductive surgery for DMPM

Variable	Actual Survivors			
-	3-year n(%)	p	5-year n(%)	p
Total (n = 50)	27(54)	-	22(44)	-
Number of abdominopelvic regions involved	-	0.332	-	0.197
≤ 10 (n = 13)	9(69)	-	8(62)	-
> 10 (n = 37)	18(49)	-	14(38)	-
Peritoneal Cancer Index	-	0.098	-	0.254
≤ 24 (n = 24)	16(67)	-	13(54)	-
> 24 (n = 36)	11(42)	-	9(35)	-
Extent of peritonectomy procedures	-	0.388	-	0.773
≤ 4 peritonectomy procedures (n = 20)	9(45)	-	8(40)	-
> 4 peritonectomy procedures (n = 30)	18(60)	-	14(47)	-
Colonic resection	-	0.254	-	0.567
No (n = 30)	14(47)	-	12(40)	-
Yes (n =20)	13(65)	-	10(50)	-
Extensive enterolysis	-	0.570	-	0.557
No (n = 23)	11(48)	-	9(39)	-
Yes (n =27)	16(59)	-	13(48)	-
Completeness of cytoreduction	-	0.003	-	0.018
Adequate (residual tumor size ≤ 2.5 cm) (n = 31)	22(71)	-	18(58)	-
Suboptimal (residual tumor size > 2.5 cm) (n = 19)	5(26)	-	4(21)	-
HIIC	-	0.183	-	0.186
No (n = 12)	4(33)	-	3(25)	-
Yes (n = 38)	23(61)	-	19(50)	-
EPIC	-	0.778	-	0.775
No (n = 29)	15(52)	-	12(41)	-
Yes (n = 21)	12(57)	-	10(48)	-
Duration of surgery (hour)	-	1.000	-	0.776
≤ 7 (n = 25)	14(56)	-	12(48)	-
> 7 (n = 25)	13(52)	-	10(40)	-
Intraoperative blood loss (cc)	-	0.021	-	0.023
≤ 500 (n = 37)	24(65)	-	20(54)	-
> 500 (n = 13)	3(23)	-	2(15)	-
Moderate perioperative adverse event	-	0.373	-	0.559
No (n = 34)	20(59)	-	16(47)	-
Yes (n = 16)	7(44)	-	6(38)	-
Severe perioperative adverse event	-	0.614	-	0.308
No (n = 46)	24(52)	-	19(41)	-
Yes (n =4)	3(75)	-	3(75)	-
Length of hospital stay (day)	-	0.733	-	0.774
≤ 21 (n = 31)	16(52)	-	13(42)	-
> 21 (n = 19)	11(58)	-	9(47)	-

HIIC: hyperthermic intraoperative intraperitoneal chemotherapy with cisplatin and doxorubicin; EPIC: early postoperative intraperitoneal chemotherapy with paclitaxel.

Multivariate Analysis for Actual 3-Year and 5-Year Survivors

All significant clinicopathologic and treatment-related parameters in univariate analysis were analyzed for their significance in multivariate analysis. Two factors were identified as independent factors predictive of 3-year survivors. They were female gender (p = 0.015; risk ratio: 0.129; 95% confidence interval: 0.25 – 0.668) and adequate cytoreduction (p = 0.005; risk ratio: 0.121; 95% confidence interval: 0.028 – 0.522).

In addition, female gender (p = 0.025; risk ratio: 0.204; 95% confidence interval: 0.051 – 0.822) and adequate cytoreduction (p = 0.018; risk ratio: 0.182; 95% confidence interval: 0.044 – 0.744) were identified as the only two factors that were independently predictive of 5-year survivors as well.

The discrepancies in actual survival results after cytoreductive surgery and perioperative intraperitoneal chemotherapy for DMPM by gender were depicted in Figure 10. It showed that the actual 3-year and 5-year survival rates in female patients were 81% and 63%, respectively, and the median survival was not reached. The actual 3-year and 5-year survival rates in male patients were 41% and 32%, respectively, with a median survival of 23 months (range 1 to 144 months).

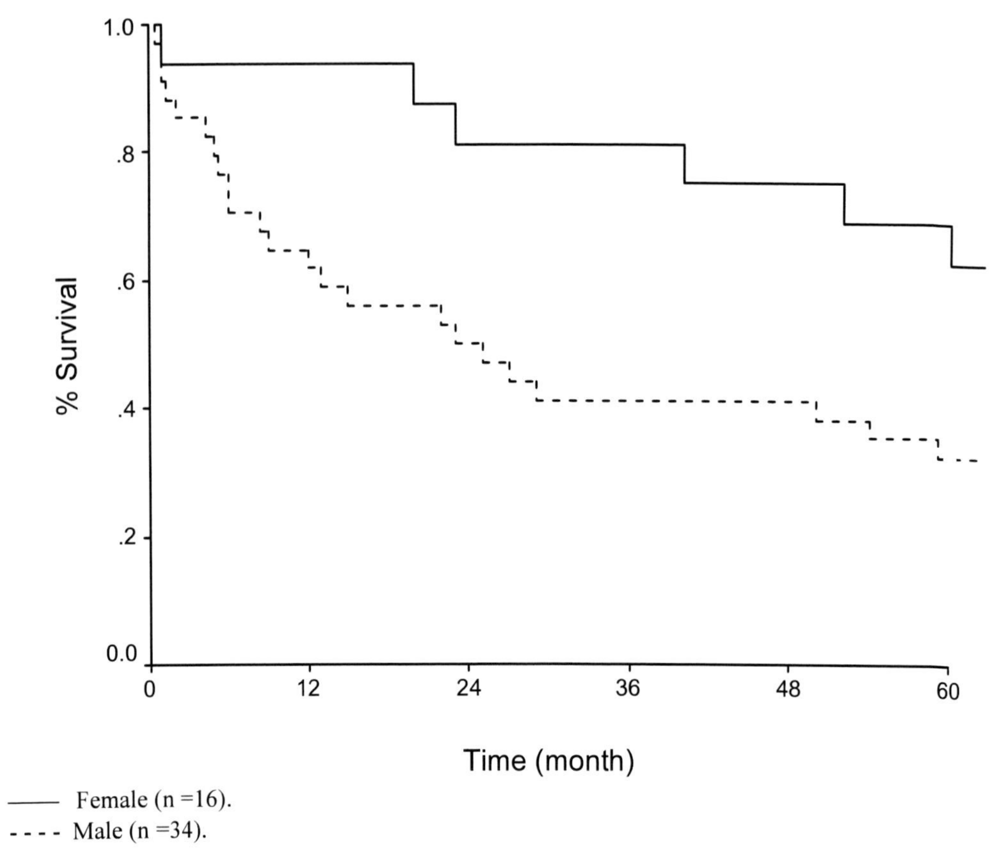

Figure 10. Actual survival results of a prospective cohort of 50 patients who underwent cytoreductive surgery for diffuse malignant peritoneal mesothelioma. Prognostic significance of gender was p = 0.012.

The discrepancies in actual survival results after cytoreductive surgery and perioperative intraperitoneal chemotherapy for DMPM by completeness of cytoreduction were depicted in Figure 11. It showed that the actual 3-year and 5-year survival rates in patients who received adequate cytoreduction were 71% and 58%, respectively, and the median survival was not reached. The actual 3-year and 5-year survival rates in patients who only received suboptimal cytoreduction were 26% and 16%, respectively, with a median survival of 12 months (range 1 to 83 months).

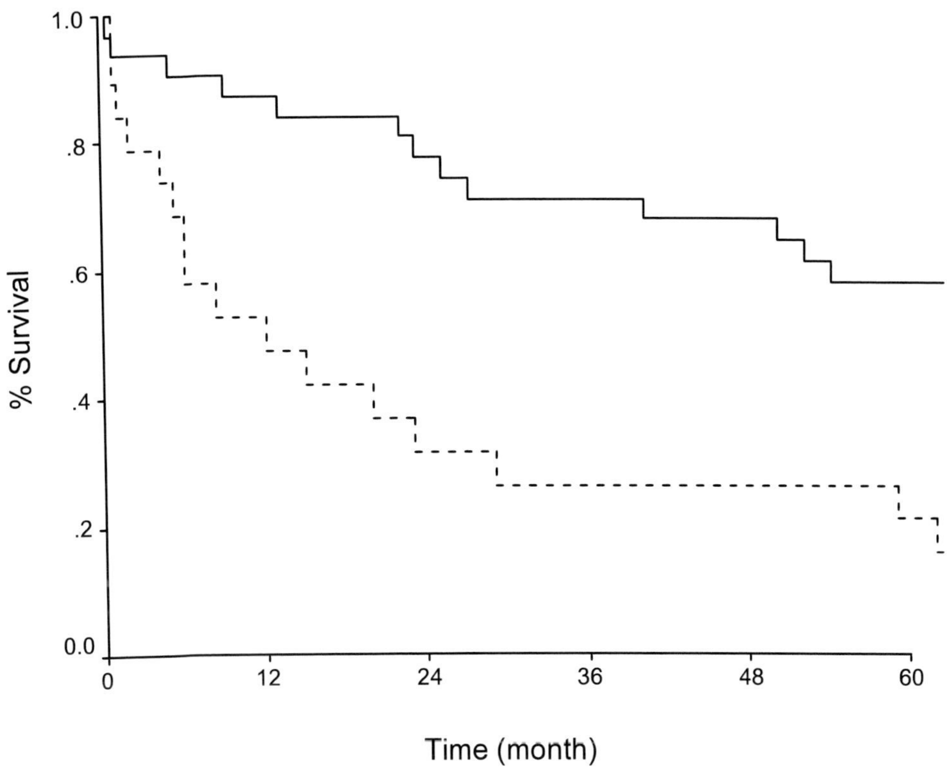

—— Adequate cytoreduction (residual tumor ≤ 2.5 cm, n = 31).
- - - - Suboptimal cytoreduction (residual tumor > 2.5 cm, n = 19).

Figure 11. Actual survival results of a prospective cohort of 50 patients who underwent cytoreductive surgery for diffuse malignant peritoneal mesothelioma. Prognostic significance of completeness of cytoreduction was $p < 0.001$.

Discussion

In the past, the median survival for patients with DMPM was no more than 12 months [3-9]. Until recently, cytoreductive surgery combined with perioperative intraperitoneal chemotherapy has shown improved survival outcomes in these patients, achieving median survival of 30 to 50 months and estimated 5-year survival of 40 to 60% in recently published series [10-18].

Alexander et al. at the National Cancer Institute, Bethesda have reported on several consecutive trials to evaluate treatment plans in DMPM patients.[10,13] The most recent report of CRS plus IPHC included patients treated with cisplatin at 250 mg/m^2.[13] At postoperative day 2 to day 10, patients received 5-flourouracil and paclitaxel as an intraperitoneal dwell. The median overall survival for the 49 patients was 92 months and the median progression for survival was 17 months. The 3-year survival was 59% [13].

Glehen's group from Lyon France recently reported 15 patients with DMPM who underwent CRS and IPHC with mitomycin C (0.5 mg/kg) and cisplatin (0.7 mg/kg) for 90 minutes. The overall median survival was 46.7 months, with 1-, 3- and 5-year survival of 71.5%, 49% and 36.8%, respectively [15].

Deraco et al. enrolled 49 patients to undergo CRS and IPHC with cisplatin (25 mg/m^2) and mitomycin C (3.3 mg/m^2) or cisplatin (43 mg/L) and doxorubicin (15.25 mg/L). The overall median survival has not been reached at the completion of the study and the progression-free survival was 40 months [16].

Taub et al. carried out a prospective single-institution phase I/II trial on 27 patients with DMPM [17]. The treatment regimen consisted of initial exploratory laparotomy with CRS and placement of indwelling intraperitoneal catheters; these were four intraperitoneal courses of doxorubicin (25 mg) alternating with four intraperitoneal courses of cisplatin (100 mg/m^2). Four intraperitoneal doses of gamma interferon were followed by a second laparotomy with biopsy verification of complete response or attempted resection of residual disease. IPHC with mitomycin (10mg/m^2) plus cisplatin (75 to 100 mg/m^2) and finally whole abdominal radiation was added to the plan of management. The overall median survival was 68 months with 3-year survival of 67% [17].

This current study of a prospective cohort of 50 patients who underwent these comprehensive treatments for DMPM, with follow-up for more than 5 years, revealed an absolute 3-year survival of 54% and an absolute 5-year survival of 44%. These survival results could serve more precise reference data for future studies pertaining the prognosis after these comprehensive treatments for DMPM.

Two most significant prognostic factors were identified for actual 3-year and 5-year survivors in both univariate and multivariate analyses and they were female gender and adequate cytoreduction. Many reports have documented an improved prognosis in female patients with DMPM [14, 18]. However, no clear causes for such a discrepancy in survival outcomes between male and female patients have been elucidated. It has been suggested though that there seems to be an epidemiological difference between male and female patients with DMPM, in that direct exposure to asbestos is definitely related to the causation of peritoneal mesothelioma in men, but is not in women [21]. It is possible that this difference in causation of the disease process is at least partly responsible for the difference in the natural history of peritoneal mesothelioma in women. Recently, Yan and colleagues have found that the histopathology of female DMPM patients showed less aggressive characteristics [22]. In addition, it might be true that women often with non-specific symptoms sought medial attention earlier or they were more likely to be investigated as part of their gynecological assessment. Early interventions may have separated this group of patients and partly account for their remarkable long-term survival results [14]. Indeed, women were found less likely to present with cachexia at time of diagnosis and with less extensive intraabdominal tumor deposits (a mean PCI of 21 in female, as compared to a mean PCI of 26 in male) and this may suggest that female patients are still at an earlier stage of their disease process at the time of definitive surgery [14]. However, in the same study, no pathological basis for such a survival difference between men and women was identified [14]

In this current series, the actual 3-year and 5-year survival rates in patients who received adequate cytoreduction were 71% and 58%, respectively. The actual 3-year and 5-year survival rates in patients who only received suboptimal cytoreduction were 26% and 16%, respectively. It is reassuring to find that the completeness of cytoreductive surgery was one of the two most significant predictors for both actual 3-year and 5-year survivors. At least, it means that as a surgeon, we can contribute a lot in the long-term outcome of a patient with DMPM, unlike gender, which is a fixed parameter. Completeness of cytoreduction was also found to be independently associated with a better survival in multivariate analysis by other major centers. Glehen and co-workers from Lyon defined an adequate cytoreduction as residual tumor nodules of ≤ 5 mm [15]. The median survival was not reached for patients with an adequate cytoreduction. It was 6.5 months for patients with suboptimal cytoreduction ($p < 0.001$ by univariate analysis) [15]. Deraco and colleagues compared the survival in patients who had optimal cytoreduction with those with a suboptimal result.[16] Optimal cytoreduction was defined as residual tumor nodules of ≤ 2.5 mm. In both univariate and multivariate analyses, CCR was a dominant treatment-related factor ($p = 0.01$ and $p < 0.001$, respectively) [16].

As indicated by a series of the CCR data, this treatment-related factor has a major impact on the benefit expected from the combined therapy. Using a radiologic test to help select patients for complete cytoreduction would be of great help to eliminate from elective treatment patients who will have suboptimal cytoreduction. In a recent study at the Washington Cancer Institute, a correlation was sought between the findings of the preoperative CT and completeness of cytoreduction [23]. Data showed that the size of the tumor mass in the epigastric region and the interpretive findings of the small bowel/mesentery strongly correlated with the outcome of the surgery, i.e. adequate versus suboptimal cytoreduction.

As indicated in Table 7, the interpretative CT appearances of the small bowel and its mesentery were categorized into four classes. Class 0 – CT showed no ascites in the region of the small bowel; the jejunal and ileal vessels appeared as round and curvilinear densities within the mesenteric fat. Class I – CT showed free intraperitoneal fluid only. The mesentery was stranded and stratified as the fluid accumulation outlined the small bowel mesentery. The small bowel vessels were easily identified within the mesenteric fat (Figure 12). Class II – CT showed tumor involvement of small bowel and/or its mesentery. The peritoneal surface was thickened and enhanced due to the presence of tumor nodules (usually half-spherical bodies) or plaques (flat implants whose diameter was greater than thickness). There may be an increased amount of ascitic fluid and the mesentery may appear stellate or pleated. The small bowel mesenteric vessels were still identifiable (Figure 13). Class III – CT showed an increased solid tumor involvement and adjacent small bowel loops were matted together in some cuts. The configuration of small bowel and its mesentery appeared distorted and thickened. Segmental small bowel obstruction might be present.

Table 7. Interpretative CT classification of small bowel and its mesentery [23]

Class	Presence of Ascites	Small Bowel and mesentery involvement	Loss of mesenteric vessel clarity	CT interpretation
0	No	No	No	Normal Appearance
I	Yes	No	No	Ascites only
II	Yes	Thickening Enhancing	No	Solid tumor present
III	Yes	Nodular thickening Segmental obstruction	Yes	Loss of normal architecture

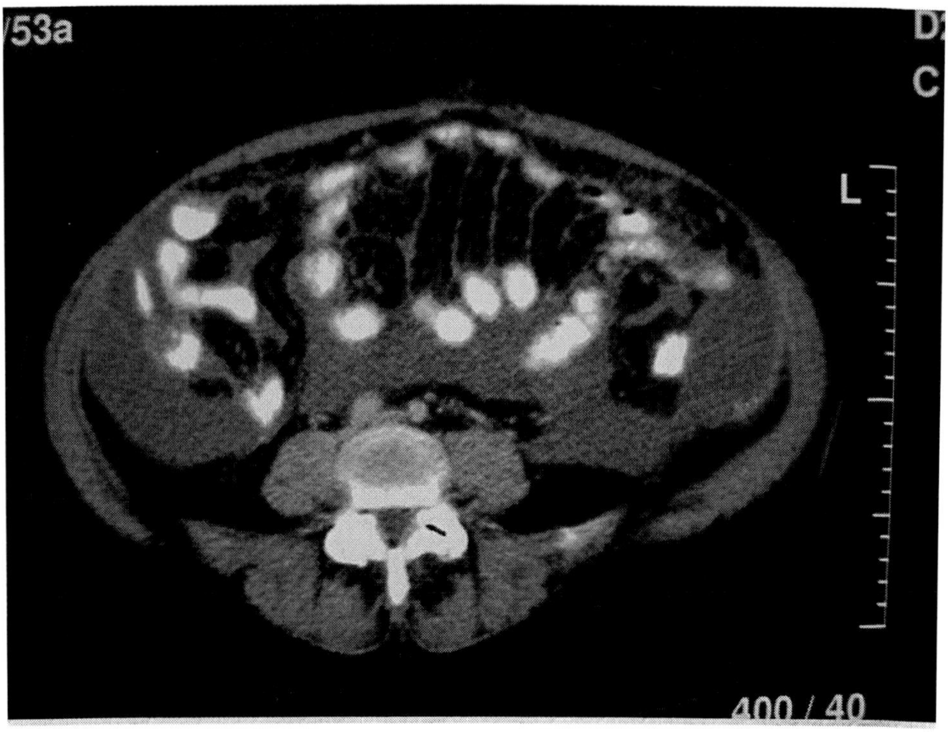

Figure 12. Interpretive CT finding of the small bowel and small bowel mesentery – Class I: CT shows free intraperitoneal fluid only. The mesentery becomes stranded and stratified as the fluid accumulation outlines the small bowel mesentery. The small bowel vessels are easily identified within the mesenteric fat.

Intraperitoneal fluid may be loculated. The small bowel mesenteric vessels were difficult to define on some cuts due to obliteration of mesenteric fat (Figure 14).

Figure 15 demonstrated the clinical pathway determined by preoperative CT for treating patients with peritoneal mesothelioma. According to this study, a patient with a tumor size > 5 cm in the epigastric region and Class III appearance of small bowel and its mesentery has a probability of 100% for a sub-optimal cytoreduction. A patient without either of these two preoperative CT findings has a 94% probability of an adequate cytoreduction [23].

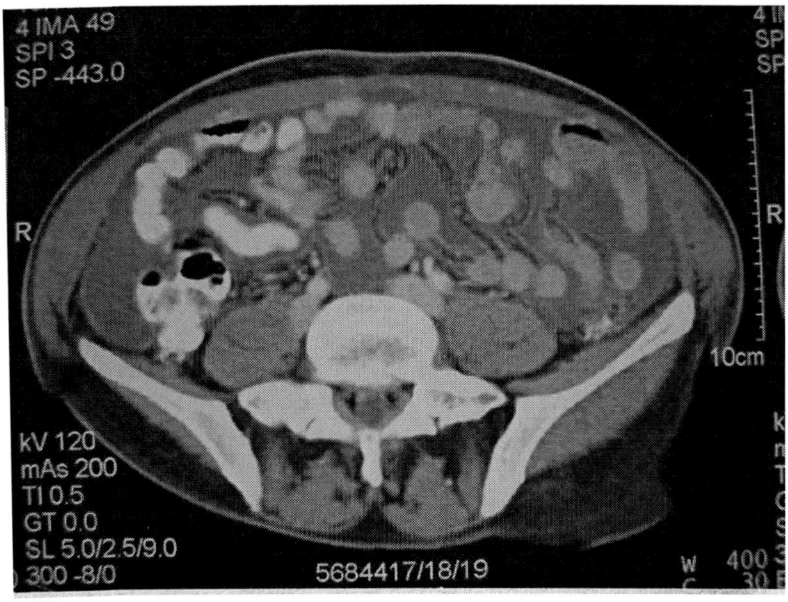

Figure 13. Interpretive CT finding of the small bowel and small bowel mesentery – Class II: CT shows tumor involvement of small bowel mesentery. The peritoneal lining is thickened and enhanced due to the presence of tumor nodules or plaques. There may be an increased amount of ascitic fluid. The small bowel mesenteric vessels are still identifiable.

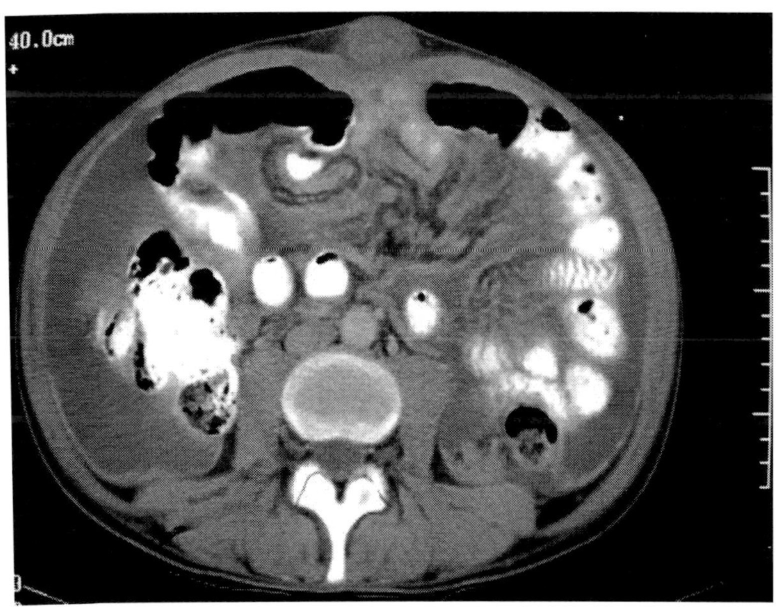

Figure 14. Interpretive CT finding of the small bowel and small bowel mesentery – Class III: CT shows an increased solid tumor involvement with adjacent bowel loops matted together; the configuration of small bowel and its mesentery appears distorted and thickened. Intraperitoneal fluid may be loculated. The small bowel mesenteric vessels are difficult to define due to the obliteration of mesenteric fat density.

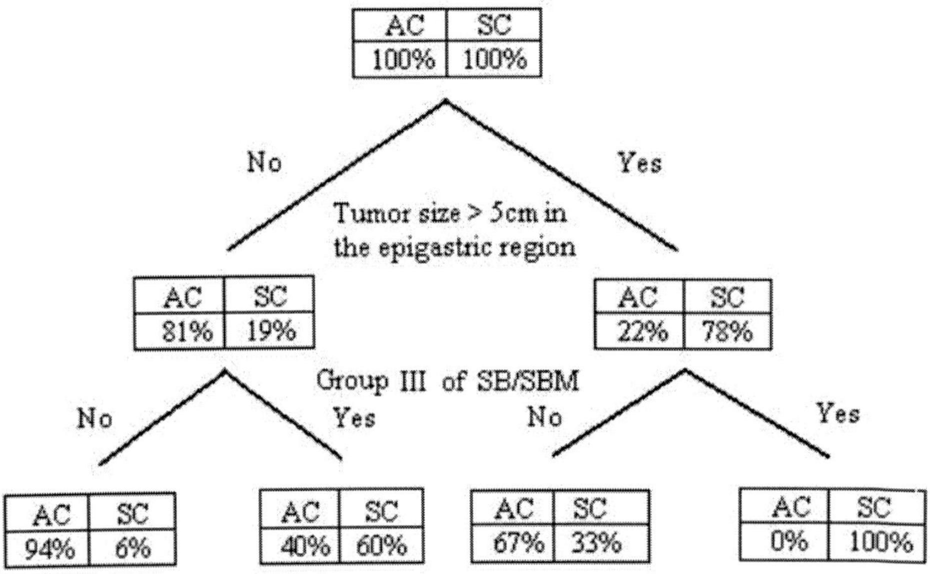

Figure 15. The predictive value of CT findings by a tree-structured diagram. AC = adequate cytoreduction; SC = sub-optimal cytoreduction; SB/SBM = small bowel and small bowel mesentery.

These data strongly suggest that preoperative abdominal and pelvic CT has an important role in the selection of patients for combined therapy.

This current study also found that less intraoperative blood loss (≤ 500 cc) was associated with both actual 3-year and 5-year survivors in univariate analysis. Cytoreductive surgery requires the complete stripping of parietal and visceral peritoneum by using electroevaporative surgery, which involves dissecting tissue by using a 0.3 cm ball-tipped diathermy with a very high electrical power between 200-250 mw [20]. This technique reduces blood loss and increases operative visibility, by sealing small vessels when it goes through the tissue planes. The ball-tipped diathermy is applied at the interface of the tumor and the normal tissue. To avoid heat damage, frequent and intermittent saline irrigation is required at the dissection site. The whole cytoreductive surgery combines one to six peritonectomy procedures into a coordinated effort and begins at the least extent of the tumor and gradually proceeds towards the greatest extent of the tumor. This so named "centripetal dissection" allows great exposure of the anatomy and is an important technique to achieve containment of the tumor and complete cytoreduction with minimal bleeding [20].

The morbidity and mortality results of these 50 patients were also reported. It showed that 38% of the patients experienced moderate or severe adverse events, requiring an interventional or a surgical treatment. Four patients (8%) died during their hospital stay. Bearing in mind that, these 50 patients were the first half of the 100 patients with DMPM underwent the comprehensive treatments at Washington Cancer Institute.

These morbidity and mortality statistics may be quite similar to those reported for CRS and PIC for peritoneal surface malignancy treatment of patients with many different diagnoses. After cytoreductive surgery and PIC, the morbidity ranges from 20-50% and mortality varies between 1-10% in most published series [24-30]. In the past, we reported a prospective morbidity and mortality analysis in the first 60 patients who underwent cytoreductive surgery and perioperative intraperitoneal chemotherapy for peritoneal carcinomatosis [24]. The Grade III/IV morbidity and in-hospital mortality rates were 35% and 5%, respectively. In 2003, the Grade III/IV morbidity and mortality rates of 68 mesothelioma patients who underwent this treatment were 23.5% and 7%, respectively.[14] The most recent prospective study on perioperative morbidity and mortality outcomes of 356 consecutive cytoreductive surgery for pseudomyxoma peritonei patients at our institution showed little overall changes in the morbidity and mortality rates [30]. This might reflect a position high on the learning curve for our group in the management of peritoneal surface malignancy. Our morbidity and mortality results may be acceptable in light of current standards for management of gastrointestinal cancer, but can be reduced with improved patient selection, technical skills intraoperatively and postoperative care.

In conclusion, this study of a cohort of 50 patients with extended follow-up period helps elucidate the long-term prognosis after cytoreductive surgery and perioperative intraperitoneal chemotherapy for DMPM by demonstrating valuable clinical data on actual 3-year and 5-year survivors. The clinicopathologic, operative, postoperative data of long-term survivors have been clarified in details and female gender and adequate cytoreduction were identified as independent predictors for both actual 3-year and 5-year survivors.

Acknowledgments

The authors thank David Chang for his expertise in statistical analysis and Tina Sugarbaker for her maintenance of the peritoneal surface malignancy database during the last 15 years.

References

[1] McDonald AD, MacDonald JC: Epidemiology of malignant mesothelioma. In: Antman K, Aisner J, ed. *Asbestos-related malignancy*. Orland, FL: Grune and Stratton, 1987: 31-35.

[2] Asensio JA, Goldblatt P, Thomford NR. Primary malignant peritoneal mesothelioma. A report of seven cases and a review of the literature. *Arch. Surg*. 1990; 125: 477-481.

[3] Chailleux E, Dabouis G, Pioche D, de Lajartre M, de Lajartre AY, Rembeaux A, et al . Prognostic factors in diffuse malignant pleural mesothelioma. A study of 167 patients. *Chest* 1988; 93: 159-162.

[4] Antman K, Shemin R, Ryan L, Klegar K, Osteen R, Herman T, et al. Malignant mesothelioma: prognostic variables in a registry of 180 patients, the Dana-Farber Cancer Institute and Brigham and Women's Hospital experience over two decades, 1965-1985. *J. Clin. Oncol.* 1988; 6: 147-153.

[5] Sridhar KS, Doria R, Raub WA Jr, Thurer RJ, Saldana M. New strategies are needed in diffuse malignant mesothelioma. *Cancer* 1992; 70: 2969-2979.

[6] Markman M, Kelsen D. Efficacy of cisplatin-based intraperitoneal chemotherapy as treatment of malignant peritoneal mesothelioma. *J. Cancer Res. Clin. Oncol.* 1992; 118: 547-550.

[7] Yates DH, Corrin B, Stidolph PN, Browne K. Malignant mesothelioma in south east England: clinicopathological experience of 272 cases. *Thorax* 1997; 52: 507-512.

[8] Neumann V, Muller KM, Fischer M. Peritoneal mesothelioma--incidence and etiology. *Pathologe* 1999; 20: 169-176.

[9] Eltabbakh GH, Piver MS, Hempling RE, Recio FO, Intengen ME. Clinical picture, response to therapy, and survival of women with diffuse malignant peritoneal mesothelioma. *J. Surg. Oncol.* 1999; 70: 6-12.

[10] Park BJ, Alexander HR, Libutti SK, Wu P, Royalty D, Kranda KC, et al. Treatment of primary peritoneal mesothelioma by continuous hyperthermic peritoneal perfusion (CHPP). *Ann. Surg. Oncol.* 1999;6:582-590.

[11] Loggie BW, Fleming RA, McQuellon RP, Russel GB, Geisinger KR, Levine EA. Prospective trial for the treatment of malignant peritoneal mesothelioma. *Am. Surg.* 2001;67:999-1003.

[12] Kerrigan SA, Turnir RT, Clement PB, Young RH, Churg A. Diffuse malignant epithelial mesotheliomas of the peritoneum in women: A clinicopathologic study of 25 patients. *Cancer* 2002;94:378-385.

[13] Feldman AL, Libutti SK, Pingpank JF, Bartlett DL, Beresney TH, Mavroukakis SM, et al. Analysis of factors associated with outcome in patients with malignant peritoneal mesothelioma undergoing surgical debulking and intraperitoneal chemotherapy. *J. Clin. Oncol.* 2003;21:4560-4567.

[14] Sugarbaker PH, Welch LS, Mohamed F, Glehen O. A review of peritoneal mesothelioma at the Washington Cancer Institute. *Surg. Oncol. Clin. N. Am.* 2003;12:605-621.

[15] Brigand C, Monneuse O, Mohamed F, Sayag-Beaujard AC, Gilly FN, Glehen O. Malignant peritoneal mesothelioma treated by cytoreductive surgery and intraperitoneal chemohyperthermia: *Results of a prospective study*. (Submitted for publication)

[16] Deraco M, Nonaka D, Baratti D, et al. *Prognostic analysis of clinicopathologic factors in 49 patients with diffuse malignant peritoneal mesothelioma treated with cytoreductive surgery and intraperitoneal hyperthermic perfusion.* (Submitted for publication).

[17] Taub RN, Hesdorffer ME, Keohan ML, et al. Combined resection, intraperitoneal chemotherapy and whole abdominal radiation for malignant peritoneal mesothelioma (MPM). (Submitted for publication).

[18] Yan TD, Sugarbaker PH. Cytoreduction and intraperitoneal chemotherapy for peritoneal mesothelioma – *Analysis of 100 consecutive patients from a prospective database.* (Submitted for publication).

[19] Glehen O, Gilly FN. Quantitative prognostic indicators of peritoneal surface malignancy: carcinomatosis, sarcomatosis, and peritoneal mesothelioma. *Surg. Oncol. Clin. N. Am.* 2003; 12: 649-671.

[20] Sugarbaker PH. Peritonectomy procedures. *Ann. Surg.* 1995; 221: 29-42.

[21] Welch LS, Acherman YIZ, Haile E, Sokas RK, Sugarbaker PH. Asbestos and peritoneal mesothelioma among college-educated men. *Int. J. Occup. Environ. Health* 2005; 11: 254-258.

[22] Yan TD, Popa E, Erwin AB, Cerruto C, Sugarbaker PH. Gender difference in diffuse malignant peritoneal mesothelioma. *Br. J. Surg.* (in press).

[23] Yan TD, Haveric N, Carmignani CP, Chang D, Sugarbaker PH. Abdominal computed tomography scans in the selection of patients with malignant peritoneal mesothelioma for comprehensive treatment with cytoreductive surgery and perioperative intraperitoneal chemotherapy. *Cancer* 2005;103:839-849.

[24] Jacquet P, Stephens AD, Averbach AM, et al. Analysis of morbidity and mortality in 60 patients with peritoneal carcinomatosis treated by cytoreductive surgery and heated intraoperative intraperitoneal chemotherapy. Cancer 1996;77:2622-9.

[25] Stephens AD, Alderman R, Chang D, et al. Morbidity and mortality of 200 treatments with cytoreductive surgery and hyperthermic intraoperative intraperitoneal chemotherapy using the Coliseum technique. *Ann. Surg. Oncol.* 1999;6(8):790-6.

[26] Elias D, Blot F, Et Otmany A, et al. Curative treatment of peritoneal carcinomatosis arising from colorectal cancer by complete resection and intraperitoneal chemotherapy. *Cancer* 2001;92:71-6.

[27] Butterworth SA, Panton ONM, Klaassen DJ, Shah AM, McGregor GI. Morbidity and mortality associated with intraperitoneal chemotherapy for pseudomyxoma peritonei. *Am. J. Surg.* 2002;183(5):529-32.

[28] Glehen O, Osinsky D, Cotte E, et al. Intraperitoneal chemohyperthermia using a closed abdominal procedure and cytoreductive surgery for the treatment of peritoneal carcinomatosis: Morbidity and mortality analysis of 216 consecutive procedures. *Ann. Surg. Oncol.* 2003;10(8):863-9.

[29] Ahmad SA, Kim J, Sussman JJ, Soldano DA, Pennington LJ, James LE, Lowy AE. Reduced morbidity following cytoreductive surgery and intraperitoneal hyperthermic chemoperfusion. *Ann. Surg. Oncol.* 2004;11(4):387-92.

[30] Sugarbaker PH, Alderman R, Edwards G, Marquardt CE, Gushchin V, Esquivel J, Chang D. Prospective morbidity and mortality assessment of cytoreductive surgery plus perioperative intraperitoneal chemotherapy to treat peritoneal dissemination of appendiceal mucinous malignancy. *Ann. Surg. Oncol.* 2005;13:1-11.

In: Mesothelioma from Bench Side to Clinic
Editor: Alfonso Baldi, pp. 469-479
ISBN: 978-1-60021-789-0

Chapter XXVIII

Reconstructive Procedures after Surgical Excision of Mesothelioma

Paolo Persichetti and Stefania Tenna
Plastic Surgery Department
"Campus Bio Medico" University - Rome, Italy

Abstract

Surgical treatment of malignant mesothelioma usually consists of wide excision resulting in large and full thickness defects to be repaired. Reconstruction can be achieved by autologous tissue, alloplastic materials or both according to extent and location of tissue loss.

The Authors describe the major techniques which can be used alone or combined, even if high complication rates, confirmed by recent literature, always suggest a meticulous patient's selection and a multidisciplinary approach.

Introduction

The appropriate management of patients with malignant mesothelioma is controversial: chemotherapy and radiation therapy are overall considered the treatment of choice but new approaches like gene therapy, immunotherapy or photodynamic therapy have been proposed as well as surgical excision combined with adjuvant therapies. A multidisciplinary approach, by means of wide surgical excision plus other therapies, showed better statistics in some leading cancer centres, even if survival rates are poor with an average expectancy of life between eight and twelve months. However comparative studies, which could suggest the best strategy to improve significantly survival or quality of life, are still limited [1].

The surgical choice is influenced by many factors including stage of cancer, localization, spread, histological type and patient's general condition; unfortunately the majority of cases, presenting with locally advanced disease or comorbid medical illness, do not benefit from surgery.

For those patients who can undergo the operation, the goal is to remove the gross disease with the knowledge that residual disease will be treated by other therapies [2].

Surgical excision must be radical according to cancer's stage, localization and infiltration in the surrounding tissues.

For pleural mesothelioma, involving the pleura only, a *pleurectomy/decortication* can be performed. In advanced stages affecting the lung a *pneumonectomy* should be advisable at the same time. The *extrapleural pneumonectomy, which* is of course the most radical approach, should be attempted, in some selective patients, by means of an "en bloc resection" of the lung, pleura, pericardium and diaphragm. Anyway this operation is often followed by a high complication rate (60 %), it is carried out in few centres just by well trained surgeons and it seems to improve the prognosis in patients with multifocal malignant mesothelioma only [3, 4].

For *peritoneal mesothelioma* peritonectomy procedures, eventually combined with visceral resections, are indicated. Peritonectomy procedures may remove the total anterior parietal peritoneum, the omentum, the right and left subphrenic peritoneum, the pelvic peritoneum, the lesser omentum and the omental bursa. Splenectomy as well as cholecystectomy are frequently performed together with a peritonectomy. In advanced stages a rectosigmoidectomy, a right colectomy, a total abdominal colectomy, a hysterectomy and a small bowel resection can also be achieved [2].

Reconstructive Procedures

Reconstruction of the defect differs according to extent and location of surgical excision. Infection and radiation injury are other important parameters to be considered but the size threshold for which a defect needs to be repaired remains unclear, except for major pneumectomy or peritonectomy where protection of visceral function is mandatory [5].

Reconstruction can be achieved by autologous tissue, alloplastic materials or both. Autologous procedures are usually preferred as they take advantage of the patient own tissue, with no risks of reactivity and low rates of infection [6-8].

The bilateral internal thoracic arteries continuing into the deep epigastric systems provide the main blood supply to the ventral aspect of the chest and the abdominal wall: this is the main system connecting the major vessels of the neck to those of the groin. Many flaps, based on this vascular supply and its branches, can then be harvested.

Pedicled and/or free flaps (using microsurgical technique to connect blood vessels), have been described for both chest and abdomen reconstruction [9-12].

To repair simple or composite tissue loss (involving one max. two stratum) grafts can be used. Sometimes autologous grafts are suitable, but these options may be limited by the dimension of the defect. On the contrary alloplastic materials are particularly indicated in case of large loss, offering a wide range of choice, each with advantages and disadvantages, according to ease of use, durability, adaptability, nonreactivity, resistance to infection and translucency to x-rays [13].

In case of full thickness defect autologous or alloplastic grafts should be combined with an autologous reconstruction performed with flaps [14].

Thorax Reconstrucion

Following a pleurectomy a graft (autologous or alloplastic) as well as a thin flap can be indicated, but in case of combined pneumectomy the residual cavity need to be packed or "stuffed" with thicker flaps. Autologous grafts include dermal or fascia. Muscle flaps are the most common choice due to their intrinsic properties of safe vascularization, resistance to infection, protective thickness and donor site complications [7,13]

Two muscle flaps, the latissimus dorsi and the rectus abdomini, are overall considered the first choice but also other flaps such as fasciocutaneous ones or omentum have been successfully used.

A brief description of the different techniques is here provided.

Flaps

Latissimus Dorsi Muscle

The latissimus dorsii (LD) is a versatile and reliable muscle. It is the largest flat muscle of the body, extending from the lower six thoracic vertebrae posteromedially, the crest of the ileum inferiorly, wrapping around with the teres major muscle anterosuperiorly and attaching to the intertubercular sulcus of the humerus. The thoracodorsal artery and vein supply the anterior two thirds of the LD, while the posterior third relies on perforator vessels. The long vascular pedicle allows a safe elevation with a wide arc of rotation covering the entire ipsilateral chest as well as the mid line and contralateral axillary fold. The flap is innervated by the thoracodorsal nerve. Minimal functional impairment is appreciated on the donor site: only forceful backward extension and adduction of the arm may be mildly-to-moderately compromised.

The LD flap can be used either pedicled or free, as a muscular flap, a muscolocutaneous flap or to compound an osteo-myocutaneous flap. It is often harvest as a muscle flap to reconstruct large soft tissue defects of both chest or abdominal wall [9, 10, 15].

Pectoralis Major Muscle

The pectoralis major (PM) is a fan-shaped muscle that covers the anterior-superior portion of the chest. The proximal attachments are the medial half of the clavicle, the anterior surface of the sternum, the six superior costal cartilages and the aponeurosis of the external oblique muscle. The lateral attachments include the lateral lip of the intertubercular groove of the humerus. Blood supply includes perforators from the internal thoracic artery, the intercostal arteries and from the thoracoacromial artery. Innervation is supplied by the lateral and medial pectoral nerves. This muscular flap is usually used for small defect of the midline of the chest and it can be considered to replace also the pericardium. Unfortunately it is sometimes damaged in case of extended thoracotomy. Skin islands also can be harvested with the muscle, leaving donor sites for primary or split-thickness skin graft closure. To minimize functional impairment in the donor site the pectoralis muscle of the nondominant chest should always be preferred [9, 10].

Serratus Anterior Muscle

The serratus anterior (SA) muscle is a small flat flap located in the lateral portion of the thorax overlying the intercostals. The attachments include distally the lateral external surfaces of ribs from the first to the eighth while proximally the medial border of the scapula. Innervation and blood supply are provided by the long thoracic nerve and artery. However the SA flap can be harvested together with the latissimus dorsii due to a branch of the thoracodorsal vessel. It has been described for small defects in the chest wall and for bronchopleural fistulas [9, 10, 16].

Rectus Abdominis Muscle

The rectus abdominis (RA) muscle is a long, broad, strap muscle and it is the principal vertical muscle of the anterior abdominal wall. The inferior origin is at the pubic symphysis and crest while the superior insertion is the xiphoid process and fifth to seventh costal cartilages. The innervation includes the ventral rami of the six inferior thoracic nerves. Blood supply depends on the inferior and superior deep epigastric arteries, supplemented by branches of the subcostal arteries. Donor site morbidity includes, in a low percentage of cases, abdominal wall herniation, especially below the arcuate line. A large skin paddle can be harvested with the muscle (vertical and transverse skin islands have been described) due to the perforator vessels passing trough the muscle and the rich net of choke vessels in the paraumbilical region which allows the communication between the deep inferior and superior epigastric arteries.

The transverse rectus abdominis myocutaneous flap (TRAM) is often indicated either pedicled or free, providing a large and thick amount of tissue with a wide arc of rotation [9, 10, 17].

External Oblique Muscle

The external oblique (EO) muscle is located in the anterolateral portion of the abdominal wall. Its origin is at the external surfaces of ribs from the fifth to the twelveth while its insertion is the linea alba, the pubic tubercle and the anterior half of the iliac crest. Innervation is supplied by the six inferior thoracic nerves, including the subcostal. Vascularization primarily involves the small arteries that arise from anterior and collateral branches of the posterior intercostal arteries in the tenth and eleventh intercostal spaces and from anterior branches of the subcostal arteries. The EO flap finds few indications due to its limited superior rotation but it may be reserved for defects below the fourth costal interspace [9, 10].

Intercostal Muscles

The intercostals muscles comprise the external, internal and innermost layers. They are located between ribs for inspiration and expiration functions. Innervation and blood supply to these muscles involve the intercostal nerves and arteries. Their use in reconstructive surgery is rare and mainly limited to bronchopleural fistulas [8].

Omentum

The omentum is located intra-abdominally and drapes off of the greater curvature of the stomach. It is a highly vascular and versatile sheet of adipose tissue supplied by the gastroepiploic arteries. The left and right gastroepiploic vessels as well as the collateral circulation via the gastroepiploic arch are all important vessels to recognize. The omental attachments to the transverse colon and greater curvature need to be taken down, rendering a bipedicle flap (both sets of gastroepiploic vessels). It is a dependable and versatile flap that allows coverage of virtually all chest wall defects and is associated with low morbidity and minimal deformity. Its pitfall primarily focuses on performing a celiotomy, yet the harvest of the omentum is routinely done laparoscopically. The omentum flap is particularly indicated in chest wall reconstruction with radiation injuries or in any case to protect visceral injuries or anastomoses as well as vascular conduits [18, 19].

Triceps Brachii

The use of the triceps brachii (TB) muscle has also been described for chest wall reconstruction especially in conjunction with partial TRAM failure even if it is rarely used.

The long head of the muscle can be harvested and rotated to cover small defect of the lateral chest. The skin island overlying the triceps is usually adequate and the functional impairment in the donor area is minimal [9, 10].

Fasciocutaneous and Cutaneous Flaps

Fasciocutaneous and cutaneous flaps are tissue paddles consisting of skin, subcutaneous tissue and eventually the fascia nourished by perforating vessels. Despite their thinness, they show some advantages including no need for repositioning the patient, direct closure of the donor site and low incidence of post-operative complications. They are usually harvested from the abdominal wall to cover chest wall defects. Dimensions can be adequate even to large tissue loss as for the "extended thoraco-abdominal Hatchet" flap but a base-to-length ratio greater than 1:3 must be carefully attempted [9, 10, 20].

Osteocutaneous Flaps

The osteocutaneous flaps include also the bone in the tissue paddle. The intercostal flap with an underlying rib based on its neurovascular pedicle may be used to close small defects and retain sensory properties. The latissimus dorsii has been described harvested together with the 11th, the 12th ribs and the posterior parietal pleura successfully [9, 10].

Grafts

To repair simple or composite tissue loss (involving one max. two stratum) grafts can be used. Autologous grafts in chest wall reconstruction are usually indicated to reconstruct bone loss and implies the use of ribs as bone grafts. New osteocytes in fact tend to replace the bone graft with new bone. Ribs can be harvested as a whole or split longitudinally. The latter option poses no defects at the donor site. Rib grafts has proven durability and should be placed overlapping as much surrounding trabecular bone as possible to prevent resorption and fibrous capsular replacement.

The disadvantages of using ribs are pain and/or instability at the donor area. Other possible sites for bone harvest are the iliac crest, the fibula and the tibia.

Limits to this technique are dimensions of the defect. A meticulous debridement of the necrotic tissue and cartilage is therefore necessary.

In case of pleural defect dermal or fascia grafts could be used but they should be combined with an autologous reconstruction performed with flaps in case of concomitant skin loss [10, 21].

Alloplastic Material

In case of large skeletal defects, diaphragmatic loss or total excision of pleura an alloplastic graft may be indicated. The choice of the most suitable material involves different considerations but first of all the defect should be clean. Stainless steel, titanium, Lucite and fibreglass can all be used, synthetic materials or composite materials are also available. Prosthetic grafts which repair fascia loss include polypropylene (Prolene, Marlex), polyethylene (Dacron), polytetrafluoroethylene (PTFE, Gore-Tex), polyester (Mersilene) and polyglactin (Vicryl, Dexon) [22-24].

Other grafts which have been experimented include AlloDerm and Sepramesh but no clinical research at the momentconclusively support their use.

Grafts combined to autologous tissue have also been indicated for skeletal patching:

- the fascia lata (prone to infection, predictable instability secondary to inherent flaccidity and pain at the donor site)
- the fascia lata with bone chips (minimal stability attained with complete bone absorption)
- the Lyodura (dura mater)
- the ox fascia (becomes flaccid with time and cannot be molded)
- the polypropylene (Marlex) sutured tightly providing a semirigid support that usually can be removed leaving the fibrous capsule as an adequate and reliable chest wall layer
- the methyl methacrylate that can be combined to Marlex mesh to decrease the tendency to fragment (remaining in the chest for 6-8 weeks allows the fibrous capsule to form)
- the absorbable polydioxanone (PDS) prosthesis.

Diaphragmatic Reconstruction

The standard procedures for diaphragm reconstruction consist of the use of biomaterials and prosthetic patches. The pedicled latissimus dorsi flap, the expanded polytetrafluoroethylene (ePTFE) sheet and the composite mesh sheet consisting of the ePTFE and 2 layers of polypropylene mesh sheets were successfully used to replace diaphragm.

Diaphragmatic replacement on the right side can be satisfactorily achieved by fixation of the liver to the thoracic wall. On the left side many homologous and heterologous tissues and prosthetic adjuncts have been suggested with varying success [9].

Abdominal Reconstruction

Abdominal wall defects following extensive resection could be reconstructed with many methods even if complication rates can be high, suggesting the importance of an accurate preoperative planning.

Small fascial deficits usually can be repaired by direct closure or with the component separation technique even if the applicability of this procedure depends on the size and location of the defect. The component separation technique introduced by Ramirez in 1990 involves the release of two separate components: longitudinally the medial edge of the external oblique aponeurosis to undermine the external oblique muscle from the internal oblique muscle, medially the medial two thirds of the posterior rectus fascia from the rectus muscle along the midline. This technique provides midline fascial advancement of 10 cm at the epigastrium, 20 cm at the waistline and 6 cm in the suprapubic area [25].

In case of large fascial defects prosthetic mesh, nonvascularized autologous graft, myocutaneous or fascial flap and tissue expansion are to be considered. When there is enough skin to close over the fascial repair, the first choice is a prosthetic mesh. The main advantage is that a larger piece of mesh avoids the dramatic increase of the intra-abdominal pressure often observed with hernia repairs. This increase of the intra-abdominal pressure can result in a decreased functional residual respiratory capacity, difficulty in weaning patients from ventilators and increased risk of hernia recurrence.

If a prosthetic material is already in the abdominal wound or extensive bowel adhesions are expected, the risk of contamination with enterotomy should always been evaluated. The existence of prosthetic mesh infection may require mesh removal and autologous reconstruction by flaps.

Myocutaneous flaps are usually a first choice as they can provide skin soft tissue and fascia to repair full-thickness abdominal wall defects. They are the preferred reconstructive option in contaminated wounds for which non-absorbable prosthetic mesh cannot be safely used.

Furthermore, they can also been indicated to "clean wounds" providing a well vascularized coverage even over a mesh.

In case of poor general conditions or following a severe infection a staged reconstruction can be useful. Staged reconstructions involve a temporary approximation of the fascia with absorbable Vicryl mesh to minimize the defect, waiting for a permanent reconstruction. Occasionally, Vicryl or Prolene meshes granulate over and allow for grafting (this occurs less commonly with Gore-Tex mesh), once the graft has matured and is separable from underlying viscera (at least after twelve months) the final reconstruction is planned according to size and location of the tissue loss.

Flaps

Rectus Abdominis Muscle

The rectus abdominis (RA) muscle is the workhorse in abdominal wall reconstruction. The RA flap can be used with or without a skin paddle to reconstruct wounds in the upper and lower quadrants of the abdomen as well as the suprapubic and umbilical area with the only exception of the epigastrium. The RA flap can be harvested either on the deep superior epigastric artery or on the deep inferior epigastric artery. The muscle averages 25 x 6 cm and provide large transverse or vertical skin components [9, 10].

Tensor Fascia Lata

The tensor fascia lata (TFL) muscle is the second option to reconstruct the umbilical, suprapubic, and lower quadrant abdominal areas. The TFL muscle is 13 cm long, 3 cm wide, and 2 cm thick. The TFL muscle originates from the anterior superior iliac spine (ASIS), the iliac crest and inserts into the iliotibial tract. The TFL flap is a myocutaneous flap based on the lateral femoral circumflex artery. The skin paddle is harvested 10 cm in width and designed over the muscle along an axis from the ASIS to the lateral tibial condyle. The inferior limit of the cutaneous territory can be extended to 6 cm above the knee and 25-35 cm in length. The flap can be made to be sensate, the rotation arc of the pedicled flap reaches the costal margin if the tensor muscle is completely detached from its origin and raised as an island flap. However, it is not useful to reconstruct defects of the upper abdomen because the distal third of the skin paddle is less reliable [9, 10].

Rectus Femori

The rectus femoris (RF) flap provide muscle and fascial coverage to the lower quadrant, umbilical, suprapubic and epigastric area. The RF muscle originates from the anteroinferior iliac spine and inserts on the patellar tendon. It is supplied by the lateral femoral circumflex vessels entering the muscle 6-8 cm below the anterior superior iliac spine or at the level of the pubic tubercle. A cutaneous paddle of 11 x 30 cm can be reliably harvested with this muscle and still allow primary closure of the donor. Functional sequelae in the donor site include weak knee extension, which can be avoided by suturing together the adjacent vastus medialis and lateralis muscle to the cut rectus femoris tendon [9, 10].

Other Flaps

Several flaps have been reported for abdominal reconstruction but their use seems to be pretty rare [9, 10]:

- the proximally based anterolateral thigh (fasciocutaneous)
- the external oblique for upper abdominal defects
- the distally based internal oblique
- the gracilis
- the vastus lateralis
- the latissimus muscles
- the groin flap (cutaneous)
- the omentum.

Graft

Autogenous nonvascularized fascial grafts have been described to repair abdominal fascial defects, even if their use seems to increase the incidence of post-operative ventral hernias. Anyway the advantage is the biocompatibility: these grafts demonstrated in fact to maintain their structural integrity. The fascia lata is a common donor site, and, if adequate soft tissue coverage is present, its use proved to be even more successful than the flap [26].

Alloplastic Materials

Polypropylene: Polypropylene is probably the most commonly used synthetic prosthetic material for abdominal fascial repair. Potential complications are wound sepsis, bowel fistula and mesh extrusion, so its use is usually reserved for clean wounds with adequate soft tissue coverage. Prolene shows greater pliability and porosity than Marlex and appears to have a lower fistula rate.

Gore-Tex mesh: Gore-Tex mesh has been shown to develop fewer adhesions to bowel than other mesh materials but poorer tissue in-growth. This results in a weaker graft to fascial interface and theoretical increased risk for recurrence at the suture line. Another concerning and frequent complication with the use of PTFE for abdominal hernia repair is seroma formation.

Polyester mesh: Polyester (Mersilene) mesh is light but strong material and conforms to contours well. Unfortunately it provokes a vigorous inflammatory response in soft tissues with contradictory results in literature for post-operative complication rates.

Absorbable polyglactin mesh: Absorbable polyglactin mesh (Vicryl, Dexon) is most suitable for temporary fascial approximation when the wound is contaminated. However, this absorbable mesh eventually must be substituted for permanent mesh or an extremely large hernia defect results.

Complications

Primary complication encountered with chest wall reconstruction is associated with infection, whether from initial wound contamination and inadequate debridement or secondary infection. Poor planning in pedicle dissection and careless sacrificing of essential arterial perforators may result in muscle flap necrosis and skin paddle epidermolysis. Closed system drains also are essential for both donor and recipient sites. Infection is controlled with wide debridement and irrigation and coverage with well-perfused viable tissue. Consequently, the incidence of infection associated with allografts and artificial material is higher. Osteomyelitis is also a difficult infection to treat and often requires debridement that may render the defect worse than the initial presentation. Removal of skeletal elements may cause an alteration in pulmonary physiology, thus resulting in respiratory compromise. Extrusion of allografts, primarily the struts and bars made of surgical steels, often is observed with time, especially when the ends of the support are placed beneath a pressure point.

Muscle flap rarely leaves the patient with debilitating functional impairment, but extensive resection together with multiple operations often result in poor outcome. Keloid scars and contractures also are observed in a small group of patients but these minor complications are usually subtle compared to the causative insult. For abdominal reconstruction hernia recurrence, fistulas or wounds dehiscence are often present [6-8, 14].

For alloplastic grafts infection is the most common complication as well as seromas that can develop around the mesh. Gore-Tex often is preferred to Marlex because of its malleability, flexibility, durability, conformability, and impermeability, but it is prone to contamination while Marlex seems to better left prevent seeding and infection. In the event of infection, the patch need to be removed: the fibrous capsule may be used as a support [26].

In conclusion it must be pointed out that complications in these patients are always more dependent on the extent of surgical excision than on the reconstructive procedure. According to the literature, complex and challenging operation such as *extra-pleural pneumonectomy* or extended peritonectomy are usually accompanied by high complication rates, confirming the importance of a meticulous patient's selection in order to identify the right group who can benefit from this kind of approach.

References

[1] Pistolesi M. and Rusthoven J Malignant Pleural Mesothelioma: Update, Current Management, and Newer Therapeutic Strategies *Chest* 2004: 126: 1318-1329.

[2] Deraco M, De Simone M, Rossi CR et al.. An Italian Multicentric Phase II study on peritonectomy and intra peritoneal hyperthermic perfusion (IPHP) to treat patients with peritoneal mesothelioma. *J. Exp. Clin. Cancer Res.* 2003 Dec;22(4 Suppl):41-5.

[3] Chang MY, Sugarbaker DJ Extrapleural pneumonectomy for diffuse malignant pleural mesothelioma: techniques and complications. *Thorac. Surg. Clin.* 2004 Nov;14(4):523-30.

[4] Lang-Ladzunski L., Tan T, Treasure T. Extrapleural pneumonectomy for malignant mesothelioma: should pericardium be resected routinely? *J Thorac Cardiovasc Surg.* 2005 May;129(5):1202.

[5] Losken A., Thourani V.H., Carlson G.W et al A reconstructive algorithm for plastic surgery following extensive chest wall resection. *Br. J. Plast. Surg.* 2004 (57): 295-302.

[6] Mansour KA, Thourani VH, Losken A, Reeves JG, Miller Jr JR, Carlson GW, Jones GE. Chest wall resection and reconstruction: a 25-year experience. *Ann. Thorac. Surg.* 2002;73:1720—26.

[7] Kroll, S. S., Schusterman, M. A., Larson, D. L., and Fender, A. Long-term survival after chest-wall reconstruction with musculocutaneous flaps. *Plast. Reconstr. Surg.* 86: 697, 1990.

[8] Arnold PG, Pairolero PC: Intrathoracic muscle flaps: a 10-year experience in the management of life-threatening infections. *Plast. Reconstr. Surg.* 1989 Jul; 84(1): 92-8; discussion 99.

[9] Edward Newsome, Camil Sader. Chest Reconstruction, Chest Wall Reconstruction *Emedicine.com* June 2006.

[10] Mathes SJ *Plastic Surgery*, Saunders 2nd Edition, Philadelphia 2006.

[11] Cordeiro PG, Santamaria E, Hidalgo D. The role of microsurgery in reconstruction of oncologic chest wall defects. *Plast. Reconstruct Surg*. 2001;108:1924–193.

[12] Hammond DC, Fisher J, Meland NB: Intrathoracic free flaps. *Plast Reconstr Surg* 1993 Jun; 91(7): 1259-64

[13] Deshamps C, Tirnaksiz BM, Darbandi R, et al. Early and long term results of prosthetic chest wall reconstruction. *J. Thorac. Cardiovasc Surg*. 1999;117:588—92.

[14] Boyd, A. D., Shaw, W. W., McCarthy, J. G., et al. Immediate reconstruction of full-thickness chest wall defects. *Ann. Thorac. Surg*. 32: 337, 1981.

[15] May, J. W., Jr., Toth, B. A., and Cohen, A. M. Teres major-latissimus dorsi skin-muscle flap for chest-wall reconstruction.*Plast. Reconstr. Surg*. 69: 326, 1982.

[16] Arnold PG, Pairolero PC, Waldorf JC: The serratus anterior muscle: intrathoracic and extrathoracic utilization. *Plast. Reconstr Surg*. 1984 Feb; 73(2): 240-8.

[17] Hemidiaphragmatic reconstruction with a transversus abdominis muscle flap after resection of a solitary diaphragmatic mesothelioma in a dog. *J. Am. Vet. Med. Assoc*. 2006 Apr 15;228(8):1204-8.

[18] Fix RJ, Vasconez LO: Use of the omentum in chest-wall reconstruction. *Surg Clin North Am* 1989 Oct; 69(5): 1029-46

[19] Jurkiewicz, M. J., and Arnold, P. G. The omentum: An account of its use in the reconstruction of the chest wall. *Ann. Surg*. 185: 548, 1977.

[20] Persichetti P., Tenna S. Cagli B., et al. "Extended cutaneous "thoraco-abdominal" flap for large chest-wall reconstruction" *Ann. Plast Surg*. 2006 Aug 57(2): 177-83.

[21] Watson, W. L., and James, A. G. Fascia lata grafts for the chest wall defects. *J. Thorac. Surg*. 16: 399, 1947.

[22] Graham, J., Usher, F. C., Perry, J. L., and Barkley, H. T. Marlex mesh as a prosthesis in the repair of thoracic wall defects.*Ann. Surg*. 151: 469, 1960.

[23] Matsui T, Kitano M, Nakamura T, et al: Bioabsorbable struts made from poly-L-lactide and their application for treatment of chest deformity. *J. Thorac. Cardiovasc. Surg*. 1994 Jul; 108(1): 162-8

[24] Hurwitz DJ, Ravitch MM, Wolmark N. Laminated Marlex-methyl methacrylate prosthesis for massive chest wall resection. *Ann. Plast. Surg*. 1980 Dec;5(6):486-90.

[25] Ramirez OM, Ruas E, Dellon AL. "Components separation" method for closure of abdominal-wall defects: an anatomic and clinical study. *Plast. Reconstr. Surg*. 1990 Sep;86(3):519-26.

[26] Matloub HS, Jensen P, Grunert BK et al. Characteristics of prosthetic mesh and autogenous fascia in abdominal wall reconstruction after prolonged implantation. *Ann. Plast. Surg*. 1992 Dec;29(6):508-11.

In: Mesothelioma from Bench Side to Clinic
Editor: Alfonso Baldi, pp. 481-500
ISBN: 978-1-60021-789-0

Chapter XXIX

A Survey on European Ongoing or Planned Clinical Trials in Malignant Pleural Mesothelioma

Adolfo Favaretto[*]
Medical Oncology Dept. Istituto Oncologico Veneto IRCCS
Via Gattamelata, 64, I - 35128 Padova, Italy

Abstract

Although malignant pleural mesothelioma (MPM) is mostly locally invasive, only a few patients can benefit by surgical resection. Among chemotherapeutic agents only antimetabolites and vinorelbine have shown response rates >20%. Two largest randomised trials in MPM showed an improved median survival with cisplatin plus pemetrexed or raltitrexed versus cisplatin alone of about 2.7 months. For the present overview about 180 requests of information were sent to the major European centres of thoracic oncology and their official web sites were checked – the US National Cancer Institute Clinicaltrials.gov included. The pharmaceutical companies interested in MPM were consulted; sponsored and non-sponsored information and brochures distributed during the major oncology conferences were analyzed. In Europe a rising interest regards trimodality treatment, with chemotherapy as preoperative treatment. At least 4 trials are running (EORTC, Denmark, Italy and Switzerland); all provide extrapleural pneumonectomy followed by 3D-conformal radiotherapy. Three international studies are Phase III randomised sponsored trials. The first compares pemetrexed plus best supportive care (BSC) versus BSC alone, the second Ranpirnase (Onconase) plus adriamycin versus adriamycin alone, and the third vorinostat (SAHA) versus placebo in MPM. Important national trials are ongoing: in the UK, the role of radical surgery (MARS Trial) and the role of chemotherapy (MS-01 trial) were challenged. Another trial tests bortezomib, a proteasome inhibitor, as first line palliative treatment. The Nordic Mesothelioma Group is conducting a study of sequential chemotherapy (pemetrexed plus carboplatin followed by Caelyx), and a phase II study of carboplatin plus Vinorelbine

[*] E-mail: adolfo.favaretto@sanita.padova.it

partly intravenously and partly orally. In Italy, a phase II multicenter trial of neoadjuvant pemetrexed plus cisplatin followed by surgery and radiotherapy is active; a second trial evaluates bevacizumab in combination with pemetrexed plus carboplatin; two other studies evaluate maintenance pemetrexed and imatinib, respectively. Two Dutch studies regard maintenance treatment with thalidomide, and vaccination with autologous Dendritic Cells in a phase I trial. Current European clinical trials cover all the major areas of interest in the treatment of MPM with many trials testing second line treatment due to the increasing number of active drugs in MPM. A long history of therapeutic nihilism has accompanied MPM management; but recent advances have put new enthusiasm on aggressive treatment in all stages of the disease.

Introduction

Malignant pleural mesothelioma (MPM) is an aggressive locally invasive malignancy with a poor prognosis. Only a minority of patients benefit of surgical resection. The median survival of patients treated with supportive care alone, without a curative resection, is about 6 months. A median survival time of 7 months was found in patients treated with chemotherapy in a series of CALGB trials. Equally disappointing were the results of radiotherapy. As single agents only antimetabolites and Vinorelbine have shown response rates >20% [1-2]. Most of the older combination regimens demonstrate response rates below 30%. The long-standing therapeutic nihilism regarding malignant mesothelioma treatment has been partially overcome after the publication of a large phase III randomized trial by Vogelzang et al.. This trial reported that the combination of pemetrexed plus cisplatin improved response (41 *vs* 17%), quality of life (QOL), time to progression (5.7 *vs* 3.9 months), and survival (12.1 *vs* 9.3 months) compared with single-agent cisplatin [3]. Another phase III trial, recently published by van Meerbeeck, has shown similar results with the raltitrexed plus cisplatin combination *vs* cisplatin alone (response rate 24 *vs* 14%, median overall survival 11.4 *vs* 8.8 months, 2-year survival rate 18.8 *vs* 10.4%) [4]. Clinical research is now mainly focusing on the best way to integrate therapies in a multimodality treatment.

Material and Methods

For the present overview on active or being activated trials in Europe, 180 requests of information were sent to the major centers dealing with thoracic oncology in 21 European countries; out of those, 60 answered. Besides, the official web sites of the major European cancer research centers and hospitals have been checked – the US National Cancer Institute Clinicaltrials.gov included. The pharmaceutical companies interested in the pathology have been consulted; sponsored and non-sponsored information and brochures distributed during the major oncology conferences have been analyzed.

Results

International Trials

EORTC Studies

The Lung Cancer Group is running a phase II feasibility trial" A Phase II Study of Neoadjuvant Chemotherapy Comprising Pemetrexed Disodium and Cisplatin Followed By Extrapleural Pneumonectomy and High-Dose Postoperative 3D-Conformal Radiotherapy in Patients With Malignant Pleural Mesothelioma" (EORTC protocol #08031).

Primary objective is to determine the feasibility of neoadjuvant chemotherapy including pemetrexed and cisplatin followed by extrapleural pneumonectomy and high-dose postoperative 3D-conformal radiotherapy, in terms of 90-day progression-free survival, in patients with malignant pleural mesothelioma. Secondary objectives are to determine the toxicity of this regimen and the progression-free survival and overall survival. This is a non-randomized, multicenter study. As neoadjuvant chemotherapy, patients receive pemetrexed 500mg/m^2 IV over 10 minutes and cisplatin 80mg/m^2 IV over 2 hours on day 1, with concomitant vitamin supplementation. Treatment repeats every 3 weeks for up to 3 courses in the absence of disease progression or unacceptable toxicity. Patients are evaluated 3 weeks after completion of neoadjuvant chemotherapy. Patients without disease progression proceed to extrapleural pneumonectomy within 21-56 days after completion of neoadjuvant chemotherapy. Thirty days after surgery, the patients are re-evaluated, and those without disease progression undergo daily high-dose 3D-conformal radiotherapy, starting 30-84 days after surgery, for 30 days. After completion of study treatment, patients are followed on days 42 and 90, every 3 months for 1 year, and then every 6 months thereafter.

Eligibility Criteria for the Study

Age up to 69 years; Histologically confirmed malignant pleural mesothelioma is required and all subtypes are allowed; Stage T1-3, N0-1, M0 disease without N2 or N3 involvement, confirmed by mediastinoscopy within 21 days before study entry; No clinical invasion of mediastinal structures (e.g., heart, aorta, spine, esophagus); no wide-spread chest wall invasion except focal chest wall lesions; no clinical or radiological evidence of shrinking hemithorax; no clinically significant third-space fluid (e.g., pleural effusions or ascites) that cannot be managed with thoracentesis or pleurodesis.

Performance status WHO 0-1, with adequate bone marrow, liver and kidney function and without pre-existing sensory neurotoxicity > grade 1 or uncontrolled infection.

No prior or concurrent melanoma, breast cancer, or hypernephroma; no other malignancy within the past 5 years except carcinoma *in situ* of the cervix or adequately treated basal cell skin cancer. No prior chemotherapy for Mesothelioma, no concurrent hormonal cancer therapy and no prior radiotherapy to the lower neck, thorax, or upper abdomen.

The study requires 52 patients and has started in July 2005. At the moment 19 patients have been included. Participating centers are in Belgium (Gent University, Antwerpen and Edegem Hospitals), Egypt (NCI, Cairo), Italy (Parma Hospital, Udine University, NCI Genoa), Nederland (Rotterdam Hospital and University, Nieuwegein Hospital, NCI Amsterdam), United Kingdom (Hull Hospital, Edinburgh Hospital).

A second trial (EORTC protocol #08052) is to be open. It is a Phase II study of bortezomib with cisplatin as first line treatment of malignant Mesothelioma. The targeted samples size is 76 patients. The Study Coordinator is M. O'Brien of the Royal Marsden Hospital, Sutton.

Industry Sponsored Trials

A randomized, prospective, multicenter and international phase-III trial (H3-MC-JMEW) compared pemetrexed plus best supportive care (BSC) versus BSC alone in previously treated patients with locally advanced or metastatic MPM. Pemetrexed 500mg/m^2 iv, day 1, every 3 weeks, with folic acid and vitamin B12 supplementation plus BSC, was compared to BSC alone. Six cycles of chemotherapy were permitted. The study, sponsored by Eli Lilly, started in June 2001 and recruited 240 patients. The study has been closed and the results will be presented at the 2006 ESMO meeting.

Two international industry-sponsored phase III trials are ongoing. The oldest is evaluating the role of Ranpirnase (Onconase) in MPM [5]: 'Onconase plus doxorubicin versus doxorubicin alone for patients with malignant pleural or peritoneal mesothelioma who have had no more than one prior chemotherapy regimen'. The study is US-based and sponsored by Alfacell (USA). This world-wide, prospective phase III trial started in 2002, and is expected to complete the accrual of at least 300 patients in the late 2006 or the beginning of 2007. Accrual seems suffering from the predominance of pemetrexed-based studies and the professional use of the pemetrexed/cisplatin combination as first line treatment. In Europe three countries are participating: Germany with Berlin, Gauting, Grosshansdorf, Hamburg and Munich hospitals; Italy with Genoa hospital; and Poland with the Warsaw, Gdansk, Poznam, and Zabrze hospitals. Eligible patients had to be inoperable and in CALGB prognostic groups 1 to 4. ECOG PS 0-1, with adequate bone marrow, liver and kidney function. It is a palliative, first or second line systemic treatment. Patients are stratified according to histology (epithelioid versus non-epithelioid) and CALGB group 1-4 and then randomized to doxorubicin 60mg/m^2 every 21 days up to 6 cycles versus doxorubicin 60mg/m^2 day 1 plus Onconase 240μgr/m^2 day 1, 8, 15 with a possible dose escalation up to 480 μgr/m^2 and up to 6 cycles. Patients demonstrating evidence of clinical response or stable disease may continue with maintenance therapy with Onconase as a single agent until disease progression.

The second international phase III trial is "Suberoylanilide Hydroxamic Acid (SAHA) versus Placebo in advanced MPM". This is a double-blind study, sponsored by Merck Sharp and Dohme, designed to determine the safety, tolerability and anti-tumor effectiveness of an oral investigational drug, vorinostat (or Suberoylanilide Hydroxamic Acid - SAHA), a histone deacetylase inhibitor, in the treatment of advanced MPM.

The primary objective is to compare the overall survival of patients with progressive or relapsed advanced MPM treated with SAHA versus placebo; and to determine the overall safety and toxicity of SAHA in these patients. Secondary objectives are to compare the overall response rate and progression-free survival of patients treated with SAHA versus placebo; compare the dyspnea score on the lung cancer symptom scale (LCSS) modified for

MPM; compare the percent change from the baseline in forced vital capacity and compare the quality of life of patients treated with these drugs.

Eligibility Criteria

Patients 18-year or older, with confirmed diagnosis of Malignant Pleural Mesothelioma, who must have failed prior chemotherapy including pemetrexed with either cisplatin or carboplatin. Patients must have adequate bone marrow, liver and kidney function; be capable of self-care and out of bed for more than 50% of waking hours; be able to complete Quality of Life questionnaires; be able to comply with follow-up requirements; have signed the written informed consent for registration; have no distant metastases. The trial, a randomized, double-blind, placebo-controlled study, is proposed in the palliative setting as second or third line systemic treatment. Patients are stratified according to histologic subtype (epithelial versus non-epithelial), Karnofsky Performance Status (70-80% versus 80-100%), and number of prior chemotherapy failures (first versus second line failures). They are randomized to one out of two treatment arms.

Arm 1: SAHA 300 mg administered orally twice daily (BID), once in the morning and once in the evening, in repeated 21-day cycles consisting of 3 days BID weekly dosing for 2 weeks followed by a 7-day rest period (on days 1-3 and 8-10).

Arm 2: placebo administered orally twice daily (BID), once in the morning and once in the evening, in repeated 21-day cycles consisting of 3 days BID weekly dosing for 2 weeks followed by a 7-day rest period (on days 1-3 and 8-10).

In both arms, courses repeat every 21 days in the absence of disease progression or unacceptable toxicity. Quality of life is assessed at baseline, every 3 weeks for up to 6 months during study treatment, within 1 month after completion of study treatment and then every 2 months thereafter. This international multicenter study started in July 2005, is ongoing and is expected to recruit 660 patients. European countries involved in the study are France, Germany, Italy (F. Grossi at INT Genoa plus 3 other centers), the Netherlands (P. Baas at NKI), Spain (Luis Paz-Ares for the Spanish Lung Cancer Group), Sweden and UK.

Independent Trials

Besides sponsored trials, some independent clinical research is being pursued. The Nordic Mesothelioma Group (Chairman G. Hillerdal) is active in Denmark, Finland, Norway, and Sweden. It is planning to perform a study comparing Pemetrexed plus Carboplatin for 6 courses versus Pemetrexed plus Carboplatin for 3 courses followed by Caelyx for 6 courses. The background is the Group's earlier experience with Caelyx, that seems to give a long period of stable disease leading to good survival [6]; the hope is to be able to combine the high Response rate of the pemetrexed-platinum combination with the prolonged disease stabilization obtained by Caelyx. This phase II randomized prospective study will hopefully start by the end of 2006.

In September 2004, "A Phase II Study of Carboplatin and Vinorelbine IV (Day 1) and Orally (Day 8) for Malignant Pleural Mesothelioma" has started. The purpose is to evaluate the activity and feasibility of a two drug regimen which is partly orally and partly intravenous in advanced pleural mesothelioma. The study covers Danish centers; the expected total enrolment is 40 patients to be recruited by January 2007.

Chemotherapy consisted of Carboplatin IV day 1 in each cycle and Vinorelbine IV day 1, and orally day 8 in each cycle. It is repeated every 3 weeks for a total of 6 cycles. The primary endpoint is response rate; secondary endpoints are survival and toxicity. Eligibility criteria for the study are:

Age 18 - 85 years and Performance status 0-2; histologically verified malignant pleural Mesothelioma; no previous chemotherapy; normal renal, liver and bone marrow function. The Principal Investigator is Jens B. Sorensen, Department of Oncology, Rigshospitalet, Copenhagen, Denmark.

Other ongoing trials are:

- A phase II trial evaluating trimodality treatment in resectable MPM. The three planned courses of neoadjuvant chemotherapy are followed by surgery (extra pleural pneumonectomy). Treatment is completed by radiotherapy at the dose of 60 Gy delivered with IMRT technique. This trial covers entire Scandinavia, i.e. includes patients from Denmark, Norway, and Sweden. All patients receive their treatment at the National University Hospital in Copenhagen, Denmark.
- The "Mesothelioma staging project" that is performed at the National University Hospital in Copenhagen, Denmark. This study provides for using PET-CT scan for the staging of all MPM patients, and performing a mediastinoscopy in resectable patients.
- A. Hjerpe is trying to combine preclinical research with the active treatment of patients. The intention is to find drugs that are active when the mesothelioma cells grow with the epithelioid morphology and when they grow with the sarcomatoid morphology, respectively, by testing it in cultured cell lines and SCID-mice. The idea is to combine such drugs to target the biphasic tumor more effectively. An interesting compound to be evaluated in mesothelioma patients is selenite, now being tested on lung cancer patients in a phase I study. A clinical study could be launched in 2008 in collaboration with the Nordic Mesothelioma Study Group.

Dean A. Fennell, of the Northern Ireland Cancer Center in Belfast, is currently the Principal Investigator on a phase II clinical trial with Bortezomib in malignant pleural Mesothelioma. This is an investigator initiated study sponsored by the Irish Clinical Oncology Research Group (ICORG) and funded by Johnson and Johnson. It is a multicenter international study (nine centers distributed in UK, Republic of Ireland, Belgium and the Netherlands).

Bortezomib is to be used either in first line or in second line. One hundred eleven patients (57 patients in the 1st line and 54 patients in the 2nd line setting) will be recruited. Patients must have an ECOG PS 0-2. Bortezomib will be administered at the dose of 1.6 mg/m^2 IV, weekly for 4 every 5 weeks. Modified RECIST criteria are used for response assessment. A thoracic and upper abdomen CT scan at 2 and 4 cycles is to be performed, with continuation of therapy until disease progression in responding patients. The trial has now commenced enrolment and should run until Dec 2007. Serum and tissue collection protocols for translational research have been included.

The European Lung Cancer Working Party (ELCWP). This international group based in Bruxelles will soon start a prospective multicenter second-line phase II study. The trial tests adriamycin (60 mg/m² every 3 weeks) plus valproate acid in patients with malignant mesothelioma relapsing or refractory to at least one prior chemotherapy regimen including platinum derivatives.

National Trials

In the UK the National Cancer Research Institute (NCRI) has approved 3 trials about the treatment of MPM. In patients fit for radical resection: the MARS trial, Chemotherapy and Radiotherapy versus Chemotherapy, Surgery and Radiotherapy.In patients requiring treatment for pleural effusion: the MesoVATS trial, Talc pleurodesis versus VATS cytoreductive pleurectomy.In patients fit for chemotherapy: the MS-01 trial, Active Symptom Control (ACS) versus ASC plus monochemotherapy versus ASC plus polychemotherapy.

The first study is the Mesothelioma and Radical Surgery (MARS) Trial, sponsored by the Institute for Cancer Research-CTSU. In the context of a trimodality treatment, radical surgery is thought to benefit patients: MARS tests this hypothesis against any and all alternative care. It is a randomized controlled trial evaluating the role of Extrapleural Pneumonectomy (EPP), as part of a trimodality treatment (chemotherapy, EPP, radical radiotherapy) of MPM.

The main trial is to be preceded by a pilot study that has to assess the treatment feasibility and acceptability in a multi-center UK-based randomized trial comparing EPP against no EPP surgery, by randomizing 50 mesothelioma patients in one year. If the pilot study is successful the main trial will be conducted Europe-wide. A multi-center European trial is needed for two reasons: first, to recruit sufficient numbers within a reasonable time; and second, to determine the results that can be achieved in a large number of specialized centers.

Potentially eligible patients will be registered at diagnosis, then randomized after chemotherapy and restaging, if still eligible for surgery. Fifty patients with T1-3, N0-1, M0 stage will be randomized to EPP or no EPP. The endpoints are peri-operative mortality, surgery effect on Quality of Life (QoL), surgery acceptability and feasibility, the proportion of randomized patients who proceed to allocated treatment and the proportion of patients considered eligible, and how this differs between centers. Moreover, all patients will be asked to complete EORTC QoL questionnaires at registration, randomization, 3, 6, 9, 12, 18, 24 months and then annually.

Eligibility Criteria at Registration: 18-year or older patients; Histologically proven mesothelioma; Patients fit to undergo EPP, as per BTS guidelines, and the planned post-operative radiotherapy; Able to complete Quality of Life questionnaires and to comply with follow-up requirements; Written informed consent for registration; No distant metastases.

Eligibility Criteria for Randomization: Still fulfill eligibility criteria for registration; Completion of 3 cycles of chemotherapy; Operable disease (T1-3, N0-1, M0); Biopsy proven malignant mesothelioma on histology and immuno-histochemistry; Normal renal function; WHO performance status 0 or 1; Written informed consent for randomization.

Exclusion criteria: Predicted post-operative FEV1 of less than 40% and TLCO of less than 40%; Significant pulmonary hypertension or cardiac ejection fraction of less than 40%.

If the feasibility study is positive, MARS will continue as a full trial whose main aims are to determine if EPP is better than no surgery in terms of survival, and to determine the effect of EPP on Quality of Life. The trial is designed as randomized, multi-center and multi-national. It requires 670 patients (stage T1-3, N0-1, M0) to be randomized to EPP or no EPP. The primary endpoint is survival. The secondary endpoint is Quality of Life to be assessed in selected centers using the EORTC Quality of Life questionnaires, whose timings have to be confirmed by the pilot study data. Local centers can choose between two regimens:

1. MVP: Mitomycin 6 mg/m^2, Vinblastine 6 mg/m^2, Cisplatin 50 mg/m^2, all day 1, every 3 weeks [7]
2. CisGem: Cisplatin 80 mg/m^2, day 1 and Gemcitabine 1250 mg/m^2 day 1 and 8, every 3 weeks. Three cycles of platinum-based chemotherapy are planned. After restaging by CT scan to assess resectability and response, the patients can be randomized to EPP versus no EPP surgery. The pilot study started in 2005 and at the moment recruited 40% of the planned sample. The planned closure date is March 2007. The MARS trial is coordinated by S. Piggott , Institute of Cancer Research - Clinical Trials and Statistics Unit (ICR-CTSU). Principal Investigators are T. Treasure, Guy's and St Thomas' Hospital, London and D. Waller, Leicester (Surgery) and K. O'Byrne, St James's Hospital, Dublin and M. O'Brien, Royal Marsden, Sutton (Oncology).

A second randomized clinical trial that is going to be concluded in UK is MS-01. It addresses the role of palliative chemotherapy in a randomized controlled trial of Active Symptom Control (ASC) with or without chemotherapy in the treatment of patients with MPM. It is an ongoing phase III trial, sponsored by MRC. It started in 1999 and planned to recruit 420 patients, until July 2006; current accrual is 403 patients. Preliminary results should be presented towards the end of 2006. The Chief Investigator is M. Muers. The primary objective is to compare the overall survival of patients treated with ASC alone, the UK recommended practice standard of care, versus ASC in addition to chemotherapy. Secondary objectives are to compare the toxic effects of these regimens, to compare symptom palliation, the Performance Status, the analgesic usage, the tumor response and progression-free survival and the Quality of Life of patients treated with these regimens.

The three options to be investigated are:

1. ASC - Active Symptom Control *versus*
2. ASC plus MVP - Mitomycin 6 mg/m^2, Vinblastine 6 mg/m^2 (max. 10 mg), Cisplatin 50 mg/m^2, every 3 weeks, for a total of 4 cycles*versus*
3. ASC plus Vinorelbine 30 mg/m^2 (max. 60 mg), 6 injections at weekly intervals, followed by a 13-day break before a further 6 injections at weekly intervals

Inclusion Criteria

Patients must fulfil all of the following criteria to be eligible for the trial:

1. Microscopically and immunohistochemically confirmed malignant pleural mesothelioma, including epithelial and other histological types. Diagnosis by immunocytochemistry on pleural fluid cell blocks is also acceptable if it is backed up with appropriate radiology, clinical evidence and history. The maximum time from diagnostic biopsy to randomization has to be 3 months.
2. Any symptomatic pleural effusions treated and brought under control by drainage, pleurodesis or pleurectomy before trial entry.
3. CT scan and/or a Chest X-Ray to be performed within a month before randomization and, whenever possible, after pleurodesis.
4. Patients who have undergone surgical resection of mesothelioma are eligible provided that 2 CT scans, 6 weeks apart, show stable or progressive disease.
5. No previous chemotherapy for mesothelioma.
6. Patients who have had local radiotherapy to a wound site after an exploratory thoracotomy are eligible.
7. No other disease or previous malignancy likely to interfere with the protocol treatments or comparisons.
8. WHO performance status 0-2.
9. Normal bone marrow function, and no clinical evidence of infection. 10) Considered medically fit to receive chemotherapy. Creatinine clearance > 50 mL/minute
10. Patient has read the patient information sheet and signed the consent form.
11. Patient has completed a Quality of Life questionnaire prior to being told the treatment allocated.

Exclusion Criteria

1. Pregnant or lactating women or women of child bearing potential not using adequate contraception
2. Under the age of 18. In 2004 the results of a randomized study to test the feasibility have been published [8]. In a trial lasting 1-year, 197 patients out of 242 registered were eligible; actually 109 were randomized. Randomization to active symptom control with or without chemotherapy was sufficiently acceptable to patients and clinicians for a large multicenter randomized trial. After the publication of the randomized pemetrexed plus cisplatin versus cisplatin study [3], there was some ethical concern about the MS-01 trial should continue; it was a debated issue but it was decided it should continue.

A third ongoing study, called MesoVATS, is a prospective randomized controlled trial of video-assisted thoracoscopic (VATS) cytoreductive pleurectomy compared to talc pleurodesis in patients with suspected or proven MPM. It is a phase III trial planned to recruit 196 patients; to date, a 25% of the sample recruitment has been pursued. The Chief Investigators are A. Ritchie and R. Winter.

Inclusion Criteria

Patients with proven or suspected mesothelioma. Suitable patients will have pleural tumour with associated pleural effusion and be fit enough for VATS pleurectomy. Patients who have had a previous malignancy for which they are no longer receiving treatment, provided they have a confirmed diagnosis of mesothelioma.

Exclusion Criteria

Patients who are unfit for a VATS procedure. Patients who have had previous attempted pleurodesis, or patients without a pleural effusion.

A fourth trial directed not only to MPM but also to NSCLC and SCLC patients with dyspnea, addresses the ability of nebulized furosemide to improve breathlessness in these patients. The study is currently open and about a third of the sample size of 30 patients has been recruited. The closure date has been planned for September 2007.

*The Inclusion criteria are:*Any cancer affecting the lungs; Moderate to severe breathlessness; Score 3-5 on Dyspnea Exertion Scale; Ability to read and exercise their arms; Medication that might affect their breathing or ability to exercise has been stable for 4 days.

The Exclusion criteria are: Treatable cause of breathlessness (eg. effusion that could be drained); Angina on exertion Heart failure; Arm or shoulder pain; Unstable COPD or other lung disease; Allergy to furosemide; Chemotherapy or radiotherapy within a month of the study. The Chief Investigator is Dr Andrew Wilcock of the University of Nottingham.

A trial addressing the specific problem of the prevention of metastatic skin nodules or tumor seeding following invasive diagnostic procedures is ongoing in Scotland. The purpose of this " Phase III Randomized Study of Radiotherapy in the Prevention of Metastatic Skin Nodules Following Invasive Diagnostic Procedures in Patients With Malignant Mesothelioma" is to determine the effectiveness of radiation therapy in preventing metastatic cancer in patients who have undergone diagnostic procedures to identify malignant mesothelioma [9]. Objectives of the study are to determine the efficacy of radiotherapy in the prevention of metastatic skin nodules or tumor seeding following invasive diagnostic procedures, such as chest drain insertion, pleural aspiration, pleural biopsy, and thoracoscopy, in patients with malignant mesothelioma; to determine whether the nodules that develop after radiotherapy are symptomatic in these patients; to compare the quality of life of patients treated with radiotherapy versus standard care alone.

Patients are randomized to 1 of two treatment arms.

Arm I: Patients receive radiotherapy on 3 consecutive days beginning within 3 weeks after chest drain insertion, pleural aspiration, pleural biopsy, or thoracoscopy and once the wounds have healed.

Arm II: Patients receive standard supportive care alone. Quality of life is assessed at baseline, and then at 1, 2, 4, 6, 9, and 12 months.

Patients are followed at 1, 2, 4, 6, 9, and 12 months.

A total of 44 patients (22 patients per arm) will be accrued for this study within 2 years.

Eligibility Criteria for the Study

Histologically proven malignant pleural mesothelioma by chest drain insertion, pleural aspiration, pleural biopsy, and/or thoracoscopy within the past 3 weeks; No Age limits or

Performance status limitation; Life expectancy of at least 3 months; No prior systemic chemotherapy for malignant mesothelioma; No prior local radiotherapy for malignant mesothelioma; No other invasive procedures to the same chest site during and for 1 year after study.

The Principal investigator is Noelle O'Rourke, MD, of the University of Glasgow. Other participating centers are the Gartnavel General Hospital and the Stobhill General Hospital, in Glasgow, Scotland.

In Switzerland the SAKK Group coordinated by W. Weder and R. Stahel, in the wake of a single-center phase II study and a successive multi-center phase II study with neoadjuvant gemcitabine plus cisplatin chemotherapy followed by EPP [10], is conducting another prospective multicenter randomized phase II study. The study "A Phase II Randomized Study of Neoadjuvant Therapy with Pemetrexed Disodium and Cisplatin Followed by Extrapleural Pneumonectomy with or without Postoperative Hemithoracic Radiotherapy in Patients with Malignant Pleural Mesothelioma" includes patients with MPM of all histologies that are treated with induction chemotherapy with 3 cycles of Cisplatin and pemetrexed followed by extrapleural pneumonectomy.

The primary objective is to evaluate the short-term outcomes and feasibility of neoadjuvant therapy with pemetrexed and cisplatin followed by extrapleural pneumonectomy in patients with malignant pleural Mesothelioma; and to evaluate the long-term outcomes and feasibility of postoperative hemithoracic radiotherapy in patients with R0 or R1 resection. Secondary objectives are to determine the quality of life of these patients; Identify predictive and prognostic markers in these patients; Determine relapse-free or progression-free survival and overall survival of these patients; Collect tissue and blood from these patients.

Patients are stratified according to participating center, histology (sarcomatoid or other versus epithelial or mixed histology), nodal status (N0-1 versus N2), and extent of disease (T1-2 versus T3).

The study is divided into two parts: The first part includes the neoadjuvant chemotherapy and surgery:

Patients receive pemetrexed IV over 10 minutes and cisplatin IV over 2 hours on day 1. Treatment repeats every 21 days for 3 courses in the absence of disease progression or unacceptable toxicity. Within 8 weeks after completion of neoadjuvant therapy, patients without progressive disease undergo extra pleural pneumonectomy.

Patients achieving R0 or R1 resection proceed to part 2 of study treatment and are randomized to 1 of 2 treatment arms. Patients with R2 resection, disease progression, or symptomatic deterioration after treatment in part 1 are taken off study.

The second part regards postoperative therapy:

Arm I (no postoperative radiotherapy): Patients do not undergo radiotherapy. Quality of life is assessed at baseline and at 6, 10, 16, and 22 weeks after randomization.

Arm II (postoperative radiotherapy): Beginning within 10 weeks after surgery, patients undergo radiotherapy to the hemithoracic region 5 days a week for approximately 5 weeks in the absence of disease progression or unacceptable toxicity. Quality of life is assessed at baseline and at 4, 8, 14, and 20 weeks after initiation of radiotherapy. (Figure 1).

After completion of study treatment, patients are followed periodically for up to 5 years after surgery.

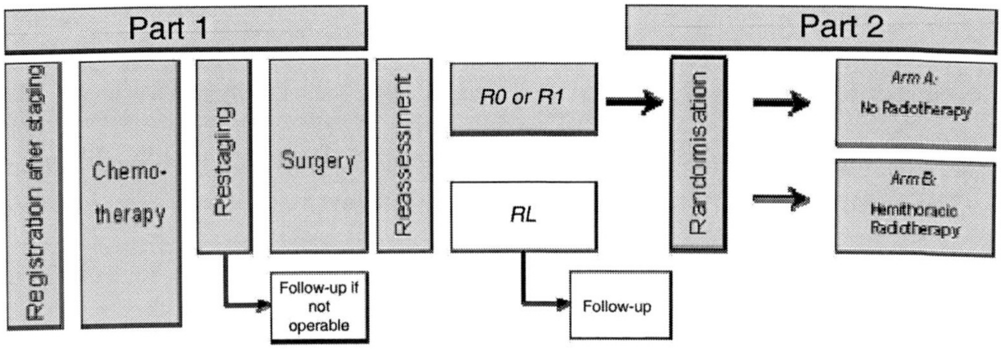

Figure 1. The SAKK study flow chart.

Eligibility criteria for the study are: Age 18-69 years and WHO performance status 0-1; Histologically or cytologically confirmed malignant pleural Mesothelioma; T1-3, N0-2, M0 disease according to International Mesothelioma Interest Group staging system; No obvious invasion of mediastinal structures, e.g. heart, aorta, spine, esophagus, by CT scan; No obvious widespread chest wall invasion, but resectable chest wall lesions are allowed; Fit for neoadjuvant therapy, surgery, and postoperative radiotherapy; adequate bone marrow, liver and kidney function; FEV1 $\geq$ 40% of predicted based on spirometry and lung perfusion scan, if necessary; No prior chemotherapy, pleurectomy or lung resection, radiotherapy of the lower neck, thorax, or upper abdomen.

A total of 155 patients will be accrued for this study. The study is open and about 15 patients have been included.

In Italy, "A phase II trial of neoadjuvant pemetrexed plus cisplatin followed by surgery and radiation in the treatment of MPM" (H3E-IT-S079), started in January 2005 (Figure 2).

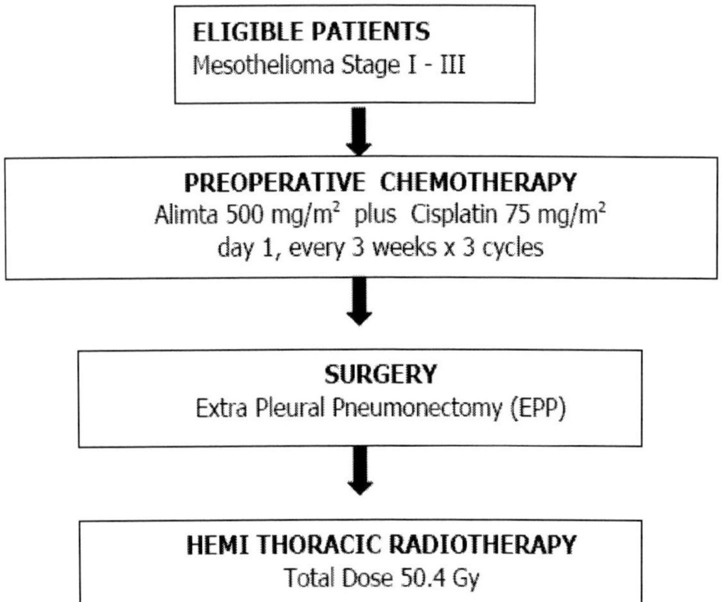

Figure 2. H3E-IT-S079 Study Flow Chart.

The primary objective is to determine the event-free survival of patients with clinical stage I, II, or III (T1-3 N0-2) mesothelioma treated with pre-operative chemotherapy (pemetrexed plus cisplatin), surgery (EPP) and hemithoracic radiation. Secondary objectives are to determine the 1- and 2-year disease-free survival, and the median survival; to determine the complete pathological response rate; to determine the clinical response rate measured by radiological assessment; to characterize the quantitative and qualitative toxicities of chemotherapy, surgery and radiation in this patient population; to determine the pattern of relapse (local versus metastatic); to measure time-to-event efficacy variables including: time to objective tumor response for responding patients, time to progressive disease. The study is designed as a Phase II, open-label, multi-center trial to determine the effectiveness and feasibility of a multi-modality approach to the treatment of MPM.

*Patient Inclusion Criteria are:*Age ≥18 years; Histological proven diagnosis of stages I to III mesothelioma of the pleura; Adequate organ function including the following: adequate bone marrow reserve, hepatic, renal, pulmonary and cardiac functions; No prior systemic chemotherapy; No previous surgical resection of mesothelioma, with the exception of previous chemical pleurodesis; No previous radiation therapy.

Exclusion Criteria are: Having received treatment within the last 30 days with a drug that has not received regulatory approval for any indication at the time of study entry; Serious concomitant systemic disorders; Second active primary malignancy; Inability or unwillingness to take folic acid, vitamin B12 supplementation, or dexamethasone.

Pathological complete response rates, clinical response rate measured by radiological assessment, disease free survival, median survival, overall toxicity will be determined for patients treated with this approach. Treatment consisted of 3 cycles of pemetrexed 500 mg/m2 plus Cisplatin 75 mg/m2 on day 1 every 3 weeks. The planned surgical procedure is Extrapleural pneumonectomy. Radiotherapy initially planned as 54 Gy has been later lowered to 50.4 Gy. The study, sponsored by Eli Lilly, is planned to recruit 53 patients by June 2008; at present, about 21 patients have been enrolled. Actively participating centers are the NCI of Rome, Milan and Padua; the centers of Naples, Turin and Venice will be activated soon; the Chief Investigator is F. Facciolo, IFO, Rome.

For inoperable patients, a new Phase II Study (ML 18791) including a new biological agent plus chemotherapy is going to start soon. G. Ceresoli, of the Department of Medical Oncology and Hematology, Istituto Clinico Humanitas IRCCS, Rozzano (Milan), has planned to combine Bevacizumab (rhuMAb VEGF) plus Pemetrexed and Carboplatin as first-line therapy in patients with MPM who have not previously received systemic treatment.

A previous experience with the pemetrexed plus carboplatin combination showed favorable results similar to those achieved with the standard regimen of pemetrexed plus cisplatin, suggesting that the carboplatin combination could be an alternative option for these patients [11]. The use of antiangiogenetic agents seems particularly appropriate in MPM, so, with the aim to improve the results of the pemetrexed plus carboplatin combination, bevacizumab was added to the combination.

The primary objective of the study is to assess the antitumor activity in terms of time to progression (TTP) of bevacizumab in combination with pemetrexed and Carboplatin.

The secondary objectives are to evaluate the objective response rate (RR) and its duration, the toxicity and the safety profile, the time to treatment failure (TTF) and the overall survival (OS) of the combination.

The study design is an open label, multicenter, phase II study; 77 patients are to be recruited in at least 10 Italian centers.

The inclusion criteria are a histologically proven diagnosis of malignant pleural mesothelioma; Inoperable disease, not pretreated with chemotherapy or patients progressed after surgery; Age ≥ 18, an ECOG Performance Status 0-1 and life expectancy of at least 12 weeks; Measurable and/or evaluable lesions according to RECIST criteria;

Laboratory requirements: normal hematological, hepatic and renal function tests; Creatinine clearance >50 mL/min, calculated according to the Cockroft-Gault formula; Written informed consent; Patients must be accessible for treatment and follow up; Patients registered on this trial must be treated and followed at the participating center.

The exclusion criteria are any prior chemotherapy for MPM including intracavitary administration; Symptomatic and/or unstable pre-existing brain metastases; Serious non-healing wound or ulcer; Evidence of bleeding diathesis, coagulopathy or uncontrolled hypertension; Clinically significant (i.e. active) cardiovascular disease, for example cerebrovascular accidents (≤6 months), myocardial infarction (≤6 months), unstable angina, New York Heart Association (NYHA) grade II or greater congestive heart failure, serious cardiac arrhythmia requiring medication; Current or recent ongoing treatment with anticoagulants for therapeutic purposes; Chronic, daily treatment with high-dose aspirin (>325 mg/day) or other medications known to predispose to gastrointestinal ulceration; Treatment with any investigational drugs within 30 days prior to enrolment; Allergy to components of the study medications; Other co-existing malignancies or malignancies diagnosed within the last 5 years with the exception of basal cell carcinoma or cervical cancer *in situ*; Major surgical procedure, open biopsy, or significant traumatic injury within 28 days prior to study treatment start.

Study Medication

Treatment will be administered on Day 1 as follows:

- Pemetrexed will be administered at the dose of 500 mg/m2 every 3 weeks.
- Carboplatin will be administered at the dose of AUC 5 every 3 weeks;
- Bevacizumab will be given by intravenous infusion at the dose of 15 mg/kg every 3 weeks.

Treatment will be continued on the basis of tumor assessment performed every 3 courses. Patients with stable disease, complete or partial response will continue treatment until progressive disease, unacceptable toxicity, patient or physician decision. For chemotherapy agents, however, a maximum of 6 cycles will be administered. Bevacizumab will be continued every 3 weeks until progression, for a maximum of 1 year. Time to progression (TTP) will be measured from the first day of treatment until to the first observation of disease progression or death due to any cause or the last date the patient was known to be progression free or alive. Response rate (RR) will be assessed according to the modified RECIST criteria for Malignant Pleural Mesothelioma [12]. Overall survival (OS) will be computed as the time between the first day of treatment and the date of death or the last date the patient was known to be alive.

The sample size was calculated on 77 patients to be accrued in 12 months and followed for a minimum follow-up time of 9 further months. For this multicenter clinical trial, about 10 centers with high MPM patients accrual will be involved.

The Protocol Board is composed by A. Santoro, Principal Investigator and G. Ceresoli, Study Coordinator, (Istituto Clinico Humanitas IRCCS, Rozzano, Milan), A. Ardizzoni (Azienda Ospedaliera, Parma), B. Castagneto (Ospedale S. Spirito, Casale Monferrato), A. Favaretto (Istituto Oncologico Veneto IRCCS, Padova), F. Grossi (Istituto Nazionale per la Ricerca sul Cancro, Genova), P. Zucali (Istituto Clinico Humanitas IRCCS, Rozzano, Milan).

Another Italian group after the recent publication of a multicenter Phase II Study of sequential chemotherapy (SITMP1) [13], proposes two phase II trials, both in the palliative setting. The first, called SITMP3, tests the combination of Pemetrexed 500 mg/m^2, on day 1 every 21 days plus Imatinib 400 mg/die. The study is designed as a multi-center phase II study. The second, called SITMP4, evaluates the combination of 'Pemetrexed plus cisplatin chemotherapy in inoperable MPM followed, in non-progressing patients, by maintenance pemetrexed'. The primary objective is evaluation of the progression-free survival. The treatment is pemetrexed 500mg/m^2, IV, plus cisplatin 75mg/m^2, IV in 1 hour, on day 1, every 3 weeks, with concomitant vitamin supplementation, for 6 courses. Patients without progressive disease have maintenance pemetrexed 500mg/m^2, day 1, every 3 weeks. Both the studies are in preparation and coordinated by C. Pinto (Bologna).

In Padua University Hospital, two carboplatin-based combinations have been studied. The results of the gemcitabine-carboplatin combination phase II trial in the palliative setting have already been published [14]. The results of the same combination in the neoadjuvant setting are going to be published (submitted to Cancer). A multicenter phase II trial with the carboplatin plus pemetrexed combination in the palliative setting have just been published [11]. The same combination of carboplatin AUC 5 plus pemetrexed 500mg/m^2, day 1, every 3 weeks for 4 cycles, has been proposed as pre-operative chemotherapy followed by surgery (EPP) and hemithoracic irradiation. The study is conducted by F. Rea, Thoracic Surgery and A. Favaretto, Medical Oncology as principal investigators, at the University Hospital and Istituto Oncologico Veneto in Padua.

At the NKI in Amsterdam, the Netherlands, based on a previous NKI-AVL experience, Thalidomide is now being evaluated as maintenance therapy after pemetrexed containing chemotherapy in a randomized phase III study of the NVALT group.

The NVALT-5 study is evaluating the role of maintenance thalidomide in non-progressing patients after the standard cisplatin-pemetrexed first line therapy is active for PS 0-2 patients with limited weight loss. Thalidomide is thought to inhibit VEGF-, tumor necrosis factor alpha-, and basic fibroblast growth factor-induced angiogenesis. The primary endpoint is time to progression. Patients are randomized to Thalidomide 200 mg daily versus observation (phase III) study. The effects of Thalidomide will also be tested in conditional knock-out MPM mouse model of MPM. Vessel density, VEGF, MMP2 and 9 and VCAM expression will serve as potential markers of the drug effect. The study has started in May 2004, is planned to recruit 216 patients and is coordinated by P. Baas.

For second line treatment, the previously cited phase II international study with Bortezomib is ongoing. Studies with chemotherapy plus bevacizumab or Zactima are supposed to begin in the near future.

At the Erasmus Medical Center in Rotterdam, a phase I study "Vaccination with Autologous Dendritic Cells Pulsed with Tumor Lysate for Treatment of Patients with Malignant Pleural Mesothelioma" has been activated in January 2006 and the expected total enrolment is 10 patients. The completion is expected for December 2010.

The purpose is exploiting the immunostimulatory capacities of dendritic cells that hold great promise for cancer immunotherapy [15]. A mouse model for malignant mesothelioma has allowed us to prove that autologous dendritic cells presenting tumor antigens were very effective by (partly) inhibiting tumor growth. This study will test the feasibility and safety of a clinical trial using autologous DC as a therapeutic adjuvant for the treatment of malignant pleural mesothelioma.

The primary outcomes are safety and tolerability. The secondary outcomes are anti-tumor responses in vitro and in vivo and clinical response evaluation. For this phase I study, patients with end-stage malignant mesothelioma and deemed to be fit enough to be treated with chemotherapy will be asked to participate in the study. Patients will first be treated with 4 courses of chemotherapy (pemetrexed plus cisplatin as standard treatment). After this chemotherapy, a leukapheresis is performed whose monocytes are used for differentiation to dendritic cells. The procedure to grow the dendritic cells in vitro and pulse them with tumor lysate is performed in a cleanroom environment. Several quality control tests will be performed before the dendritic cells are ready for re-injection. Three doses of properly pulsed autologous dendritic cells are then re-injected every two weeks. Using the proper procedure in mesothelioma patients, minor side effects are expected. Ten patients will be treated by this procedure to define the safety and toxicity of immunization and to observe anti-tumoral immune responses.

Inclusion Criteria for the study: Patients with clinically and histological or cytological confirmed newly diagnosed mesothelioma, that can be measured in two dimensions by a radiological imaging study. Patients must be at least 18 years old and must be able to give written informed consent. Patients must be ambulatory (Karnofsky scale >70, or WHO-ECOG performance status 0-2) and in stable medical condition. The expected survival must be at least 4 months. Patients must have normal organ function and adequate bone marrow reserve. Positive delayed type hypersensitivity skin test (induration >2 mm after 48hrs) against at least one positive control antigen of Multitest CMI (Pasteur Merieux). Stable disease or response after chemotherapy.

Exclusion Criteria: Conditions that make the patient unfit for chemotherapy or progressive disease after 4 cycles of chemotherapy. Pleurodesis at the affected side before the pleural fluid is obtained. Medical or psychological impediment to probable compliance with the protocol. Patients on steroid (or other immunosuppressive agents) are excluded on the basis of potential immune suppression. Patients must have had 6 weeks of discontinuation and must stop of any such treatment during the time of the study. No prior malignancy is allowed except for adequately treated basal cell or squamous cell skin cancer, superficial or in-situ cancer of the bladder or other cancer for which the patient has been disease-free for five years. Serious concomitant disease, no active infections. Patients with a history of autoimmune disease or organ allografts, or with active acute or chronic infection, including HIV and viral hepatitis. Patients with serious intercurrent chronic or acute illness such as pulmonary (asthma or COPD) or cardiac (NYHA class III or IV) or hepatic disease or other illness considered by the study coordinators to constitute an unwarranted high risk for investigational Dendritic Cell treatment.

The principal investigator is Joachim G. Aerts, Department of Pulmonary Medicine at Erasmus Medical Center, Rotterdam. The study is presently open for inclusion.

In France, Nicolas Vénissac of the Hospital of Nice is conducting a phase I-II multicenter study on the multimodal treatment of malignant pleural mesothelioma. The study combines neoadjuvant chemotherapy (2 cycles of cisplatin 80 mg/m² day 1 and gemcitabine 1250 mg/m² days 1 and 8), extrapleural pneumonectomy plus intra-thoracic hyperthermic (42°C) cisplatin 100mg/m² and gemcitabine 1250 mg/m², and postoperative radiotherapy (65 Gy). The study started in January 2005.

Spain has an active participation in the previously cited phase III SAHA trial and in a second trial starting soon. The University Hospital in Madrid will participate in a phase II trial of a PDGFR/VEGFR/KIT inhibitor sponsored by Amgen.

In Turkey, H. Batirel of the Department of Thoracic Surgery at Marmara University is conducting a prospective trimodality trial on the treatment of malignant pleural mesothelioma. This prospective, Phase II study, tests the feasibility of trimodality treatment in Turkey. After having been treated with extrapleural pneumonectomy, patients receive adjuvant therapy consisting of high dose hemithoracic irradiation followed by 3 cycles of platinum based chemotherapy.

Patients with Stage I-III MPM, radiologically resectable disease on chest CT and MRI are eligible. No routine preoperative mediastinoscopy is planned; PET scan only if suitable.

The study started in January 2003 and is planned to end in December 2006. Centers involved in the study are Marmara University, Istanbul (Department of Thoracic Surgery: H.Batirel, M. Yuksel; Radiotherapy: H. Caglar and Medical Oncology), and Osmangazi University, Eskisehir (Department of Chest diseases: M. Metintas).

Twenty patients are planned to be enrolled. So far, 14 patients have been recruited: 12 with epithelial, 2 with mixed histology. One perioperative death occurred. All patients had EPP, 10 patients completed radiotherapy and chemotherapy. Four patients could not complete radiotherapy and chemotherapy due to postoperative complications in 3 patients and early hepatic recurrence (at 2 months) in 1 patient. Three patients are alive without recurrence at 31, 26 and 8 months; 7 patients who completed trimodality treatment recurred (2 distant-abdomen, 2 distant-abdomen plus local-chest wall, 3 local-chest wall). All cases were due to environmental asbestos (n=11 patients) or erionite (n=3 patients) exposure.

Conclusion

MPM is becoming a huge problem both in industrialized countries and in developing countries. Major results are far to be reached, but some improvements have been achieved.

Moreover, pharmaceutical companies are taking MPM into more consideration, investing in large phase III studies on specifically MPM oriented drugs. After the publication of the results of the first large phase III trial by Vogelzang [3], the pemetrexed-cisplatin combination has become the standard treatment in most countries. Among the countries where it is not accepted, a particular case is given by the UK where, apart from the specific combination, both chemotherapy and surgery are challenged as standard treatment. And such doubts are the object of two British studies the MARS and the MS-01.

Compared to a previous survey conducted in 2004 [16], one can see that the overwhelming predominance of pemetrexed in the studies conducted under the Extended Access Program (EAP) has been substituted by the professional use of the pemetrexed-cisplatin combination in the first line palliative setting or as part of a trimodality treatment in the preoperative setting. Since then, two important studies have been published. A randomized phase III trial by the EORTC [4] has shown that the raltitrexed plus cisplatin combination is more effective than cisplatin alone. The results are consistent with the Vogelzang trial [3], making sounder the evidence that polychemotherapy is better than monochemotherapy also in MPM. The second is an Italian study that tested the pemetrexed-carboplatin combination [11]. A phase II study recruiting more than one hundred patients, it showed that substituting cisplatin with carboplatin did not worsen the efficacy of treatment although activity was compromised. On the contrary, the combination tolerability seems better.

Current European clinical trials cover all the major areas of interest in the treatment of MPM: multimodality treatment, first- and second-line or maintenance treatment, new drugs. A rising interest is in trimodality treatment, but using chemotherapy first, as preoperative treatment. Trials are running within EORTC and in Denmark, Italy and Switzerland. All provide extrapleural pneumonectomy followed by 3D-conformal radiotherapy, which should yield a better local control through a higher dose of radiotherapy.

As first line palliative treatment, there is bortezomib — a proteasome inhibitor that induces apoptosis or enhances the apoptotic effect of chemo- and radiotherapy in cancer cells —, alone, in a UK study, or in combination with cisplatin in a EORTC study. A randomized trial still ongoing, but almost concluded, is the international trial with Onconase, an antineoplastic ribonuclease derived from frog eggs, which has shown antitumor activity in mesothelioma. A sequential chemotherapy approach, pemetrexed plus carboplatin followed by Caelyx, is going to be tested in a comparative way by the Nordic Mesothelioma Group. A similar but not randomized experience has been recently published [13] and showed favorable results in terms of disease control and survival.

Due to the increasing number of active drugs in MPM, many trials are testing second line treatment. The JMEW randomized study, evaluating BSC *versus* BSC plus pemetrexed, is concluded and the results are to be published soon. Both Onconase and bortezomib are tested also in the second line setting. Finally, vorinostat (SAHA) is a new interesting histone deacetylase inhibitor, evaluated in a randomized study in second or third line, that is administered orally.

Often treatment compliance and tolerability are greater with oral drugs, and this may be useful in a disease like MPM where symptom palliation is a major objective. Other trials using orally administrable drugs are ongoing: a Danish trial uses Vinorelbine partly orally and partly intravenously, and an Italian trial that tests the use of imatinib.

Two studies dealing with maintenance therapy are ongoing: one at the Dutch National Cancer Institute is testing thalidomide, a now rediscovered old drug, and the second in Italy will test pemetrexed. Both studies provide pemetrexed plus cisplatin as the standard first line chemotherapy.

Finally, new anticancer non-chemotherapeutic drugs are being tested. Besides mentioned imatinib and bortezomib trials, two other studies are ongoing: one in Italy tests the anti-VEGF drug bevacizumab together with the pemetrexed–carboplatin combination, and one in the Netherlands is a phase I trial of vaccination with autologous dendritic cells.

Despite the long history of therapeutic nihilism that has accompanied MPM management —actually no patient with unresectable disease appears to be cured, and overall median survival time is still poor — recent advances have put new enthusiasm on aggressive treatment of the disease in all stages. The recent phase III trials of cisplatin plus pemetrexed or raltitrexed have shown that chemotherapy is beginning to have a clinical impact in MPM, both on survival and on symptom control. Biological agents, vaccines and immunotoxins, are being tested too.

The understanding of MPM biology has rapidly increased. The continuous research on new molecular targets and their respective targeted therapies is becoming more and more important to further improve the disease outcome, and the prospect of a molecular-tailored therapy is becoming a realistic hope for a step forward in the struggle against MPM.

References

[1] Tomek S, Emri S, Krejcy K, Manegold C. (2003) Chemotherapy for malignant pleural mesothelioma: past results and recent developments. *Br. J. Cancer* 88:167–174.

[2] Vogelzang NJ, Porta C, Mutti L. (2005). New agents in the management of advanced mesothelioma. *Semin. Oncol.* 32:336-350.

[3] Vogelzang NJ, Rusthoven JJ, Symanowski J, Denham C, Kaukel E, Ruffie P, Gatzemeier U, Boyer M, Emri S, Manegold C, Niyikiza C, Paoletti P. (2003) Phase III study of pemetrexed in combination with cisplatin versus cisplatin alone in patients with malignant pleural mesothelioma. *J. Clin. Oncol.* 21:2636-2344.

[4] van Meerbeeck JP, Gaafar R, Manegold C, Van Klaveren RJ, Van Marck EA, Vincent M, Legrand C, Bottomley A, Debruyne C, and Giaccone G. (2005) Randomized Phase III Study of Cisplatin With or Without Raltitrexed in Patients With Malignant Pleural Mesothelioma: An Intergroup Study of the European Organisation for Research and Treatment of Cancer Lung Cancer Group and the National Cancer Institute of Canada. *J. Clin. Oncol.* 23:6881-6889.

[5] Mikulski SM, Costanzi JJ, Vogelzang NJ, McCachren S, Taub RN, Chun H, Mittelman A, Panella T, Puccio C, Fine R, Shogen K. (2002) Phase II trial of a single weekly intravenous dose of ranpirnase in patients with unresectable malignant mesothelioma. *J. Clin. Oncol.* 20:274-281.

[6] Hillerdal G, Sundstrom S, Sorensen JB, for the Nordic Mesothelioma Group. (2003) Malignant pleural mesothelioma treated with a combination of pegylated liposomal doxorubicin, carboplatin and gemcitabine: The CCG study. *Proc. ASCO* 22: abstr 2534.

[7] Andreopoulou E, Ross PJ, O'Brien MER, Ford HER, Priest K, Eisen T, Norton A, Ashley S, Smith IE. (2004). The palliative benefits of MVP (mitomycin C, vinblastine and cisplatin) chemotherapy in patients with malignant Mesothelioma. *Ann. Oncol.* 15:1406–1412.

[8] Muers MF, Rudd RM, O'Brien MER, Qian W, Hodson A, Parmar MKB, Girling DJ, on behalf of the British Thoracic Society Mesothelioma Group. (2004) BTS randomised feasibility study of active symptom control with or without chemotherapy in malignant pleural mesothelioma: ISRCTN 54469112. *Thorax* 59:144–148.

[9] O'Rourke N, Paul J, Hill J (2000) Radiotherapy to mesothelioma drain sites may not be worthwhile: interim report of a randomized study. *Lung Cancer* 29(suppl 2): 168.

[10] Weder W, Kestenholz P, Taverna C, Bodis S, Lardinois D, Jerman M, Stahel R. (2004) Neoadjuvant Chemotherapy Followed by Extrapleural Pneumonectomy in Malignant Pleural Mesothelioma. *J. Clin. Oncol.* 22:3451-3457.

[11] Ceresoli GL, Zucali PA, Favaretto AG, Grossi F, Bidoli P, Del Conte G, Cerebelli A, Bearz A, et Al. (2006) Phase II study of pemetrexed plus carboplatin in malignant pleural mesothelioma. *J. Clin. Oncol.* 24:1443-1448.

[12] Byrne MJ, Nowak AK: Modified RECIST criteria for assessment of response in malignant pleural mesothelioma *Ann. Oncol.* (2004) 15: 257–260.

[13] Pinto C, Marino A, De Pangher Manzini V, Benedetti G, Galetta D, Mazzanti P, Del Conte G, dell'Amore D, Piana E, Giaquinta S, Lopez M, Martoni A. (2006) Sequential chemotherapy with cisplatin/gemcitabine (CG) followed by mitoxantrone/ methotrexate/ mitomycin (MMM) in patients with malignant pleural mesothelioma. A multicenter Italian Phase II Study (SITMP1). *Lung Cancer* 52:199-206.

[14] Favaretto AG, Aversa SM, Paccagnella A, de Pangher-Manzini V, Palmisano V, Oniga F, Stefani M, Rea F, Bortolotti L, Monfardini S. (2003) Gemcitabine combined with carboplatin in patients with malignant pleural mesothelioma: a multicentric phase II study. *Cancer* 97:2791—2797.

[15] Hegmans JP, Hemmes A, Aerts JG, Hoogsteden HC, Lambrecht BN. (2005) Immunotherapy of murine malignant mesothelioma using tumor lysate-pulsed dendritic cells. *Am. J. Respir. Crit. Care Med.* 171:1168-1177.

[16] Favaretto AG (2005) Overview on ongoing or planned clinical trials in Europe. *Lung Cancer* 49 (Suppl 1), s117-s121.

In: Mesothelioma from Bench Side to Clinic
Editor: Alfonso Baldi, pp. 501-519

ISBN: 978-1-60021-789-0

Chapter XXX

Clinical Trials in Mesothelioma: Australia

Anna K. Nowak**[1], Malcolm Feigen[2] and Nick Pavlakis[3]

[1]Department of Medicine and Pharmacology, University of Western Australia,
4th Floor, G block,
Sir Charles Gairdner Hospital. Hospital Avenue,
Nedlands, WA 6009 Australia
[2]Radiation Oncology Centre, Heidelberg Repatriation Hospital,
Austin Health PO Box 5444, Heidelberg West,
Victoria 3081 Australia
[3] Department of Medical Oncology,
Royal North Shore Hospital (University of Sydney),
St Leonards, NSW, 2065, Australia

Abstract

Australia has one of the highest incidences of malignant mesothelioma in the developed world, due to asbestos mining and production, and occupational use of this fiber. Although the population of Australia is relatively small, health care resources are concentrated in the major capital cities, allowing tertiary referral centres to develop interest and expertise in rare tumours such as mesothelioma. Several Australian centres have active investigator-initiated clinical trial programs in this disease. Current research programs encompass the use of radiotherapy in mesothelioma, second line systemic therapy with novel agents, maintenance therapy after first-line treatment, and study of clinical trial endpoints and imaging in mesothelioma. The clinical trials currently underway in Australia are described and discussed.

* Corresponding author: Dr Anna Nowak, Department of Medicine and Pharmacology, 4th Floor, G block, Sir Charles Gairdner Hospital. Hospital Avenue, Nedlands, WA 6009 Australia. Email: anowak@cyllene.uwa.edu.au. Fax: +61 8 9346 3390. Phone: +61 8 93463841.

Keywords: *Malignant Mesothelioma, Antineoplastic agents, Clinical trials, Radiotherapy.*

Introduction

The mineral resources of Australia include rich natural deposits of asbestos, which were mined for domestic use and export for over 100 years, between 1880 and 1983. Asbestos production increased over the first half of the 20th century, and crocidolite asbestos became the most important fiber mined with the opening of the Wittenoom mine in the north of Western Australia in 1937. Wittenoom closed in 1967, but mining of crocidolite asbestos continued at other sites, and chrysotile asbestos was mined until 1983[1]. The legacy of asbestos exposure amongst miners, mill-workers, wharf workers Wittenoom residents and their children remains (Figure 1), with one of the highest mesothelioma incidence rates in the world, almost 60 per million per year in males[1]. Whilst Western Australia has the highest incidence of mesothelioma in Australia (7.9 per 100,000 population in males), larger numbers arise in the eastern states of Australia, with their numerically larger populations (181 new cases in NSW in 2001, 4.8 per 100,000 in males). In 2001, there were 567 diagnoses of mesothelioma reported Australia-wide [2].

Healthcare delivery in Australia is concentrated in the state capitals in much of the country, with limited tertiary hospital care and oncology expertise in rural areas. This means that despite relatively small patient numbers, the majority of patients with mesothelioma can expect to be referred to a respiratory physician or medical oncologist with expertise and a large caseload of patients with mesothelioma.

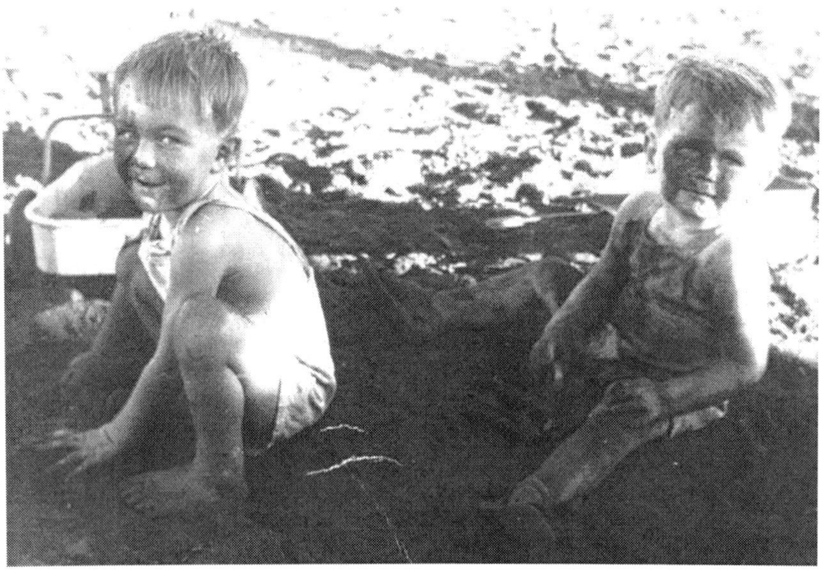

Figure 1. Children playing in crocidolite asbestos tailings, Wittenoom, Western Australia. Both subsequently died of malignant mesothelioma in adulthood.

The availability of financial compensation for many Australian patients with malignant mesothelioma [3] is another reason why a relatively small number of physicians are involved with the management of this disease. This concentration of patients in relatively few centres around the country is clearly beneficial for the development of clinical trials at individual sites, and co-operatively Australia-wide.

Perth is the capital city of Western Australia with a population of approximately 1.5 million. It is the closest major city to the mining town of Wittenoom. There has been no asbestos mining in Wittenoom since 1967, and the population of that town has dwindled to a small number of people who choose to stay despite the known health risks. However, the population of often unskilled and itinerant workers with anywhere from a few weeks to a few years exposure to asbestos has spread throughout the state. Exposure in the building industry, dockyards, or Navy and merchant navy is also common in the Western Australian population. The majority of patients with mesothelioma are referred to clinician members of the Perth Mesothelioma Group, an informal consortium of clinicians and researchers predominantly based at Sir Charles Gairdner Hospital. This group is active in clinical and preclinical research in this disease. Previous clinical trials from this group include reports of the use of cisplatin and gemcitabine in mesothelioma [4, 5], and trials of immunotherapy, gene therapy, and chemo-immunotherapy approaches [6-9].

Co-Operative Group Clinical Trials in Mesothelioma in Australia

The conduct and planning of clinical trials in mesothelioma in Australia will be greatly facilitated by the recent formation of the Australasian Lung cancer Trials Group (ALTG). The inaugural meeting of the group was in Sydney in February 2004. Full membership is open to medical and non-medical persons active in and interested in the conduct of Australian clinical trials in lung cancer. The mission statement of the ALTG is to "reduce the incidence, morbidity and mortality of lung cancer in Australia and New Zealand through the co-ordination and facilitation of high quality clinical research". The group meets twice yearly for submission, scientific review and discussion of potential investigator-initiated projects and identification and formulation of important clinical research questions. The ALTG will also co-ordinate and develop accepted multi-centre trials, collaborate with national and international clinical trials groups, and give strategic assistance in obtaining funding. The objectives of the ALTG include improving patient access to clinical trials and educating patients with lung cancer and mesothelioma about the role of clinical trials in clinical care. This new group is likely to play an important role in clinical trials in mesothelioma in this region.

The discussion below covers current clinical trials and investigational approaches to the clinical management of mesothelioma in Australia.

Clinical Trials of Radiotherapy for Mesothelioma in Australia

The role of radiotherapy in the management of mesothelioma in Australia has followed practices in the larger institutions in the United Kingdom and North America, as local clinicians adopted standards detailed in oncological textbooks, journals and conference presentations. Two reviews of the experience from the Peter MacCallum Cancer Institute in Melbourne during the 1980s reflect this approach [10, 11]. The majority of patients are treated with a palliative intent to small volumes over one or two weeks, without a coordinated plan involving the other specialties of surgery and medical oncology. No survival benefit was demonstrated for radical radiotherapy, but short courses produced useful palliation in occasional patients [12]. Standard treatment modalities included orthovoltage, megavoltage and electron beam radiotherapy, but in well-meaning attempts to enhance the poor responses from conventional radiotherapy, various innovative practices were evaluated, including moving strip radiotherapy, brachytherapy and UHF microwave radiation [13], without success.

In 1997 a randomised trial of prophylactic electron beam irradiation for thoracic drainage of thoracoscopy sites was initiated in Perth. No benefit was found for a single fraction of 10 Gy using 9 MeV electrons to 58 chest wall sites, with three subcutaneous masses in the control arm and two in the prophylactic radiotherapy arm [14].

In December 2002 Perth was host to the 6th International Mesothelioma Interest Group meeting, recognising the high incidence of the disease and research contributions from Australia. Following a presentation by Dr Craig Stevens, a radiation oncologist from the MD Anderson Cancer Center in Houston, Texas in which he described a novel radiotherapy technique using intensity modulated radiation therapy (I.M.R.T.) for postoperative treatment following extrapleural pneumonectomy (EPP) with excellent locoregional control, a new approach to managing mesothelioma patients was considered by staff at the Austin Hospital in Melbourne. Stevens reported on the radiosensitivity of mesothelioma cell-lines [15] and the importance of targeting a large volume including the full hemithorax after radical surgery, guided by close interaction with the surgical team to define the surgical bed and include the insertion of the diaphragm prior to resection and replacement by a synthetic membrane [16].

A pilot study was subsequently undertaken in Melbourne to treat regions of gross residual disease in patients who had undergone pleurectomy/decortication with phototherapy [17] using 3D-conformal radiotherapy to high doses, limited by the need to observe tolerances of adjacent normal organs including the intact ipsilateral lung. IMRT had been instituted for selected patients with prostate and head and neck cancers at a few radiation oncology centres in Victoria and New South Wales, but with the much larger target volumes and complexity involved in limiting the dosage to multiple adjacent organs for treating mesothelioma cases, available resources necessitated preliminary development at a single Australian centre. The Austin Hospital had the advantages of a dedicated team of thoracic surgeons committed to the multidisciplinary management of thoracic tumours with a technologically advanced radiotherapy department and Australia's largest PET Centre, which acquired a PET/CT scanner in 2003. A feasibility proposal for the study was presented at the annual meeting of TROG, the Trans-Tasman Radiation Oncology Group which conducts most of the Australasian clinical trials in radiotherapy, in April 2004, and discussed with other interested centres at various national conferences of radiation, medical and surgical oncologists, all agreeing on the single centre policy. In April 2004 a team from the Austin Radiation Oncology Centre visited Dr Stevens at MD Anderson for training in mesothelioma IMRT, confirming that the early results were maintained and that side effects were tolerable [18].

The vast majority of patients with mesothelioma present with local symptoms confined to one hemithorax, and most recur after surgery in the same area, despite intraoperative or postoperative chemotherapy and conventional radiotherapy [19]. The establishment and maintenance of local control is therefore a major goal of treatment, and until more effective systemic agents become available, the local therapies of radical surgery followed by targeted large field postoperative radiotherapy are essential components for cure. Although extrapleural pneumonectomy followed by IMRT encompassing all sites of microscopic residual disease is highly successful, only a small proportion of mesothelioma patients are suitable to undergo this radical procedure. Those who are older with reduced respiratory reserves and comorbidities are eligible for the shorter operation of pleurectomy/decortication, and we are therefore attempting to develop a modified form of IMRT which spares more of the ipsilateral lung than the MD Anderson technique. This approach is being investigated at other centres, with little success to date [20]. Problems to be considered include treating the diagonal interlobar fissures, margins for respiratory movement and disease progression outside the planned target volume in the interval between surgery and the completion of radiotherapy. This interval frequently exceeds four months in order to incorporate time for surgical recuperation, wound healing, pain control, radiotherapy planning, ability to remain immobilised during simulation and for 45 minutes per fraction over six weeks.

Potential solutions to these difficulties are currently being assessed. We hope that the inclusion of intraoperative phototherapy will improve sterilisation of microscopic residual mesothelioma cells at the margins of surgical resection, including the interlobar fissures. Hematoporphyrin derivative (HpD) is a first generation photosensitiser which has been used in 140 patients at the Austin since 1989 without any significant toxicity. The use of. neoadjuvant chemotherapy may retard short-term tumour progression following surgery in addition to improving operability by shrinking large masses of tumour [21, 22]. Most normal tissues can be spared excessive radiation by adopting IMRT, but the lung becomes the dose-limiting structure. The removal of all macroscopic disease at pleurectomy by performing when appropriate chest wall resection, lymphadenectomy and reconstruction of the diaphragm and pericardium (as is standard for EPP) will reduce the radiation dose required, but it remains very difficult to spare lung in the centre of a large tumour volume with current techniques. A recent report from Sugarbaker's group in Boston has warned of the high risk of acute pneumonitis following IMRT irradiation to the contralateral lung in patients who have undergone pneumonectomy and adjuvant chemotherapy, with six fatalities in their first thirteen cases [23]. To reduce the risk of pneumonitis one other option is to consider amifostine, a radioprotectant which in a recent meta-analysis of randomized trial data was found to raise the threshold for acute radiation pneumonitis and oesophagitis, while enhancing tumour response rates from radical radiotherapy [24]. This agent, in common with premetrexed, is not subsidised for this indication in Australia and is seldom used.

We have completed postoperative radiotherapy using high dose 3D-conformal radiotherapy on 13 patients between July 2003 and February 2006. Eleven have been referred following surgery by pleurectomy/decortication with intraoperative phototherapy using HpD at the Austin Hospital, and a further two patients were resected elsewhere by EPP and radical pleurectomy that resulted in complete macroscopic disease resection. Radiation doses ranged from 45 to 60 Gy in 25 to 30 fractions, using a complex arrangement of 7-21 beams to meet the planning constraints set by Stevens et al [18]. Treatment plans were based on simulation CT scans fused with PET scans where available, using CMS planning software. This technology has enabled us to assess whether any relapses have occurred within the planned target volume (PTV) at followup.

Nausea and vomiting experienced by our early cases have been almost completely controlled with prophylactic 5HT3 receptor antagonist antiemetics, with most patients experiencing grade II radiation dermatitis, tiredness and weight loss. All have completed treatment on schedule and recovered their previous performance status in all but one case, who died 2 months after radiotherapy after pneumonia. No patient has had any grade 3 or 4 toxicities following radiotherapy, and in particular none have required steroids for pneumonitis. There has been one case of partial liver necrosis which completely resolved within three months. Median followup is six months post-radiotherapy.

Regular clinical, CT scan and PET scan assessments and serum mesothelin assays have been performed. Of 12 assessable patients, six patients have died, five with recurrent mesothelioma outside the irradiated field and one from a late surgical complication with no disease recurrence at nine months. Five are alive with progressive disease and one is alive with no recurrence at 13 months. Followup PET scans have shown significantly reduced FDG-avidity in all irradiated areas at assessment 3 months post-treatment, with progressive disease at sites beyond the planned targets in six cases (Figure 2).

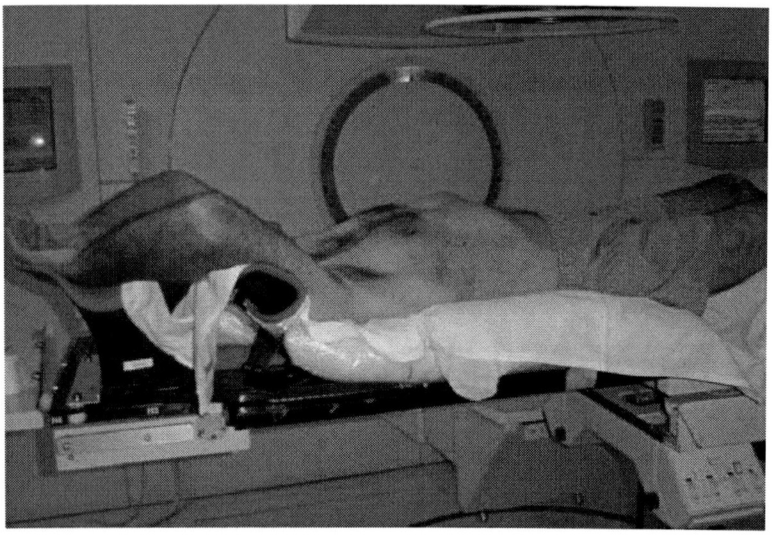

Figure 2. Patient positioned for IMRT with immobilisation support, showing skin reaction on last day of treatment.

Patients have experienced lengthy delays between surgery and radiotherapy to allow time for surgical recuperation, wound healing, pain control, radiotherapy planning and ability to lie immobilised for 1 hour treatments and we have not repeated their imaging studies after simulation to incorporate new sites of disease in the PTVs.

Time taken to produce an acceptable treatment plan often exceeded one month due to difficulties in satisfying normal tissue tolerance constraints in the presence of unresected gross disease, and in the majority of cases we have compromised our target volume in order to reduce the risk of radiation toxicity, primarily to the lung. In one case who had received chemotherapy before resection in order to downstage disease, we recommended further combination chemotherapy in the planning interval following surgery to reduce the volume of active disease. Our compromised plans were unsuitable for an IMRT approach as the added complexities increased the daily fraction times from ten to forty minutes, and only one patient had the full hemithorax irradiated.

We succeeded in treating our first suitable patient with IMRT in May 2006. A dose of 50-60 Gy in 25 fractions was delivered through 6 fields to the lower hemithorax and upper abdomen after a PET/CT scan detected recurrence following PD and phototherapy one year previously. A concomitant boost was used (Figure 3), allowing of shortening the treatment time to five weeks instead of six, and all of the planning targets received doses which met the standard constraints (Figures 4,5).

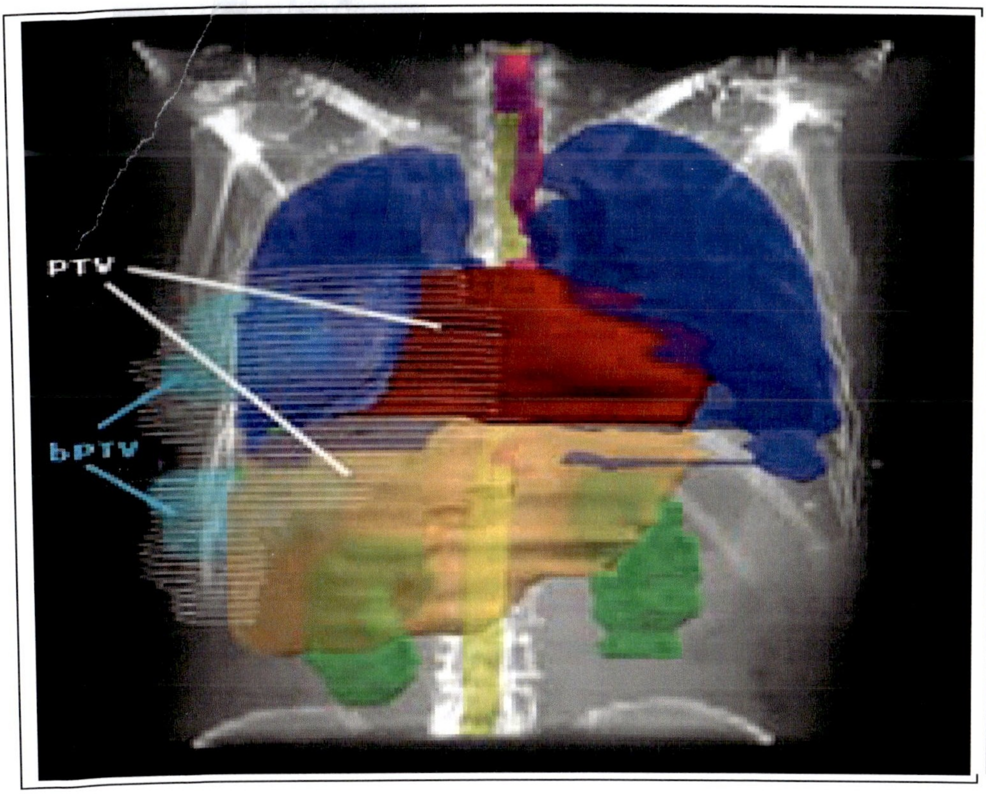

Figure 3. Digital reconstruction radiograph showing organs at risk with planning target volume (PTV, delineated by white wired volume, and boost planning target volume (bPTV) treated to 50 Gy and 60 Gy respectively in 25 fractions.

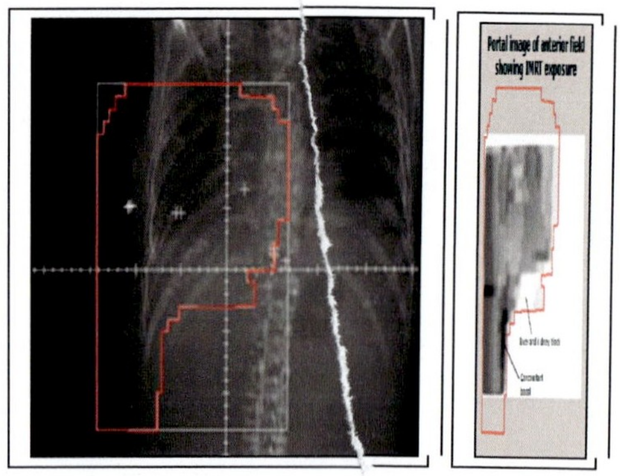

Figure 4. Digital reconstruction radiograph of anterior IMRT field, with electronic portal image of treatment exposure showing intensity modulation of beamlets delivering varying doses over the treatment volume, allowing protection of organs at risk. The full length of this field is too long to fit on the standard viewer.

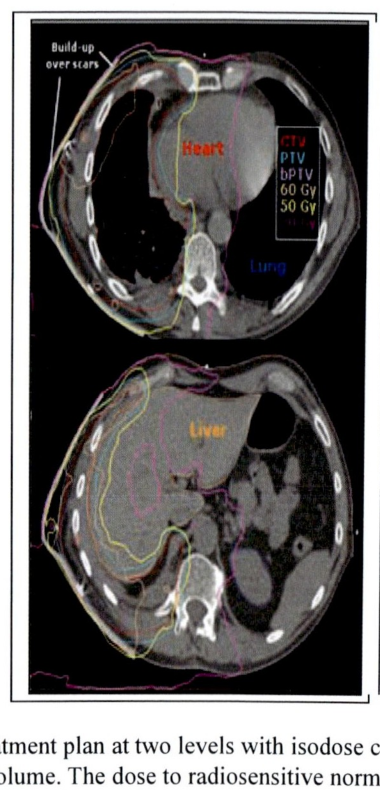

Figure 5. Transverse cuts of treatment plan at two levels with isodose contours for 20, 50 and 60 Gy, encompassing planning target volume. The dose to radiosensitive normal tissues including contralateral lung, heart, liver and spinal cord are within tolerance limits.

Future proposals include considering neoadjuvant chemotherapy with four cycles of cisplatin and pemetrexed in fully staged patients before surgery, and adopting more aggressive approaches to tumour resection. We will refine our IMRT technique with fused PET/CT scans performed at the time of simulation incorporating full immobilisation in the treatment position.

acceptable toxicity profile with grade 3 fatigue (8%), neutropenia (8%) and gastrointestinal toxicity (2%) the most prominent side effects [40]. In a recent phase III study in patients with renal carcinoma, sunitinib demonstrated a a highly clinically and statistically significant advantage in progression-free survival and response rate over interferon-alpha [41], and this drug is quickly moving into the therapeutic armamentarium in this disease. Sunitinib also shows activity in patients with previously treated metastatic breast cancer [42], and is US FDA approved for Imatinib-resistant gastrointestinal stromal tumours (GIST) and renal cell carcinoma [43].

Its oral availability, acceptable toxicity profile and multi-targeted spectrum of receptor tyrosine kinase inhibition suggested its potential for significant anti-tumour activity in mesothelioma. This is a non-randomised single centre phase II study of single-agent sunitinib as second line therapy in mesothelioma, underway at Sir Charles Gairdner Hospital in Western Australia. Eligibility requirements are for a histologically or cytologically confirmed diagnosis of pleural malignant mesothelioma, previous therapy with at least one cycle of a platinum analogue and an antimetabolite with documented progression on or after completion of first-line therapy, an ECOG performance status of 0-1, measurable disease, a life expectancy >12 weeks, adequate organ function, and written informed consent. Exclusion criteria are standard, with the exception that patients with a prior talc pleuradesis are excluded. Patients with prior talc pleuradesis are ineligible as this renders changes on PET scan, a response criterion, more difficult to interpret reliably, due to residual pleural inflammation from the procedure.

The primary endpoint of the trial is objective response rate as assessed by the Modified RECIST Criteria [44] and by response on PET scan. Secondary endpoints include time to tumour progression, time to treatment failure, overall survival, change in lung function tests, toxicity, and change in serum mesothelin levels. In addition to objective tumour response, visual and quantitative assessment of the change in tumour metabolism after one cycle of treatment will be assessed by serial [F-18] FDG PET scans. Quantitative indices of total glycolytic volume (TGV) and tumour volume (TV) have been related to tumour response to chemotherapy in a first line treatment setting in patients with MPM [45, 46].Changes in the standard uptake value (SUV) as measured with PET have previously been used as an index of antitumour activity with sunitinib [47].

All patients will receive sunitinib 50 mg daily orally for four weeks, followed by two weeks off treatment each 6-week cycle. Dose modifications are specified for toxicity. Most endpoints are assessed 6 weekly. The sample size has been calculated using Simon's optimal two-stage design, with an initial 23 patients and a maximum of 51 patients recruited assuming a response rate of 20% to be of interest and a response rate of 5% to be of no interest. Recruitment over approximately two years is anticipated. The study commenced recruiting in June 2006.

A conventional phase II study design using single-agent sunitinib as second line therapy may reveal activity in this patient population, however prolongation of time to progression may also indicate potential for sunitinib following response to first-line chemotherapy or following multimodality therapy including surgical resection for early stage mesothelioma. Any activity would justify the early development of protocols in a first line setting.

The MATES Study – Maintenance Thalidomide in Mesothelioma

Thalidomide, a sedative first used in pregnancy in the late 1950s with subsequent devastatingly detrimental effects on embryogenesis, was re-discovered in the 1990s as an anticancer agent after being shown to inhibit bFGF and VEGF mediated angiogenesis together with it's cytokine modulatory properties, in particular involving interleukin-6 and tumour necrosis factor alpha [48-50]. Two Phase II clinical trials involving thalidomide have been reported. In the first published Phase II study conducted in the Netherlands (N = 42, 20 received prior chemotherapy), thalidomide up to 400 mg daily did not produce any tumour responses however 11 of the 40 patients (27.5%) could be treated with the drug for 6 months or longer showing stabilization of the disease [51]. Side effects were manageable and consisted of sleepiness, constipation and in two patients neurological toxicity grade 2 and 3 was observed.

In Australia, a parallel design Phase II study was conducted investigating the activity of thalidomide in combination with cisplatin/gemcitabine (C/G) chemotherapy (Arm A) or alone (Arm B) in patients with advanced malignant pleural mesothelioma [52]. Thalidomide was administered alone (arm B) (100 – 500 mg p.o./d), or in combination with weekly i.v. C (25 mg/m^2)/G (800 mg/m^2) chemotherapy (D1, 8,15 Q4 weekly) (arm A). The primary objective was response rate (PR = partial response, PD = progressive disease, SD = stable disease). Eligibility criteria included no prior chemotherapy (arm A) or prior chemotherapy or medically unsuitable for chemotherapy (arm B). 63 patients were enrolled: 34 in arm A, 29 in arm B (9 (31%) having prior chemotherapy); 7 female and 27 male (A); 4 female and 25 male (B); median age 59 (A) and 67 (B). In the combination arm there were only 3 PR (14%) whilst in the thalidomide alone arm 8 patients (27%) had stable disease for > 6 months. Median tolerated thalidomide dose was 200 mg (both arms). Common toxicities from thalidomide included mild constipation, dry mouth, fatigue, dizziness and parasthesiae (B). Exploratory analysis of serum VEGF indicated a possible prognostic role with worse survival associated with high baseline serum VEGF. These results confirmed the findings from the Netherlands Cancer Institute Phase II study and raised the hypothesis that thalidomide may delay disease progression.

Based on these Phase II findings, an Open label Randomized Phase III study of Thalidomide as maintenance therapy in non-progressing patients after first line Alimta based chemotherapy was commenced in the Netherlands in 2004 (The NVALT5 Study, Dr P Baas). A similarly designed study was proposed in Australia by the ALTG and the two groups agreed to co-operate in the one study. The Australian study includes two sub-studies: one addressing QoL, using several established tools, and the other exploring the predictive/prognostic value of a series of serum biomarkers, including VEGF, mesothelin and osteopontin: The Mates study -M*a*intenance *T*halidomide's *E*ffectiveness, *S*afety, and *Q*uality of *L*ife after chemotherapy for m*e*sothelioma.

Participation in International Pharmaceutical Industry Initiated Clinical Trials

Australian sites participate in international clinical trials initiated by the pharmaceutical industry. Participation in other international industry-initiated clinical trials of novel agents is currently under discussion.

SAHA Second Line in Mesothelioma

Histone deacetylase (HDAC) is an enzyme involved in removing acetyl groups from histones and other proteins. An imbalance in histone acetylation may lead to transcriptional dysregulation of genes involved in the control of cell cycle progression, differentiation, and apoptosis [53]. HDAC inhibitors are a novel class of agents shown to induce tumor cell growth arrest, differentiation, or apoptosis in vitro and inhibit tumor growth in animals [53]. A number of HDAC inhibitors have entered clinical trials [53]. Among these agents, Suberoylanilide Hydroxamic Acid – SAHA (L-001079038) is a potent inhibitor of HDAC that can be administered orally with good bioavailability.

In a Phase I study of oral L-001079038 in patients with advanced solid tumors and hematologic malignancies, 13 patients with mesothelioma who had failed front-line therapy were enrolled. Two patients responded with decreases in tumor mass and pleural effusion and improvement of tumor-related pain or shortness of breath.

Based on this finding and the unmet need for exploration of novel therapies beyond pemetrexed and cisplatin for mesothelioma patients, an international Phase III study has been initiated by Merck: A Phase III, Randomized, Double-Blind, Placebo-Controlled Trial of Oral Suberoylanilide Hydroxamic Acid (L-001079038) in Patients With Advanced Malignant Pleural Mesothelioma Previously Treated With Systemic Chemotherapy. Several centres in Australia are participating in this study.

Clinical Trial Methodology Studies in Australia

Measurement of response for clinical trials of mesothelioma has been an active area of research in Australia. Malignant mesothelioma grows as a 'rind' around the thoracic cavity, rather than in a roughly spherical fashion like many other neoplasms. This made measurement by the WHO criteria and, more recently, the RECIST criteria, difficult to perform and to reproduce between centres and investigators. The Modified RECIST Criteria [44] are now in widespread use in mesothelioma clinical trials, and go some way towards addressing these problems. Partial response as assessed by the Modified RECIST Criteria correlates with relief of symptoms, improvement in lung function tests and health-related quality of life, and patient survival. However, application of these modified criteria is still time consuming, and inter-observer reliability has not been validated. Furthermore, it is often not clear whether patients are responding to chemotherapy until several cycles of treatment have been given. In a previous study, we found that of those patients achieving a partial response, only 47% did so after one treatment cycle, and the median time taken to achieve a radiological partial response was four cycles [5]. Clearly, this means that many patients are exposed to more cycles of chemotherapy and thus more toxicity, when they may not be deriving benefit from treatment. If patients could be identified early as unlikely to benefit from treatment, they could be spared further side-effects, and potentially enrolled in clinical trials of second-line therapy whilst their performance status was preserved.

Use of FDG PET in the Assessment of Tumour Extent and Tumour Response in Pleural Mesothelioma

The considerations discussed above led to work investigating the use of FDG PET to stage mesothelioma at presentation, and to assess response to chemotherapy. ^{18}F FDG PET scans measure the metabolic activity, and therefore the viability, of tumour cells. Serial changes in ^{18}F FDG uptake can predict response in other tumour types after just one cycle of chemotherapy [54-56]. Mesothelioma has been demonstrated to be FDG PET avid [57-59]. This ongoing single-centre prospective cohort study at Sir Charles Gairdner Hospital in Western Australia has accrued over 50 eligible patients to date for assessment of staging of disease and, in those patients who go on to have chemotherapy as part of their routine clinical care, for assessment of response to treatment. Eligible consenting patients have confirmed malignant pleural mesothelioma, and those on the response study are planned to have chemotherapy as part of their routine clinical care. The important exclusion criterion is past pleuradesis, which renders PET scans difficult to interpret even many months after the procedure [60]. The staging study aims to define the PET appearance in patients with masses visible on CAT scan and those with effusion only, to examine the incidence and extent of cryptic metastatic disease demonstrated by PET scan compared to routine CAT scanning, to assess the relationship of the PET appearance to the histological subtype of mesothelioma, and to evaluate whether the PET appearance provides prognostic information. The response study aims to assess the sensitivity and specificity of FDG PET scan changes after one cycle of chemotherapy to predict ultimate response to chemotherapy, time to progression and overall survival, and to assess the relationship between HRQL changes and tumour volume and PET scan changes.

There are no formal guidelines for measurement of response to chemotherapy using ^{18}F FDG PET in solid tumours, and other authors have used visual analysis, maximum standardised uptake values (SUVmax), or mean standardised uptake values (SUVmean) to assess response. However, as well as posing challenges for measurement of radiological response, mesothelioma also brings particular challenges for measurement of response by PET scanning. The disease is often diffuse and heterogenous, and it is difficult to select a representative site as SUVmax. Furthermore, SUVmax represents only one pixel of the often large and complex tumour mass. Novel semi-automated software has been developed for this study, which uses a region-growing algorithm to define the 3-dimensional boundaries of the tumour, giving a measure of the total glycolytic volume (TGV) of the mass [45]. This software shows excellent inter-observer reliability and is simple to use [46]. Preliminary results have been reported for the response study, showing that ^{18}F FDG PET response after one cycle of chemotherapy is a better predictor of survival outcomes than CT scan response at this time [45, 46]. This technique appears promising as a surrogate measure of clinical benefit, and as an outcome measure in future clinical trials in mesothelioma.

Conclusion

Despite the small population of Australia, the high incidence of malignant mesothelioma and the concentration of healthcare resources and expertise in major population centres has led to considerable activity in mesothelioma research. Working within limitations in research funding, investigators continue to develop clinical trials and clinical trials methodology. Furthermore, the small number of investigators and concentration of patients with mesothelioma at relatively few sites make Australia a favourable country for activity by the pharmaceutical industry. Results from ongoing clinical trials described should be available within the next few years, and will hopefully make a substantial contribution to the body of knowledge in this devastating disease.

References

[1] Leigh, J., P. Davidson, L. Hendrie, and D. Berry, Malignant mesothelioma in Australia, 1945-2000. *Am. J. Indust. Med.* 2002; 41: 188-201.

[2] Australian Institute of Health and Welfare (AIHW) and Australasian Association of Cancer Registries (AACR) 2004. *Cancer in Australia 2001.* AIHW cat. no. CAN 23. Canberra: AIHW (Cancer Series no. 28).

[3] Burton, B., Asbestos company is forced to fund compensation shortfall. *BMJ* 2005; 330: 62.

[4] Byrne, M.J., J.A. Davidson, A.W. Musk, J. Dewar, G. van Hazel, M. Buck, N.H. de Klerk, and B.W. Robinson, Cisplatin and gemcitabine treatment for malignant mesothelioma: a phase II study. *J. Clin. Oncol.* 1999; 17: 25-30.

[5] Nowak, A.K., M.J. Byrne, R. Williamson, G. Ryan, A. Segal, D. Fielding, P. Mitchell, A.W. Musk, and B.W. Robinson, A multicentre phase II study of cisplatin and gemcitabine for malignant mesothelioma. *Br. J. Cancer* 2002; 87: 491-6.

[6] Robinson, B.W., S.A. Mukherjee, A. Davidson, S. Morey, A.W. Musk, I. Ramshaw, D. Smith, R. Lake, T. Haenel, M. Garlepp, J. Marley, C. Leong, I. Caminschi, and B. Scott, Cytokine gene therapy or infusion as treatment for solid human cancer. *Journal of Immunotherapy* 1998; 21: 211-7.

[7] Davidson, J.A., A.W. Musk, B.R. Wood, S. Morey, M. Ilton, L.L. Yu, P. Drury, K. Shilkin, and B.W. Robinson, Intralesional cytokine therapy in cancer: a pilot study of GM-CSF infusion in mesothelioma. *Journal of Immunotherapy* 1998; 21: 389-98.

[8] Upham, J.W., A.W. Musk, G. van Hazel, M. Byrne, and B.W. Robinson, Interferon alpha and doxorubicin in malignant mesothelioma: a phase II study. *Aust. NZ. J. Med.* 1993; 23: 683-7.

[9] Christmas, T.I., L.S. Manning, M.J. Garlepp, A.W. Musk, and B.W. Robinson, Effect of interferon-alpha 2a on malignant mesothelioma. *Journal of Interferon Research* 1993; 13: 9-12.

[10] Davis, S.R., L. Tan, and D.L. Ball, Radiotherapy in the treatment of malignant mesothelioma of the pleura, with special reference to its use in palliation. *Australasian Radiology* 1994; 38: 212-4.

[11] Ball, D.L. and D.G. Cruickshank, The treatment of malignant mesothelioma of the pleura: review of a 5-year experience, with special reference to radiotherapy. *American Journal of Clinical Oncology* 1990; 13: 4-9.

[12] Chin, Y.S., R. Yeghaian-Alvandi, and M. Noel, Radiotherapy for the palliation of high-volume pleural effusion in malignant mesothelioma: case report. *Palliative Medicine* 2002; 16: 63-4.

[13] Review Committee on Microwave Cancer Therapy, *Review of the use of microwave therapy for the treatment of patients with cancer.*, in *National Health and Medical Research Council report.* 2005.

[14] Bydder, S., M. Phillips, D.J. Joseph, F. Cameron, N.A. Spry, Y. DeMelker, and A.W. Musk, A randomised trial of single-dose radiotherapy to prevent procedure tract metastasis by malignant mesothelioma. *Br. J. Cancer* 2004; 91: 9-10.

[15] Carmichael, J., W.G. Degraff, J. Gamson, D. Russo, A.F. Gazdar, M.L. Levitt, J.D. Minna, and J.B. Mitchell, Radiation sensitivity of human lung cancer cell lines. *European Journal of Cancer and Clinical Oncology* 1989; 25: 527-34.

[16] Ahamad, A., C.W. Stevens, W.R. Smythe, A.A. Vaporciyan, R. Komaki, J.F. Kelly, Z. Liao, G. Starkschall, and K.M. Forster, Intensity-modulated radiation therapy: a novel approach to the management of malignant pleural mesothelioma. *International Journal of Radiation Oncology, Biology, Physics* 2003; 55: 768-75.

[17] Clarke, C.P., S.R. Knight, F.J. Daniel, and S. Seevanayagam, Management of malignant mesothelioma by decortication and adjunct phototherapy. *Asian Cardiovasc. Thorac. Ann.* 2006; 14: 206-9.

[18] Stevens, C.W., K.M. Forster, W.R. Smythe, and D. Rice, Radiotherapy for mesothelioma. *Hematology - Oncology Clinics of North America* 2005; 19: 1099-115.

[19] Janne, P.A. and E.H. Baldini, Patterns of failure following surgical resection for malignant pleural mesothelioma. *Thoracic Surgery Clinics* 2004; 14: 567-73.

[20] Gupta, V., B. Mychalczak, L. Krug, R. Flores, M. Bains, V.W. Rusch, and K.E. Rosenzweig, Hemithoracic radiation therapy after pleurectomy/decortication for malignant pleural mesothelioma. *International Journal of Radiation Oncology, Biology*, Physics 2005; 63: 1045-52.

[21] Opitz, I., P. Kestenholz, D. Lardinois, M. Muller, V. Rousson, D. Schneiter, R. Stahel, and W. Weder, Incidence and management of complications after neoadjuvant chemotherapy followed by extrapleural pneumonectomy for malignant pleural mesothelioma. *European Journal of Cardio-Thoracic Surgery* 2006; 29: 579-84.

[22] Flores, R., L. Krug, K.E. Rosenzweig, E. Venkatraman, E. Vincent, R. Heelan, T. Akhurst, and V.W. Rusch, Induction chemotherapy, extrapleural pneumonectomy, and postoperative high-dose radiotherapy for locally advanced malignant pleural

mesothelioma: a phase II trial. *J. Thoracic Oncol. 2006. J. Thoracic. Oncol.* 2006: 289-95.

[23] Allen, A.M., M. Czerminska, P.A. Janne, D.J. Sugarbaker, R. Bueno, J.R. Harris, L. Court, and E.H. Baldini, Fatal pneumonitis associated with intensity-modulated radiation therapy for mesothelioma. *International Journal of Radiation Oncology, Biology, Physics* 2006; 65: 640-5.

[24] Sasse, A.D., L.G. Clark, E.C. Sasse, and O.A. Clark, Amifostine reduces side effects and improves complete response rate during radiotherapy: results of a meta-analysis. *International Journal of Radiation Oncology, Biology, Physics* 2006; 64: 784-91.

[25] Vogelzang, N.J., J.J. Rusthoven, J. Symanowski, C. Denham, E. Kaukel, P. Ruffie, U. Gatzemeier, M. Boyer, S. Emri, C. Manegold, C. Niyikiza, and P. Paoletti, Phase III study of pemetrexed in combination with cisplatin versus cisplatin alone in patients with malignant pleural mesothelioma. *J. Clin. Oncol.* 2003; 21: 2636-44.

[26] Gralla, R.J., P.J. Hollen, A.M. Liepa, J. Symanowski, M. Boyer, R. Abraham, J. Rusthoven, L. Paz-Ares, and N.J. Vogelzang, Improving quality of life in patients with malignant pleural mesothelioma: Results of the randomized pemetrexed + cisplatin vs. cisplatin trial using the LCSS-meso instrument. *Proc. Am. Soc. Clin. Oncol.* 2003; 22: 621(abstr 2496).

[27] van Meerbeeck, J., C. Manegold, R. Gaafar, R.J. van Klaveren, M. Vincent, C. Legrand, C. Debruyne, and G. Giaccone, A randomized phase III study of cisplatin with or without raltitrexed in patients (pts) with malignant pleural mesothelioma (MPM): An intergroup study of the EORTC Lung Cancer Group and NCIC. *Proc. Am. Soc. Clin. Oncol.* 2004; 23: (abstr 7021).

[28] Fizazi, K., H. Doubre, T. Le Chevalier, A. Riviere, J. Viala, C. Daniel, L. Robert, P. Barthelemy, A. Fandi, and P. Ruffie, Combination of raltitrexed and oxaliplatin is an active regimen in malignant mesothelioma: results of a phase II study. *J. Clin. Oncol.* 2003; 21: 349-54.

[29] Porta, C., M. Zimatore, L. Bonomi, I. Imarisio, C. Paglino, A. Sartore-Bianchi, and L. Mutti, Raltitrexed-Oxaliplatin combination chemotherapy is inactive as second-line treatment for malignant pleural mesothelioma patients. *Lung Cancer* 2005; 48: 429-34.

[30] Giaccone, G., M.E. O'Brien, M.J. Byrne, M. Bard, E. Kaukel, and B. Smit, Phase II trial of ZD0473 as second-line therapy in mesothelioma. *European Journal of Cancer* 2002; 38: S19-24.

[31] Masood, R., A. Kundra, S. Zhu, G. Xia, P. Scalia, D.L. Smith, and P.S. Gill, Malignant mesothelioma growth inhibition by agents that target the VEGF and VEGF-C autocrine loops. *Int. J. Cancer* 2003; 104: 603-10.

[32] Strizzi, L., A. Catalano, G. Vianale, S. Orecchia, A. Casalini, G. Tassi, R. Puntoni, L. Mutti, and A. Procopio, Vascular endothelial growth factor is an autocrine growth factor in human malignant mesothelioma. *J. Pathol.* 2001; 193: 468-75.

[33] Konig, J., E. Tolnay, T. Wiethege, and K. Muller, Co-expression of vascular endothelial growth factor and its receptor flt-1 in malignant pleural mesothelioma. *Respiration* 2000; 67: 36-40.

[34] Langerak, A.W., P.A. De Laat, C.A. Van Der Linden-Van Beurden, M. Delahaye, T.H. Van Der Kwast, H.C. Hoogsteden, R. Benner, and M.A. Versnel, Expression of

platelet-derived growth factor (PDGF) and PDGF receptors in human malignant mesothelioma in vitro and in vivo. *J. Pathol.* 1996; 178: 151-60.

[35] Attanoos, R.L., A. Griffin, and A.R. Gibbs, The use of immunohistochemistry in distinguishing reactive from neoplastic mesothelium. A novel use for desmin and comparative evaluation with epithelial membrane antigen, p53, platelet-derived growth factor-receptor, P-glycoprotein and Bcl-2. *Histopathology* 2003; 43: 231-8.

[36] Hanahan, D. and R.A. Weinberg, The hallmarks of cancer. *Cell* 2000; 100: 57-70.

[37] Gale, N.W. and G.D. Yancopoulos, Growth factors acting via endothelial cell-specific receptor tyrosine kinases: VEGFs, angiopoietins, and ephrins in vascular development. *Genes and Development* 1999; 13: 1055-66.

[38] Ferrara, N., Molecular and biological properties of vascular endothelial growth factor. *Journal of Molecular Medicine* 1999; 77: 527-43.

[39] Laird, A.D., J.G. Christensen, G. Li, J. Carver, K. Smith, X. Xin, K.G. Moss, S.G. Louie, D.B. Mendel, and J.M. Cherrington, SU6668 inhibits Flk-1/KDR and PDGFRbeta in vivo, resulting in rapid apoptosis of tumor vasculature and tumor regression in mice. *FASEB Journal* 2002; 16: 681-90.

[40] Beaumont, J., D. Cella, J. Li, R. Motzer, B. Rini, D. Michaelson, S. Kim, and C. Baum, Patient reported outcomes in a phase 2 trial of SU11248 for metastatic renal cell carcinoma. *Proc. Am. Assoc. Cancer Res.* 2005; 24: Abstr 8167.

[41] Motzer, R.J., T.E. Hutson, P. Tomczak, M.D. Michaelson, R.M. Bukowski, O. Rixe, S. Oudard, S.T. Kim, C.M. Baum, and R.A. Figlin, Phase III randomized trial of sunitinib malate (SU11248) versus interferon-alfa (IFN-α) as first-line systemic therapy for patients with metastatic renal cell carcinoma. *Journal of Clinical Oncology, 2006 ASCO Annual Meeting Proceedings* Part I. Vol 24, No. 18S (June 20 Supplement), 2006: LBA3.

[42] Miller, K.D., H.J. Burstein, A.D. Elias, M.A. Rugo, M.A. Cobleigh, M.D. Pegram, P.D. Eisenberg, M. Collier, B.J. Adams, and C.M. Baum, Phase II study of SU11248, a multitargeted receptor tyrosine kinase inhibitor, in patients with previously treated metastatic breast cancer. *Proc. Am. Assoc. Cancer Res.* 2005; 24: Abstr 563.

[43] Demetri, G.D., A. Van Oosterom, M. Blackstein, C. Garret, M. Shah, M.C. Heinrich, G. Mc Arthur, I. Judson, C. Baum, and P.G. Casali, Phase 3, mulitcenter, randomized, double-blind, placebo-controlled trial of SU11248 in patients following failure of imatinib for metastatic GIST. *Proc. Am. Assoc. Cancer Res.* 2005: Abst 4000.

[44] Byrne, M.J. and A.K. Nowak, Modified RECIST criteria for assessment of response in malignant pleural mesothelioma. *Ann. Oncol.* 2004; 15: 257-60.

[45] Francis, R.J., A.A. van der Schaaf, and M.J. Byrne, A prospective study of FDG PET to assess response to chemotherapy in patients with malignant pleural mesothelioma. *J. Nucl. Med.* 2005; 46: 102.

[46] Byrne, M.J., R.J. Francis, A.A. van der Schaaf, J. Boucek, A.K. Nowak, M. Phillips, R. Price, A. Patrikeos, A.W. Musk, and M. Millward, Early prediction of response to chemotherapy and survival in malignant pleural mesothelioma using a novel semi-aitomated 3D volume-based analysis of serial FDG PET scans. In Press *J Nuclear Med*, 2007.

[47] Toner, G., P. Mitchell, R. De Boer, P. Gibbs, R. Hicks, A. Scott, G. Mc Arhtur, N. Brega, G. Massimini, and P. Scigalla, PET imaging study of SU11248 in patients with advanced malignancies. *Proc. ASCO* 2003; 22: 191.

[48] D'Amato, R.J., M.S. Loughnan, E. Flynn, and J. Folkman, Thalidomide is an inhibitor of angiogenesis. *Proc. Natl. Acad. Sci.* 1994; 91: 4082-5.

[49] Quiltz, R., Thalidomide in Oncology: The peril and the Promise. *Cancer Control*; *JMCC* 1999; 6: 483-495.

[50] Corral, L.G. and G. Kaplan, Immunomodulation by thalidomide and thalidomide analogues. *Annals of the Rheumatic Diseases* 1999; 58 Suppl 1: I107-13.

[51] Baas, P., W. Boogerd, O. Dalesio, A. Haringhuizen, F. Custers, and N. van Zandwijk, Thalidomide in patients with malignant pleural mesothelioma. *Lung Cancer* 2005; 48: 291-6.

[52] Pavlakis, N., R. Abraham, R. Harvie, C. Brock, D. Bell, and H. Wheeler, Thalidomide alone or in combination with cisplatin/Gemcitabine in malignant pleural mesothelioma (MM); Interim results from two parallel non randomized phase II studies. *Lung Cancer* 2003; 41: S11.

[53] Johnstone, R.W., Histone-deacetylase inhibitors: novel drugs for the treatment of cancer. *Nature Reviews Drug Discovery* 2002; 1: 287-99.

[54] Dose Schwarz, J., M. Bader, L. Jenicke, G. Hemminger, F. Janicke, and N. Avril, Early prediction of response to chemotherapy in metastatic breast cancer using sequential 18F-FDG PET. *J. Nuc. Med.* 2005; 46: 1144-50.

[55] Pio, B.S., C.K. Park, R. Pietras, W.A. Hsueh, N. Satyamurthy, M.D. Pegram, J. Czernin, M.E. Phelps, and D.H. Silverman, Usefulness of 3'-[F-18]fluoro-3'-deoxythymidine with positron emission tomography in predicting breast cancer response to therapy. *Molecular Imaging and Biology* 2006; 8: 36-42.

[56] Romer, W., A.R. Hanauske, S. Ziegler, R. Thodtmann, W. Weber, C. Fuchs, W. Enne, M. Herz, C. Nerl, M. Garbrecht, and M. Schwaiger, Positron emission tomography in non-Hodgkin's lymphoma: assessment of chemotherapy with fluorodeoxyglucose. *Blood* 1998; 91: 4464-71.

[57] Flores, R.M., T. Akhurst, M. Gonen, S.M. Larson, and V.W. Rusch, Positron emission tomography defines metastatic disease but not locoregional disease in patients with malignant pleural mesothelioma. *J. Thorac. Cardiovasc. Surg.* 2003; 126: 11-6.

[58] Benard, F., D. Sterman, R.J. Smith, L.R. Kaiser, S.M. Albelda, and A. Alavi, Prognostic value of FDG PET imaging in malignant pleural mesothelioma.[see comment]. *J. Nuc. Med.* 1999; 40: 1241-5.

[59] Benard, F., D. Sterman, R.J. Smith, L.R. Kaiser, S.M. Albelda, and A. Alavi, Metabolic imaging of malignant pleural mesothelioma with fluorodeoxyglucose positron emission tomography.[see comment]. *Chest* 1998; 114: 713-22.

[60] Kwek, B.H., S.L. Aquino, and A.J. Fischman, Fluorodeoxyglucose positron emission tomography and CT after talc pleurodesis. *Chest* 2004; 125: 2356-60.

In: Mesothelioma from Bench Side to Clinic
Editor: Alfonso Baldi, pp. 521-536

ISBN: 978-1-60021-789-0

Chapter XXXI

US Trials in Mesothelioma

Tom Routledge and Raja Flores
Department of Thoracic Surgery,
Memorial Sloan-Kettering Cancer Center,
1275 York Avenue, New York, NY 10021, USA

Abstract

The US clinical data on management of malignant pleural mesothelioma are reviewed. The review examines data on chemotherapy as sole modality treatment. The observed success with pemetrexed doublets is discussed. We go on to discuss multimodality treatment outcomes, largely focusing on the ongoing output of the US academic centers with longstanding interest in mesothelioma. Although randomized data is still lacking, the increasing weight of prospective observational data supporting a benefit offered by surgical treatment in combination with chemotherapy and radiotherapy for selected patients is described.

Introduction

This chapter will examine the recent United States literature on treatments for malignant mesothelioma. The discussion is divided into sections on chemotherapy as sole treatment, then on multi-modality treatments (involving surgery in association with other local and systemic treatments).

Chemotherapy

There have been a number of Phase II trials of single-agent therapy for mesothelioma involving most available agents. The majority of these have been small, heterogenous as to stage, pathologic subtype, and patient performance status. It is, thus, invalid to draw conclusions about relative efficacy between agents. The responses are universally limited with no proof that chemotherapy offers either improved survival or quality of life over best supportive care [1].

Doxycycline

This is the most studied single agent. The ECOG series reported a response rate of 14% and median survival of 7.3 months [2].

Cisplatin

In a SWOG study, a similar response rate of 14% and median survival of 7.5 months was seen [3]. A similar response rate has been reported using carboplatin in US Phase II study with possibly improved tolerability [4]. Cisplatin has formed the control arm of the largest Phase III studies [5].

Anti-Metabolites

Drugs that block nucleotide synthesis or nucleotide analogues, such as gemcitabine, have shown activity but toxicity (edatrexate) [6]. Pemetrexed (a combination enzyme inhibitor - see below) as a single agent has a moderate affect – response rate 14% and median survival 10.7 months [7]. The amelioration of toxicity by folate and B12 supplementation was also established.

Regarding the nucleoside analogue gemcitabine, a CALGB multi-center Phase II study found no evidence of single agent activity [8]; likewise capecitabine [9]. Studies performed outside of the US have shown promise with doublets containing gemcitabine, particularly with cisplatin [10].

Vinorelbine

This agent has been studied with some promise outside the US [11].

Topoisomerase Inhibitors

For irinotecan, a recent CALGB Phase II study found no evidence of activity and considerable toxicity [12]. This is similar for topotecan.

Many combinations of the agents showing modest activity in monotherapy Phase I trials have been investigated in Phase I / II studies. In general, slight increases in response rates are seen in Phase II studies of combination chemotherapy over single agent regimes. However, data on median survival show no benefit over single agent treatment [1]. The important exception is pemetrexed and cisplatin (and later raltitrexed and cisplatin, tested in Phase III trials outside the US [13])

Pemetrexed-Cisplatin

This doublet was first studied in a Phase I trial in 1999 when it was observed to produce a response in 5 out of 11 mesothelioma patients. Although small numbers, this was a response rate much in excess of previously studied combinations. A Phase II trial demonstrated efficacy of this doublet, and it was known to be acceptable from a toxicity point of view from studies in non-small cell lung cancer. It has been studied in the largest Phase III randomized controlled trial of therapy for mesothelioma [5]. Pemetrexed is a novel multi-targeted, anti-folate agent inhibiting three enzymes involved in both purine and pyrimidine synthesis (thymidylate synthase, dihydrofolate reductase and glycinamide ribonucleotide formyl transferase). Four hundred and forty-eight patients were randomized to cisplatin or cisplatin plus pemetrexed. The stated primary outcome was survival. During the study it became evident that the severe bone marrow suppression seen in the doublet arm could be ameliorated by folic acid and B12 supplementation and this was added to both arms of the ongoing study.

The median survival in the doublet group was significantly although modestly better (12.1 months vs. 9.3 months, p=0.02), with significant survival benefit at 18 but not at 24 months. Benefit in median time to disease progression was also reported (6.1 months vs. 3.9 months). Despite supplementation, major hematological toxicity was more common in the doublet group (grade ¾ neutropenia 28%). Quality of life (QOL) data showed benefit in terms of dyspnea and pain, and also objective pulmonary function (both reported in abstract-form only). This doublet has also been shown to be active in peritoneal mesothelioma [14].

Of note, pemetrexed should not be used in patients with severely impaired renal function [15]. It can accumulate in large pleural fluid collections, increasing the likelihood of toxicity.

This trial led to the cisplatin-pemetrexed doublet being the only FDA approved treatment for malignant mesothelioma. It is widely considered standard first-line treatment for mesothelioma in patients not suitable for multi-modality treatment. It is being currently studied as a neoadjuvant regime in US trials of multi-modal treatment.

The study has been criticized for claiming to show overall QOL benefit for pemetrexed-cisplatin, when no control group of pleural effusion treatment only was available for comparison. A major symptomatic advantage of the studied doublet was improved dyspnea, and it has been argued that even better dyspnea control might be obtained by talc pleurodesis alone in those without a trapped lung. There are data suggestive that effusion control alone might have a survival advantage. Certainly the benefits of pemetrexed-cisplatin are modest, although clinically meaningful and similar in magnitude to those seen in treating stage IV non-small cell lung cancer. However, the toxicity of this best available systemic therapy remains considerable and the question of whether similar benefit could be obtained by simple pleurodesis in some patients remains important. Of note, a currently open United Kingdom (UK) Phase III protocol will compare chemotherapy (although not pemetrexed-cisplatin) with supportive treatment alone.

There are few data on second-line treatments. There have been no dedicated Phase II trials of second line chemotherapy performed in the US, and only one worldwide (studying a cisplatin analog and reporting no major evidence of benefit [16]). A few Phase II trials have enrolled both pre-treated and chemo-naïve patients, with some evidence of efficacy for a number of single and combination agents.

The trialists studying pemetrexed-cisplatin vs cisplatin analyzed their data on post-study (ie. second line) chemotherapy [17]. Forty-two percent of the patients in the Phase III trial received post-study chemotherapy (more in the cisplatin only arm: 37.2% vs 47.3%). Gemcitabine was the most commonly used agent. The use of second-line chemotherapy was used as a variable in a retrospective multivariate analysis, and found to be associated with survival benefit. As the authors state, it is difficult to conclude real evidence of benefit from these data as it is likely that a considerable degree of unaccounted for selection went into determining who received second line treatment.

Ranpirnase

This is a novel, injectable ribonuclease, with *in vitro* cytostatic and cytotoxic effects in a variety of cell-lines. It is a peptide, first extracted from Northern Leopard frog oocytes. It has been studied in a Phase II trial in mesothelioma, in which 105 patients were enrolled. Thirty-seven percent had received prior chemotherapy. The data showed little radiological regression of disease but a possible effect on halting progression, including those with prior chemotherapy [18]. A subsequent small Phase III study (154 patients, abstract only [19]) of ranpirnase vs doxorubicin showed no survival advantage, although there was an excess of poor prognostic factors in the ranpirnase group. There is an ongoing multi-center trial of ranpirnase- doxorubicin vs ranpirnase alone [20].

Targeted Agents: VEGF and EGFR

VEGF has been shown to be involved in mesothelioma biology [21]. Bevacizumab is a recombinant humanized anti-VEGF monoclonal antibody that blocks the binding of VEGF to its receptor. There is an ongoing US trial (University of Chicago, clinicaltrials.gov) of gemcitabine-cisplatin plus or minus bevacizumab vs placebo. Interim analysis of this data shows that higher serum VEGF correlates to worse survival, supporting the hypothesis that it is a valid therapeutic target. There are ongoing US (at the University of Texas–Southwestern and the University of Chicago, clinicaltrials.gov) Phase II trials of bevacizumab as addition to the now standard pemetrexed-cisplatin, and also of bevacizumab as second-line therapy.

Gefitinib (an EGFR tyrosine kinase inhibitor) has been studied in a Phase II trial and found not to be active in mesothelioma, despite high levels of EGFR over-expression in tumor tissue [22].

Given the at best minimal effect that systemic treatment alone has on malignant mesothelioma, attention has focused on combined modalities. Local control is particularly important with mesothelioma, as local progression is responsible for most symptoms and often for death. The anatomy of mesothelioma would require a large radiation field, with toxicity to a number of vital structures. Thus, attention has focused on surgery as the primary method of local control, even though complete extirpation of the tumor is often not possible.

Multi-Modality Treatments

Given the clear importance of local control in mesothelioma treatment, and the at best one year median survival achieved with optimal chemotherapy, surgery has been investigated by a number of US groups as part of multi-modality treatment. Surgery alone is unlikely to achieve complete microscopic extirpation of the disease given the broad based anatomy of the tumor and its widely infiltrative nature. Earlier US experience with surgery alone was universally poor, with frequent local recurrence in the ipsilateral hemithorax. Thus, local adjuvant treatments such as radiotherapy, photodynamic therapy and intra-pleural chemotherapy have been studied to try and improve local control. Local treatments have been combined with neoadjuvant and adjuvant systemic treatment both to further treat the primary tumor and reduce the risk of distant recurrence, which has been increasingly observed as local treatment becomes more radical and more effective.

There are almost no US randomized controlled trials between multi-modal regimes involving surgery, so it is difficult to draw clear conclusions about which operation and which adjuvant treatments might be better, or even whether there is certain benefit to a surgical approach at all. This is because the disease is rare and the prognosis so desperate that patients and doctors are unwilling to enter trials in which they may be denied treatments perceived as their only chance. The best data are prospective Phase II trials, with no internal control groups. The worse are retrospective case series, often spanning many years. The difficulty in interpreting such data is increased by the lack of clear data on the prognosis of the studies patients without treatment.

Granted the limitations of the US literature to date, what information can be gained?

Prognostic Features

Prognosis is of great importance in selecting patients with generally limited lifer expectancy for treatment that carries a very significant toxicity. The risk of using up a patient's remaining months with toxic, and possibly lethal, medical intervention of uncertain benefit is very real. Information in selecting who will do best with multimodality treatment is of paramount usefulness. However, are they doing well *because* of or *in spite of* our treatments? Certainly, medium term survival without multimodality treatment seems almost unheard of, whereas it is at least a possibility with treatment. The impressive recent survival data from prospective series of patients with early stage disease treated with resection and adjuvant treatment strongly suggest benefit. This is the argument on which proponents of radical treatment must currently hang their hats.

Efficacy of Treatments

Treatment efficacy is reported as survival data predominantly, with little data on symptom control being available. Survival data is difficult to interpret due to inevitable strong selection bias and no gold standard of natural history for the studied sub-set of patients being available. The risk is of not comparing apples to apples. Given that even in the most optimistic estimates medium term survival is unlikely, the effects of treatment on symptom control and quality of life are important to understand. Yet most studies do not report this.

Within the context of multi-modality treatment, uni- and multivariate analyses of observational data have yielded a number of sets of prognostic factors in patients undergoing surgical treatment of mesothelioma. A few factors are consistent across data sets.

In 1999 Dr Valerie Rusch et al. analyzed the Memorial Sloan-Kettering Cancer Center, New York prospective data base for prognosis [23]. The series spans 15 years and 231 patients. It is a surgical series with 75 % undergoing macroscopic complete resection (2/3 with EPP and 1/3 with pleurectomy). This ensures excellent data on pathological stage. The remaining 25% were explored with a view to resection but deemed unresectable. On univariate analyses, IMIG T stage was found to predict survival (although the small numbers of T1 tumors meant the T1 vs T2 comparison was non-significant), as did N0 vs N1+, and also numbers of involved nodes. IMIG stage group was also a significant prognostic factor, confirming the validity of the staging system. Of note the median survival of stage I disease was 29.9 months, strikingly more than data from other series of unresected patients, implying although not proving a benefit from surgery. Equally, the results in high stage / non-epithelioid tumors remained poor despite complete resection and adjuvant treatment, underlining the need to exclude such patients from radical therapy. Epithelioid histology, female gender, but not platelet count, were prognostic. Other investigators have found platelet count to be prognostic. Of treatment factors, adjuvant treatment (predominantly radiotherapy in this series) was associated with a better prognosis. In comparison of EPP vs pleurectomy, no survival advantage was seen. It would be wrong to conclude that more radical surgery is thus unjustified. The EPP group had more advanced disease by definition (i.e. it was not possible to achieve complete macroscopic clearance with a lesser resection), so would be expected to do worse, but may have been fitter in order for EPP to be deemed appropriate (selection bias). The tentative conclusion is that being able to completely resect the tumor (by whatever procedure is required) is the critical thing, with EPP entailing a slightly higher operative mortality (5.2% vs 3.5% in this series) and a higher morbidity (other series). On multivariate analysis, all these factors remained significant.

Of note, although extra-pulmonary nodal disease (mediastinal, internal mammary) is recognized as a poor prognostic factor, mediastinoscopy is less useful as a staging tool than in lung cancer. This is because 25% of all mesothelioma nodal metastases are missed at mediastinoscopy [23]

In 1999 Sugarbaker et al. published the analysis of prognostic factors from the other large US series of surgically-treated mesothelioma, from the Brigham and Women's Hospital, Boston [24]. The series included 183 patients. Unlike the Memorial series, they all underwent extrapleural pneumonectomy, followed by adjuvant chemotherapy (varying regimes) and radiotherapy. Details of the parameters used to select patients for their trimodality therapy are given, allowing others to ascertain how applicable the results might be to their own patients. Also, operative morbidity as well as mortality (3.8%) is discussed. They found age, smoking status and asbestos exposure history to be non-prognostic. Gender (female being an advantage) was weakly prognostic. Epithelial histology was prognostic- survival data given at 2 and 5 years being 52% and 21% vs. 16% and 0%. An attempt was made to assess margins. This is clearly difficult given the large surface area of the resection specimen, any part of which could be positive, with macroscopic appearance being a poor guide. A method of systematic sampling was developed to address this, but it can only be a compromise, an estimate of microscopic completeness of resection at best. However, a prognostic advantage of negative margins is reported (2 and 5 year survival being 44% and 22% vs 33% and 9%), confirming belief that adequacy of local control is vital in this locally aggressive disease. The presence of disease in extrapleural or peridiaphragmatic nodes also conferred a strong survival disadvantage 93% vs 42% at 2 years). The figure from Sugarbaker's series, most touted by enthusiasts for radical mesothelioma surgery, is the survival in the 31 patients with all the good prognostic features – epithelial, node negative and margins negative: 51 months median survival, 46% 5 year survival. Although how much of this impressive outcome is a result of treatment rather than mere selection is impossible to say, it seems likely that some part is played by surgery.

The current T stage descriptors in the IMIG staging system depend significantly on an intra-operative assessment of invasiveness, and thus clinical (pre-operative) T stage is necessarily rather imprecise. An attempt to address this has been made using the data from a trial of intra-operative photodynamic therapy performed by Pass et al.[25]. The trial itself is discussed below. The trialists also made tumor volume estimates from pre- and post-treatment CT scans and looked for correlation with survival and nodal status (from resected tissue). A pre-treatment volume of >100cc (or post-treatment >9cc) was associated with significantly worse survival. Of more general relevance is that tumour volume correlated well with pathological T stage, suggesting it may be an accurate way of clinically staging patients before treatment. Likewise greater volume of tumor correlated with an increased nodal stage.

The degree of FDG avidity of many cancers has been correlated with outcome, as has the reduction in glucose avidity in response to (induction) treatment. A high SUV has been found to predict N2 status but not T status [26]. It has also been correlated with survival [27]. In a series of 137 patients, an SUV of above or below 10 was found to be the best cut-off. The hazard ratio for an SUV of greater than 10 was 1.9m making it as important a predictor as clinical stage. Of those with SUV<10 (and epithelial histology) 20% were alive at 5 years, whereas those with an SUV >10, non were alive at 2 years.

Trials of Surgery as Sole Treatment

A number of earlier US series reported results of EPP or pleurectomy without adjuvant treatment. Patient numbers were small (20-40 for EPP series, 30- 60 for pleurectomy). Median survival was poor, 9-13 months (no different from that of unresected patients) [28].

More radical surgery did not seem to confer better outcome, and thus many inferred that surgery had no role in mesothelioma treatment at all. Others focused on combining surgery with other local and systemic treatments. All recent surgical treatment (other than purely palliative pleurodesis) has involved multimodality treatment.

Is EPP Superior to Pleurectomy Alone?

There are no randomized comparisons to answer this question. In series including both procedures, local recurrence is typically more common after pleurectomy and distant recurrence (abdomen or chest) after extra-pleural pneumonectomy [29].

Perhaps the clearest data on this come from the small Lung Cancer Study Group trial on EPP [28]. Of the 83 eligible patients, only 17 underwent EPP and survived (with no adjuvant treatment permitted). Of the remaining patients, 25 underwent pleurectomy (some with adjuvant treatment). Of the EPP group, 11 of the 17 recurred at a distant site (65%) whereas 64% of the pleurectomy group recurred locally first.

This is interpreted as better local control with more radical surgery. However, it could merely be that those with a more infiltrative tumor phenotype are not found at surgery not to be amenable to EPP and so get a lesser procedure and more local recurrence. Alternatively, those requiring EPP may have a more advanced disease and thus be more at risk of systemic metastasis.

An advantage of EPP is that it permits high doses (54 Gy) of post-operative radiotherapy. This combination is associated with very low rates of local recurrence. This observation has led some US groups, including Memorial Sloan-Kettering, to adopt this strategy for early stage mesothelioma. See below for further discussion.

What Are the Risks of Mesothelioma Surgery?

Extra-pleural pneumonectomy is clearly a major procedure, entailing considerable morbidity and mortality. The need to minimize this is particularly acute for two reasons: firstly, most patients are not cured and so quality of life is critical; secondly, it is increasingly recognized that adjuvant treatments are important, and the patient must not be rendered so unwell by surgery that they are unable to receive such therapy. The most detailed report of the morbidity of extra-pleural pneumonectomy is from Sugarbaker's group [24]. In the report of their first 183 patients undergoing trimodality (including EPP) treatment, they divide morbidity into major (prolonging hospital stay) and minor. They report a major complication rate of 24.5% and an overall complication rate of 50%. The commonest type of complications was pulmonary (respiratory failure, aspiration, pulmonary emboli), followed by cardiovascular (cardiac arrest, ventricular failure), technical (bleeding, patch disruption, cardiac herniation) and then infectious. Of minor complications, atrial fibrillation was the most prominent (37%).

The peri-operative mortality after EPP in recent series from large US centers is routinely 3-5%, which is itself an impressive achievement [23, 24].

Studies of *Local* Adjuvant Treatments

Local recurrence remains the most likely outcome of even the most radical surgery in early stage disease, focusing attention on local adjuvant treatments to obliterate tumor remaining at the margins. A number of modalities have been used, with the best results seeming to be obtained with high dose radiation (permitted only after extra-pleural pneumonectomy). But as ever, the lack of randomized head-to head comparisons makes it difficult to be sure how much *apparent* efficacy is down to case selection.

Radiation

Earlier data on adjuvant radiation were not promising. In a 1984 series from Memorial Sloan-Kettering, 45 patients between 1976 and 1982 underwent pleurectomy accompanied by varying methods of intra-operative/brachytherapy (with iodine or iridium) and post-operative external beam radiotherapy [30]. Median survival was good – 21 months. But the local recurrence rate was 71%.

A single-center retrospective review of 123 patients treated with pleurectomy and radiotherapy (mean 42.5 Gy external beam, with 54 patients also receiving brachytherapy) was published in 2005[31]. This reported an overall mean survival of 13.5 months, with actuarial one-year local recurrence of 58%. Trials of radiation after pleurectomy are limited in the possible radiation dose by pulmonary toxicity, and thus the efficacy in improving local control is disappointing.

However after EPP, the risk of ipsilateral pulmonary toxicity has been (literally) removed and much higher doses are permitted. The most impressive data on this are from 2001, a phase II trial investigating the feasibility and outcomes of *high* dose post operative adjuvant radiation in the context of resection [32]. This was a single center study in which 88 patients underwent surgery followed 3 to 5 weeks later by 54 Gy external beam radiation delivered in 30 daily fractions. The initial protocol included 10-15Gy of intra-operative radiation delivered as iridium. This prolonged operative time to an unacceptable extent and in the first few patients undergoing extra-pleural pneumonectomy was associated with a high incidence of empyema [33]; intra-operative radiation treatment was dropped from the revised protocol. Of the 88 patients enrolled, 60 underwent complete resection. The histology was about two thirds epithelial. They were evenly distributed between N0-1 and N2, and were mostly T2-3, and so were well representative of typical surgical mesothelioma series. All but three of these were able to receive the adjuvant radiation. This was well-tolerated, the only grade IV toxicity being a late esophago-pleural fistula that eventually required esophagectomy. In total 54 patients were treated with EPP and radiation.

Overall survival was a mean of 17 months; 33.8 months for IMIG I-II and 10 months for III-IV. Even more impressive was the data on sites of recurrence. Only 3 (5.5%) had local (within the treated hemithorax) recurrence. The commonest sites of distant recurrence were peritoneal and contralateral thorax, more rarely osseus. It was not clear if the peritoneal recurrences were confluent with the resected pleural disease across the diaphragm (in which case some would class it as loco-regional). This represents the best published local control data.

Sugarbaker's rolling case series, although not a trial, also represents valuable data on this topic [34]. Adjuvant radiation is part of the Brigham trimodality approach. Their radiation protocol varies, with a mean of 31Gy, and additional boosts of treatment given to areas considered at high clinical risk of recurrence. They report a 35% local failure rate. The comparison with Rusch's high dose data suggests there may be a critical required dose of radiation needed to augment local control after EPP.

The recent phase II trial of trimodality treatment from Memorial Sloan-Kettering [35]formally assessed the feasibility and safety of induction chemotherapy (cisplatin gemcitabine, as the trial was designed prior to Vogelzang et al. key phase III cisplatin-pemetrexed study), extra-pleural pneumonectomy and subsequent hemithoracic radiation (54 Gy). The study population was notable as being stage III-IV patients, who are known to do poorly in most treatment protocols. Nineteen patients received chemotherapy, with nine going on to surgery (the remaining patients excluded because of progression of disease). All patients undergoing resection tolerated radiotherapy 6 weeks later. The median survival of those who did not progress on chemotherapy (about half of those enrolled) had a median survival of 33.5 months. This trial showed that induction chemotherapy did not increase surgical morbidity and mortality unacceptably, and that critically those who did not progress were able to tolerate the subsequent local control modalities shown to be so effective in previous studies [32]. While it remains a small phase II study, the results in this poor-prognosis and prospectively studied group are encouraging. The median survival for stage III-IV in this previous trial of surgery plus radiation was less than a year, due to overwhelming distant metastases.

A similarly designed contemporaneous Swiss study showed that induction chemotherapy could be used in stage I-II disease with encouraging results [36].

There is a currently-recruiting international multi-center protocol testing pemetrexed-cisplatin induction followed by extra-pleural pneumonectomy and adjuvant radiotherapy. This is nearing completion in 2006.

New radiation oncology technologies (such as combining electron and photon intensity modulated radiotherapy) will allow deliver a high dose to the target field, while minimizing expose of the (remaining) at-risk viscera (spinal cord, heart, liver) [37,38].

Photodynamic Therapy

Several groups around the world have used photodynamic therapy (PDT) after debulking surgery to improve local control. The best-designed US study of this technique was a small, randomized Phase III study published in 1997[29]. 63 patients were enrolled, but in 15 it was not possible to resect all tumor tissue down to less than 5 mm thickness (an inclusion criterion based on the maximum effective depth of the PDT used). All patients received an investigational adjuvant regime consisting of cisplatin, interferon and tamoxifen. Patients were randomized to PDT or no PDT having undergone sufficiently successful partial extirpation. The PDT involved pre-operative administration of an intravenous porphyrin-based first generation photosensitizer (Photofrin II) and then application of 630nm laser light intra-operatively.

The patients were well-matched for TNM stage and pre-operative tumor volume (as assessed by CT). Equal numbers in each arm underwent extra-pleural pneumonectomy or pleurectomy to achieve debulking. The results showed no difference between arms in either median overall survival (about 14 months) or progression free survival (about 8 months). Operative morbidity and mortality was similar between the two groups.

From this small but carefully conducted randomized controlled trial it seems that PDT has little role in mesothelioma treatment.

A US case series of PDT as an adjunct to surgery for mesothelioma was published the following year [39]. The series was of 40 patients, with 6 years follow up. They reported median survivals of 36 months for stage I-II patients and 10 months for stage III-IV. PDT dose was reported as an independent predictor of survival on their multi-variate analysis. Although these observational data in isolation might suggest a possible benefit for PDT, they must be considered in the light of a negative contemporary randomized trial.

There remains ongoing US interest in PDT for mesothelioma. In 2003 a phase I dose escalation study of intra-operative PDT using a newer sensitizer (Foscan) in 20 patients was reported [40]. This established a maximum tolerated dose, although of course no data on efficacy were produced.

Intrapleural Chemotherapy

Intrapleural cytotoxics have been studied as an intra-operative adjunct to debulking surgery and as sole therapy [41] (see section on single-agent cisplatin chemotherapy). Early feasibility [42] and pharmacokinetic [43] studies suggested it may be useful treatment, following success in intra-peritoneal malignancies (ovarian and mesothelioma). There was more systemic absorption than in peritoneal lavage [43], raising concern about renal toxicity and meaning most investigators have limited the dose of cisplatin used to less than 100 mg/m2. The requirement for vigorous peri-operative hydration to ameliorate renal toxicity has mostly limited its use to the context of pleurectomy rather than extra-pleural pneumonectomy.

In 1995 the UCLA experience in intra-pleural post-debulking chemotherapy was published [44]. They gave 100 mg/m2 of cisplatin, with cytosine, to 15 patients. The patients received various adjuvant treatments in addition, some systemic chemotherapy and some radiotherapy. The median survival of just 11.5 months and high local recurrence rate led them to see no merit in further investigation of the technique.

The MSKCC group who had performed the pilot and pharmacokinetic studies went on to publish a Phase II trial in 1994[45]. They studied patients who had had all visible gross disease resected by pleurectomy (27 patients in all) and administered initially 100 mg/m2 then 75 mg/m2 of cisplatin, with mitomycin. The patients then received adjuvant systemic cisplatin starting 3 to 5 weeks post-operatively. They observed an encouraging median overall survival of 18.3 months, with only one serious toxicity episode. Progression-free survival was 13 months. Overall morbidity was 55% and mortality 3.7%. However, the authors reported that local recurrence remained a dominant problem (17 out of 27 patients).

The other US group with an interest in intra-pleural chemotherapy as an operative adjunct is that in Boston. The hypothesized that the failure of previous investigators to gain significant local control or survival benefit by this approach might be because of inadequate dosing. In 2006 they published the results of a combined dose escalation and phase II study of hyperthermic (42 degree C) cisplatin pleural lavage following debulking pleurectomy [46]. They used intravenous thiosulphate as renal protection, as well as careful hydration, avoidance of NSAIDS, and hemodynamic optimization. They studied 44 patients, initially to determine the maximum tolerated dose. The second part of the study was to deliver this dose to a further ten patients to investigate efficacy as well as dose tolerability.

The dose-limiting toxicity is reported at 250 mg/m2 of cisplatin, so the maximum tolerated dose was taken as 225 mg/m2. This is more than twice the dose used in previous studies. However, of the 5 patients who died during the study, four received the maximum dose. The complication rate was significant with 25% major complications (not including atrial fibrillation at 32%). 57% of patients suffered some degree of renal impairment, which led to dialysis dependency in one patient (who subsequently died). 9% suffered a deep venous thrombosis. The overall mortality was 11%. However the median survival in the group receiving 225 mg/m2 was 18 months vs 6 months in the lower dose group. Local recurrence was far from obliterated in the high dose group: 75% of all patients recurred, and 75% of these recurrences were in the ipsilateral hemithorax. This was not different between dosage groups. However, higher dose was associated with a significantly longer time to first recurrence noted in this (non-randomized) study: 9 months vs 4 months. The authors accept the limitations of the study design in providing clear evidence of efficacy but the results are provocative as to whether such high doses may offer advantage.

Conclusion

Mesothelioma remains a very difficult disease to treat, and the prognosis of those with advanced disease remains dismal. However, the trials discussed have led to the development of successful multimodality treatment for both early and advanced stage mesothelioma. There is no longer a ground for therapeutic nihilism about mesothelioma, with Phase II data suggesting a median survival of several times that seen a decade ago with modern multimodality programs.

This has been achieved by a number of successes. The risks of radical surgery in experienced centers in now low, with a mortality of 6%. The problem of local control has been effectively addressed by a combination of radical surgery and high dose hemithoracic radiation. The remaining major problem is distant metastases, underlining the need for more effective systemic treatments. While recent successes with pemetrexed (or raltitrexed) and cisplatin are a notable positive result, our ability to control metastatic mesothelioma lags behind improvements in local control.

Trimodality treatment remains applicable to a minority of mesothelioma patients, with many unfit for such aggressive treatment, and others progressing during chemotherapy. This is further grounds for the need for more effective chemotherapy.

The role for pleurectomy remains ill-defined. It may be that if the tumor is technically resectable without extra-pleural pneumonectomy then this remains an equally effective alternative. However, pleurectomy alone does not allow adjuvant high dose radiotherapy and hence local control may be less effective. At the least it may have a role in those unfit for extra-pleural pneumonectomy.

A legitimate criticism of the current mesothelioma literature is that few randomized trials exist, and the current trimodality trials do not compare treatments head to head. This is true, but the apparent success of trimodality treatment in Phase II studies makes any study randomizing patients to less intensive treatments likely to fail, given the perceived (by physicians and patients) lack of equipoise.

There is no one size fits all treatment for mesothelioma. Individual cases must be judged on their merits, and it is likely that, analogous with non-small cell lung cancer, treatment will be driven by stage and co-morbidity.

References

[1] Krug LM. An overview of chemotherapy for mesothelioma. *Hematol. Oncol. Clin. North Am*. 2005; 19:117-36.

[2] Belani CP, et al. Docetaxel for malignant mesothelioma: phase II study of the Eastern Cooperative Oncology Group. *Clin. Lung Cancer* 2004; 6:43-47.

[3] Zidar BL, et al. A phase II evaluation of cisplatin in unresectable diffuse malignant mesothelioma: a Southwest Oncology Group Study. *Invest New Drugs* 1988; 6:223-226.

[4] Vogelzang NJ, et al. Carboplatin in malignant mesothelioma: a phase II study of the Cancer and Leukemia Group B. *Cancer Chemother Pharmacol* 1990 27:239-242.

[5] Vogelzang NJ, et al. Phase III study of pemetrexed in combination with cisplatin versus cisplatin alone in patients with malignant pleural mesothelioma. *J. Clin. Oncol*. 2003; 21: 2636-2644.

[6] Kindler HL, et al. Edatrexate (10-ethyl-deaza-aminopterin) (NSC #626715) with or without leucovorin rescue for malignant mesothelioma. Sequential phase II trials by the cancer and leukemia group B. *Cancer* 1999;86:1985-1991.

[7] Scagliotti GV, et al. Phase II study of pemetrexed with and without folic acid and vitamin B12 as front-line therapy in malignant pleural mesothelioma. *J. Clin Oncol*. 2003;21:1556-1561.

[8] Kindler HL, et al. Gemcitabine for malignant mesothelioma: A phase II trial by the Cancer and Leukemia Group B. *Lung Cancer* 2001;31: 311-317.

[9] Otterson GA, Herndon JE, Watson D, Green MR, Kindler HL. Capecitabine in malignant mesothelioma: a phase II trial by the Cancer and Leukemia Group B (39807). *Lung Cancer* 2004; 44:251-259.

[10] Byrne MJ, et al. Cisplatin and gemcitabine treatment for malignant mesothelioma: a phase II study. *J. Clin. Oncol.* 1999; 17:25-30.

[11] Steele JP, et al. Phase II study of vinorelbine in patients with malignant pleural mesothelioma. *J. Clin. Oncol.* 2000;18: 3912-3917.

[12] Kindler HL, Herndon J E. Zhang C, Green MR Irinotecan for malignant mesothelioma. A phase II trial by the Cancer and Leukemia Group B. *Lung Cancer* 2005; 48:423-428.

[13] van Meerbeeck, J. P. et al. Randomized phase III study of cisplatin with or without raltitrexed in patients with malignant pleural mesothelioma: an intergroup study of the European Organisation for Research and Treatment ofCancer Lung Cancer Group and the National Cancer Institute of Canada. *J. Clin. Oncol.* 2005;23, 6881-6889.

[14] Janne PA. et al. Open-label study of pemetrexed alone or in combination with cisplatin for the treatment of patients with peritoneal mesothelioma: outcomes of an expanded access program. *Clin. Lung Cancer* 2005; 7: 0-46.

[15] Mita AC, et al. Phase I and pharmacokinetic study of pemetrexed administered every 3 weeks to advanced cancer patients with normal and impaired renal function. *J. Clin. Oncol.* 2006; 24:552-562.

[16] Giaccone G, et al. Phase II trial of ZD0473 as second-line therapy in mesothelioma. *Eur. J. Cancer* 2002; 38 Suppl. 8:S19-24.

[17] Manegold C, et al. Second-line (post-study) chemotherapy received by patients treated in the phase III trial of pemetrexed plus cisplatin versus cisplatin alone in malignant pleural mesothelioma. *Ann. Oncol.* 2005;16:923-927.

[18] Mikulski SM, et al. Phase II trial of a single weekly intravenous dose of ranpirnase in patients with unresectable malignant mesothelioma. *J. Clin. Oncol.* 2002; 20:274-281.

[19] Vogelzang N, Taub R, Shin D. Phase III randomized trial of onconase vs doxorubicin in patients with unresectable malignant mesothelioma. *Proceedings of the American Society of Clinical Oncologists* 2002; 19:557a.

[20] Pavlakis N, Vogelzang N J Ranpirnase--an antitumour ribonuclease: its potential role in malignant mesothelioma. *Expert Opin. Biol. Ther.* 2006; 6:391-399.

[21] Masood R, et al. Malignant mesothelioma growth inhibition by agents that target the VEGF and VEGF-C autocrine loops. *Int. J. Cancer* 2003; 104:603-610.

[22] Govindan R. et al. Gefitinib in patients with malignant mesothelioma: a phase II study by the Cancer and Leukemia Group B. *Clin. Cancer Res.* 2005; 11: 300-2304.

[23] Rusch VW, Venkatraman ES. Important prognostic factors in patients with malignant pleural mesothelioma, managed surgically. *Ann. Thorac. Surg.* 1999; 68:1799-1804.

[24] Sugarbaker DJ. et al. Resection margins, extrapleural nodal status, and cell type determine postoperative long-term survival in trimodality therapy of malignant pleural mesothelioma: results in 183 patients. *J. Thorac. Cardiovasc Surg* 1999; 117:54-63; discussion 63-5.

[25] Pass HI, Temeck BK, Kranda K, Steinberg SM, Feuerstein IR. Preoperative tumor volume is associated with outcome in malignant pleural mesothelioma. *J. Thorac. Cardiovasc. Surg.* 1998; 115:310-7; discussion 317-8.

[26] Flores RM, Akhurst T, Gonen M, Larson SM, Rusch VW. Positron emission tomography defines metastatic disease but not locoregional disease in patients with malignant pleural mesothelioma. *J. Thorac. Cardiovasc. Surg.* 2003; 126:11-16.

[27] Flores RM, et al. Positron emission tomography predicts survival in malignant pleural mesothelioma. *J. Thorac. Cardiovasc. Surg.* 2006; 132: 763-768.

[28] Rusch VW, Piantadosi S, Holmes E C. The role of extrapleural pneumonectomy in malignant pleural mesothelioma. A Lung Cancer Study Group Trial. *J. Thorac. Cardiovasc. Surg.* 1991;102:1-9.

[29] Pass H I, et al. Phase III randomized trial of surgery with or without intraoperative photodynamic therapy and postoperative immunochemotherapy for malignant pleural mesothelioma. *Ann. Surg. Oncol.* 1997;4:628-633.

[30] Hilaris BS, Nori D, Kwong E, Kutcher GJ, Martini N. Pleurectomy and intraoperative brachytherapy and postoperative radiation in the treatment of malignant pleural mesothelioma. *Int. J. Radiat. Oncol. Biol. Phys.* 1984; 10:325-331.

[31] Gupta V, et al. Hemithoracic radiation therapy after pleurectomy/decortication for malignant pleural mesothelioma. *Int. J. Radiat. Oncol. Biol. Phys.* 2005; 63:1045-1052.

[32] Rusch VW, et al. A phase II trial of surgical resection and adjuvant high-dose hemithoracic radiation for malignant pleural mesothelioma. *J. Thorac. Cardiovasc. Surg.* 2001; 122:788-795.

[33] Rosenzweig KE, et al. A pilot trial of high-dose-rate intraoperative radiation therapy for malignant pleural mesothelioma. *Brachytherapy* 2005; 4:30-33.

[34] Baldini EH, et al. Patterns of failure after trimodality therapy for malignant pleural mesothelioma. *Ann. Thorac. Surg.* 1997; 63:334-338.

[35] Flores RM, Krug LM, Rosenzweig KE, Venkatraman E, Vincent A, Heelan R, Akhurst T, Rusch VW. Induction chemotherapy, extrapleural pneumonectomy, and postoperative high dose radiotherapy for locally advanced malignant pleural mesothelioma. A phase II trial. *J. Thor. Onc.* 2006; 1:289-295.

[36] Weder W, et al. Neoadjuvant chemotherapy followed by extrapleural pneumonectomy in malignant pleural mesothelioma. *J. Clin. Oncol.* 2004; 22: 3451-3457.

[37] Chan M F. et al. A novel radiation therapy technique for malignant pleural mesothelioma combining electrons with intensity-modulated photons. *Radiother. Oncol.* 2006; 79: 218-223.

[38] Yajnik S et al. Hemithoracic radiation after extrapleural pneumonectomy for malignant pleural mesothelioma. *Int. J. Radiat. Oncol. Biol. Phys.* 2003; 56:1319-1326.

[39] Moskal T L, et al. Operation and photodynamic therapy for pleural mesothelioma: 6-year follow-up. *Ann. Thorac. Surg.* 1998; 66:1128-1133.

[40] Friedberg J S et al. A phase I study of Foscan-mediated photodynamic therapy and surgery in patients with mesothelioma. *Ann. Thorac. Surg.* 2003; 75:952-959.

[41] Lu C, et al. Phase II study of a liposome-entrapped cisplatin analog (L-NDDP) administered intrapleurally and pathologic response rates in patients with malignant pleural mesothelioma. *J. Clin. Oncol.* 2005; 23:3495-3501.

[42] Rusch VW, Figlin R, Godwin, D, Piantadosi S. Intrapleural cisplatin and cytarabine in the management of malignant pleural effusions: A Lung Cancer Study Group trial. *J. Clin. Oncol.* 1991; 9: 313-319.

[43] Rusch V, et al. Intrapleural cisplatin and mitomycin for malignant mesothelioma following pleurectomy: pharmacokinetic studies. *J. Clin. Oncol.* 1992; 10: 1001-1006.

[44] Lee JD, Perez S, Wang HJ, Figlin RA, Holmes EC. Intrapleural chemotherapy for patients with incompletely resected malignant mesothelioma: the UCLA experience. *J. Surg. Oncol.* 1995; 60: 262-267.

[45] Rusch V, et al. A phase II trial of pleurectomy/decortication followed by intrapleural and systemic chemotherapy for malignant pleural mesothelioma. *J. Clin. Oncol.* 1994; 12:1156-1163.

[46] Richards WG, et al. Phase I to II study of pleurectomy/decortication and intraoperative intracavitary hyperthermic cisplatin lavage for mesothelioma. *J. Clin. Oncol.* 2006; 24: 1561-1567.

In: Mesothelioma from Bench Side to Clinic
Editor: Alfonso Baldi, pp. 537-546

ISBN: 978-1-60021-789-0

Chapter XXXII

Canine Mesothelioma: An Epidemiological and Preclinical Model

***Enrico P. Spugnini*[1], *Bruce Keene*[2], *Gabriela Seiler*[3] and *Gennaro Citro*[1]**

[1]S.A.F.U. Department, Regina Elena Cancer Institute, Rome, Italy
[2]Department of Clinical Sciences, North Carolina State University, College of Veterinary Medicine, Raleigh, NC, USA
[3]Department of Clinical Studies, School of Veterinary Medicine, University of Pennsylvania, Philadelphia, PA, USA

Abstract

The authors review the most important characteristics of canine mesotheliomas. In particular, the clinical, histological, and instrumental diagnosis of this neoplasm in dogs is described, as well as the most recent therapeutical protocols.

Epidemiology

Malignant mesotheliomas (MM) are uncommon tumors originating from the ectodermal cells that line the serosal surfaces of canine body cavities. MM have been described in the pleura, pericardium, peritoneum and tunica vaginalis [1]. Mesothelioma of the pleura and pericardium are more frequently reported than those originating in the peritoneum. These neoplasms are usually described in aged individuals (average age of onset 8 years), [2] but occasional cases of MM in juvenile dogs (<6months old) have been reported, [3, 4] thus suggesting that a congenital variant of the pathology may affect dogs. Some breeds such as Irish Setters and German Shepherd appear to be at increased risk; male dogs seem to be more prone to develop this cancer than their female counterparts.

Epidemiological and experimental studies of MM suggest that potential causative factors include urban environments, exposure to asbestos, pesticides, and cigarette smoke [5-7]. In particular, crocidolite (blue asbestos) has been experimentally shown to induce bronchitis and focal granulomas containing asbestos fibers both free within the granuloma as well as phagocyted by foreign body giant cells. More asbestos bodies (chrysotile) and ferruginous bodies (asbestos fibers mixed with ferritin and amorphous protein) have been isolated from dogs with mesothelioma than from control dogs.

Histology and Gross Features

Normal mesothelial cells are flattened, but become cuboidal or even columnar when they react to inflammatory stimuli. There is not a characteristic cytological feature that allows reliable discrimination between reactive and neoplastic mesothelium, and neither histochemistry nor immunocytochemistry provide much help in diagnosing MM.

Grossly, MM most often present as papillated, nodular or, rarely, cystic masses involving serosal surfaces; these masses can merge to form diffuse granular or velvety plaques [8-10]. MM is characterized by a diffuse growth pattern that leads to the formation of proliferations in the visceral layer of the serosa. Lymph node metastases have been reported, but distant metastases are uncommon. Sometimes when patients have widespread involvement of the abdominal cavity it is impossible to ascertain whether the widespread involvement is the result of diffusion of a focal tumor, or of multifocal origination of the disease. Microscopically, mesotheliomas in pets can be epithelial, fibrous (sarcomatoid) or a combination of the two (also known as biphasic), with a predominance of epithelial patterns with papillary foci [11-13]. The epithelioid elements have a variable size but are generally bigger than reactive mesothelial cells. Nuclei appear larger, centrally located, with hyperchromasia, pleomorphism and presence of nucleolar organizer regions. Frequently it is possible to identify binucleated cells while, on the other hand, mitotic figures are scarce. Sometimes it is difficult to differentiate such tumors from carcinomatosis, however MM do not react with mucicamine or periodic acid-Schiff staining, since they lack the neutral mucosubstances usually detected in epithelial malignancies.

Clinical Presentation and Diagnostic Workup

Mesotheliomas induce the formation of significant cavitary effusions that lead to tumor cell exfoliation and diffusion throughout the affected body cavity. Clinical signs develop secondarily to the fluid accumulation and consist most often of dyspnea in case of pleural effusion, or abdominal distension with peritoneal MM. In cases of pericardial mesothelioma, the signs are caused by the compression of the heart by the pericardial effusion (tamponade) leading to clinical signs of weakness, exercise intolerance, collapse, or right heart failure (fluid accumulation (transudation) in the abdomen or pleural space) [14, 15]. The sclerosing variant of mesothelioma is usually non-effusive. These cases most often present as diffuse thickenings within the pleural or peritoneal cavity, with clinical signs associated with the resultant strangulation of organs within the tumor folds leading to vomiting or intestinal or urinary tract obstruction (Figure 1 and 2).

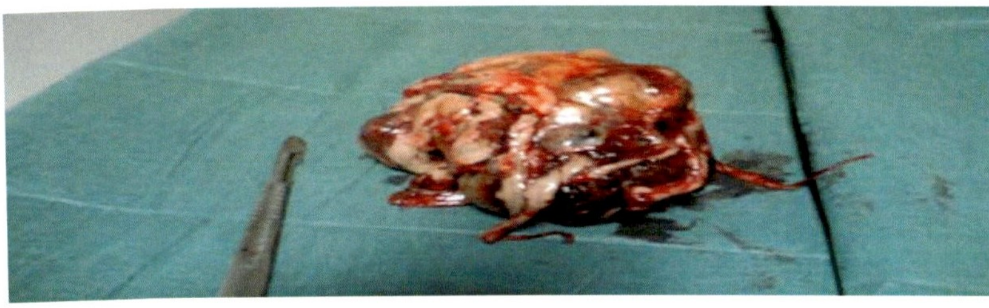

Figure 1. A large sclerosing mesothelioma (mixed type) invading the abdominal cavity of a 13 year-old male Siberian husky. The tumor weighed 700 grams (Courtesy of Dr. Paola Willy, Rome, Italy).

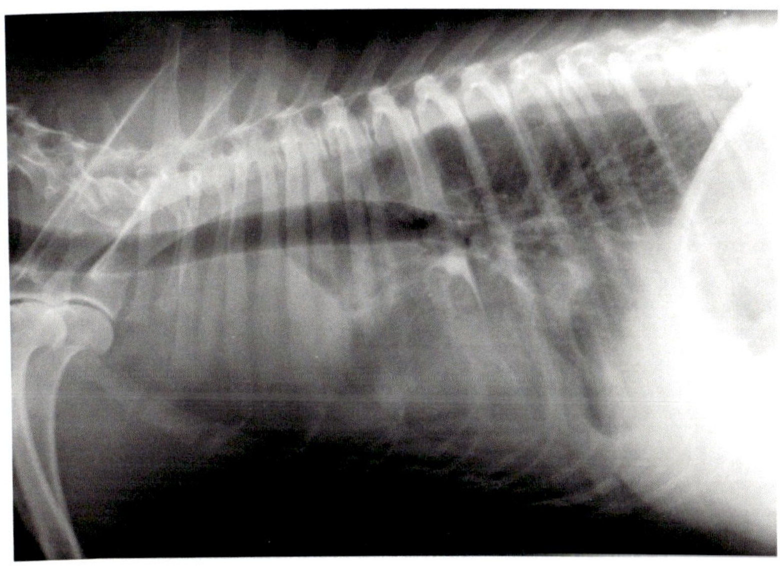

Figure 2. Lateral thoracic radiograph of an 8 year old, female spayed Mixbreed dog with thoracic mesothelioma. A moderate amount of pleural effusion is present, obscuring the cardiac silhouette. There is an increased opacity present in the cranial mediastinum with mild dorsal elevation of the trachea and caudal displacement of the cranial lung lobes. A suspicion of cranial mediastinal mass was confirmed with thoracic ultrasound.

The main finding in diagnostic imaging is pleural or peritoneal effusion using radiographic techniques (Figure 3). Ultrasonographic examination additionally reveals focal or diffuse thickening of the pleura, pericardium or peritoneum, sometimes with a hypoechoic, nodular appearance (Figure 4 and 5).

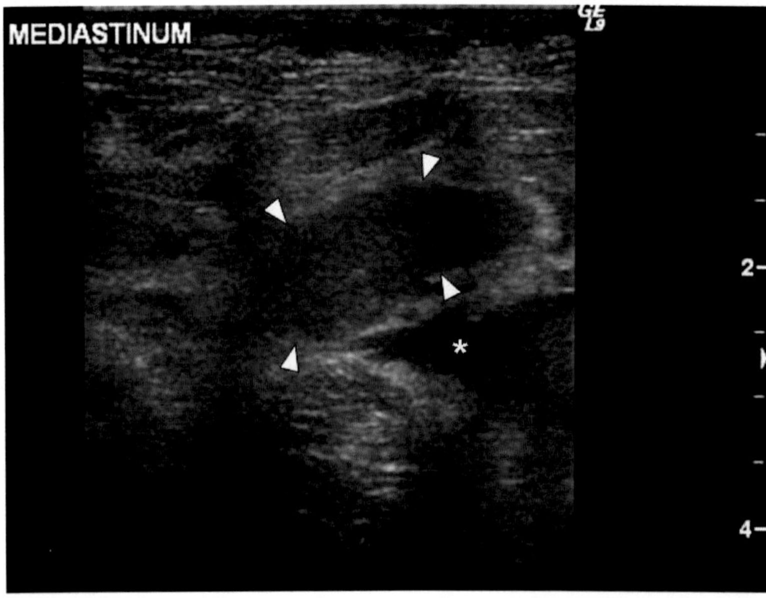

Figure 3. Parasternal long axis view of the cranial thorax of an 8 year old female spayed Mixbreed dog with thoracic mesothelioma. Cranial is to the left. Pleural effusion is present seen as a triangular anechoic space (*). Arrowheads outline an oval hypoechoic cranial mediastinal lymph node.

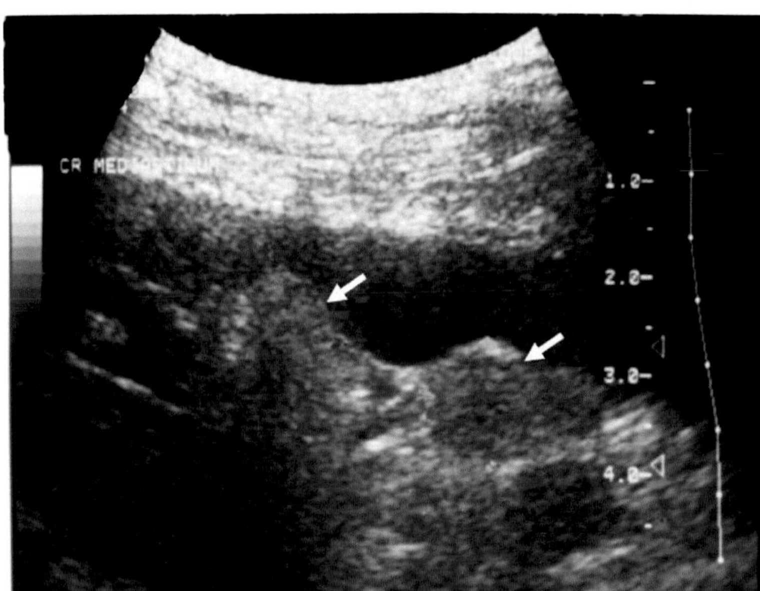

Figure 4. Parasternal long axis view of a 7 year old, male castrated Golden Retriever with thoracic mesothelioma. Cranial is to the left. The outline of the mediastinum is very irregular with a nodular appearance (arrows).

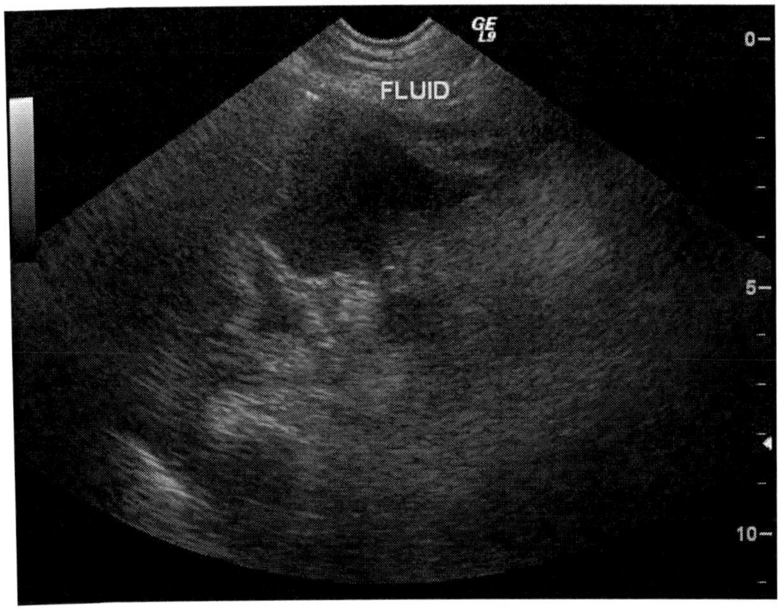

Figure 5. Short axis (intercostal) view of the left caudal thorax of a 12 year old female Mixbreed dog with thoracic mesothelioma. Ventral is to the left. There is a large amount of pleural effusion present with multiple irregular linear structures, likely representing thickened mediastinum.

These nodules or masses can get quite large and present as solitary or multiple pleural masses. Lymph node enlargement can be associated with mesothelioma, seen as round, hypoechoic structures within the hyperechoic mediastinal fat. In the cranial mediastinum it can be difficult to differentiate between enlarged lymph nodes and foci of tumor. Invasion of the lung seen as hypoechoic nodules within the lung lobes is possible [16]. The effusion often has a cellular appearance and may contain linear echoes representing thickened pleura or mediastinum. However, fibrin tags have a similar appearance and can be seen in many other diseases with associated chronic effusion.

Differentials for such findings include granulomatous disease such those caused by mycotic infections. Pericardial mesothelioma can appear as sonolucent stripes of tissue lining the pericardium; in many cases however, pericardial effusion is the only sonographic finding without discernible pericardial thickening (Figure 5 and 6) [17]. In cases of pericardial effusion, cardiac auscultation often reveals muffled heart sounds, while electrocardiography may reveal low voltage QRS complexes with or without electrical alternans or arrhythmias (Figure 7). Echocardiography in these cases reveals pericardial effusion, generally without evidence of a discreet mass, although some cases have an obviously thickened and irregular pericardium (Figure 8). Caution is indicated in interpreting the pericardial thickness echocardiographically, since the pericardium may appear abnormally echogenic or "bright" and more prominent than normal in the presence of pericardial effusion from any cause. Computed tomography can provide a better imaging of pleural effusions revealing nodular thickening of the serosal surface (Figure 9).

Examination of the cavitary effusion may provide additional insights. Cytological analysis can help to rule out some of the other cancers affecting the district such as lymphoma, however the features of MM cells such as phagocytic transformation, binucleation or multinucleation are not distinctive and are shared also by reactive mesothelium.

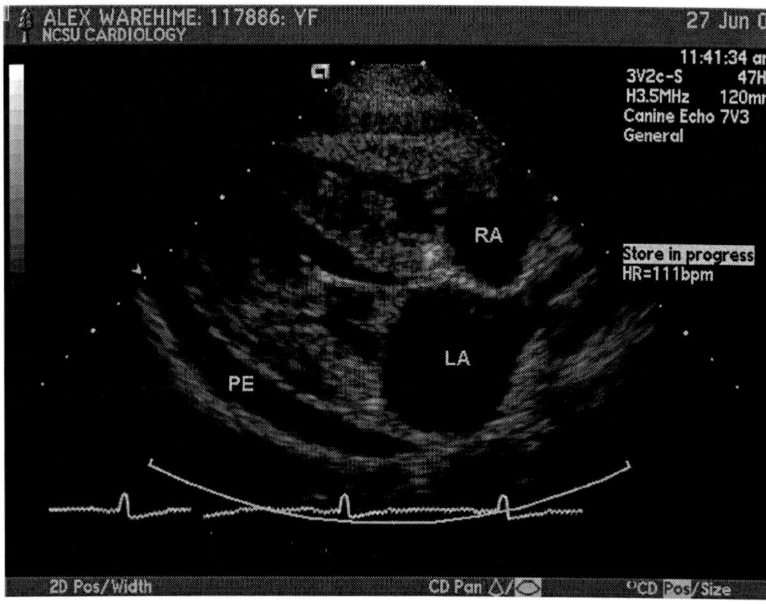

Figure 6. Cardiac ultrasonographic exam of a dog with pericardial mesothelioma showing pericardial effusion.

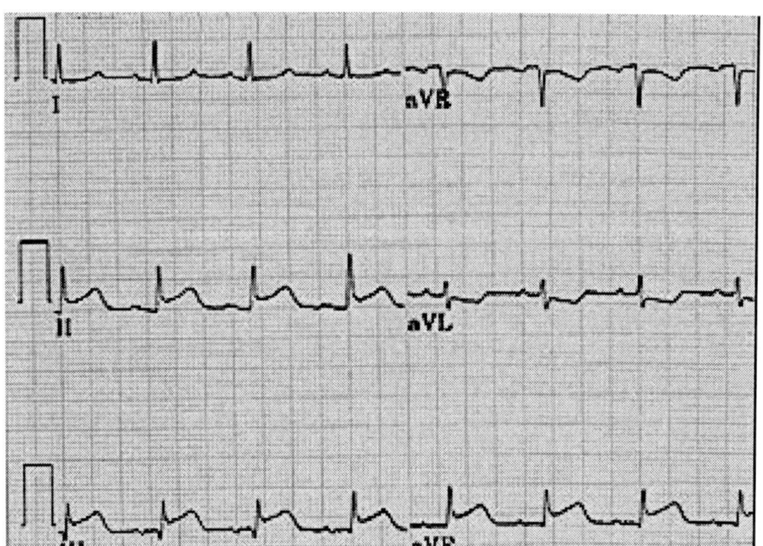

Figure 7. ECG from a dog with pericardial effusion showing typical changes, including low voltage QRS complexes, ST segment elevation in the caudal leads (II, III, aVf) associated with epicardial injury. Although difficult to appreciate in this abbreviated format, subtle electrical alternans is also present.

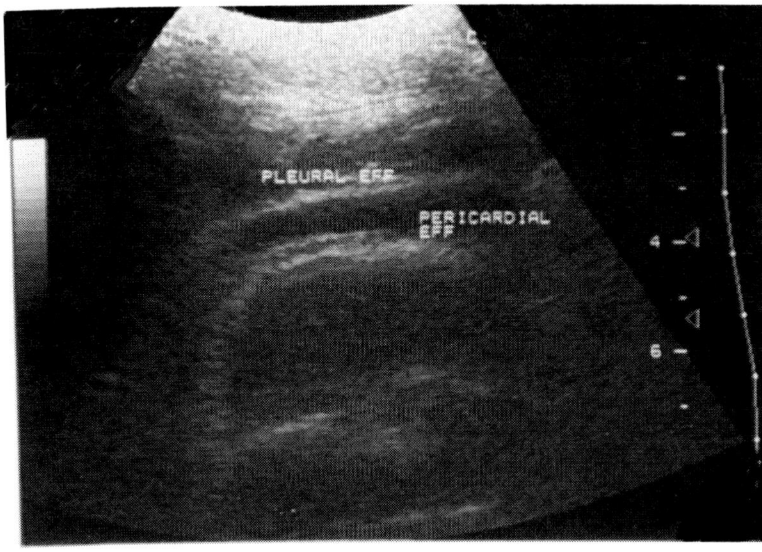

Figure 8. Left parasternal short axis view of a 7 year old, male castrated Golden Retriever with thoracic mesothelioma. There is pleural and also pericardial effusion present.

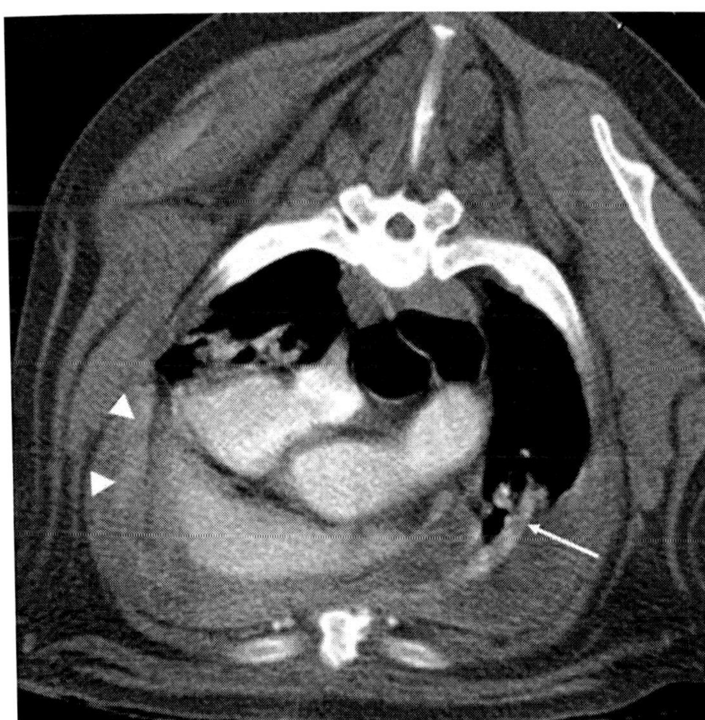

Figure 9. Axial CT scan of the cranial thorax of a 9 year old male castrated Golden Retriever with thoracic mesothelioma. Iodinated contrast medium was injected previous to the scan. There is pleural effusion present in the ventral thorax, the lung lobes are collapsed (arrow). Along the right chest wall there is irregular contrast-enhancing tissue visible (arrowheads), likely representing thickened pleura.

In one study cytology was capable of correctly diagnosing MM in only one out of six examined cases [12]. Mesotheliomatous effusions are typically hemorrhagic, sterile and nonclotting similar to those induced by a broad spectrum of neoplastic and nonneoplastic disorders such as hemangiosarcoma, carcinoma, and, (for pericardial MM only) idiopathic pericardial hemorrhage or pericarditis, disseminated intravascular coagulation (DIC), coagulation disorders, and atrial rupture. While the pH of the pericardial effusion has been investigated (among other factors) as a means of distinguishing malignant from nonmalignant effusions, recent studies suggest that while there are statistically significant differences in pH, glucose concentration and lactate concentration in animals with malignant versus nonmalignant effusions, the variability of those differences is too great to provide definitive diagnostic aid. MM can apparently be excluded from the diagnostic algorithm if the levels of fibronectin are not increased while the pH values have been shown to be not clinically useful [18, 19]. In conclusion a definitive diagnosis is dependent on the demonstration that the neoplasm is confined to the coelomic cavity lining and on performing a significative biopsy for histopathological analyis.

Therapy

As with humans, dogs cannot be cured of MM. As with humans with down-staged mesothelioma at the time of diagnosis, surgical excision cannot be successfully performed in dogs. The only exception to this rule may be pericardial MM, where successful palliation can sometimes be achieved by total or partial pericardiectomy, relieving the hemodynamic problems caused by tamponade [20, 21]. Systemic chemotherapy using mitoxantrone or doxorubicin has been limited to case reports or to small series. Its effectiveness has been limited when used as single modality, while its use as an adjunct to cytoreduction (especially pericardiectomy) has led to reports of prolonged tumor control [22-24]. Probably the best use of chemotherapy for canine mesothelioma is confined to palliation for advanced disease by means of intracavitary instillation. This approach is well tolerated and is capable of significantly decrease the amount of fluid released by the mesothelioma, furthermore it seems to induce tumor shrinking for a limited amount of time. In a small cohort of 6 dogs, treatment with intracavitary cisplatin resulted in survival times approaching one year in 5 patients [25]. Unfortunately the low penetration of the drug within the mesothelial layers (2-3 mm in depth) limits its usefulness in case of bulky disease. The use of other drugs such as tetracycline, talk, or bleomycin (Spugnini EP, personal observation) to induce pleurodesis has been unrewarding [26, 27].

In conclusion, there are not established chemotherapy protocols for dogs with MM and, in view of the many similarities shared with humans, canine patients should be considered valuable models for the study of novel approaches such as chemosensitizers, immune modulators, imaging studies and new delivery systems for loco-regional therapy. However results should be evaluated with caution since it's likely that MM has a more benign biological course in dogs than it does in people and this has to be considered in evaluating uncontrolled case reports of 1 year survival in the dog.

References

[1] Morrison WB. Nonpulmonary intrathoracic cancer. In: Morrison WB (Ed) *Cancer in dogs and cats,* 1st edition, Baltimore, Williams and Wilkins, 1998, pp 537-550.

[2] Ogilvie GK, Moore AS. Clinical briefing: tumors of the body cavities. In: Ogilvie and Moore (Eds) *Managing the veterinary cancer patient,* 1st edition, Trenton, Veterinary Learning Systems Co., Inc, 1995, pp 441-444.

[3] Leisewitz AL, Nesbit JW. Malignant mesothelioma in a seven-week-old puppy. *J. S. Afr. Vet. Assoc.* 1992, 63: 70-73.

[4] Kim JH, Choi Y-K, Yoon HY, Kweon O-K, Kim DY. Juvenile malignant melanoma in a dog. *J. Vet. Med. Sci.* 2001, 64: 269-271.

[5] Humphrey EW, Ewing SL, Wrigley JV, Northrup WF, Kersten TE, Mayer JE, Varco RL. The production of malignant tumors of the lung and pleura in dogs from intratracheal asvestos instillation and cigarette smoking. *Cancer* 1981, 47: 19994-1999.

[6] Harbison ML, Godleski JJ. Malignant mesothelioma in urban dogs. *Vet. Pathol.* 1983, 20: 531-540.

[7] Glickman LT, Domanski LM, MacGuire TG, Dubielzig RR, Churg A. Mesothelioma in pet dogs associated with exposure of their owners to asbestos. *Environ. Res.* 1983, 32: 305-313.

[8] Brunner P. Papillary polypous mesothelioma of the pericardium of a dog. *Virchows Arch. Pathol. Anat. Physiol.* 1972, 357: 275-280.

[9] Dubielzig RR: Sclerosing mesothelioma in five dogs. *J. Am. An. Hosp. Assoc.* 1979, 15: 745-748.

[10] DiPinto MN, Dunstan RW, Lee C. Cystic, peritoneal mesothelioma in a dog. *J. Am. An. Hosp. Assoc.* 1995, 31: 385-389.

[11] HarbisonML, Godleski JJ: Malignant mesothelioma in urban dogs. *Lab. Invest.* 1982, 46: 34A.

[12] Thrall DE, Goldshmidt MH. Mesothelioma in the dog: six case reports. *J. Am. Vet. Radiol. Soc.* 1978, 19: 107-114.

[13] Trigo FJ, Morrison WB, Breeze RG. An ultrastructural study of canine mesothelioma. *J. Comp. Pathol.* 1981, 98. 531-537.

[14] Cobb MA, Brownlie SE. Intrapericardial neoplasia in 14 dogs. *J. Small Anim. Pract* .1992, 33: 309-316.

[15] McDonough SP, MacLachlan NJ, Tobias AH. Canine pericardial mesothelioma. *Vet. Pathos.* 1992, 29: 256-260.

[16] Carreras JK, Sorenmo KU. Neoplasms of the cranial mediastinum and pleura. In: King LG (ed.) *Textbook of Respiratory Disease in Dogs and Cats*, 1st edition, WB Saunders, USA 2004.

[17] Mattoon JS, Nyland TG. Thorax. In: Nyland / Mattoon (eds.) *Small animal diagnostic ultrasound.* 2nd edition, WB Saunders, USA 2002.

[18] de Laforcade AM, Freeman LM, Rozanski EA, Rush JE. Biochemical analysis of pericardial fluid and whole blood in dogs with pericardial effusion. *J. Vet. Intern. Med.* 2005 Nov-Dec;19(6):833-6.

[19] Hirschberger J, pusch S. Fibronectin concentrations in pleural and abdominal effusions in dogs and cats. *J. Vet. Intern. Med.* 1996, 10: 321-325.

[20] Kerstetter KK, Krahwinkel DJ, Millis DL, et al. Pericardiectomy in dogs: 22 cases (1986-1996). *J. Am. Vet. Med. Assoc.* 1997, 211: 736-740.

[21] Jackson J, Richter K, Launer D. Thoracoscopic partial pericardiectomy in 13 dogs. *J. Vet. Intern. Med.* 1999, 13: 529-533.

[22] Ogilvie, GK, Obradovich JE, Emslie RE, et a. Efficacy of mitoxantrone against various neoplasms in dogs. *J. Am. Vet. Med. Assoc.* 1991, 198: 1618-1621.

[23] Ogilvie GK, Reynolds HA; Richardson RC, et al. Phase II evaluation of doxorubicin for treatment of various canine neoplasms. *J. Am. Vet. Med. Assoc.* 1989, 195: 1580-1583.

[24] Stepien RL, Whitley NW, Dubielzig RR. Idiopathic or mesothelioma-related pericardial effusion: clinical findings and survival in 17 dogs (1983-1996). *J. Small Anim. Pract.* 2000, 41: 342-347.

[25] Moore AS, Kirk C, Cardona A. Intracavitary cisplatin chemotherapy experience with six dogs. *J. Vet. Intern. Med.* 1991, 5: 227-231.

[26] Gallagher LA, Birchard SJ, Weisbrode SE. Effects of tetracycline hydrochloride on pleurae in dogs with induced pleural effusion. *Am. J. Vet. Res.* 1990, 51: 1682-1687.

[27] Birchard SJ, Gallagher L. Use of pleurodesis in treating selected pleural diseases. *Compend. Contin. Educ. Pract. Vet.* 1988, 10: 826-832.

In: Mesothelioma from Bench Side to Clinic
Editor: Alfonso Baldi, pp. 547-554

ISBN: 978-1-60021-789-0

Chapter XXXIII

Medico-Legal and Economic Aspects of Mesothelioma

Naumann Moazzam and Robert A. Kratzke
University of Minnesota Medical School
Section of Hematology, Oncology, and Transplant

Early Asbestos Litigation in the United States

The major economic costs associated with asbestos exposure arise from the consequent diagnoses of mesothelioma or asbestosis. Asbestos associated mesothelioma has accounted for the largest series of past and ongoing lawsuits involving contamination or exposure. The majority of experience with litigation regarding asbestos exposure has been presented in North American courts, although there is increasing case law originating from Australia and Europe [1]. This chapter will review both the history and magnitude of legal action regarding asbestos exposure and mesothelioma in North American courts. Asbestos litigation has been associated with a lengthy history of case law resulting in significant financial liability. Although a connection between asbestos and pulmonary disease was well established by the early 1960's, there was little significant case law in the United States involving asbestos exposure until later in the same decade. Asbestos litigation started increasing dramatically in the late 1960's and early 1970's starting with a series of lawsuits filed in Texas [1, 2]. One of earliest asbestos product lawsuits was filed by an asbestos worker named Claude Tomplait in December 1966. The suit was filed in Beaumont, Texas, against eleven manufacturers of asbestos-containing insulation products including Johns-Manville, Fibreboard, and Owens-Corning Fiberglas. Tomplait had been diagnosed with asbestosis in July of 1966. The case proceeded to trial on May 12, 1969 and a week later the verdict was returned in favor of the manufacturers.

In October 1969, a similar case was filed for one of Mr. Tomplait's co-workers, a man named Clarence Borel. Much like Tomaplait, Borel was suffering from asbestos-related pulmonary disease. Again, numerous asbestos manufacturers were the defendants [3]. Unlike the Tomplaint case, the jury returned a verdict for Mr. Borel in the amount of approximately $80,000. This verdict was appealed, but the ruling was upheld in 1973. With the success of this case, legal battles on behalf of asbestos victims shifted to other parts of the United States. By the early 1970's, cases involving litigation associated with disease following asbestos exposure were rapidly being filed in a wide variety of jurisdictions in the United States.

As a result of the increase in both lawsuits and subsequent verdicts involving asbestos related litigation, Johns-Manville filed for bankruptcy protection in 1982 to avoid paying compensation to the growing number of victims of diseases caused by exposure to its asbestos products [1,2]. This is thought to be the first time a Fortune 500 company was driven into bankruptcy by litigation involving personal injury. A number of other asbestos manufacturing and processing companies including Eagle Picher, UNARCO, Amatex, H.K. Porter, Carey Canada, and Celotex, followed Johns-Manville into insolvency. Within a few years, the entire asbestos textile industry was in bankruptcy, as were several major asbestos insulation manufacturers. The capacity for an environmental pathogen to drive these major corporations into bankruptcy was unprecedented in the history of litigation. We will now examine some of the individual lawsuits that established this case law.

Critical Asbestos Related Lawsuits

As previously described, in 1969, Clarence Borel asked Ward Stephenson, an attorney in Orange, Texas, to bring suit against eleven asbestos manufacturers (2). This was the first major case resulting in significant economic liability resulting from asbestos exposure. Borel v. Fibreboard Paper Products Corporation was filed in the District Court for the Eastern District of Texas and was influential in that it changed significantly the way litigation would progress in the future. Ward Stepehnson, a Texas attorney, was to play a central role in the rapid proliferation of asbestos related litigation that followed in the early 1970's. Borel was the first case in the nation that recognized the manufacturer's duty to warn of asbestos dangers. It became a case that provided a basis for future developments in asbestos litigation. On September 10, 1973, Judge John Minor Wisdom issued the opinion of the United States Court of Appeals for the Fifth Circuit in Borel v. Fibreboard Paper Products Corporation. The opinion extended the doctrine of strict product liability to asbestos-related disease caused by the use of insulation materials. As a result, a wave of person injury litigation flooded the American court system. Less than ten years later, over 16,000 asbestos-related personal injury cases had been filed in the U.S. and had become the largest area of product liability litigation.

Several of the major cases establishing monetary damages for asbestos related injuries have involved the diagnosis of asbestosis rather than malignant mesothelioma. Asbestosis is a non-malignant but progressively fatal disease of the lung that follows asbestos exposure. In many patients a diagnosis of asbestosis can precede the eventual development of mesothelioma, although this is not always the case. An early example of compensation for asbestos related disease, Drake v. Raybestos-Manhattan, involved a woman diagnosed with asbestosis in 1958. She worked for Raybestos-Manhattan for 30 years from 1924 to 1954 [4].

By 1958, she was completely disabled due to her disease. In 1958 she filed a workmen's compensation claim for benefits asserting she had an occupation associated disease. She was awarded compensation at the relative modest rate of $23.01 per week. Although not a subject of open litigation, this case raised the notion that compensation was appropriate for total disabilities due to asbestos exposure. In a similar case, John Karjala was diagnosed with asbestosis in 1966 after working as an asbestos insulation installer from 1948 to 1966 [3]. He filed the law suit against several manufacturers of asbestos insulation in 1971. Karjala's suit was successful resulting in an award of $200,000 in damages. Although the defendant appealed, the appellate court held that defendants could be held to the knowledge and skill of an expert and could be found liable if it did not disclose to the public those dangers inherent in its products.

In 1974, there was filed a civil lawsuit on behalf of the defendant Reba Rudkin. Rudkin had developed asbestosis after working for 29 years at the Johns-Manville manufacturing plant in Pittsburg, California [1, 2]. This case was precedent-setting because the company would normally be protected from such a lawsuit since workers' compensation was considered the exclusive remedy for an employee suing an employer. However, Karzan and associates argued that Johns-Manville and its executives should not be shielded from fraud and conspiracy charges. During the lawsuit it became clear the defendants had committed fraud and conspiracy when it was discovered that these companies conspired to suppress knowledge about the hazards of asbestos since the 1930s. The case was decided in favor of Rudkin. A major victory on the behalf of victims of asbestos was won when the California Supreme Court upheld the ruling against Johns-Manville establishing the principle that workers had the right to sue their employers [2]. In the aftermath of this precedent setting case, additional employees were free to proceed with their cases in civil court against Johns-Manville. Robert Speake, a co-worker of Reba Rudkin, won a verdict and was awarded a $150,000 payment from Johns-Manville for its role in contributing to Speake's asbestos related deteriorating health. The ruling allowing employees and former employees to sue Johns-Manville was to have long reaching consequences for the asbestos industry and for Johns-Manville in particular. In 1982, Johns-Manville filed for bankruptcy as a result of litigation arising from asbestos exposure.

A truly landmark case involving asbestosis was that of Waters v. W.R. Grace and Company [5]. Thomas Waters filed for action seeking compensatory and punitive damages against several asbestos manufacturers, one of which being W. R. Grace and Company. Waters worked as a tile setter from the late 1950s until 1988. He alleged that he developed asbestosis as a result of exposure to Grace's products at various work sites. In the first court, the decision required that Grace pay the compensatory damages but struck the punitive damages claim because Grace had to pay punitive damages in previous cases. When brought to an appeal, the second court ruled that Grace did have to pay the compensatory damages, and also ruled that the first court should not have taken out the punitive damages claim. The question was then raised, "Are successive claims of punitive damages against the same defendant fair?" Grace asked for leniency because it had already been punished for those damaged and warned the court about "overkill" and not advancing the spirit behind "punishment and deterrence".

Surprisingly, the court recognized that multiple punitive damages claims on the same defendant would put that company at a disadvantage. However, the court also held that the punishment for previous punitive damages should not affect successive ones. W. R. Grace was required to pay both the compensatory and punitive damages in the Waters case. The court would not grant leniency and put a limit on punitive damage claims just because the company would be repeatedly charged for the same claims by various plaintiffs because of the company's own negligence. Upon appeal, the Supreme Court of the United States ruled that in punitive damage cases, the jury should hear evidence on negligence, compensatory damages, and liability for punitive damages in phase one of the trial. The same jury should determine the amount of punitive damages in phase two. Dividing litigation in this manner would always result in a jury being questioned about and hearing evidence of, alleged willful conduct in the same phase of the trial in which the jury is required to assess compensatory damages.

Although cases involving asbestosis have been important in establishing the precedents of asbestos exposure, many of the largest settlements have involved asbestos related cancers including mesothelioma and lung cancer. An important case in asbestos litigation involving mesothelioma was the Case of Union Carbide Corp v. Kavanaugh [7]. Dennis Kavanaugh, a West Palm Beach carpenter, claimed that inhaling asbestos fibers in drywall joint compound during the 1970s led to mesothelioma 30 years later. Kavanaugh eventually died of his cancer. The 4th District Court of Appeal upheld a jury's initial $1.153 million award to a gastric cancer victim, ruling that Union Carbide Corp. didn't fully disclose the product's hazards or warn users about it. Union Carbide mined asbestos and supplied it to manufacturers for use as a binder in the joint adhesive. Kavanaugh sued several manufacturers, including Georgia-Pacific Corporation, but a jury found only Union Carbide 100 percent at fault in May, 2003. The company appealed, saying it had fulfilled its duty by putting warning labels on bags of raw asbestos sold to manufacturers and that it had no way of warning "ultimate users" not to breathe drywall dust. It also said Circuit Judge Timothy McCarthy erred in not dismissing the case before it went to the jury. In December, the court ruled that Union Carbide was 90 percent liable for a $1.8 million verdict won by the Broward County drywall worker.

In 2001 the case of Bell v. Dresser Industries was brought to court [6]. A group of Alabama plaintiffs claimed that a former employer allowed them to be exposed to dangerous levels of asbestos. The five men, all laborers or millwrights, said they contracted asbestosis when exposed to the asbestos in the spray products mixed by U.S. Pipe, their Alabama employer. They also alleged that Dresser Industries, an asbestos manufacturer that sold asbestos byproducts, had known for many years that asbestos was a carcinogen yet failed to warn of the danger. The equipment they used at U.S. Pipe was from Dresser Industries and the plaintiffs claimed that they were defective products with inadequate warnings. The defendants, Dresser Industries, contested that the men were never exposed to their products and that the products in question were never sold to U.S. Pipe.

However, the exposure was fatal: all five of the men were diagnosed with asbestosis. Two also had lung cancer and two others had colon cancer. The two with colon cancer died of their conditions and their widows presented claims of loss of consortium and household services. The jury, in an 11 to 1 vote, awarded the plaintiffs $130 million after finding negligence, defective products and inadequate warnings as to each defendant. The surviving employees each received $4 million in the past and $2 million in future damages. The estates of the deceased were each rewarded $4 million and the two widows were each awarded $2 million. The Bell v. Dresser Industries case was one of the largest asbestos verdicts in the United States.

One of the largest cases of asbestos related liability involved Travelers Property Casualty Corporation. For more than 30 years Travelers insured Johns-Manville Corporation while it produced and sold asbestos. As previously noted, Johns-Manville filed for bankruptcy protection in 1982 to deal with billions of dollars in asbestos claims. Because of this, more than 600,000 claims were filed against Travelers, according to court papers. Travelers offered $500 million dollars in settlement to litigants against Johns Manville. Under the proposal, about $445 million would go to the individuals and families who filed wrongful death and personal injury claims against Travelers for insuring Johns-Manville and not disclosing that asbestos was hazardous. Another $57 million was used to cover legal fees.

Economic Cost of Asbestos Litigation

As outlined in the previous section, there has been an increasing cascade of asbestos related lawsuits in North America since the early 1970's. It is difficult to calculate the total amount of money that has been spent to date on asbestos claims. In the history of United States, asbestos litigation is the longest-running mass tort litigation [2]. The RAND Corporation publishes the most accurate estimates on the total cost of asbestos litigation in 2005 [8]. Approximately 730,000 people had filed an asbestos claim through 2002. In the past few years, the number of claims filed annually has increased sharply, probably because of increased public awareness. The defendants who were receiving 10,000 to 20,000 claims per year in the early 1990s were receiving three to five times as many claims per year by the year 2000 according to the RAND study. In the recent years, claimants with nonmalignant injuries account for most of the growth in claims. During the early parts of asbestos litigations, claims of all types grew at approximately the same rate. In the early 1990s, the number of people asserting a nonmalignant injury, including those with little or no current functional impairment, grew much faster than the annual number of new claimants asserting some form of cancer. Nonmalignant claims accounted for roughly 80 percent of all claims entering the system through the 1980s. Rand also reports that number of claimants with mesothelioma has been increasing in recent years. Although the absolute numbers of claims for mesothelioma are very small, they have been growing. Since 1994, more of such claims have been filed each year, resulting in a doubling of mesothelioma claims in the eight-year period to 2002. According to RAND survey, at least 8,400 entities have been named as asbestos defendants through 2002. Defendants are distributed across most U.S. industries, but most of the litigation is concentrated in eight industries.

One estimate of the total costs of asbestos litigation in United States is around 70 billion dollars [8]. This total cost can be divided into defense transaction cost of around 21 billion dollars and gross compensation of around 49 billion dollars. Out of the gross compensation of 49 billion dollars, it is estimated that around 19 billion dollars were claimant's transaction cost. Thus the net compensation for asbestos cases in US was around 30 billion dollars, which is about 42 percent of total spending. In summary, only forty-two cents of every dollar spent on asbestos litigation actually go to asbestos victims. The rest of the money is split between plaintiff and defense attorneys fees. Specifically, thirty one cents of every dollar goes to defense costs while twenty seven cents to plaintiff attorneys.

The first bankruptcy filed in the US due to asbestos litigation was in 1976. According to the RAND report, 19 bankruptcies were filed in the 1980s and 17 in the 1990s. Between 2000 and mid-2004, there were 36 bankruptcy filings, more than in either of the prior two decades [9]. At least 73 firms that had been named on a substantial number of asbestos claims had filed for bankruptcy through mid-2004. It is estimated that bankruptcy reorganization can be a major drain on defendants' resources and the cost of reorganization is equal to about 3 percent of the average firm's book value or about 6 percent of a firm's market value. Insurance companies are required to list their cumulative net paid losses, including loss adjustment expenses, in their annual statements. The prominent insurance industry analyst, A. M. Best, collects and collates these data. They report that U. S. insurers have spent about $21.6 billion on asbestos claims to date [9].

The Projected Costs of Future Mesothelioma Cases

Up to 2000 new cases of mesothelioma are diagnosed in the U.S. each year, according to the National Cancer Institute. Internationally, the incidence is approximately 9 cases per every 1 million persons. Using mesothelioma incidence data covering the period between 1973 and 2000 released by the Surveillance, Epidemiology, and End Results Program in April 2003, it can be estimated whether the parameters of a birth-cohort and age model on previously reported patterns of mesothelioma in the United States have changed [10]. Compared with analyses based on data through 1992, a slower decline was found in male cases of mesothelioma immediately after a peak in between 2000 and 2004, but no other notable changes in the time pattern were detected. This analysis confirmed that the annual number of male mesothelioma cases, which increased steeply from the 1970s through the mid-1990s, has leveled off in terms of both the age-adjusted rate and the absolute numbers of cases [11]. After a peak of approximately 2,000 cases, a return to background levels is expected by 2055. Based on these estimates, the total projected number of male mesothelioma cases in the period between 2003 and 2054 will be approximately 71,000. Using the previous estimates of litigation costs between 1973 and 2003, it can be projected that at least 125 to 150 billion dollars in expense will arise from mesothelioma and asbestosis litigation over the next 50 years in the United States alone. These projections do not include the costs of asbestos removal and remediation that are almost certain to rise as older buildings are demolished or remodeled. The world wide costs over the next 50 years are incalculable, but will certainly exceed 1 trillion dollars if current policies and trends continue. One estimate holds that a projected 10 million asbestos induced cancer deaths will occur worldwide before asbestos control is implemented thought the world [14]. Even this estimate may be conservative in light of the slow progress made in asbestos control policies outside of the developed world.

In light of these staggering costs, many have proposed a legislative answer involving a unified and standard approach to compensating patients with asbestos associated diseases. In the United States, one proposed solution has involved The Fairness in Asbestos Resolution (FAIR) Act of 2005. The FAIR Act states "The tens of thousands of asbestos claims filed every year have overwhelmed the ability of the courts to provide fair, individualized justice in a timely manner [12]." Opinions regarding this bill vary wildly. Many feel the result could be problematic for deserving claimants and defendants alike, while others feel it could make for a fair solution to the looming crisis in litigation. Sponsors of the FAIR Act maintain the current system is unfair to both claimants and defendants. For claimants, the large number of pending cases can mean delay, inequitable compensation, and increasing uncertainty that the defendants responsible for their injury will remain solvent and able to compensate their claims. Meanwhile, for defendants the overwhelmed tort system has caused companies, many of whom never even manufactured asbestos, to face the possibility of devastating liabilities against which they may have little practical defense. The FAIR Act of 2005 proposes taking asbestos claims out of the existing system and processing them through a federally administered trust fund that compensates current and future asbestos claimants on a no-fault basis according to standardized medical criteria and corresponding claims awards. The bill currently remains under consideration in the United States Senate.

Conclusion

In the history of United States, asbestos litigation is the longest-running mass tort litigation with enormous impact on the United States economy. Currently, it is estimated over 70 billion dollars in litigation is complete or pending in the United States alone. The costs of worldwide efforts at asbestos remediation and removal are virtually incalculable. Clearly, asbestos contamination has cast a massive monetary shadow over and above the loss of human life from the medical manifestations of disease. The explosion of litigation in the past 30 years, in addition to the incredible medical costs associated with asbestosis and mesothelioma, calls for the examined application of scientific fact to public policy. Asbestos related litigation outside of North America has lagged by about a decade, but is gaining momentum rapidly [1]. The worldwide costs of asbestos contamination, both monetary and medical, are almost impossible to calculate and almost certain to rise [14-16].

References

[1] Bale A The American compensation phenomenon. *International Journal of Health Services*. 1990. 20(2):253-275.

[2] Rosenberg, D. The dusting of America: A story of asbestos-carnage, cover up, and litigation. *Harvard Law Review*. 1986. 99(7):1693-1706.

[3] Borel vs Fibreboard *Paper Products Corporation*, 493 F.2d 1076 (1973).

[4] Karjala vs Johns-Manville *Products Corporation*, 523 F.2d 155, Minn., 8th Circle (1975).

[5] Drake vs Raybestos-Manhattan, Inc., 127 S.E. 2d 288 (1962).

[6] http://www.asbestosresource.com/litigation/waters.html.

[7] http://www.asbestosresource.com/litigation/bell.html.

[8] *Union Carbide Corp. v. Kavanaugh*, 879 So. 2d 42 (Fla. 4th DCA 2004).

[9] Stephen J. Carroll, Deborah Hensler, Jennifer Gross et al. *Asbestos Litigation*. RAND Institute for Civil Justice. 2005.

[10] Plevin and Kalish, What's Behind the Recent Wave of Asbestos Bankruptcies?, *Mealey's Litigation Report: Asbestos*, April 20, 2001.

[11] United States Cancer Statistics 2002 Incidence and Mortality. US Department of Health and Humar Sevices, 2005.

[12] Price B, Ware A. Mesothelioma trends in the United States: an update based on Surveillance, Epidemiology, and End Results Program data for 1973 through 2003. *Am. J. Epidemiol.* 2004 Jan 15;159(2):107-12.

[13] *Fairness in Asbestos Injury Resolution Act of 2005* (H.R. 1360, 109th Congress).

[14] LaDou J. The asbestos cancer epidemic. *Environ. Health Perspect.* 2004 Mar;112(3):285-90.

[15] Castleman BI, Vera Vera MJ. Impending proliferation of asbestos. *International Journal of Health Services* 1980;10(3):389-403.

[16] Kjellstrom TE. The epidemic of asbestos-related diseases in New Zealand, *Int. J. Occup. Environ. Health.* 2004 Apr-Jun;10(2):212-9.

Index

A

B

C

D

E

F

G

H

I

J

K

L

M

O

P

Q

R

S

T

U

V

W

X

Y

Z